MW01118248

Parasitic Infections
in the Compromised Host

INFECTIOUS DISEASE AND THERAPY

Series Editors

Brian E. Scully, M.B., B.Ch.

College of Physicians
and Surgeons
Columbia University
New York, New York

Harold C. Neu, M.D.

College of Physicians
and Surgeons
Columbia University
New York, New York

Volume 1 Parasitic Infections in the Compromised Host,
edited by Peter D. Walzer and Robert M. Genta

Additional Volumes in Preparation

Parasitic Infections in the Compromised Host

edited by

PETER D. WALZER and ROBERT M. GENTA

Cincinnati Veterans Administration Medical Center and
University of Cincinnati College of Medicine
Cincinnati, Ohio

MARCEL DEKKER, INC.　　　New York and Basel

Library of Congress Cataloging-in-Publication Data

Parasitic infections in the compromised host / edited by Peter D.
Walzer and Robert M. Genta.
     p.   cm. -- (Infectious disease and therapy series)
   Includes bibliographical references and index.
   ISBN 0-8247-7943-6
   1. Parasitic diseases--Pathogenesis. 2. Host-parasite
relationships.   3. Immunological deficiency syndromes--Complications
and sequelae. I. Walzer, Peter D.,   . II. Genta, Robert
M.,   . III. Series.
QR201.P27P37 1989
616.9'6--dc19   88-25614
                                     CIP

MARCEL DEKKER, INC.
270 Madison Avenue, New York, New York 10016

Current printing (last digit):
10 9 8 7 6 5 4 3 2 1

PRINTED IN THE UNITED STATES OF AMERICA

To Kathy and Marcia
for their support, love, and patience

Series Introduction

Marcel Dekker, Inc., has for many years specialized in the publication of high-quality monographs in tightly focused areas in a variety of medical disciplines. These have been of great value to both the practicing physician and the research scientist as sources of detailed and up-to-date information presented in an attractive format. During the last decade, there has been a veritable explosion in knowledge in the various fields related to infectious diseases and clinical microbiology. Antimicrobial resistance, antibacterial and antiviral agents, AIDS, Lyme disease, infections in immunocompromised patients, and parasitic diseases are but a few of the areas in which an enormous amount of significant work has been published. This new Infectious Disease and Therapy series will cover carefully chosen topics which should be of interest and value to the practicing physician, the clinical microbiologist, and the research scientist.

Brian E. Scully, M.B., B.Ch.
Harold C. Neu, M.D.,

Preface

A parasite is defined by *Stedman's Medical Dictionary* as "an organism that lives on or in another and draws nourishment therefrom." Parasites range from protozoa with simple modes of transmission to multicellular helminths with complex life cycles involving several intermediate hosts. Parasites have often been considered exotic organisms which cause disease only in tropical or developing countries. Since parasitology occupies a very small place in American medical school and residency curricula, physicians are generally insufficiently informed about the natural history of parasitic diseases, methods of diagnosis, and treatment.

Over the past 10–15 years, the medical importance of parasites in this country has increased considerably. *Giardia lamblia* has emerged as a major public health problem, and surveys have revealed that large areas of the southeastern United States and Appalachia remain highly endemic for intestinal parasites. The rise in the use of day-care centers, changes in sexual practices, and other alterations in our life-style have created new opportunities for parasitic transmission and clinical disease. The increase in international travel and influx of refugees have brought parasitic infections of other lands to the attention of primary-care physicians.

One of the most important clinical challenges in parasitology today involves the immunocompromised host. Increasing numbers of people are being kept alive by cytotoxic or immunosuppressive therapy for the treatment of cancer, organ transplantation, and collagen vascular disorders. Some parasites which cause mild or self-limited illness in the normal host cause severe and life-threatening disease in the compromised host. *Strongyloides stercoralis*, a soil-transmitted nematode, typifies these opportunistic pathogens. Infection is usually acquired in childhood, but *S. stercoralis* can persist in the host for decades after leaving the host; with corticosteroid or other immunosuppressive therapy, the parasite disseminates widely throughout the body, causing systemic disease.

The 1980s have witnessed the emergence of the acquired immunodeficiency syndrome (AIDS), which has confronted society with health problems on an unprecedented scale. Parasites are a major cause of morbidity and mortality in AIDS. *Pneumocystis carinii*, the most common pathogen, causes pneumonia in more than 60% of AIDS patients and has served as a major epidemiological marker for this disorder. *Toxoplasma gondii*, an intracellular protozoan, causes serious central nervous system infections. The genus *Cryptosporidium*, which only recently has been found to be a human pathogen, causes unremitting choleralike diarrhea. *G. lamblia* and *Entamoeba histolytica* are highly prevalent among homosexual men, the major population group at risk for AIDS; these organisms have manifestations ranging from mild or asymptomatic infection to severe gastrointestinal disease.

Parasitic infections in persons with AIDS and other immunosuppressed patients are characterized by their chronicity and refractoriness to standard forms of therapy. These features have prompted renewed interest in the immunobiology of these organisms and in host defense mechanisms. Knowledge about parasitic infections in the immunocompromised host has been obtained in a fragmented manner from a diverse group of sources. There appeared to be a need for a book that provided an in-depth analysis of both host-parasite relationships and clinical disease problems.

The present text has been designed with these considerations in mind. Our approach has not been to include all possible parasites; rather, we have focused our attention on organisms which are of major medical importance in this country or which have contributed to our understanding of pathogenic mechanisms. The authors of the chapters are all experts in their fields and have a broad view of basic science concepts and clinical applications.

The book is divided conceptually into two broad areas. Chapter 1 deals with the specific types of immune defects in the compromised host and how they predispose to infection with different organisms. Chapter 2 focuses on host defenses against intracellular protozoa using *Leishmania* as a model. Chapter 8 covers host defenses against helminths.

The remaining chapters deal with specific parasitic infections and follow a similar format. Chapter 3 deals with *P. carinii*; Chapter 4 with *T. gondii*; Chapter 5 with *Cryptosporidium* spp.; Chapter 6 with *G. lamblia*; Chapter 7 with *E. histolytica*; Chapter 9 with *S. stercoralis*.

We believe this book will be of interest to physicians, parasitologists, micro-biologists, immunologists, and other scientists and health professionals. We hope it will be of value to anyone who is involved in the care of immunosuppressed patients.

Peter D. Walzer
Robert M. Genta

Contributors

William L. Current   Animal Research Laboratories, Lilly Research Laboratories, A Division of Eli Lilly and Company, Indianapolis, Indiana

Melanie T. Cushion   Cincinnati Veterans Administration Medical Center and Division of Infectious Diseases, Department of Internal Medicine, University of Cincinnati College of Medicine, Cincinnati, Ohio

Robert M. Genta   Cincinnati Veterans Administration Medical Center and Department of Pathology and Laboratory Medicine, University of Cincinnati College of Medicine, Cincinnati, Ohio

C. Kurtis Kim   Cincinnati Veterans Administration Medical Center and Department of Pathology and Laboratory Medicine, University of Cincinnati College of Medicine, Cincinnati, Ohio

Benjamin J. Luft   Division of Infectious Diseases, Department of Medicine, Health Sciences Center, State University of New York at Stony Brook, Stony Brook, New York

Henry Masur   Department of Critical Care Medicine, Clinical Center, National Institutes of Health, Bethesda, Maryland

Thomas B. Nutman   Laboratory of Parasitic Diseases, National Institutes of Health, Bethesda, Maryland

Richard D. Pearson Division of Geographic Medicine, Section of Infectious Diseases, Departments of Medicine and Pathology, University of Virginia School of Medicine, Charlottesville, Virginia

William A. Petri, Jr. Divisions of Infectious Diseases and Geographic Medicine, Departments of Internal Medicine and Microbiology, University of Virginia School of Medicine, Charlottesville, Virginia

Jonathan I. Ravdin Divisions of Clinical Pharmacology, Geographic Medicine, and Infectious Diseases, Departments of Internal Medicine and Pharmacology, University of Virginia School of Medicine, Charlottesville, Virginia

Phillip D. Smith Laboratory of Immunology, NIDR, National Institutes of Health, Bethesda, Maryland

Peter D. Walzer Cincinnati Veterans Administration Medical Center and Division of Infectious Diseases, Department of Internal Medicine, University of Cincinnati College of Medicine, Cincinnati, Ohio

Mary E. Wilson* Division of Geographic Medicine, Departments of Medicine and Pathology, University of Virginia School of Medicine, Charlottesville, Virginia

---

Present affiliation: Division of Infectious Diseases, Department of Internal Medicine, University of Iowa, Iowa City, Iowa.

Contents

1
The Compromised Host: AIDS and Other Diseases

HENRY MASUR
Clinical Center, National Institutes of Health, Bethesda, Maryland

I. INTRODUCTION

Patients who lack normal resistance to infection because of a deficiency in any of their multifaceted host defense mechanisms are referred to as "compromised hosts." In the 1980s physicians have been confronted with a rapidly expanding population of patients who fit into the category of compromised hosts. Compromised hosts are increasing in numbers because the medical sciences are employing more aggressive surgical and medical techniques to control or cure previously hopeless diseases including congenital immunodeficiencies, malignant neoplasms, and end-stage cardiac, hepatic, or renal failure. In addition, their number is increasing because of exposure to environmental hazards such as that which occurred at Chernobyl but more dramatically because of infection with human immunodeficiency virus (HIV, previously known as HTLV–III or LAV or ARV). Clinicians have made rapid strides over the last two decades in managing the hemorrhagic and metabolic disorders that formerly were lethal for many of these patients. Now, to an ever-increasing degree, infection is the major factor that limits the quality and duration of life for many of these populations.

In North America and Western Europe, where sanitation and arthropod control are well-developed public health priorities, most clinicians give scant consideration to protozoan and helminthic organisms. For physicians dealing with immunocompetent patients, protozoans and helminthic diseases are rarely considered and even more rarely recognized. However, a large percentage of the population is exposed to such organisms and may harbor them for life. About 15–40% of the North American population become infected with *Toxoplasma gondii*, for example, and have viable cysts in their muscle and brain for their lifetime after acute infection (1,2). About 4-7% of visitors to certain endemic areas in the United States are infected with *Babesia microti* (3). *Giardia lamblia* is present in 20-50% of children in some day care centers and in high fractions of residents of certain areas with contaminated water supplies (4). Homosexual men are likely to have *Entamoeba histolytica* or *G. lamblia* in their stool in 30-40% of cases depending on their sexual activity and city of residence (4-6). *Strongyloides stercoralis* is endemic in many parts of the southern United States and has been reported to be frequent in certain institutionalized populations (7). As a final example, the frequency of *Pneumocystis* pneumonia in all groups of North American patients who develop AIDS suggests that this protozoan is ubiquitous in North America. Since each of these protozoan and helminthic organisms requires immunological and nonimmunological host defense mechanisms to protect the exposed host from serious disease, and since host defense mechanisms are, to an increasing degree, being seriously compromised by environmental, infectious, and iatrogenic processes, it is not surprising that clinicians are recognizing more and more protozoan and helminthic diseases in their patient populations.

The epidemic of HIV infection in North America has provided a graphic demonstration of the precarious balance between human beings in North America and the protozoa in their microbial environment. The immunological defect that is central to AIDS appears also to be central to much of antiprotozoan host defense. As a result, protozoan diseases such as pneumocystosis, toxoplasmosis, cryptosporidiosis, and isosporiasis are major causes of serious morbidity and death in this population.

For compromised patients who live in tropical ares or who have emigrated to North America or Western Europe, the problem of protozoan and helminthic infection is clearly magnified, since exposure to *Plasmodia, Trypanosoma, Leishmania, E. histolytica, G. lamblia,* and *S. stercoralis* is so common. Each geographical area has its unique protozoan and helminthic ecology that demands special consideration. In many parts of North America where refugees from tropical areas are concentrated, where the indigenous population travels or lives abroad for business or pleasure, or where foreign nationals come seeking health care, protozoan and helminthic diseases are increasingly important considerations.

The focus of this chapter is to provide an overview of protozoan and helminthic diseases as one component of the interrelationship between the compromised host and his or her microbial environment.

II. HOST DEFENSE MECHANISMS

For patients whose host defense mechanisms are less capable than normal, a variety of terminologies are loosely used, including "compromised host," "abnormal host," "immunocompromised patient," and immunosuppressed host."

It is important to recognize that although some of these terms can be used interchangeably, the latter two refer specifically to those patients whose immunological or inflammatory defense mechanisms are compromised, while the former terms refer to patients who might be deficient in any of their physical, chemical, inflammatory, or immunological defenses. For protozoa and helminths, compromise of immunological defense mechanisms is the major predisposition to life-threatening disease, in contrast to ther microbial pathogens, such as bacteria, for which physical and chemical and inflammatory barriers have more importance.

Host defense mechanisms against microbial agents are an increasingly important issue. Medical science has made rapid strides in artifical joint construction, cardiac valve replacement, organ transplatnation, thermal injury rescue, and treatment of inflammatory and neoplastic diseases. Many of these advances depend on the use of aggressive surgical techniques that breach physical barriers and that often insert foreign bodies into the patient. Many of these advances also utilize increasingly potent anti-inflammatory and cytotoxic pharmacological agents. Noninfectious complications such as hemorrhage, uremia, electrolyte disorders, endocrinological dysfunction, and organ rejections are being managed with increasing success. Infection is becoming the major threat to the quality and duration of patient survival. Bacterial and fungal infections continue to be the major causes of morbidity and mortality. Rapid advances are being made in the management of bacterial processes; it seems likely that fungal, viral, and protozoal problems will become increasingly important. Moreover, in parts of the world where protozoan and helminthic diseases are highly endemic and where these aggressive immunosuppressive techniques are introduced, protozoan and helminthic diseases will almost certainly increase as serious clinical problems.

Antimicrobial defense mechanisms consist of complex and interacting systems that protect the host from endogenous and exogenous microorganisms (Table 1). The degree to which a patient becomes abnormally susceptible to infection depends on (1) which mechanisms are affected, (2) the severity of the derangement, and (3) the interaction of affected mechanisms if more than one are simultaneously diminished. Which mechanism is affected determines the constellation of organisms that will have increased pathogenicity for the host. The severity of the derangement is clearly important, since a decrease in neutrophil count from $3000/mm^3$ to $1000/mm^3$ will likely have no importance for the host, while a decrease to $150/mm^3$ will most likely result in a higher number of bacterial infections and in bacterial infections of greater severity. The interaction of diminished host resistance is also important. A neutropenia of $500/mm^3$ or a third-degree thermal injury to 50% of the body surface might be manageable individually. If both defects were present simultaneously for an extended period of time, however, survival would be unlikely.

Table 1   Mechanisms of Host Defense

Physical and chemical barriers
  Skin and mucous membranes
  Sphincters
  Epiglottis
  Normal secretory and excretory flow
  Endogenous microbial flora
  Gastric acidity
Inflammatory response
  Circulating phagocytes
  Complement
  Other humoral mediators (bradykinins, fibrinolytic systems, arachidonic acid cascade)
Reticuloendothelial system
  Tissue phagocytes
Immune response
  T lymphocytes and their soluble products
  B lymphocytes and immunoglobulins

A. Physical and Chemical Barriers

Physical and chemical barriers (Table 1) are part of a complex and interacting system of nonspecific host defense mechanisms that are responsible for preventing the introduction of endogenous and exogenous microorganisms into the host. These barriers protect the host by a variety of mechanisms. An intact mucosa prevents oral, gastrointestinal, or respiratory flora from invading the lymphatics or the bloodstream. Localized anatomical barriers such as the epiglottis, the sphincter of Oddi, and the urethral sphincter prevent flora from being introduced into normally sterile areas. The flushing action of intestinal peristalsis or of normal urine flow helps keep intestinal microorganisms stable and assists in ridding the bladder of introduced bacteria or fungi. Sloughing of cutaneous mucosal epithelial cells has a similar effect.

    Chemical barriers include gastric acidity, which kills a variety of bacteria and fungi although not spores or certain cysts. These barriers also include the high alkalinity of biliary and pancreatic fluids, which have similar effects, and a complex matrix of antibacterial properties of the skin including the presence of fatty acids, relative dryness, and pH. The urine contains substances that have mild antimicrobial effects; urea, certain solutes, and the extremes of pH contribute to this antimicrobial effect.

Another important part of the physical and chemical barrier is the presence of "normal" host flora. The presence of relatively less virulent organisms in the gastrointestinal tract and on the skin provides competition for space and nutrients with introduced flora that might be more pathogenic. This flora is important; its elimination allows more resistant and virulent organisms to colonize the host and take advantage of other defects in host antimicrobial defense mechanisms, such as mucosal or cutaneous erosions.

Physical and chemical barriers play relatively minor roles for most protozoan and helminthic diseases, most of which gain access to the host by penetration of intact skin (e.g., *S. stercoralis* or schistomal cercaria or hookworm), by arthropod vectors (*Babesia, Leishmania, Trypanosoma, Plasmodia*), by resistance to chemical insults in the stomach (*G. lamblia, Cryptosporidium sp, Isospora, E. histolytica, T. gondii*), or by respiratory droplets (probably *P. carinii*).

B. Inflammatory Response

From the bone marrow arise circulating phagocytes, which include neutrophils, monocytes, eosinophils, and basophils. Upon the appropriate signal, these cells enter the peripheral circulation and are distributed to tissue sites where they are the major component of inflammatory responses. The recruitment of phagocytes from the bloodstream is a complex process that involves phagocyte aggregation, adherence to vascular endothelium, migration through endothelial spaces, and migration to local tissue sites. In order for an inflammatory response to be effective, the phagocyte must adhere to a surface, deform, be able to have random locomotion, but also respond to a chemical signal with directed movement. The locomotion of the phagocyte is guided by a complex array of soluble factors including complement components, the arachidonic acid cascade, kinin-generating systems, and the products of such cellular elements as fibroblasts, neutrophils, lymphocytes, macrophages, and microorganisms. Once the phagocyte arrives at the focus of infection, it can adhere to the microorganism, ingest it, and digest it, particularly if the organism has been opsonized by immunoglobulin or complement. A wide variety of gram-positive bacteria, gram-negative bacteria and fungi are killed by neutrophils in the schema. Protozoa are generally not as influenced by this system as by lymphocyte- and macrophage-mediated immune response and the reticuloendothelial system.

C. Reticuloendothelial System

Tissue phagocytes that are derived from circulating phagocytes are capable of clearing circulating organisms from the blood. These tissue phagocytes reside in the liver (Kupffer cells), spleen, lymph node, lungs (alveolar macrophages), and brain (microglial nodules). Their antimicrobial properties are strongly influenced by opsonins such as IgG and C3b as well as a large variety of mononuclear leukocyte-produced soluble mediators. The efficacy of tissue phagocytes in clearing the blood stream of organisms is dependent on the ability of microorganisms to resist specific steps necessary for antimicrobial activity. *Cryptococcus neoformans* is able to inhibit the phagocytosis; *T. gondii* is able to avoid destruction by inhibiting phagosome-lysosome fusion; *Leishmania* are resistant to the degradative effects of lysosomal products; *Trypanosoma* are able to avoid remaining in the phagosome and escape into the cytoplasmic substance.

D. Immune Response

The major cellular components of the immune response are T lymphocytes and B lymphocytes. These cells are distributed throughout the body in the bloodstream and at tissue sites. They interact in a highly complex fashion among themselves and with monocytes, macrophages, immunoglobulins, and the complement cascade. T lymphocytes are the major cellular component of the cell-mediated immune system. They secrete a multitude of soluble products that influence the functional status of other T lymphocytes, B lymphocytes, monocytes, and macrophages. B lymphocytes and plasma cells secrete specific antibodies that have important roles in eradicating certain infections such as those caused by *P. carinii, Babesia,* and *Plasmodia.* As noted above, the ability of the monocytes and macrophages to ingest and kill a wide variety of bacteria, fungi, and protozoa is dependent on the ability of the T lymphocyte to activate these cells. Any process that requires opsonization with antibody, such as the phagocytosis of *Pneumocystis carinii* by fresh macrophages, can also be profoundly influenced by the regulatory effect of T lymphocytes on B lymphocytes.

III. ETIOLOGY AND PATHOGENESIS OF INFECTION

In compromised hosts, the occurrence of infectious diseases reflects the interaction of impaired immunological and nonimmunological host defense mechanisms with the host's endogenous and exogenous microbial environment (8-12). Potentially pathogenic microorganisms may arise from the host's endogenous flora as well as from the patient's external environment. Thus, factors that change either the internal or external microbial flora have an important impact on the organisms that are likely to cause disease. Such factors include antimicrobial therapy, nonsterile invasive procedures or trauma, ingestion or inhalation of infected material, and hospitalization itself.

Infectious diseases in compromised patients are more often related directly to alterations in host defense mechanisms than to changes in the microbial flora, although both factors are undoubtedly important. Numerous processes can predispose to serious infection by compromising the anatomical and physical barriers of host defense. For example, the skin and mucous membranes can be breached by conditions such as tumor invasion, tumor necrosis, or vascular insufficiency induced by arteritis or athersclerosis; by injury such as burns, pressure, or trauma; by therapy such as radiation or cytotoxic chemotherapy; by a drug-induced cutaneous slough; and by procedures such as venipuncture or surgery. The respiratory tract can become the site of infection when its anatomical barriers are disrupted: The epiglottis may fail to protect the lower tract when the patient's consciousness is impaired or when he is subjected to intubation or bronchoscopy. The patient's ability to expel organisms may be adversely affected if he is unable to cough due to infection, tumor, or drugs that alter the state of consciousness; if his mucociliary transport is disrupted by a congenital disorder of cilial subunits (such as Kartagener's syndrome) or by smoke or other inhaled toxins, anesthetic agents, or cytotoxic therapy; or if an airway is obstructed by a tumor, a foreign body, or lymph node enlargement. The gastrointestinal tract can become a less effective barrier against the entry of organisms if gastric acidity is abolished by a surgical procedure or antacid therapy (infection with *Salmonella* and *Myobacteria* are particularly important in this regard) or if its mucosa is eroded by tumor or cytotoxic therapy, especially in neutropenic patients. Obstruction of the intestinal or biliary tract by a tumor, a stricture, or a stone also allows endogenous or introduced flora to gain access to capillary and lymphatic systems. The genitourinary tract can become a portal of entry for infections if its mucosa is eroded by tumor, irradiation, or cytotoxic therapy. Obstruction of urine flow by tumor, strictures, stones, or prostatic hypertrophy also allows organisms to multiply and gain access to the capillaries and lymphatic systems. Renal failure associated with oliguria or anuria deprives the genitourinary system of the ability to flush out microorganisms and obviates the antimicrobial effects of urine itself. The insertion of foreign bodies into the urethra during catheterization or cystoscopy is an iatrogenic cause of exogenous organisms being introduced into this system. Any locus in the body can become the site of infection if devitalized tissue or foreign bodies are seeded by bacteria or introduced by direct penetration. Spontaneous or traumatic hematomas, necrotic tissue, infarcts, calcified heart valves, and prosthetic devices (joints, heart valves, semipermanent intravascular access devices, or central nervous system appliances) are particularly prone to infection.

Defects in inflammatory and immune function may permit infections that would normally be promptly eradicated to progress and cause clinically important disease. These quantitative or qualitative defects may be related to a congenital disorder, an underlying acquired disease, or drug therapy. Substantial abnormalities in measured in vitro immunological function can also be produced by protozoa themselves such as *T. gondii, Leishmania, Schistosoma,* or *Plasmodia.* In addition, the consequences of protozoan disease such as malnutrition (from giardiasis or amebiasis) may alter immune function. These alterations in measured immune function are not usually associated with clinical susceptibility to opportunistic pathogens, however, although they may contribute to poor host response to conventional pathogenic organisms. Several specific types of therapy or underlying disease-related defects are associated with particularly frequent or severe infectious complications.

A. Leukocyte Disorders

The clinical consequences of leukocyte disorders depend on which subpopulation of leukocytes are numerically or functionally affected, and how prolonged the dysfunction is (Table 2). Neutropenia (less than 3000 neutrophils per cubic millimeter) is the most commonly encountered defect in inflammatory host defense mechanisms. As the neutrophil count falls below 100 cells/mm^3, there is a progressive increase in susceptibility to bacterial and fungal infections and a progressive decrease in the clinical signs and symptoms of inflammation that ordinarily provide clinical clues to the location of the infection (8,10). Susceptibility to bacterial and fungal infection (but not protozoan or helminthic disease) increases dramatically when the peripheral neutrophil count falls below 500 cells/mm^3 and increases even more markedly when the count falls below 100 cells/mm^3. The rate of decline and the duration of neutropenia are also important parameters that influence the clinical consequences. Neutropenia can occur because of bone marrow failure, peripheral destruction of cells, or pooling or sequestration of cells. The most common causes of neutropenia are neoplastic invasion of the bone marrow, aplastic anemia, and idiosyncratic drug reactions.

Neutrophil dysfunction can also result in a substantial predisposition to serious bacterial and fungal infection (8). Dysfunction may be a manifestation of a congenital disorder such as chronic granulomatous disease or Chediak-Higashi syndrome. Neutrophil dysfunction can also be a consequence of drug therapy, e.g., corticosteroids. Thus, certain multidrug chemotherapeutic regimens may alter both the number and the fucntion of circulating neutrophils.

Lymphopenia in adults is defined as less than 1000 lymphocytes/mm^3 (9). The clinical consequences of lymphopenia depend on which subsets are affected; regardless of the total lymphocyte count, severe infections of various types may occur if profound deficiencies of either B lymphocytes or T lymphocytes are present. Substantial reductions in helper T lymphocytes have particularly

Table 2 Infections Associated with Common Defects in Inflammatory or Immunological Response

Host defect	Examples of diseases or therapies associated with defects	Common etiological agents of infection
Inflammatory response		
Neutropenia	Hematological malignancies	Gram-negative bacilli
	Cytotoxic chemotherapy	*Staphylococcus aureus*
	Aplastic anemia	*Candida* species
		Aspergillus species
Chemotaxis	Chediak-Higashi syndrome	*Staphylococcus aureus*
		Streptococcus pyogenes
	Job's syndrome	*Staphylococcus aureus*
		Hemophilus influenzae
	Protein calorie malnutrition	Gram-negative bacilli
Phagocytosis (cellular)	Systemic lupus erythematosus	*Streptococcus pneumoniae*
	Chronic myelogenous leukemia	*Hemophilus influenzae*
	Megaloblastic anemia	
Microbicidal defect	Chronic granulomatous disease	Catalase-positive bacteria and fungi: Staphylococci *Escherichia coli* *Klebsiella* species *Pseudomonas aeruginosa* *Candida* species *Aspergillus* species *Nocardia* species
	Chediak-Higashi syndrome	*Staphylococcus aureus* *Streptococcus pyogenes*
Complement system		
C3	Congenital	*Staphylococcus aureus*
	Liver disease	*Streptococcus pneumoniae*
	Systemic lupus erythematosus	*Pseudomonas* species
		Proteus species

Table 2 Infections Associated with Common Defects in Inflammatory or Immunological Response (Continued)

Host defect	Examples of diseases or therapies associated with defects	Common etiological agents of infection
C5	Congenital	*Neisseria meningitides* gram-negative rods
C6, C7, C8	Congenital Systemic lupus erythematosus	*Neisseria meningitides* *Neisseria gonorrhea*
Alternative pathway	Sickle-cell disease Splenectomy	*Streptococcus pneumoniae* *Salmonella* species
Immune response		
T-lymphocyte deficiency	Thymic aplasia Thymic hypoplasia Hodgkin's disease Sarcoid Lepromatous leprosy	*Listeria monocytogenes* *Mycobacterium* species *Candida* species *Aspergillus* species *Cryptococcus neoformans* *Herpes simplex* *Herpes zoster* *Strongyloides stercoralis*
	Acquired immunodeficiency syndrome	*Pneumocystis carnii* Cytomegalovirus *Herpes simplex* *Mycobacterium avium-intracellulare* *Cryptococcus neoformans* *Candida* species
T lymphocyte	Mucocutaneous candidiasis	*Candida* species
	Purine nuceloside phosphorylase deficiency	Fungi Viruses
B-cell deficiency/ dysfunction	Bruton's x-linked agammaglobulinemia Agammaglobulinemia Chronic lymphocytic leukemia Multiple myeloma Dysglobulinemia	*Streptococcus pneumoniae* Other streptococci *Hemophilus influenzae* *Neisseria meningitidis* *Staphylococcus aureus* *Giardia lamblia* *Pneumocystis carinii* Enteroviruses

Host defect	Examples of diseases or therapies associated with defects	Common etiological agents of infection
	Selective IgM deficiency	*Streptococcus pneumoniae* *Hemophilus influenzae* *Escherichia coli*
	Selective IgA deficiency	*Giardia lamblia* Viral hepatitis *Streptococcus pneumoniae* *Hemophilus influenza*
Mixed T- and B-cell deficiency/dysfunction	Common variable hypo-gammaglobulinemia	*Pneumocystis carinii* Cytomegalovirus *Streptococcus penumoniae* *Hemophilus influenzae* *Staphylococcus aureus* Rubella *Giardia lamblia*
	Served combined immunodeficiency	*Candida albicans* *Pneumocystis carinii* Varicella Rubella Cytomegalovirus
	Wiscott-Aldrich	Infections seen in T- and B-cell abnormalities

important consequences in terms of susceptibility to protozoan and helminthic infection. The most common causes of lymphopenia are hematological malignancies, corticosteroid therapy, antilymphocyte globulines, cytotoxic drugs, and infection with certain viruses such as cytomegalovirus and HIV. Congenital lymphopenias can also have severe consequences.

Lymphocyte dysfunction can predispose to life-threatening infection even if lymphocyte number is normal. Lymphocyte dysfunction is most often a consequence of corticosteroids or of cytotoxic antineoplastic or anti-inflammatory therapy or of HIV infection.

B. Immunoglobulin Disorders

A profound decrease in the ability to synthesize functional immunoglobulin, particularly IgG, can cause a marked increase in susceptibility to infections caused by *P. carinii, Plasmodia, Babesia,* and *G. lamblia.* Patients with significant reduction in IgG (usually less than 200-300 mg/dl) characteristically have recurrent infections due to encapsu'ated bacteria, particularly *Streptococcus pneumoniae, Hemophilus influenzae,* and *Neisseria meningitidis,* and to certain protozoa (*Pneumocystis carinii* and *Giardia lamblia*). Selective IgA deficiency, when severe, can be associated with similar infections, particularly those due to *Giardia lamblia,* as well as severe viral hepatitis. The few documented cases of significant selective IgM deficiency have also been associated with severe infections, particularly those associated with gram-negative organisms such as *Neisseria meningitidis.* Causes of clinically important immunoglobulin deficiency or dysfunction include both congenital and acquired disorders, malignancies (multiple myeloma, chronic lymphocytic leukemia), sickle cell disease, and childhood splenectomy (Table 2).

C. Complement Disorders

The consequences of total absence of functional complement proteins depends on which of the specific components are deficient (Table 2) (11). Deficiencies of the early components (C1, C4, C2) have been associated with pneumococcal infections, while deficiencies of C3, C5, C6, C7, or C8 may lead to relapsing *Neisseria meningitidis* or *Neisseria gonorrhea* infections. The majority of severe deficiencies are reported with inherited disorders, although there are reports relating significant deficiencies to systemic lupus erythematosus, cirrhosis, and splenectomy. Complement disorders are not directly important factors with respect to the frequency or severity of protozoan or helminthic processes.

D. Splenectomy

The spleen is a major site for T-cell-independent immune responses, and large numbers of B lymphocytes reside there, as do monocytes and macrophages. The spleen has an important role in the phagocytosis of circulating opsonized organisms. Following splenectomy, young children are at high risk for fulminant infections due to *Streptococcus pneumoniae, Hemophilus influenzae,* and

Neisseria meningitidis. In contrast, when otherwise healthy adults undergo splenectomy they probably are at only modestly increased risk for these infections, especially during the first three years post surgery. Malaria appears to be more severe after splenectomy in several reported cases, and babesiosis as a clinical illness seems to occur with unusually high frequency in individuals who have had splenectomies. The clinical importance of splenectomy for other protozoan and helminthic infections is less clear. Pneumocystis pneumonia, for example, has not been reported in individuals whose only risk factor was splenectomy. Similarly, giardiasis does not appear to be more frequent or severe after splenectomy even though humoral immunity is clearly an important component of host defense mechanisms against *G. lamblia.*

The specific host defense mechanisms listed in Table 1 are all important for protecting the host against endogenous and exogenous flora. The physical and chemical barriers are probably more important for bacterial and fungal organisms that for protozoa, or helminths. For example, the filariform larvae of *S. stercoralis* can penetrate intact mucosal and cutaneous barriers, respectively, in contrast to bacteria and fungi. Similarly, although the sphincter of Oddi protects the biliary system from the entire range of microbial flora in the gastrointestinal tract, the aerobic and anaerobic flora are much more plentiful and more likely to cause biliary disease if the sphincter barrier is breached than are *Cryptosporidium sp, G. lamblia,* or *E. histolytica.* However, intestinal protozoa may on rare occasion be associated with biliary disease. Gastric acidity is probably less important for protecting the host against protozoan cysts than for protection against bacteria and fungi.

Recognition of which specific and nonspecific host defenses are compromised is essential to developing an effective strategy for prevention, early recognition, and prompt therapy of the etiological agents that are most likely to cause infectious diseases. Such an understanding thus enhances the quality and duration of patient survival. Faced with an immunocompromised patient with a febrile illness, some clinicians feel overwhelmed by the breadth of possibilities and either become nihilist or try to start therapy with a vast array of the newest, most toxic, or most expensive agents. In fact, understanding which host defense mechanisms are compromised is an important first step to developing a rational plan of medical management. Such an understanding is particularly important with regard to protozoan and helminthic infections, since most clinicians do not routinely order the appropriate diagnostic tests for these diseases and most broad-spectrum regimens do not include antiprotozoan or antihelminthic coverage. The understanding of mechanisms of host defense must be supplemented by practical experience with the patient population. Immunological or inflammatory parameters measured in the laboratory may not be a precise measure of host susceptibility because of subtle differences that are beyond the discriminant capabilities of current tests. For instance, patients with Hodgkin's disease, CMV hepatitis, and AIDS all have superficially similar in vitro abnormalities in T-lymphocyte function. The clinical experience with susceptibility to infection shows major differences, however: AIDS patients are much more likely to become infected with an opportunistic pathogen than are patients with untreated Hodgkin's disease. Patients who appear to be immunosuppressed because of CMV disease alone do not appear to develop opportunistic infections despite sometimes impressive laboratory abnormalities. Despite the importance of observing the clinical behavior of specific patient populations, separation of defects into the categories listed in Table 1 and matching these defects with common causative organisms (Table 2) are useful in giving the clinican a starting point for designing diagnostic and therapeutic work-ups.

When categorizing defects in host defense mechanisms, it is important to recognize that most patients have defects in more than one host defense mechanism. There are some patients, it is true, who have only one defective antimicrobial defense mechanism. Examples would include a postgastrectomy patient who has lost the chemical barrier of gastric acidity or a patient with a small third-degree burn (whose immune function and nutrition are not altered) who has lost only part of the physical barrier of intact skin. A patient with untreated acute myelocytic leukemia may have a defect only in his inflammatory defense mechanism by virtue of severe neutropenia, and another with untreated Hodgkin's disease may have a defect only in cell-mediated immune mechanisms. After each patient is started on cytotoxic therapy, however, both are likely to have erosions of physical and chemical barriers due to the therapy and iatrogenic procedures. The Hodgkin's disease patient may become neutropenic because of chemotherapy, and the leukemic patient may develop defective cell-mediated immunity due to corticosteroid therapy or malnutrition. Thus, the clinician must keep in mind that many forces are likely to be compromising several defense mechanisms simultaneously. As a result, most patients fit into several categories simultaneously.

IV. PROTOZOA AND HELMINTHS IN COMPROMISED
PATIENTS

Everyone who lives in North America is likely to be exposed to protozoa or helminths at some juncture in his or her life. For some of the microorganisms listed in Table 3 there are good serological tests for assessing the frequency of infection; for others, the evidence for exposure in North America is based on surveys of stool examination or autopsy records. Exposure to *P. carinii,* as the first example, must be very common. There is no sensitive and specific serology to detect *P. carinii* infection, so prevalence in North America must

Table 3   Protozoan and Helminthic Organisms of Special Importance to
Compromised Patients

| | Neutropenia | Enhanced importance in compromised patient populations | |
		Deficient humoral immunity	Deficient cell-mediated immunity
Protozoans			
Pneumocystis carinii	−	+	+
Toxoplasma gondii	−	−	+
Cryptosporidia	−	−	+
Giardia lamblia	−	+	−
Entamoeba histolytica	−	−	+/−
Free living amoeba (*Acanthamoeba*)	−	−	+/−
Babesia species	−	+	+
Isospora belli	−	−	+
Plasmodia species	−	+/−	+/−
Leishmania species	−	−	+
Trypanosoma species	−	−	−
Helminths			
Strongyloides stercoralis	−	+/−	+
Filaria species	−	−	+/−

be estimated. Transmission is thought to be by a respiratory route (13,14). When any subpopulation with AIDS is examined retrospectively at autopsy there is a high frequency of *P. carinii* pneumonia regardless of whether the population consists of males, females, homosexuals, drug abusers, hemophiliacs, or heterosexual recipients of blood products (15-21). This suggests either that primary exposure occurs frequently during the period of immunosuppression or, more likely, that most of the population has a history of exposure and subclinical infection at a young age and that reactivation occurs during appropriate immunosuppression. Thus, indirect evidence suggests that *P. carinii* is a ubiquitous pathogen in North America.

Toxoplasma gondii has been shown by reliable serological techniques to be present in 20-70% of North Americans, who appear to acquire infection by consuming inadequately cooked meat or by exposure to the feces of cats producing oocysts in their gastrointestinal mucosa (1,2,22,23). Some disease in immunocompromised patients may be due to primary infection. Serological data suggest that most toxoplasmosis in immunocompromised patients represents reactivated latent infection. In some western countries such as France, *T. gondii* infection is even more common than in the United States, occurring in 87% of Parisians 30-40 years old (22).

E. histolytica and *G. lamblia* are common worldwide, including North America. They are transmitted by fecal-oral spread that occurs due to fecally contaminated food and water or because of fecal contamination due to sexual practices or poor hygiene (4-6). *Giardia lamblia* is the most commonly recognized cause of waterborne diarrheal disease and is the most commonly recognized intestinal protozoan in the United States (4,30-31). In some studies, as many as 20-50% of children in day care centers are infected. The prevalence of *Entamoeba histolytica* in the United States for the population as a whole is less than 1%, although there are higher prevalence rates in institutionalized individuals and in specific subpopulations (32). *E. histolytica* is not commonly encountered in heterosexual North Americans, but homosexually active individuals have a high prevalence. Either *G. lamblia* or *E. histolytica* is present in 30-50% of the homosexual males in some cities (6). Other intestinal protozoa are less common in North America. The occurrence of occasional disease due to *Isospora belli* and *Cryptosporidium* indicate that these protozoans are also present in the environment, but they appear to be quite rare compared to *G. lamblia* and *E. histolytica* (33-39). As more refugees and emigrants from tropical areas are seen in the United States, more such protozoan disease will be encountered.

Free-living ameba, particularly *Acanthamoeba*, are present in soil and freshwater and can be found in human oral cavities. *Acanthamoeba* are ubiquitous, but it is difficult to assess what fraction of North Americans are colonized with them (40-42).

Babesia species infect North Americans who visit Nantucket, Martha's Vineyard, and other geographical locations where the appropriate vector and animal reservoirs are present. As many as 7% of individuals active outdoors in Nantucket become seropositive (3,43). How long the parasitemia persists in seropositive individuals has not been clearly delineated (43). The duration of persistence of parasitemia has obvious relevance to the potential for subsequent immunosuppression to cause active disease.

Plasmodia, Trypanosoma, and *Leishmania* are not likely to be acquired within the United States. *Trypanosoma cruzi* or *Plasmodia* or *Leishmania* could be acquired during travel. Alternatively, *T. cruzi* and *Plasmodia* can be acquired by blood transfusion in the United States, although this is a very rare occurrence. Parasitemia with some of these organisms (e.g., *Plasmodium malariae*) can persist for years after initial infection (44,45).

Strongyloides stercoralis is common in many parts of the United States; a prevalence rate of 0.4–4% is estimated for some southern states, including 3% of children in Clay County, Kentucky (7,46). In some institutions, prevalence rates of 5–35% have been reported. Humans are infected by infective filariform larvae, which can penetrate intact skin of individuals walking barefoot. An internal cycle of autoinfection also occurs since the eggs excreted by adult worms can transform into filariform larvae in the intestine and produce the autoinfective cycle (47). This cycle permits persistence of viable organisms for decades after initial exposure, a relevant issue even for North American urban dwellers who have previously been exposed during residence in endemic areas domestically or abroad.

These epidemiological features suggest that an individual residing in the United States has a substantial chance of being infected with several protozoans or ameba during his lifetime. Since many of these protozoans and helminths persist in the human as viable organisms for years or decades or a lifetime (especially *P. carinii, T. gondii,* and *S. stercoralis*), it is not surprising that an alteration in host defense mechanisms could result in clinically important protozoan or helminthic disease.

Alteration in host defense mechanisms has dramatically different implications for the various protozoans and helminths listed in Table 3. There is no evidence that alteration in physical or chemical mechanisms will increase the frequency of infection for any of these entities, unlike the case of *Mycobacterium tuberculosis* or *Salmonella* with regard to gastrectomy or unlike the case of bacterial sepsis associated with extensive alterations in cutaneous or mucosal barriers. Depression in inflammatory or immunological function does alter the expression of some of these protozoan and helminthic infections, however. For some, such as *T. gondii, P. carinii, Cryptosporidium sp,* and *S. stercoralis* alteration in cell-mediated immunity has profound effects on the ability and frequency with which latent (and probably primary) infection causes disease. For others such as *G. lamblia, Babesia,* and probably *Plasmodia,* alteration in humoral immunity influences the frequency and severity of clinical disease. For organisms such as *Trichomonas* alterations in inflammatory and immunological mechanisms do not appear to influence the expression or frequency of clinical disease although immunological mechanisms do appear to have a role in host defense against the organisms.

V. SPECIAL PATIENT POPULATIONS

Protozoan and helminthic infections clearly occur in immunocompetent as well as immunocompromised patient populations. Life-threatening disease due to any of the organisms listed in Table 3 was a rarity at most medical centers, however, until the early 1980s and the advent of AIDS. Pneumocystis pneumonia was the only life-threatening protozoan or helminthic infection seen with any regularity at most medical centers. The Centers for Disease Control estimated annual attack rates to be 0.01–1.1% from 1967 to 1970 in a variety of populations with congenital and acquired immunodeficiencies (45). Few centers, even those with active oncology and transplant units, probably documented more than one to three cases per year of cerebral or disseminated toxoplasmosis, disseminated strongyloidiasis, chronic crytposporidiosis, or cases of amebiasis, malaria, or giardiasis that were unusually severe because of immunodeficiency (48–51). The other organisms listed in Table 3 were rarely seen in North America as causes of life-threatening disease, with the possible exception of *Babesia* species at certain hospitals in special endemic areas.

The epidemic of AIDS in North America and worldwide has resulted in an explosion in the number of cases of life-threatening protozoan diseases. Table 4 shows the frequency of specific infectious complications in AIDS patients reported to the Centers for Disease Control. Since most of these patients were

Table 4   Opportunistic Infections Among 16,500 AIDS Cases at Time of Report to Centers for Disease Control June 1981–January 1986

Opportunistic infection	Percent of AIDS cases
Pneumocystosis	63%
Candida esophagitis	14%
Cytomegalovirus disease	7%
Cryptococcosis	7%
Mucocutaneous herpes simplex	4%
Cryptosporidiosis	4%
Toxoplasmosis	3%
Other	3%

Source: Adapted from Ref. 15.

Table 5   Immediate Cause of Death in 110 Autopsied AIDS Patients

Cause of death	Percent of patients
Infections	88
CMV disease	24
Pneumocystosis	24
Toxoplasmosis	15
Cryptococcosis	6
Bacterial infections	5
Mycobacterium avium-intracellulare	1
Multiple and other infections	6
Malignant neoplasms	7
Kaposi's sarcoma	5
Lymphoma	2
Other	5

Source: Adapted from Refs. 16 and 19.

reported soon after initial diagnosis, these figures undoubtedly are substantial underestimates of true frequency (15). Table 5 lists the immediate cause of death in patients with AIDS (16-21). The data in these two tables combined with U.S. Public Health Service projections for 175,000–235,000 cumulative AIDS cases in the United States by 1991 demonstrate that life-threatening protozoan infections will be frequent causes of morbidity and mortality in the United States over the next five years unless a method to prevent the progressive immunological decline induced by HIV is found.

   The dramatic frequency of protozoan infections in AIDS presents an important lesson about the interrelationship between protozoans or helminths and cellular immunity. AIDS is only one of many diseases that are associated with defective cell-mediated immunity because of the underlying disease or because of therapy. Patients with Hodgkin's disease, other lymphomatous leukemias, or a variety of congenital disorders including DiGeorge's syndrome and patients receiving corticosteroids all have defective cellular immune mechanisms, but none has the extraordinary and dramatic predisposition to clinically important and life-threatening protozoan processes that characterize AIDS. Interestingly, disseminated strongyloidiasis has been a relatively rare occurrence in AIDS, suggesting either a discordance between the geographical occurrences of AIDS and *S. stercoralis* or an immunological defect that does not involve those specific and subtle mechanisms that control *S. stercoralis* in contrast to certain protozoans. The relationship between the immune response in AIDS and protozoan disease is especially important because of the high prevalence of many protozoan infections for certain groups of AIDS patients. Enteric organisms such as *Entamoeba histolytica, Giardia lamblia,* and more recently *Isospora belli* and cryptosporidia are well known to be common in homosexual males who are sexually active (6,33–35). *E. histolytica* or *G. lamblia* can be found in 30–50% of certain subpopulations of homosexual males and are well-recognized components of the "gay bowel syndrome" (4–6). *Cryptosporidium* and *Isospora* can be isolated but are much less common. It is an important observation relating to important aspects of HIV-induced immunodeficiency (in contrast with other immunosuppressive disorders) that *Entamoeba histolytica* and *Giardia lamblia* do not appear to cause unusually severe disease in AIDS patients in contrast to *Cryptosporidium, Isospora, P. carinii,* and *T. gondii* (52–65). Whether common protozoans such as *Trypanosoma, Leishmania,* or *Plasmodia,* or helminthic diseases will produce unusually severe clinical disease in AIDS in Africa and South America remains to be seen (59–65). As HIV disease is studied more intensively in these areas, it may become apparent that susceptibility to severe, reactivated malaria, leishmaniasis, or trypanosomiasis may complicate the clinical course of AIDS. Similarly, as AIDS cases increase in number, it remains to be determined. whether ubiquitous protozoans such as *Acanthamoeba* or geographically restricted organisms such as *Babesia* species will become more important clinical problems. Thus, the details of the immunological abnormalities in AIDS have important implications for assessing which specific defense mechanisms are important for specific organisms and what immunomodulating therapy might be beneficial in the future.

HIV infection is one of many diseases that are characterized by defective cell-mediated immunity. The most striking immunological consequence of HIV infection is diminution in the number and function of the helper/inducer subset of T lymphocytes, and abnormality that has ramifications for other aspects of immunological and inflammatory host defense (64,65). T lymphocytes in HIV-infected patients demonstrate enhanced in vivo activation without stimulation, as evidenced by increased spontaneous incorporation of [^{3}H] thymidine. Mitogenic and specific antigen-induced responsiveness of unfractionated T cells are reduced in HIV-infected patients. When purified T-cell populations are examined, mitogen responsiveness appears to be normal, in contrast to antigen-induced responsiveness, which remains markedly abnormal. This inability of T4 cells to respond to soluble specific antigen appears to be one of the earliest defects in the immunological responsiveness of HIV-infected individuals. This has obvious implications relevant to the frequency of opportunistic infections in this patient population.

Functionally, T4 cells have been shown to be a poor source of help to B cells. The ability of T4 cells to produce soluble mediators that influence phagocytic cells is also markedly defective. Gamma interferon production has been shown to be markedly reduced or absent. Gamma interferon has particular importance because of its recognized role in inducing effective intracellular killing of intracellular protozoans such as *T. gondii* and *Leishmania* (72–76).

T4-lymphocyte number and function appear to correlate with the susceptibility to infection and life expectancy for groups of HIV-infected individuals (69,70). Groups with relatively longer life expectancy such as those with Kaposi's sarcoma (without opportunistic infection) and generalized lymphadenopathy have more T4 cells than patients who have had opportunistic infections. Similarly, unpublished observations would suggest that HIV-infected individuals with greater than 200/mm^3 T4 lymphocytes rarely develop life-threatening opportunistic infection. The function of T4 lymphocytes also correlates with outcome: Antigen-stimulated lymphocyte proliferation and gamma interferon production are absent or barely measurable in HIV-infected individuals in whom AIDS develops on short-term follow-up. In contrast, patients whose T4 lymphocytes are better able to respond to antigen stimulation and produce gamma interferon are less likely to have AIDS-defining events. It is important to recognize, however, that these correlations of in vitro function and clinical status are valid for groups of patients but that within each group there is some heterogeneity. Thus, these in vitro parameters are not absolute predictors for individual patients. Several patients with no T4 lymphocytes and markedly reduced production of gamma interferon have survived for 12–24 months without serious infections, suggesting that there are subtle differences in host defense mechanisms that are not delineated by currently available laboratory tests.

In addition to abnormalities in helper/inducer T4 lymphocytes, HIV-infected individuals manifest quantitative and qualitative abnormalities in cytotoxic/ suppressor T8 lymphoctyes. T8 lymphocyte numbers may be elevated, normal, or depressed. Qualitatively, responses mediated by T8 cells such as cytotoxic responses against CMV-infected syngeneic targets. This cytotoxic responsiveness correlates with poor clinical outcome for CMV-infected organ transplant recipients (75). Its importance for protozoan infections is uncertain, although bone marrow and kidney transplant recipients with defective cytotoxic responsiveness to CMV-infected targets do not have simultaneous clinical problems with *P. carinii* or *T. gondii* that are nearly as frequent and severe as their clinical problems due to CMV.

HIV-infected individuals have abnormalities in humoral response as well as cell-mediated response (76). They characteristically have normal or elevated serum immunoglobulin levels.Their B cells are intensely polyclonally activated. B lymphocytes fail to react to normal signals for B-cell activation. Patients have diminished capability to respond to immunization by mounting antigen-specific antibody. It seems likely that these B-cell abnormalities are due to viral transformation in the absence of a normal T-cell regulatory environment. The relevance of these B-cell abnormalities to clinical susceptibility to disease is uncertain. There are some data suggesting that AIDS patients have enhanced susceptibility to bacterial pathogens such as *Streptococcus pneumoniae*. Whether this is a real association when other factors are considered is uncertain. The role that deficient quantity or quality of immunoglobulin plays in predisposing to bacterial or protozoan disease is uncertain.

Monocytes and macrophages are essential for controlling protozoan diseases. In HIV-infected patients the number of circulating monocytes appears to be normal. These monocytes are functionally abnormal, however, as manifested by defective chemotaxis. The ability of HIV-infected monocytes to perform phagocytosis and intracellular killing appears to be normal. If gamma interferon is present, AIDS monocytes produce normal quantities of hydrogen peroxide and have normal cytotoxic potential. As noted above, however, HIV-infected individuals are often unable to produce normal quantities of gamma interferon. AIDS monocytes and macrophages also appear to have defective Fc receptor-mediated clearance as assessed by clearance of ^{51}Cr-labeled antibody-coated erythorcytes, a potentially important issue for protozoans present in the peripheral circulation.

These immunological abnormalities in HIV-infected individuals are qualitatively and quantitatively so severe that they render the individual far more susceptible to opportunistic infection than any other population of immunologically abnormal patients. Some infectious diseases such as pneumocystosis and toxoplasmosis occur far more frequently in AIDS patients than in any other population recognized. *P. carinii,* for example, appears to have an annual attack rate of 35-70% in AIDS patients, in contrast to 0.01-1.1% for other patient population studies 10–15 years ago. Toxoplasmosis, *Mycobacterium avium* infection, cryptosporidiosis, and candidiasis are other examples of infections that occur far more frequently in AIDS patients than in any other immunosuppressed population currently dealt with (65). The immunological defect in AIDS does not produce clinical susceptibility to all pathogens that depend on cell-mediated immunity for host defense, however. Organisms such as *Listeria* and *Nocardia* are common in organ transplant recipients and patients with lymphomas but are almost never seen in patients with HIV infection. Strongyloidiasis has only rarely been reported in association with HIV infection, as is true of clinically severe or invasive amebiasis or giardiasis. Thus the immunological defect in AIDS is selective. This selectivity should be a productive avenue to explore in order to elucidate precise determinants of susceptibility to individual pathogens.

Information about immune defects in AIDS and other immunological disorders would be expected to have therapeutic implications as recombinant immunomodulators become available and bone marrow transplantation is attempted. Unfortunately, no one has yet demonstrated that administration of recombinant gamma interferon, alpha interferon, or interleukin 2 can improve immunological function or prevent or treat opportunistic infection. Identical twin nonablative bone marrow transplantation has also failed to restore immunocompetence or prolong survival. These failures may relate to the doses, schedules, or precise products used. Clearly, however, more research is needed before these immunological lessons gleaned from AIDS can be translated into effective immunoadjuvant therapy for patients with serious protozoan or helminthic disease, many of whom have immunological lesions induced by the parasite or by the underlying disease that share many of the immunological abnormalities induced by HIV.

VI. CONCLUSION

From the data presented in this chapter, it should be clear that exposure to protozoans and helminths is not uncommon in the United States. Moreover, physicians in this country are seeing an expanding number of travelers, immigrants, and refugees who may have been heavily exposed to a wide variety of organisms prior to arriving in the United States for residence or for medical care. The antimicrobial mechanisms most responsible for protecting the host against severe or life-threatening processes are immunological mechanisms. As more and more patients are being immunosuppressed to treat tumors and inflammatory diseases and for organ transplants, and as more and more individuals are infected and immunosuppressed by HIV infection, an increasing number of life-threatening protozoan and helminthic diseases are being seen. Why certain protozoan diseases are so extraordinarily frequent in HIV-infected patients compared to the other groups with deficient cell-mediated immunity is not clear. Investigations of those aspects of host defense in HIV-infected individuals, which allows pneumocystosis, toxoplasmosis, and cryptosporidiosis to be so common and so severe while strongyloidiasis, amebiasis, and giardiasis are clinically less remarkable will do much to improve our understanding of immune response to these organisms. Such studies may also point toward promising strategies for therapeutic immunomodulation.

For physicians caring for immunosuppressed patients, a strategy is necessary for preventing disease before it occurs. For certain populations, screening for *E. histolytica, G. lamblia, S. stercoralis,* and *Plasmodia* could be useful and cost-effective. Eradicating *E. histolytica* and *G. lamblia* from homosexual males before debilitating diarrhea becomes a clinical problem has merit for certain high-risk homosexual groups. Screening immigrants from countries where malaria is endemic to assess the presence of parasitemia or screening their stools for *S.*

Table 6 Diagnostic Tests to Recognize Clinical Disease Due to Protozoa and Helminths in Compromised Patients

Microorganism	Diagnostic test
Protozoa	
Pneumocystis carinii	Special stain (e.g., toluidine blue O, methanamine silver, Gimesa) of pulmonary secretion or lung tissue
Toxoplasma gondii	Special stain (e.g., Giesma) of tissue biopsy, serology
Cryptosporidia	Stool (or other fluid) examination using special stain (e.g., modified acid fast)
Giardia lamblia	Stool examination or duodenal aspiration
Entamoeba histolytica	Stool examination, colonic biopsy, serology
Free-living ameba	Tissue biopsy with special stain (e.g., Giemsa)
Babesia species	Peripheral smear with special stain (e.g., Giemsa or Wright's)
Isospora belli	Stool examination
Plasmodia species	Peripheral smear with special stain (e.g., Giemsa or Wright's)
Leishmania species	Tissue biopsy with special stain (e.g., Giemsa)
Trypanosoma species	Peripheral smear or CSF examination using special stain (e.g., Giemsa)
Helminths	
Strongyloides stercoralis	Direct examination of stool, duodenal contents, sputum, CSF
Filaria species	Tissue biopsy or peripheral smear using special stain (e.g., Giemsa)

stercoralis could provide an opportunity to treat subclinical infection before life-threatening disease occurs.

For immunosuppressed patients who develop a life-threatening helminthic or protozoan disease, a major impediment to successful outcome is that physicians often do not consider such infections as diagnostic possibilities. Thus, the correct diagnostic studies, listed in Table 6, are often unordered since they are not part of the routine fever work-up for immunosuppressed patients. Moreover, many laboratories lack expertise in detecting these organisms. Physicians may be increasingly sophisticated about pneumocystosis and toxoplasmosis in AIDS, but in other settings diagnostic evaluations and empirical therapies often overlook these possibilities.

Protozoans and helminths are important components of our microbial flora. Migration, travel, sexual practices, the use of day care centers, combined with aggressive immunosuppressive medical therapies and the HIV epidemic are providing physicians in the United States with rapidly increasing clinical experience with severe protozoan and helminthic diseases. This experience should mandate more emphasis on these infectious processes in terms of diagnosis, therapy, and prevention if morbidity and mortality due to these processes are to be reduced.

REFERENCES

1. Feldman, H. A., and Miller, L. T. Serological study of toxoplasmosis prevalence. *Am. J. Hyg. 64*:320 (1956).
2. Feldman, H. A. A nationwide serum survey of United States military recruits; VI toxoplasma antibodies. *Am. J. Epidemiol. 81*:305–391 (1965).
3. Ruebush, T. K., Juranek, D. D., Chisholm, E. S., et al. Human babesiosis on Nantucket Island—evidence of self-limited and subclinical infections. *New Engl. J. Med. 297*:825–827 (1977).
4. Hill, D. R. Giardiasis. In *Principles and Practice of Infectious Diseases*, 2nd ed. (G. L. Mandell, R. G. Douglas, and J. E. Bennett, eds.). Wiley, New York, 1985, pp. 1552–1556.
5. Ravdin, J. I., and Jones, T. C., *Entamoeba histolytica* (amebiasis). In *Principles and Practice of Infectious Diseases*, 2nd ed. (G. L. Mandell, R. G. Douglas, and J. E. Bennett, eds.). Wiley, New York, 1985, pp. 1506–1511.
6. William, D. C., High rates of enteric protozoal infections in selected homosexual men attending a venereal disease clinic. *Sex Transm. Dis. 6*:155 (1978).
7. Walzer, P. D., Milder, J. E., Banwell, J. G., Kilgore, G., Klein, M., and Parker, R. Epidemiologic features of *Stronglyloides stercoralis* infection in an endemic area of the United States. *Am. J. Trop. Med. 31*:313–319 (1982).
8. Gallin, J. I., and Fauci, A. S. *Advances in Host Defense Mechanisms*. Vol. 1. *Phagocytic Cells*. Raven Press, New York, 1982.
9. Gallin, J. I., and Fauci, A. S. *Advances in Host Defense Mechanisms*. Vol. 2. *Lymphoid Cells*. Raven Press, New York, 1983.
10. Bodey, G. P., Buckley, M., Sathe, Y. S., and Freireich, E. J. Quantitative relationships between circulating leukocytes and infection in patients with acute leukemia. *Ann. Intern. Med. 64*:328 (1966).

11. Ross, S. C., Densen, P. Complement deficiency states and infection. Epidemiology, pathogenesis and consequences of neisserial and other infections in an immune deficiency. *Medicine 63*:243 (1984).
12. Tramont, E. C. General or non-specific host defense mechanisms. In *Principles and Practice of Infectious Diseases*, 2nd ed. (G. L. Mandell, R. G. Douglas, and J. E. Bennett, eds.). Wiley, New York, 1985 pp. 25–31.
13. Walzer, P. D., Schnelle, V., Armstrong, D., et al. Nude mouse: a new experimental model for *Pneumocystis carinii* infection. *Science 197*:177 (1977).
14. Singer, C., Armstrong, D., Rosen, P. P., and Schottenfeld, D. *Pneumocystis carinii* pneumonia: a cluster of eleven cases. *Ann. Intern. Med. 82*:772–777 (1975).
15. CDC. Update: acquired immunodeficiency syndrome. *MMWR 35*:17–21 (1986).
16. Moskowitz, L., Hensley, G. T., Chan, J. C., and Admas, K. Immediate causes of death in acquired immunodeficiency syndrome. *Arch. Pathol. Lab. Med. 109*:735–738 (1985).
17. Guarda, L. A., Luna, M. A., Smith, J. L., Jr., Mansell, P. W. A., et al. Acquired immune deficiency syndrome: postmortem findings. *AJCP, 81*: 549–557 (1984).
18. Neidt, G. W., and Schinella, R. A. Acquired immunodeficiency syndrome: clinicopathologic study of autopsies. *Arch. Pathol. Lab. Med. 109*:727–734 (1985).
19. Joshi, V. V., Oleske, J. M., Saad, S., et al. Pathology of opportunistic infections in children with acquired immunodeficiency syndrome. *Pediatr. Pathol. 6*:145–150 (1986).
20. Pitchenik, A., Fischl, M., Dickinson, G. M., Becker, D. M., et al. Opportunistic infections and Kaposi's sarcoma among Haitians: evidence of a new acquired immunodeficiency state. *Ann. Intern. Med. 98*:277–284 (1983).
21. Niedt, G. W., and Schinella, R. A. Acquired immunodeficiency syndrome—clinicopathologic study of 56 autopsies. *Arch. Pathol. Lab. Med. 109*: 727–734 (1985).
22. Couvreur, J., and Desmonts, G. Congenital and maternal toxoplasmosis. A review of 300 congenital cases. *Develop. Med. Child Neurol. 4*:519–530 (1962).
23. Kean, B. H., Kimball, A. C., and Christenson, W. N. An epidemic of acute toxoplasmosis. *JAMA 208*:10002 (1969).
24. Vietzke, W. M., Gelderman, A. H., Grimley, P. M., et al. Toxoplasmosis complicating malignancy—experience at the National Cancer Institute. *Cancer 21*:816 (1968).
25. Carey, R. M., Kimball, A. C., and Armstrong, D. Toxoplasmosis: clinical experiences in a cancer hosptial. *Am. J.Med. 54*:30–38 (1973).
26. Ruskin, J., and Remington, J. S. Toxoplasmosis in the compromised host. *Ann. Intern. Med. 84*:193–199 (1976).
27. Wong, B., Gold, J. W. M., Brown, A. E., et al. Central nervous system toxoplasmosis in homosexual men and drug abusers. *Ann. Intern. Med. 100*:36–42 (1984).

28. Mills, J. *Pneumocystis carinii* and *Toxoplasma gonii* infections in patients with AIDS. *Rev. Infect. Dis. 8*:1001–1011 (1986).
29. Rosenberg, S., Lopes, M. B., and Tsanaclis, A. M. Neuropathology of acquired immunodeficiency syndrome. Analysis of 22 Brazilian cases. *J. Neurol. Sci. 76*:187–198 (1986).
30. Craun, G. F. Waterborne giardiasis in the United States: a review *Am. J. Pub. Health 69*:817 (1979).
31. Sullivan, R., Linneman, C. C., Clark, C. S., and Walzer, P. D. Seroepidemiologic study of giardiasis patients and high risk groups in a midwestern city in the United States. *Am. J. Public Health 77*:960–963 (1987).
32. Krogstad, D. J. Amebiasis and amebic meningoencephalitis. In *Cecil Textbook of Medicine*. (J. B. Wyngaarden and L. H. Smith, eds). W. B. Saunders, Philadelphia, 1985, pp. 1799–1802.
33. Navin, T. R., and Juaranek, D. D. Cryptosporidiosis: clinical epidemiologic and parasitologic review. *Rev. Infect. Dis. 6*:313–327 (1984).
34. Soave, R., Danner, R. L., Ma, P., Hart, C., et al. Cryptosporidiosis in homosexual men. *Ann. Intern. Med 100*:504–511 (1984).
35. Current, W. M., Reese, N. C., Ernest, J. V., Bailey, W. S., et al. Human cryptosporidiosis in immunocompetent and immunodeficient persons. *New Engl. J. Med. 308*:1252–1257 (1983).
36. Henry, M. C., DeClerq, D., Lokombe, B., et al. Parasitologic observations of chronic diarrhea in suspected AIDS adult patients in Kinshasha (Zaire). *Trans. R. Soc. Trop. Med. Hyg. 80*:309–310 (1986).
37. Schneiderman, D. H., Cello, J. P., and Laing, F. C. Papillary stenosis and sclerosing cholangitis in the acquired immunodeficiency syndrome. *Ann. Intern. Med. 106*:546–549 (1987).
38. DeHovitz, J. A., Pape, J. W., Boncy, M., and Johnson, W. D., Jr. Clinical manifestations and therapy of *Isospora belli* infection in patients with the acquired immunodeficiency syndrome. *New Engl. J. Med. 315*:87–90 (1986).
39. Restrepoc, C., Macher, A. M., and Radany, E. H. Disseminated extraintestinalisosporiasis
40. Martinez, A. J. Is acanthameba encephalitis an opportunistic infection? *Neurology 30*:567 (1980).
41. Gonzales, M. M., Gould, E., Dickinson, G., Martinez, J. A., et al. Acqired immunodeficiency syndrome associated with acathamoeba infection and other opportunistic organisms. *Arch. Pathol. Lab. Med. 110*:749–751 (1986).
42. Wiley, C. A., Safrin, R. E., Davis, C. E., et al. Acanthameba meningoencephalitis in a patient with AIDS. *J. Infect. Dis. 155*:130–133 (1987).
43. Ruebush, T. K., Juranek, D. D., Apielman, A., et al. Epidemiology of human babesiosis on Nantucket Island. *Am. J. Trop. Med. Hyg. 30*:937 (1981).
44. Tapper, M. L., and Armstrong, D. Malaria complicating neoplastic disease. *Arch. Intern. Med. 136*:807 (1976).
45. Walzer, P. D., Gibson, J. J., and Schultz, M. G. Malaria fatalities in the United States. *Am. J. Trop. Med. Hyg. 23*:328 (1974).

46. Mahmoud, A. A. F. Intestinal nematodes (roundworms). In *Principles and Practice of Infectious Diseases*, 2nd ed. (G. L. Mandell, R. G., Douglass, and J. E. Bennett, eds.). Wiley, New York, 1985, pp. 1563–1568.

47. Neva, F. Biology and immunology of human strongyloidiasis. *J. Infect. Dis.* *153*:397–406 (1986).

48. Ruskin, J. Parasitic diseases in the compromised host. In *Clinical Approaches to Infection in the Compromised Host* (R. H. Rubin and L. S. Young, eds.). Plenum Medical, New York, 1981, pp. 269–334.

49. Walzer, P. D., Perl, D. P., Drogstad, D.J., Rawson, P. G., and Schultz, M. G. *Pneumocystis carnii* pneumonia in the United Stated. Epidemiologic, diagnostic, and clinical features. *Ann. Intern. Med.* *80*:83–93 (1974).

50. Igra-Siegman, Y., Kapila, R., Sen, P., Kaminsi, Z. C., and Louria, D. B. Syndrome of hyperinfection with *Strongyloides stercoralis*. *Rev. Infect. Dis. 3*:397–407 (1981).

51. Scowden, E. B., Schaffner, W., and Stone, W. I. Overwhelming strongyloidiasis. *Medicine 57*:85 (1978).

52. Trissl, D. Immunology of *Entamoeba histolytica* in human and animal hosts. *Rev. Infect. Dis. 4*:1154–1184 (1982).

53. Eisert, J., Hannibal, J. E., Jr., and Sanders, S. L. Fatal amebiasis complicating corticosteroid management of pemphigus vulgaris. *New Engl. J. Med. 261*:843–845 (1959).

54. El-Hennawyn, M., and Abd-Rabbo, H. Hazards of cortisone therapy in hepatic ameobiasis. *J. Trop. Med. Hyg. 81*:71–73 (1978).

55. Salata, R. A., and Ravdin, J. I. Review of the human immune mechanisms directed against *Entamoeba histolytica*. *Rev. Infect. Dis. 8*:261–272 (1986).

56. Zinneman, H. H., and Kaplan, A. P. The association of giardiasis with reduced intestinal secretory immunoglobulin. *Am. J. Dig. Dis. 17*:793 (1972).

57. LoGalbo, P. R., Sampson, H. A., and Buckley, R. H. Symptomatic giardiasis in three patients with x-linked aggamaglobulinemia. *J. Pediatr. 101*:78 (1982).

58. Hartong, W. A., Gourley, W. K., and Arvanitakis, C. Giardiasis: clinical spectrum and functional-structural abnormalities of the small intestinal mucosa. *Gastroenterology 77*:61–66 (1979).

59. Badaro, R., Carvalho, E. M., Rocha, J., Queiroz, A. C., and Jones, T. C. *Leishmania donovani*: an opportunistic microbe associated with progressive disease in three immunocompromised patients. *Lancet, i*:647–648 (1986).

60. Ma, D. D. F., Concannon, A. J., and Hayes, J. Fatal leishmaniasis in renal transplant patients. *Lancet ii*:311–312 (1979).

61. DeLetona Martinez, J. L. Masa Vasquez, C., and Perez Maestu. Visceral leishmaniasis as an opportunistic infection. *Lancet, ii*:1094 (1986).

62. Clavel, J. P., Couderc, L. J., Belmin, J., et al. Visceral leishmaniasis complicating AIDS. *Trans. R. Soc. Trop. Med. Hyg. 80*:1010–1011 (1986).

63. Nistal, M., Santana, A., Paniaqua, R., and Palacios, J. Testicular toxoplasmosis in two men with acquired immunodeficiency syndrome. *Arch. Pathol. Lab. Med. 110*:744–746 (1986).

64. Parke, D. W., and Font, R. L. Diffuse toxoplasmic retinochoroiditis in a patient with AIDS. *Arch. Ophthalmol. 104*:571-575 (1986).
65. Blaser, M., and Cohn, D. L. Opportunistic infections in patients with AIDS: clues to the epidemiology of AIDS and the relative virulence of pathogens. *Rev. Infect. Dis. 8*:21-30 (1986).
66. Ledford, D., Overman, M., AmericoGonzalvo, M., Cali, A. Mester, E. W., et al. Microsporidiosis myositis in a patient with the acquired immunodeficiency syndrome. *Ann. Intern. Med. 102*:628-630 (1985).
67. Desportes, I., le Charpentier, Y., Galian, A., et al. Occurrence of a new microsporidian enterocytozoan bieneusi n.g., n.sp., in the enterocytes of a human patient with AIDS. *J. Protozoas 32*:250-254 (1985).
68. Simmons, C., Jr., Winter, H. S., Berde, C., Scrater, C., et al. Zoonotic filariasis with lymphedema in an immunodeficient infant. *New Engl. J. Med. 310*:1243-1244 (1984).
69. Lane, J. C., and Fauci, A. S. Immunologic abnormalities in the acquired immunodeficiency syndrome. *Ann. Rev. Immunol. 3*:477-500 (1985).
70. Roger, H. D., and Remherz, E. L. Current concepts—T lymphocytes and ontogeny, function, and relevance to clinical disorders. *New Engl. J. Med.* 1136-1142 (1987).
71. Murray, H. W., Hillman, J. K., Rubin, B. Y., et al. Patients at risk for AIDS related opportunistic infections—clinical manifestations and impaired gamma interferon production. *New Engl. J. Med. 313*:1504-1510 (1985).
72. Murray, H. W., Berish, Y., Rubin, S. C., and Acosta, A. M. Reversible defect in antigen-induced lymphokine and of interferon generation in cutaneous leishmaniasis. *J. Immunol. 133*:2250-2254 (1984).
73. Carvalho, E. M., Badaro, R., Reed, S., Jones, T. C., and Johnson, W. D., Jr. Absence of gamma interferon and interleukin 2 production during active visceral leishmaniasis. *J. Clin. Invest. 76*:2066-2069 (1985).
74. Murray, J. W., Berish, Y. R., and Rothermal, C. D. Killing of intracellular *Leishmania donovani* by lymphokine-stimulated human mononuclear phagocytes. *J. Clin. Invest. 72*:1506-1510 (1983).
75. Quinnan, G. V., Kirmani, N., Rook, A., et al. Cytotoxic T cells in cytomegalovirus infection: HLA restricted T lymphocyte and non-T lymphocyte cytotoxic responses correlate with recovery from cytomegalovirus in bone marrow transplant recipients. *New Engl. J. Med. 307*:7-13 (1982).
76. Lane, H. C., Masur, H., Edgar, L. C., et al. Abnormality of B cell activation and immunoregulation in patients with the acquired immunodeficiency syndrome. *New Engl. J. Med. 309*:453-458 (1983).

2

Host Defenses Against Prototypical Intracellular Protozoans, the *Leishmania*

RICHARD D. PEARSON and MARY E. WILSON*
University of Virginia School of Medicine, Charlottesville, Virginia

I. INTRODUCTION

Parasitic diseases have been a scourge of mankind since antiquity. In developing areas of the world, malaria alone is estimated to cause more than 1.5 million deaths per year, and schistosomiasis another 500,000 (1). In the industrialized countries of North America, Europe, Australia, and Asia, the implementation of public health measures, the availability of antiparasitic chemotherapy, and the development of generally high standards of personal hygiene have resulted in a progressive reduction in the incidence of serious parasitic diseases since the turn of the century. However, the 1980s have witnessed a reversal in this trend. The rapid spread of HIV infection and the use of immunosuppressive chemotherapy for organ transplantation and the treatment of neoplasms, collagen vascular disease, and other diseases have resulted in increasing numbers of immunocompromised persons who are susceptible to life-threatening opportunistic parasitic infections.

Parasitism can be broadly defined as the intimate association in which one species depends on another for its existence. The consequences for the host vary and are contingent in part on the number of parasitic organisms, their tissue tropism, and the specific mechanisms by which they mediate tissue damage (2). Equally important are the efficacy of the host's innate defenses and the humoral and cell-mediated immune responses that develop.

Protozoans are unicellular organisms that often have multiple sexual and asexual developmental stages. Pathogenic protozoans are capable of multiplying within their human hosts, whereas helminths (worms) generally are not. The

---

Present affiliation: University of Iowa, Iowa City, Iowa.

inoculation of even a single protozoan can in many instances produce life-threatening infection. Although overlap exists, protozoans can be broadly classified into intestinal pathogens, which spend most of their life in the lumen of the gut, and blood and tissue parasites. Worldwide the most important blood and tissue protozoal diseases are malaria (*Plasmodium* species), leishmaniasis (*Leishmania* species), African trypanosomiasis (*Trypanosoma brucei gambiense* and *T. brucei rhodesiense*), Chagas' disease (*Trypanosoma cruzi*), toxoplasmosis (*Toxoplasma gondii*), and *Pneumocystis carinii* pneumonia. Important intestinal protozoans include *Entamoeba histolytica*, which on occasion has extraintestinal manifestations, *Giardia lamblia,* and *Cryptosporidium*.

Protozoal pathogens pose a formidable challenge to the immune system because of their multiple stages and antigenic diversity. The relative contributions of humoral and cellular responses in controlling or preventing infection vary among the parasites. For example, in the case of *Trypanosoma brucei*, antibody responses against variant surface glycoproteins are dominant; humoral immunity is also of great importance in malaria. The association of *Pneumocystis carinii* pneumonia and central nervous system toxoplasmosis with HIV infection and immunosuppressive chemotherapy point to the importance of cell-mediated responses in controlling these particular organisms.

Exciting new insights into the immunobiology of systemic protozoal diseases have come from the study of *Leishmania* species (3-6). The *Leishmania* are particularly attractive model systems for the study of cellular immunology. The parasites reside only in mononuclear phagocytes in mammals; control of infection appears to be solely by cell-mediated mechanisms; animal models of infection are well characterized and readily available; the organisms are easily propagated; and parasite-phagocyte interactions can be studied in vitro. Studies of leishmaniasis have been particularly helpful in characterizing (1) the steps involved in activation of macrophages to kill intracellular microbes, (2) the genetic determinants of cell-mediated immune responses, (3) the mechanisms that mediate antigen-specific immunosuppression during intracellular infection, and (4) the contributions of immune responses to the clinical manifestations of disease. The focus of this chapter is on aspects of the immunobiology of leishmaniasis that have provided the greatest insights into the general principles of cellular immunology.

II. THE PARASITE

Leishmania species exist in two basic morphological forms during their life cycle (3). In humans and animals, they are found within mononuclear phagocytes as oval intracellular amastigotes that are 2-3 μm in length and lack an exteriorized flagellum (Fig. 1). In Giemsa or Wright-Giemsa stained preparations, the nucleus appears relatively large and red. The kinetoplast, a specialized mitochondrial

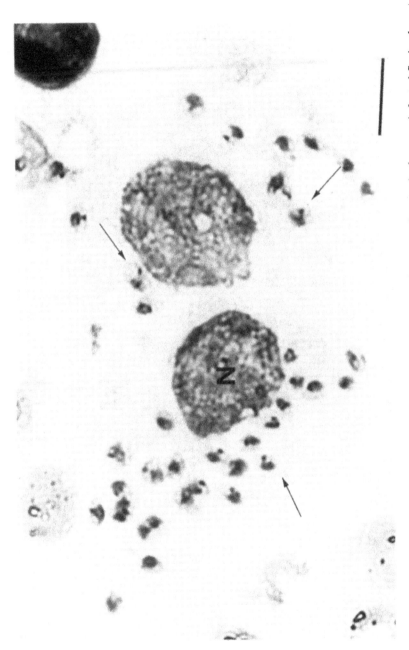

Figure 1 *Leishmania donovani* amastigotes (arrows) are seen in a touch preparation made from an infected Syrian hamster spleen (Wright-Giemsa stain). Amastigotes are 2–3 μm in diameter and have an eccentrically located nucleus and dense-staining, rod-shaped kinetoplast. Nuclei (N) of host mononuclear phagocytes are also seen. The bar represents 10 μm. [Pearson, R. D., et al. *Rev. Infect. Dis. 5:*907–926 (1983); used with permission.]

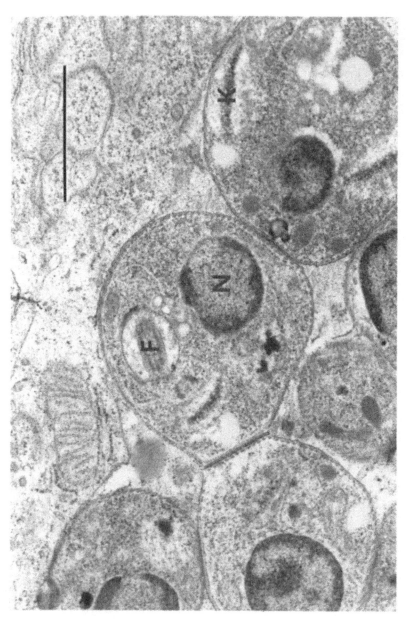

Figure 2 Transmission electron micrograph of an *L. donovani* amastigote showing the parasite nucleus (N), flagellum (F), and kinetoplast (K). A dividing parasite is present. The bar represents 1 μm. [Pearson, R. D., et al. *Rev. Infect. Dis. 5*:907–926 (1983); used with permission.]

structure that contains extranuclear DNA, stains intensely red and appears as a distinctive rod-shaped body. *Leishmania* multiply by fission (Fig. 2). The amastigote converts to and multiplies as a flagellated, extracellular promastigote in the gut of its arthropod vector, the sandfly (Figs. 3 and 4). Promastigotes are pleomorphic and vary in size as they mature. They have pear- or spindle-shaped bodies approximately 10–15 μm in length and 1.5–3.5 μm in width, with a flagellum that is 15–28 μm long. A number of culture media support the growth of promastigotes in vitro (7).

Although minor ultrastructural differences exist, it is impossible to reliably differentiate between *Leishmania* species on the basis of promastigote or amastigote morphology (8–14). Consequently, the original classification of species was based on the clinical syndrome produced in humans, epidemiological differences, geographical distribution, involvement of specific animal reservoirs, and transmission by different sandfly species. Several biochemical methods subsequently became available: isoenzyme pattern (15–19), buoyant density analysis of nuclear or kinetoplast DNA (16,20), radiorespirometry (21), and antigenic

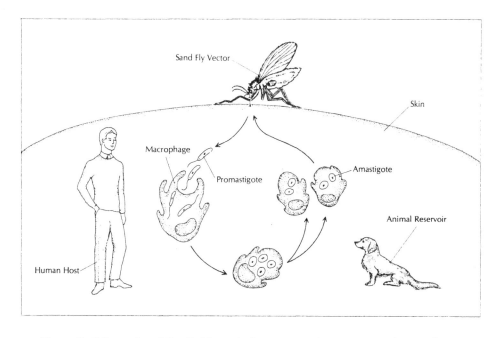

Figure 3 Life cycle of the *Leishmania* from reservoir to vector to human host. In the digestive tract of the arthropod vector, the sandfly, organisms exist as flagellated, extracellular promastigotes. In the mammalian host, parasites are found within mononuclear phagocytes as amastigotes. [Pearson, R. D. *Hospital Practice 19*:100e–100x (1984); used with permission.]

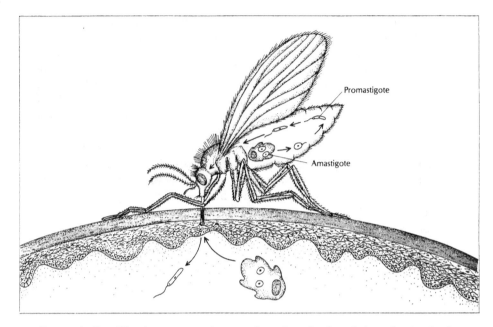

Figure 4 Sandflies ingest amastigotes when they feed on infected animals. In the insect gut, parasites convert to promastigotes and multiply. When sandflies attempt to take their next blood meal, promastigotes are inoculated. [Pearson, R. D. *Hospital Practice 19*:100e–100x (1984); used with permission.]

differences in promastigotes or their excreted factors (22,23). Isoenzyme analysis has been one of the most widely used. Species-specific monoclonal antibodies (24) and restriction endonucelase analysis or hybridization of kinetoplast DNA (24–27) have recently emerged as effective methods of speciation. Although there is no consensus as to the best method for speciation, there has been general agreement among the various biochemical methods. Recently, pulsed field gradient gel electrophoresis has been used to fractionate chromosomes of *Leishmania* species (28), and the karyotypes of species have been found to differ (29).

Cutaneous leishmaniasis is usually caused by *L. major*, *L. aethiopica*, or *L. tropica* (Africa, Asia, Middle East), the *L. mexicana* complex (Central and South America), or the *L. braziliensis* complex (Central and South America). The *L. donovani* complex is the most common cause of visceral disease (South and Central America, Africa, Mediterranean littoral, India, and China). Under certain conditions, the *L. donovani* complex involves the skin. When development of skin lesions follows chemotherapy, the syndrome is termed post-kala-azar dermal leishmaniasis. Conversely, *L. mexicana* and *L. tropica* have been isolated on occasion from patients with typical visceral leishmaniasis.

In most areas, leishmaniasis is a zoonosis; that is, it is primarily a disease of animals, and humans are incidental hosts (3-6). The major exceptions are *L. donovani* infection in India, where no animal reservoir has been found, and possibly in East Africa; and cutaneous leishmaniasis due to *L. tropica*. Sandflies of *Lutzomyia* and *Psychodopygus* species transmit leishmania in the Western hemisphere. *Phlebotomus* species are responsible elsewhere.

III. GENETIC DETERMINANTS OF RESISTANCE

Tremendous progress has been made in the past decade in defining the immuno-genetics of the leishmaniases using murine models. Inbred strains of mice vary dramatically in their susceptibility to infection with various *Leishmania* species. These murine models have proven particularly useful in defining the genetic determinants of susceptibility to infection (30-39).

A. Murine *L. donovani* Infection

Bradley and co-workers were the first to observe that some inbred strains of mice such as BALB/c or C57BL/10 were highly susceptible to infection with *L. donovani* whereas others like C3H/HeJ were resistant (30,34,36). Within a given mouse strain, there was little variation in susceptibility. However, the course of visceral leishmaniasis in susceptible mice differs from that in humans in that mice do not usually die of *L. donovani* infection, even though they develop high parasite burdens. Bradley and co-workers found that susceptibility in mice was mediated by a single gene, termed *Lsh*, located on chromosome 1, and not by the major histocompatibility complex. The regulator(s) of resistance to two other intracellular pathogens, *Salmonella typhimurium* (*Ity*) and *Mycobacterium bovis* (*Bcg*) are seemingly identical to *Lsh* (37). The leishmania-resistant allele (*Lsh^r*) behaves as an incomplete dominant, and the leishmania-sensitive allele (*Lsh^s*) as a recessive.

In vitro and in vivo studies suggest that the *Lsh* gene product is expressed at the level of the liver macrophage (Kupffer cell) (35). Liver macrophages from *Lsh^s* mice support the growth and division of amastigotes, whereas *Lsh^r* cells limit parasite proliferation after 2 days. This lag period may be the time it takes for expression of the *Lsh^r* gene product. Similarly, infection of *Lsh^s* mice is associated with rapid proliferation of amastigotes in liver Kupffer cells, but *Lsh^r* strains limit amastigote growth after a brief period of multiplication. This lag time in *Lsh^r* mice is unaltered after lethal irradiation, suggesting that the effect is independent of T cells.

Among *Lsh^s* strains, some retain high parasite burdens indefinitely, while in others the parasite burden eventually declines. With the use of congeneic mice, which differ from the parent strain only at a small segment of a chromosome, it has been possible to systematically study the genetic determinants responsible for this "curing" pattern. Blackwell used congeneic mice on a B10 background (C57BL/10) that differed only at the chromosome containing the H-2 complex (34). Mice homozygous for H-2^b were found to cure, while those homozygous for H-2^d behaved as noncure. Study of other H-2 haplotypes indicated that H-2^s and H-2^r cleared their infections more rapidly than H-2^b (early versus late cure). These differences between cure and noncure were verified in congeneic mice of different backgrounds (e.g., BALB or CXB), but it was observed that the rate of recovery varied as a function of the background. Finally, studies with recombinant haplotypes carried at either end of the H-2 complex localized control of the response to the K end of H-2. Subsequent studies have revealed that the H-2 differences are dose-dependent and that alleles at the H-11 locus can override the H-2^b response. Both H-2- and H-11-linked genes influence the course of *L. donovani* infection in Lsh^s mice (39). As will be discussed in detail later, the late cure or noncure of Lsh^s strains is probably dependent on a complex interaction between cell-mediated helper and disease-enhancing elements.

B. Murine *L. major* Infection

The susceptibility of mice to *L. major** is also under genetic control, but the genes involved are distinct from *Lsh* (31–33) and attempts to map them have given variable results (28). The strains susceptible to *L. major* do not parallel those susceptible to *L. donovani*, although some strains are resistant or susceptible to both pathogens. Strains of mice susceptible to *L. major*, such as BALB/c, develop progressive cutaneous infection that disseminates widely and eventually leads to death. In contrast, B10 mice and other resistant strains have localized, self-curing ulcers.

Studies using radiation chimeras indicate that susceptibility to *L. major* is determined by descendants of donor hematopoietic bone marrow cells (40). Susceptibility depends on both a "permissive" macrophage and defective T-cell response (41). In general, macrophages from susceptible strains of mice allow extensive intracellular amastigote growth in vitro (42). Macrophages from some resistant mouse strains do not support amastigote growth, whereas macrophages from other resistant strains permit replication. Recent studies indicate that progressive disease in genetically susceptible BALB/c mice is due to the induction of disease-enhancing T-cell subpopulations and/or the failure of protective T-cell clones to proliferate (43). This will be discussed in detail later.

Blackwell and colleagues found, using congeneic mice, that polymorphism in structural genes encoding class II molecules of the major histocompatibility complex, H-2, which can have a profound effect on the course of *L. donovani*

Leishmania major has been widely studied in experimental models. Many older reports refer to it as *Leishmania tropica major* or merely as *Leishmania tropica. Leishmania major* should be distinguished from true *Leishmania tropica*, previously termed *Leishmania tropica tropica*.

infection, have little effect on the development of *L. major* or *L. mexicana mexicana* skin lesions (28). H-11-linked differences affect cutaneous disease due to *L. major* and visceralization and metastatic lesion development with *L. mexicana mexicana* (39). Thus, the H-11-linked gene seems to control one or more mechanisms central to the development of resistance to both visceral and cutaneous disease. Another gene, *Scl-1*, which on recent evidence maps to mouse chromosome 8, is another determinant of *L. major* infection. The *Scl-1* gene also exerts influence over *L. mexicana mexicana.* The gene products of H-11 and *Scl-1* have not yet been identified.

C. Human Leishmaniasis

Clinical observations suggest that people differ in their susceptibility to *Leishmania* species, but the genetics of human leishmaniasis have not been thoroughly studied. In areas where *L. mexicana* subspecies or *L. aethiopica* are endemic, the majority of victims develop localized cutaneous ulcers that heal spontaneously, but some people go on to develop progressive, nonulcerating diffuse cutaneous leishmaniasis, which is an anergic variant. It is tempting to ascribe this to genetic differences among humans, but the parasite strain, size of the infecting inoculum, site of inoculation, concurrent immunosuppression such as that associated with malnutrition or other infection (e.g., measles), or other factors might be important variables. Similar arguments can be made with respect to *L. donovani*, which appears to produce progressive disease in only a minority of infected patients (44). Finally, in a study in the eastern Andes of Bolivia, extreme facial mutilation due to mucocutaneous leishmaniasis was observed almost exclusively in residents of African ancestry, even though more cases of cutaneous leishmaniasis were observed in endogenous Indians (45). Blacks tended to have larger, more severe reactions to intradermally administered leishmanial antigen, suggesting that their mutilating, mucocutaneous lesions were due to exaggerated, but ineffective, hyperergic immune responses. It is again tempting to ascribe this to genetic differences, but alternative explanations are plausible.

IV. EARLY EVENTS

The events that follow inoculation of promastigotes by an infected sandfly can be divided into two segments: the brief period in which promastigotes encounter humoral and phagocytic host defenses and convert to amastigotes, and the remainder of infection in which amastigotes proliferate in macrophages. Studies of the initial stage of leishmanial infection have focused on (1) the histological response that follows experimental inoculation of axenically grown promastigotes into humans or susceptible animals, (2) the interaction of promastigotes with humoral factors, and (3) the attachment to, ingestion by, and fate of promastigotes within mononuclear and polymorphonuclear leukocytes.

Leishmania promastigotes grow in vitro in any of several media. Their morphology and infectivity are dependent in part on their growth cycle. Sacks and co-workers (46,47) have shown in studies of promastigotes derived from sandflies or axenic culture that dividing logarithmic-phase *L. major* promastigotes are noninfectious, whereas a subset of stationary-phase, nondividing "metacyclic" promastigotes are infectious, both for susceptible mice and for macrophages cultured in vitro. Earlier, Giannini (48) observed that the infectivity of *L. donovani* promastigotes for Syrian hamsters increased with culture age.

Sacks et al. (46,47) found that logarithmic *L. major* promastigotes were agglutinated by peanut agglutinin but that the 50% of stationary-phase organisms, which were infective, were not. They then used peanut agglutinin to effectively purify infective, stationary-stage, metacyclic *L. major* promastigotes. A monoclonal antibody raised against peanut agglutinin-negative infective promastigotes was found to recognize a surface antigen not present on logarithmic, noninfective promastigotes. Unfortunately, peanut agglutinin does not differentiate between noninfective and infective promastigotes of all other *Leishmania* species.

The precise sequence of events following inoculation of promastigotes into mammals by sandflies has not been determined. Sandflies are modified pool feeders; that is, they form a pool of blood and extracellular fluid by repeatedly probing with their proboscises. *Leishmania*-infected sandflies are unable to aspirate blood because their proboscises are occluded by promastigotes. Promastigotes are thought to be released into the pool of blood and extracellular fluid as the sandflies attempt to feed.

Wilson et al. (49) studied the early histological responses following experimental inoculation of stationary-phase *L. donovani* promastigotes into the skin of highly susceptible Syrian hamsters. Within 1 hr of parasite inoculation, a mixed polymorphonuclear and mononuclear phagocyte response was noted. Parasites were observed within both types of phagocytes. They appeared to be degraded within polymorphonuclear leukocytes but assumed amastigote morphology within mononuclear phagocytes. Over the next 48 hr the percentage of identifiable parasites in polymorphonuclear leukocytes fell to zero, but intact amastigotes remained in mononuclear phagocytes. The number of intracellular parasites increased dramatically over the subsequent 2 weeks of infection. These in vivo findings suggest that polymorphonuclear leukocytes are capable of ingesting and killing promastigotes whereas at least some mononuclear phagocytes permit their intracellular conversion to amastigotes and support subsequent parasite multiplication.

A. Promastigote–Mononuclear Phagocyte Interactions

The interactions of promastigotes of many *Leishmania* species with peritoneal macrophages, human monocytes, and monocyte-derived macrophages, as well as nonprofessional phagocytes, have been studied extensively in vitro (50–66). Attachment of promastigotes to mononuclear phagocytes occurs in the absence of serum (56,61–64). The initial interaction can occur at either the flagellar or aflagellar poles of the parasite (Fig. 5). Flagellum-first attachment has predominated in most studies, possibly because the parasite is pulled forward by its flagellum. Macrophage pseudopodia develop in response to attachment and progressively advance around the parasite (59). Electron microscopic studies suggest that contact occurs at discrete points at the parasite-phagocyte interface (52). Eventually the parasite is engulfed, often after it has been trapped between adjacent phagocytes (59). The ingestion of promastigotes by macrophages is saturable, and the attachment to macrophages exhibits characteristics

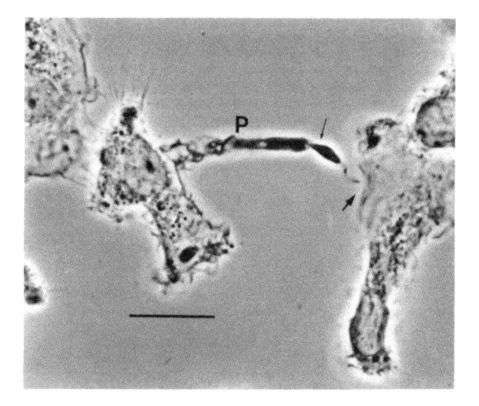

Figure 5 A *Leismania donovani* promastigote that has attached to a human monocyte-derived macrophage by its aflagellar pole. A long pseudopod (P) has formed from the macrophage on the left in response to attachment (small arrow). The parasite's flagellum extends to the macrophage on the right (large arrow). Bar = 10 μm. [Pearson, R. D., et al. *Infect Immun. 40*:411–416 (1983); used with permission.]

of a receptor–ligand interaction (56,60). Klempner et al. demonstrated that attachment of membrane vesicles prepared from human mononuclear cells to *L. tropica* promastigotes exhibited specificity, saturability, and competitive inhibition (65). Promastigote attachment to mononuclear cells was dependent on calcium (55,56) and sensitive to the action of trypsin on the phagocyte but not on the parasite surface (61,66). These observations suggested that the serum-independent attachment of promastigotes to mononuclear phagocytes was a receptor-mediated event and led to the search for relevant macrophage receptors and parasite ligands.

Early competitive binding studies indicated that several monosaccharides including D-glucose, D-mannose, and their derivatives could partially inhibit promastigote ingestion by hamster peritoneal macrophages (55,56). Lectin-binding studies further revealed that promastigotes of multiple *Leishmania* species displayed an array of glycoconjugates on their surfaces and in particular appeared to be rich in exposed surface mannose (67–75). Biochemical studies of *L. donovani* and *L. mexicana mexicana* confirmed that mannose was a major constituent of surface membrane proteins (75,76).

Independently, it was observed that macrophages possess one or more receptors for mannose-terminal glycoconjugates, termed mannose/fucose receptors, that mediate the attachment and ingestion of yeast zymosan (77,78). Macromolecular ligands of these receptors inhibit attachment of *L. donovani* promastigotes to murine peritoneal and human macrophages (66,79–81). The use of mannan, a mannose polymer derived from yeast cell walls, or the neoglycoprotein mannose-bovine albumin, inhibited the attachment and ingestion of *L. donovani* promastigotes by macrophages by approximately 40–60%. The monosaccharide mannose, which is a poor inhibitor of the mannose/fucose receptor, had little effect on promastigote attachment. These data suggest that macrophage mannose/fucose receptors play an important role in parasite attachment.

A mannose-containing ligand from promastigotes, which is involved in promastigote attachment, has subsequently been isolated from *L. mexicana mexicana* and other *Leishmania* species (82–85). Initial examination of promastigote surface proteins by radiolabeling and two-dimensional polyacrylamide gel electrophoresis revealed an abundant polypeptide of molecular weight 63 kD (gp63). Lectin-binding studies indicated that it was a glycoprotein that contained mannose, *N*-acetylglucosamine, and *N*-acetylgalactosamine residues. The gp63 was found to be distributed over the entire promastigote plasmalemma, and anti-gp63 antibodies reduced promastigote binding to macrophages by 65–70% (84). Additional evidence for the involvement of gp63 in parasite-macrophage interactions was provided by studies in which gp63 was incorporated into proteoliposomes. Liposomes containing gp63 were phagocytosed by macrophages, and uptake was inhibited by more than 90% by both anti-gp63 F(ab) fragments and mannan. These results suggest that the abundant gp63 is a ligand for the macrophage mannose/fucose receptor (Fig. 6). Recent studies indicate that this major integral membrane protein is a protease (83). A water-soluble form of the protease is obtained following digestion with the phospholipase C responsible for the release of variant surface glycoprotein from *Trypanosoma brucei* (83).

Recently, attention has turned to the novel glycoconjugates on the cell surface of *Leishmania* termed lipophosphoglycans (LPG). Structurally, LPG from *L. donovani* contain a repeating phosphorylated unit of $PO_4 \rightarrow 6Gal\beta1$-4 Manα1 (76,86-88). This unit is attached via a carbohydrate core to a unique lipid anchor lysoalkylphosphatidylinositol. Gp-63 appears to have the same type of anchoring system. The role that LPG plays in parasite–phagocyte interactions and in the immunology of leishmaniasis is of intense interest. The studies of Handman and Mitchel in BALB/c mice infected with *L. major* suggest that LPG plays an important role in immune responses, as will be discussed.

The failure of mannan and mannose-bovine albumin to completely inhibit *L. donovani* promastigote attachment to and ingestion by macrophages and the finding that promastigotes attach to human monocytes, which do not display mannose/fucose receptors, suggested that other receptor system(s) might be involved. Recently published data indicate that the macrophage type 3 complement receptor (CR3), which binds C3bi, a cleavage product of the third component of complement, also mediates promastigote attachment (80,81,89, 90). Using monoclonal antibodies directed against the mouse macrophage CR3 (anti-Mac-1) or against the human macrophage CR3 (anti-mo1), it has been possible to inhibit the attachment of promastigotes to human monocyte-derived or murine peritoneal macrophages even in the absence of serum (Fig. 7).

Leishmania species are known to activate complement by the alternative pathway (89). In addition, *L. donovani* can activate the classical pathway when incubated with nonimmune or patient serum (91). In the presence of serum, complement components, including C3b, are deposited on the parasite surface; C3b is rapidly cleaved to C3bi. Binding and ingestion of promastigotes by macrophages can be inhibited by anti-CR3 antibodies. Even in the absence of exogenous serum, antibodies against CR3 decrease promastigote binding and ingestion. There is evidence that promastigotes are opsonized locally by complement components secreted by macrophages (92).

Studies of *L. major* suggest that macrophage fibronectin receptors (93) are also involved in parasite–macrophage interactions. The various receptor systems may promote parasite attachment in an additive manner, like sequential teeth in a zipper, or it is possible that they modulate one another's activity, as has been previously demonstrated in studies of fibronectin and complement receptors in which ligation of fibronectin receptors induced a reversible alteration in the function of complement receptors (94).

A promastigote that attaches to a macrophage is progressively engulfed by the

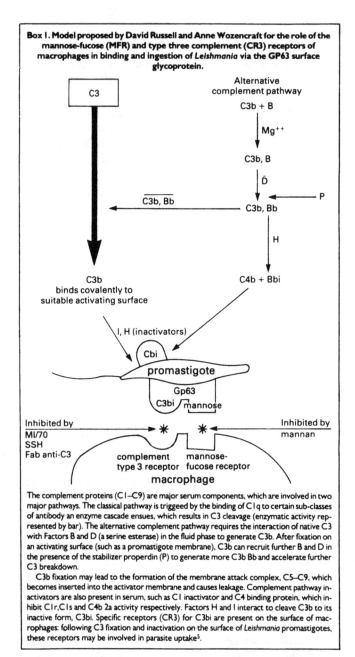

Box I. Model proposed by David Russell and Anne Wozencraft for the role of the mannose-fucose (MFR) and type three complement (CR3) receptors of macrophages in binding and ingestion of *Leishmania* via the GP63 surface glycoprotein.

The complement proteins (C1–C9) are major serum components, which are involved in two major pathways. The classical pathway is triggeed by the binding of C1q to certain sub-classes of antibody an enzyme cascade ensues, which results in C3 cleavage (enzymatic activity represented by bar). The alternative complement pathway requires the interaction of native C3 with Factors B and D (a serine esterase) in the fluid phase to generate C3b. After fixation on an activating surface (such as a promastigote membrane), C3b can recruit further B and D in the presence of the stabilizer properdin (P) to generate more C3b Bb and accelerate further C3 breakdown.

C3b fixation may lead to the formation of the membrane attack complex, C5–C9, which becomes inserted into the activator membrane and causes leakage. Complement pathway inactivators are also present in serum, such as C1 inactivator and C4 binding protein, which inhibit C1r,C1s and C4 2a activity respectively. Factors H and I interact to cleave C3b to its inactive form, C3bi. Specific receptors (CR3) for C3bi are present on the surface of macrophages: following C3 fixation and inactivation on the surface of *Leishmania* promastigotes, these receptors may be involved in parasite uptake[5].

Figure 6 Postulated role of the macrophage mannose/fucose receptor (MFR) and type 3 complement receptor (CR3) in the binding of *Leishmania* promastigotes to macrophages. [Blackwell, J., McMahon-Pratt, D., and Shaw, J. *Parasitology Today* 2:45–53 (1986); used with permission.]

macrophage (59), and the parasite ultimately comes to lie within a vacuole (52,57). Parasite antigens are displayed on the surface of the infected macrophage (50,51). The majority of *L. donovani* promastigotes survive ingestion by human monocyte-derived macrophages, convert to amastigotes as determined by morphological criteria, and then multiply. Human macrophages undergo a phagocytic oxidative burst when ingesting promastigotes, but it is small, and macrophages lack lysosomal myeloperoxidase. In contrast, peripheral blood monocytes are capable of a larger oxidative burst, have lysosomal myeloperoxidase, and kill the majority of ingested promastigotes (60). Promastigotes are very sensitive to the phagocytes' hydrogen peroxide-peroxidase-halide microbicidal mechanism (95-102). The survival of promastigotes in monocytes from donors with chronic granulomatous disease of childhood, which are unable to mount an oxidative burst, has provided direct evidence that oxidative microbicidal mechanisms are involved in the killing of promastigotes by normal monocytes (60,102). Murine peritoneal macrophages also kill *L. donovani* promastigotes by oxidative microbicidal mechanisms, but promastigotes survived well in a clone of a murine macrophage tumor cell line that was not capable of producing a phagocyte oxidative response (103). It has been postulated that oxidatively weak dermal macrophages provide a sanctuary in which promastigotes convert to the more resistant amastigote form.

B. Promastigote-Polymorphonuclear Leukocyte Interactions

In the experimental hamster model of *L. donovani* infection, polymorphonuclear leukocytes were observed in lesions for 48-72 hr after inoculation of promastigotes (49). Polymorphonuclear leukocytes contained degenerating parasites, suggesting that they might be involved in host defense against promastigotes. In vitro studies indicate that human polymorphonuclear leukocytes have the capacity to ingest and kill *L. donovani* promastigotes that are opsonized with complement (97). Few promastigotes were ingested in the absence of opsonization. Promastigotes elicited a phagocytic oxidative burst, and parasites were killed by oxidative microbicidal mechanisms; no killing of ingested promastigotes was observed in polymorphonuclear leukocytes from a donor with chronic granulomatous disease. The histological studies suggest that polymorphonuclear leukocytes migrate to the site of experimental promastigote inoculation, and the in vitro data indicate that they are capable of killing complement-opsonized promastigotes.

C. Interaction of Promastigotes with Serum Factors

Both immune and nonimmune human serum can kill promastigotes (89,91, 104-112). Promastigotes of many *Leishmania* species have been shown to be susceptible to killing by the complement membrane attack complex (C5b-C9). The mechanism of complement activation varies: *L. major* and *L. enriettii* promastigotes activate complement via the alternative pathway (89), while *L. donovani* promastigotes also activate it via the classical pathway (91). Fixation of complement on the parasite surface results in opsonization with C3b and then C3bi and death of the organism if the membrane attack complex is activated. Stationary-phase promastigotes are more resistant to complement-mediated killing than logarithmic-stage parasites (112). In the *L. major* system, log-phase organisms activate complement with deposition of covalently bound C3b on their surface. They are killed by the membrane attack complex. Stationary-phase infective promastigotes bind C3b but not covalently and are not killed (113). Developmentally regulated LPG appears to be a major C3 receptor on both types of promastigotes (113). When polymorphonuclear leukocytes are present, ingestion of complement-opsonized promastigotes may result in parasite death (97). Conversely, complement-mediated ingestion of promastigotes by oxidatively weak macrophages may facilitate entry of the parasite into a sanctuary where it can convert to its amastigote form. Activation of complement by promastigotes may also result in macrophage chemotaxis toward the parasite (114). It has also been postulated that promastigotes may be inoculated by sandflies into the skin at a site where complement is not active or, more likely, that proteases in sandfly saliva might inactivate complement, protecting the parasite from the lethal effects of the membrane attack complex.

The role of antileishmanial antibodies in defense against promastigotes is uncertain. Pretreatment of *L. major* (115) or *L. mexicana* (116) promastigotes with monoclonal antibodies prior to inoculation has at least partially protected experimental animals from disease. However, passive transfer of immune serum to naive recipients has not been shown to be protective, and the high titers of antileishmanial antibodies present during progressive visceral leishmaniasis do not result in resolution of infection.

V. LATER EVENTS

Once *Leishmania* have successfully transformed to amastigotes, the outcome of infection is determined principally by cell-mediated immune mechanisms (117). Amastigotes are adapted to survival within mammalian mononuclear phagocytes, but they can be killed by macrophages that have been "activated" by lymphocytes, either through production of soluble lymphokines such as interferon-gamma or by direct contact. The outcome of infection depends on a complex interplay between helper and disease-enhancing cell-mediated immune elements. In certain instances, the *Leishmania*, despite high parasite burdens, fail to induce antigen-specific immunity. In order to understand the sequence of events that results in clinically apparent leishmaniasis, the following areas will be reviewed:

(1) the interactions of amastigotes with mononuclear phagotcytes, (2) the role of lymphocyte activation of macrophages in amastigote killing, (3) the failure of *Leishmania*-specific immunity in progressive disease, and (4) the contribution of immune responses to the pathophysiology of leishmaniasis.

A. Amastigote-Phagocyte Interactions

Studies of the interaction of mammalian cells with amastigotes have focused on peritoneal macrophages from laboratory rodents (118-126), human peripheral blood monocytes and monocyte-derived macrophages (57-60,63,127), and tumor cell lines (54,128-130). Amastigotes, like promastigotes, bind readily to mononuclear phagocytes in the absence of serum (57-60). Although not as thoroughly studied, it is likely that attachment is mediated by mannose/fucose receptors, CR3 receptors, and/or fibronectin receptors as discussed in reference to promastigotes (81-85,89,92). Furthermore, antileishmanial antibodies are present in the skin during cutaneous leishmaniasis (131) and circulate during visceral disease. They too may contribute to attachment of amastigotes to macrophages via macrophage Fc receptors. The relative contributions of these various receptor-ligand systems to amastigote attachment and ingestion have not been determined.

Antibodies against *Leishmania* have been shown to affect the interaction of amastigotes with macrophages in vitro, possibly by shifting the mechanism of parasite attachment from serum-independent receptor-ligand interaction (e.g., binding of parasites to mannose/fucose receptors, CR3 receptors, or fibronectin receptors) to one mediated by Fc receptors. In one study, rabbit antibodies against amastigotes inhibited attachment of amastigotes to human monocytes (132). In another study, C57BL/6J mice were infected with *L. donovani*, rechallenged after 60 days, and then bled 10-11 days later (133). Their sera contained cytophilic antibodies and opsonins for *L. donovani* amastigotes and promastigotes that resulted in enhanced binding and ingestion of parasites by elicited and "activated" macrophages. Theoretically, enhanced amastigote attachment could be either beneficial or detrimental to the host, depending on the ultimate intracellular fate of the parasite.

Studies of *L. major* suggest that amastigotes actively participate in the attachment process (63). Pretreatment of amastigotes with microfilament inhibitors such as cytochalasin B or D significantly reduced parasite attachment to human monocytes in vitro (63). Once attachment has taken place, however, the macrophage appears to be responsible for the ingestion of amastigotes.

Amastigotes are resistant to killing by circulating human monocytes, monocyte-derived macrophages, and rodent peritoneal macrophages. Both amastigotes and promastigotes possess an iron-containing superoxide dismutase (95). Amastigotes elicit a smaller phagocyte oxidative response (60,79,101). This may be due in part to their smaller surface area. There is also evidence to suggest that a leishmanial membrane-associated acid phosphatase is capable of inhibiting the macrophage respiratory burst (134,135). Finally, amastigotes contain more catalase and glutathione peroxidase than promastigotes and are less susceptible to oxidants such as hydrogen peroxide (60,136,137). Once inside macrophages, amastigotes do not stimulate a continuous oxidative response, and they can decrease the oxidative response to subsequent stimuli.

Amastigotes reside in parasitophorous vacuoles that fuse with lysosomes as evidenced by both in vitro and in vivo studies (63,119-126,138). *Leishmania* thus resemble *Mycobacterium lepraemurium* (139), which permits phagosome-lysosome fusion in macrophages, but differ from viable *Mycobacterium tuberculosis* (140) and *Toxoplasma gondii* (141), whose survival within macrophages seems to be related to their capacity to inhibit phagosome–lysosome fusion. The *Leishmania* also differ from *Trypanosoma cruzi*, which escapes into the cytoplasm of the host cell (142).

The pH of the parasitophorous vacuole, at least in the case of *L. mexicana*, is in the range of pH 5.0 (143). The amastigote seems to be adapted for survival under these conditions. Amastigote membrane transport of glucose and amino acids is optimal at pH 5, whereas promastigotes have optimal function at approximately pH 7 (144). *Leishmania* have a membrane proton translocating ATPase that contributes to the acidic pH within the phagolysosome (28,145). Chang (52) observed that debris trapped in the phagolysosome at the time of amastigote ingestion was degraded over time. This observation suggests that amastigotes do not inactivate macrophage lysosomal enzymes in the parasitophorous granule. The swelling of *L. mexicana*-containing phagolysosomes after treatment with a weak base such as leucine *O*-methyl ester further suggests that substances are hydrolyzed in the phagolysosome (146). Finally, amastigotes are adapted for mammalian temperatures, whereas promastigotes grow at ambient temperatures of 24-26°C. Heat-shock genes may play a role in interconversion between the two parasite stages (147).

Human polymorphonuclear leukocytes are capable of ingesting and killing amastigotes in vitro (148), but polymorphonuclear leukocytes are not thought to play an important role in the resolution of disease. The histopathology of established leishmaniasis is a granulomatous response (131,149); polymorphonuclear leukocytes are not a prominent finding.

Circulating antibodies do not lead to resolution of infection. In general, the magnitude of the circulating antileishmanial antibody response is inversely proportional to the extent and progression of disease in both humans and animals (117,150,151). High antileishmanial antibody titers are found in patients with visceral leishmaniasis, while specific antibodies are absent or at low titer in patients with localized, self-healing cutaneous lesions. Passive transfer of serum has failed to protect animals against amastigote challenge (117,152,153). It is possible, however, that antibodies present during progressive leishmaniasis are not directed against protective parasite epitopes. Interestingly, immune sera from convalescent animals have been shown to augment the level of adoptive immunity expressed in recipient animals when administered concurrently with immune T cells (117).

The effect of complement on amastigotes varies with the *Leishmania* species. *Leishmania donovani* amastigotes are relatively resistant to killing by complement (91). Conversely, *L. major* amastigotes are killed after alternative pathway activation of the complement cascade (154,155). The entire membrane attack complex (C5b-C9) need not be intact for death to occur (156). The relative resistance of *L. donovani* amastigotes to complement killing may contribute to their ability to spread widely throughout the reticuloendothelial system. In contrast, the susceptibility of *L. major* amastigotes may inhibit their visceral dissemination.

B. Lymphocyte Activation of Macrophages in the Killing of *Leishmania*

Clinical experience, evidence from animal models, and in vitro studies indicate that resolution of leishmaniasis depends primarily on the ability of lymphocytes to activate macrophages to kill amastigotes (117,152,153,157–163). One of the best-studied early model systems of cutaneous leishmaniasis was *L. enriettii* infection of guinea pigs (164–169). Just as in humans, spontaneous healing of cutaneous *L. enriettii*-induced lesions occurred only after development of DTH and lymphoproliferative responses to leishmanial antigens. Circulating anti-leishmanial antibodies were present during disease, but they did not correlate with resolution of the lesions. Suppression of cell-mediated responses by the use of antithymocyte antisera increased the severity of the lesions, suggesting that T cells played a critical role in control of infection. Similarly, CBA mice, which self-cure *L. major* infection, developed progressive disease after thymectomy and irradiation (170,171). Mononuclear cells from spleen, peritoneal exudates, or lymph nodes of healed CBA mice conferred protection to syngeneic recipient mice challenged with *L. major*. Comparable findings were reported from animal models of *L. donovani* infection (153,172,173).

These early animal studies pointed to the central role of T cells in the control of leishmanial infection and stimulated in vitro studies of lymphocyte–macrophage interactions. Multiple groups have shown that exposure of murine macrophages or human monocyte-derived macrophages to antigen- or mitogen-elicited lymphocyte supernates (lymphokines) under the proper in vitro conditions resulted in the inhibition or death of intracellular amastigotes (174–191). The *Leishmania* have subsequently emerged as model systems for the study of the mechanisms involved in macrophage activation.

Murray and co-workers (102,187) reported that concanavalin A–elicited lymphokines could activate human monocyte-derived macrophages to kill *L.*

donovani amastigotes. Antibodies against interferon-gamma abrogated this macrophage activating factor (MAF) activity. They then demonstrated that exposure of human macrophages to recombinant interferon-gamma also resulted in intracellular killing of *L. donovani* amastigotes, and concluded that interferon-gamma was primarily responsible for MAF activity in their system (187). The importance of interferon-gamma in activating macrophages to kill *Leishmania* has been confirmed by many groups (188–192). Carvalho et al. (193) subsequently demonstrated that production of interferon-gamma and interleukin 2 in response to leishmanial antigens was absent during active visceral leishmaniasis but was restored after chemotherapy. The failure of T cells to produce interferon-gamma in response to *L. donovani* is thought to represent a key defect in the immune response during visceral leishmaniasis.

Nacy and co-workers (179–183) examined the process of macrophage activation that led to the killing of *L. major* by murine macrophages in suspension culture. They found that macrophage activation involved both priming and triggering signals. When macrophages were infected with *L. major* and then treated with lymphokines, potent leishmanicidal activity was observed. Murine macrophages exposed to lymphokines before incubation with *L. major* unexpectedly took up fewer amastigotes but killed those parasites that were ingested. Subsequent studies indicated that lymphocyte supernates contained interferon-gamma and at least one other molecule capable of priming and triggering macrophages (192). Furthermore, different *Leishmania* isolates vary in their susceptibility to lymphokine-activated macrophages (181,194).

Nacy's studies of a T-cell line (phorbol myristate acetate–stimulated EL-4 thymoma cells) indicate that T cells can also secrete soluble factors capable of preventing macrophage priming by lymphokines (183). Of note, EL-4 supernates blocked lymphokine-induced macrophage killing of *L. major* without affecting macrophage killing of extracellular tumor targets. Thus, T cells have the potential to activate or to inhibit activation of macrophages by secretion of soluble factors. There is also evidence that accessory factors in lymphocyte supernates may amplify the effects of interferon-gamma or other macrophage activating factors without themselves priming or triggering macrophages.

Exposure of macrophages to mitogen-elicited lymphokines or recombinant interferon-gamma in vitro results in an increase in their oxidative potency. This correlates with the acquisition of leishmanicidal activity (185,187,191,195). It is likely that oxidative microbicidal mechanisms contribute to the killing of amastigotes by macrophages. There is also evidence that nonoxidative microbicidal mechanisms are important. First, a macrophage cell line, IC-21, which is oxidatively impotent, has been activated by lymphokines to kill intracellular *L. donovani* amastigotes (196). In addition, monocytes from patients with chronic granulomatous disease, which are unable to mount an oxidative burst, have been activated by lymphokines or recombinant gamma-interferon to kill amastigotes (103). It was not clear whether the killing of amastigotes by these oxidatively impotent cells was due to an active microbicidal process or to changes in macrophage metabolism that resulted in starvation of parasites. Pfefferkorn observed that interferon-gamma treatment of infected fibroblasts blocked the growth of *Toxoplasma gondii* by inducing host cells to degrade tryptophan (197), but this does not appear to play a role in the control of leishmania by lymphokine-treated macrophages. Oxidative and nonoxidative microbicidal mechanisms are not exclusive; both probably contribute to the intracellular death of amastigotes after lymphokine or recombinant interferon-gamma treatment of macrophages.

Although much of the early attention focused on the effects of soluble lymphokines, Wyler and co-workers (198–201) have found that Lyt 1^+2^- lymphocytes* obtained from mice that had self-cured *L. major* infection exerted antileishmanial activity in vitro that required direct contact with amastigote-infected macrophages. Macrophage activation was leishmanial antigen specific and was I–A restricted. Soluble factors were clearly not involved, and the macrophages were not killed. The mechanism by which macrophages are activated through direct contact with Lyt 1^+2^- lymphocytes to kill intracellular amastigotes remains to be defined but appears to be entirely independent of lymphokines. It is noteworthy that maximal lymphokine-mediated antileishmanial activity is substantially reduced at 34°C, which is close to skin temperature, whereas cell contact is effective at both 34 and 37°C. Finally, cell contact has been shown to activate macrophages to kill an *L. mexicana* isolate that is resistant to killing by lymphokine-activated macrophages.

The development of *Leishmania*-specific T-cell responses appears to be critical for spontaneous resolution of cutaneous leishmaniasis, but the appearance of antigen-specific DTH and lymphoproliferative responses of circulating mononuclear cells to parasite antigens do not correlate well with healing. In one laboratory-acquired case of human *L. tropica* infection, sequential bioassays of cell-mediated responses were performed during the development of a cutaneous lesion (202). Peripheral blood lymphocyte proliferation and production of interleukin 2 in response to parasite antigens reached maximal levels coincident with cutaneous ulceration. Thereafter, the magnitude of both in vitro responses diminished as healing occurred.

Additional information about human cutaneous leishmaniasis can be gleaned from the histopathological responses (131). In a minority of acases, intact macrophages assumed epitheloid morphology as amastigotes were eliminated, suggesting activation of macrophages by lymphocyte-derived factors. In the rest of the cases, parasites were eliminated as an apparent result of lysis of infected macrophages, either individually or in small clusters, or, more commonly, by focal necrosis of a mass of parasitized cells. However, there has been no evidence

---

*Lyt-1^+2^- and L3T4$^+$, refer to antigens on the T-cell surface which are found to be either present (+) or absent (–) by monoclonal antibody binding. Lymphocyte surface antigens sometimes correlate with function of the lymphocyte subset.

of lysis of *Leishmania*-infected macrophages in vitro after lymphokine exposure. Eradication of amastigotes during human cutaneous leishmaniasis may involve more than simple macrophage activation by lymphocytes.

The role of cytotoxic mononuclear cells in the death of amastigotes or amastigote-infected macrophages is uncertain. Involvement of natural killer (NK) cells in defense against *L. donovani* was suggested by studies using homozygous beige C57BL/6J mice, which are a homologue of the human Chediak-Higashi syndrome and have an NK cell defect (203). Homozygous beige mice developed a higher splenic burden of *L. donovani*, but not of *L. major*, than control wild type or heterozygous mice. This raised the possibility that NK cells might contribute to control of *L. donovani* infection. In addition, earlier in vitro studies with *L. enriettii* suggested that mononuclear cells could exert a direct cytotoxic effect against guinea pig macrophages that had been coated with *L. enriettii* antigen or contained amastigotes (164,165). Although these observations are intriguing, they have yet to be confirmed in other in vitro or in vivo systems (204,205), and the role of cytotoxic mononuclear cells in control of *Leishmania* remains speculative.

The actual sequence of immune events in vivo is no doubt complex and influenced by multiple variables. Subpopulations of macrophages differ in their ability to bind and ingest amastigotes and to support amastigote replication (206). Furthermore, mononuclear cells of different ages or obtained from different sites such as the peritoneum, liver (Kupffer cells), or skin may vary in their susceptibility to *Leishmania* (81), their ability to respond to lymphokines, their expression of histocompatibility antigens (207), and their efficacy in activating helper rather than disease-enhancing T cells (208). The various *Leishmania* species also differ in their susceptibility to killing within activated macrophages (181,196,209). Finally, macrophage activation by lymphokines appears to be less effective at skin temperature than at 37°C, and this may contribute to the chronicity of cutaneous lesions (210). Despite major advances in our understanding of host–parasite interactions, important questions remain about the variables that influence the course of infection in vivo.

C. Failure of *Leishmania*-Specific Cell-Mediated Immune Responses to Develop During Progressive Leishmaniasis

1. Murine Leishmaniasis: The Role of T Cells

A central question in leishmaniasis is that of why effective cell-mediated responses develop so slowly in cutaneous leishmaniasis or not at all in progressive visceral or diffuse cutaneous disease. Over the past few years, studies of the cellular immunology of murine *L. major* infection have provided critical new insights into this area (211–224). Howard, Liew, and co-workers (28,211–217) observed that sublethal irradiation of genetically susceptible BALB/c mice, at levels of radiation known to deplete precursors of functionally suppressive T lymphocytes, resulted in resolution of infection at the same rate as in genetically resistant mice (211,213). T cells from irradiated BALB/c mice that had cleared *L. major* infection were protective when transferred to naive BALB/c recipients. However, when the irradiated mice were reconstituted with T cells from normal BALB/c donors, *L. major* infection again progressed to death, suggesting that one or more subsets of *Leishmania*-specific T cells arose and overcame protective antigen-specific T cells. The outcome of *L. major* infection in BALB/c mice appears to depend on which T-cell subpopulations dominate.

Further evidence for this hypothesis comes from studies of BALB/c nude mice, which, like normal BALB/c mice, develop progressive *L. major* infection. When nude BALB/c mice were given a limited number of Lyt 1^+2^- T cells from normal BALB/c donors, the partially reconstituted nude mice displayed self-resolving *L. major* infection (218). In contrast, reconstitution with a larger number of T cells was accompanied by progressive disease. Again, the observations suggested the presence of potentially protective and disease-enhancing T-cell subsets. The protective T cells seem to be present in higher frequency in naive mice than the disease-enhancing T cells.

It was subsequently shown that mice genetically susceptible or resistant to *L. major* would develop immunity against an *L. major* challenge if immunized with live-irradiated, heat-killed, or sonicated promastigotes as long as the antigen was administered by intravenous or intraperitoneal routes with an adjuvant (214). Immunity could be secondarily transferred to naive, syngeneic mice by Lyt 1^+2^- T cells from immunized animals but not by transfer of immune serum.

Surprisingly, it was observed that subcutaneous administration of the same antigen preparations with an adjuvant actually inhibited self-cure in genetically resistant mice (217,218). This disease-enhancing activity could be transferred to naive recipients by Lyt 1^+2^- T cells. Furthermore, the disease-enhancing cells recovered from subcutaneously immunized mice abrogated the transfer of protection mediated by T cells from sublethally irradiated mice that had self-cured, or by T cells from intravenously immunized mice, when disease-enhancing and protective cells were injected together into naive BALB/c recipients. Recent studies indicate that susceptible BALB/c mice treated prophylactically with cyclosporin A develop smaller lesions in response to *L. major*, presumably because disease-enhancing T cells are inhibited (219–221).

Surprisingly, the disease-enhancing Lyt 1^+2^- T cells that arose following subcutaneous immunization of BALB/c mice "helped" *Leishmania*-specific antibody production and transferred DTH responses to naive BALB/c mice. Furthermore, these Lyt 1^+2^- disease-enhancing cells were of the L3T4$^+$ (helper/inducer) phenotype. Thus there appear to be multiple Lyt 1^+2^- T-cell subsets that determine the outcome of murine cutaneous leishmaniasis, and T-cell function cannot be predicted by Lyt on L3T4 phenotype in murine cutaneous leishmaniasis. Liew and co-workers observed a correlation between the capacity of Lyt 1^+2^- populations to produce MAF, as assessed in tumoricidal assays, and their capacity to transfer protection against *L. major*. They postulated that protective T-cell subsets produce MAFs that activate macrophages to kill amastigotes, while disease-enhancing subsets do not (28).

Titus et al. (222) successfully isolated an Lyt 1^+2^-, L3T4$^+$ T-cell line that proliferated in response to leishmanial antigen and provided specific helper activity for antileishmanial antibody production. Transfer of these cells to syngeneic mice resulted in acquisition of DTH responses to leishmanial antigen but also resulted in the development of larger skin lesions after challenge with *L. major*.

Based on cell transfer experiments and studies in which anti-L3T4$^+$ monoclonal antibodies (GK 1.5) were administered to mice to deplete L3T4$^+$ T cells (222,223), Titus and colleagues hypothesized that the ratio of Lyt 2^-, L3T4$^+$ *Leishmania*-specific T cells to Lyt 2^+, L3T4$^-$ cells was critical in determining the outcome of infection. The ratio was relatively high in BALB/c mice in comparison to genetically resistant mice (224) and increased as *L. major* disease progressed. When the ratio was low, as in BALB/c mice treated with anti-L3T4$^+$ antibodies or in genetically resistant CBA mice, disease resolved. However, when nearly complete eradication of L3T4$^+$ cells was achieved, progressive *L. major* infection occurred. The T-cell line of Titus et al. was similar in Lyt and L3T4 phenotype, ability to help *Leishmania*-specific antibody production, and disease-enhancing characteristics to the disease-enhancing T cells that arose after subcutaneous immunization in the studies of Liew et al. (215,216). The major difference was that Titus et al.'s (222) T-cell line produced MAF in response to leishmanial antigens, as assessed in a tumoricidal assay, whereas disease-enhancing T-cell subsets from subcutaneous immunized BALB/c mice in Liew et al.'s studies did not. One possible explanation for this apparent discrepancy is that the T-cell line may have contained multiple subpopulations; the T cells that enhanced disease may not have been responsible for the production of MAF. In summary, it appears that functionally different T-cell subpopulations of helper/inducer phenotype arise during infection with *L. major* or after immunization. Depending on the genetic background of the animal, the route of immunization, and possibly the parasite strain, protective or disease-enhancing T cells come to dominate. The findings are consistent with recent reports of a split within the CD4 T-cell subset. On the basis of profiles of lymphokine activities and secreted proteins, Mossman et al. (225) and Marvel et al. (226) have divided CD4 cells into two groups: Th1, which secretes interleukin 2, interferon-gamma, interleukin 3, and GM-CSF; and Th2, which secretes interleukin 3, interleukin 4, and interleukin 5 as well as GM-CSF. Th1 would seem to be responsible for control of intracellular pathogens, whereas Th2, by virtue of interleukin 4, upregulates both IgE synthesis and mast cell proliferation. Although yet to be studied, the function and interaction of Th1 and Th2 may be important in the evolution of cutaneous leishmaniasis.

What factors determine whether protective or disease-enhancing T-cell populations come to predominate? Handman and co-workers (227–229) isolated and characterized an amphipathic membrane glycolipid from *L. major*, which has recently been identified as an LPG, and its delipidated, water-soluble residue that is derived by enzymatic cleavage. They have postulated that this LPG is involved in eliciting protective Lyt 2⁻ T cells, whereas the delipidated residue contributes to proliferation of disease-enhancing Lyt 2⁻ T cells (228). LPG is displayed on the surface of *L. major* and serves as a ligand for binding of *L. major* promastigotes to macrophage receptors. It is susceptible to phospholipase CIII, which cleaves the carbohydrate portion from the lipid. The delipidated portion binds to macrophages but not to T or B cells and is found in abundance in promastigote culture supernates. It was previously isolated, characterized, and termed "excreted factor." As discussed earlier, excreted factors have been used as the basis for a serotyping system for *Leishmania* (230–234).

LPG administered intravenously with *Corynebacterium parvum* or Freund's complete adjuvant protected both genetically susceptible BALB/c and resistant C3H/He mice against an *L. major* challenge. Mitchell and Handman postulated that the LPG, when anchored by its lipid moiety in the proper orientation with class II major histocompatibility molecules on the surface of macrophages, was an effective inducer of protective T cells (228) (Fig. 7). In contrast, disease-enhancing T cells were thought to proliferate in response to the delipidated carbohydrate portion when it was bound to the macrophage membranes.

Mitchell and Handman have offered possible explanations as to why disease-enhancing T cells come to predominate in BALB/c and other susceptible mice but not in genetically resistant mice (228). One possibility is that *Leishmania*-infected BALB/c macrophages present a reduced number of MHC molecules on their surfaces, or that these molecules are structurally different, and that this contributes to differential proliferation of certain T-cell subsets.

Studies by Sacks et al. (235) indicate that B cells may also play a role in the development of disease-enhancing T-cell subsets. BALB/c mice that were chronically treated with anti-IgM antibodies to deplete B cells were found to be resistant to infection with *Leishmania major*. These effects were not merely due to the abrogation of antibody production, because normal susceptibility was restored to anti-IgM-treated mice by transfer of T cells from normal mice under conditions in which there was no restoration of antibody synthesis. The findings indicate that B cells, but not antileishmanial antibodies, contribute to the development of disease-enhancing T cells, possibly by virtue of their antigen-presenting capacity. Subsequent studies by Scott et al. indicate that B lymphocytes are also involved in the generation of T cells that mediate healing of cutaneous leishmaniasis in resistant mice (236). Chronic treatment with anti-IgM antibodies to deplete B cells rendered genetically resistant mice susceptible to *L. major*.

One of the interesting findings that has emerged from studies of murine *L.*

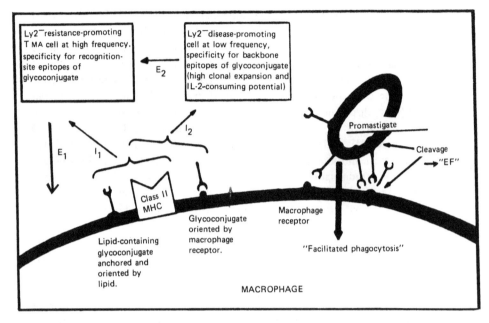

Figure 7 Sequence of events postulated by Mitchell and Handman, which results in induction (I) and expression (E) of resistance-promoting and disease-enhancing immune responses during murine cutaneous leismaniasis due to *L. major*. Induction is class II MHC restricted in both cases (I1 and I2). E1 represents macrophage activation through MAF such as interferon-gamma, and E2 represents inhibition of resistance-promoting T cells. EF = excreted factor. [Diagram modified from Mitchell, G. F., and Handman, E. *Parasitology Today* *1*:61–63 (1985); used with permission.]

major infection has been the lack of a correlation between the ability of T-cell subsets to transfer DTH responsiveness and their ability to protect against disease (215,216,237). The Lyt 1^+2^- disease-enhancing line of Titus et al. transferred DTH responses to recipient mice. In Liew et al.'s studies, disease-enhancing Lyt 1^+2^- cells from subcutaneously immunized mice also bestowed DTH responses to syngeneic recipients, whereas protective Lyt 1^+2^- cells from intravenously immunized animals did not (215,216). Intravenous immunization of BALB/c mice was subsequently shown to result in expansion of a Lyt 1^+2^+, $L3T4^+$ subpopulation that suppressed the development of *Leishmania*-specific cutaneous DTH responses without abrogating protective immunity against a parasite challenge (238).

Studies of *Leishmania*-specific T-cell responses during murine *L. donovani* infection have not been as extensive as those with *L. major*. An antigen-specific Lyt 1^+2^- T-cell line has been isolated from genetically resistant C57BL/6 mice that self-cured their infection (239). The parent cell line and some clones transferred *Leishmania*-specific DTH responses to syngeneic recipients, and in vitro they proliferated and secreted lymphokines in response to leishmanial antigens capable of activating macrophages to kill amastigotes. In *L. donovani* susceptible mice visceral leishmaniasis is characterized by the emergence of a Lyt 1^+2^- *Leishmania*-specific, disease-enhancing T-cell population just as in the case of *L. major* infection (240).

2. Murine Leishmaniasis: The Role of Macrophage Factors

Studies of murine leishmaniasis indicate that mononuclear phagocytes can also have an immunosuppressive effect. Adherent splenic mononuclear cells from *L. major*-infected BALB/c mice produced a nonspecific reduction in the proliferative responses of normal spleen cells to concanavalin A (241). This suppression was abrogated in vitro by indomethacin. Although the spleen cell population responsible for suppression was not specifically identified, the data suggested that macrophages were responsible. Studies of BALB/c mice infected with *L. donovani* also indicated a reduction in spleen cell lymphoproliferative responses and lymphokine production after stimultion with phytohemagglutinin and concanavalin A (242). These reductions could not be attributed to a decrease in the number of splenic T cells, and the suppressive, indomethacin-sensitive, adherent spleen cells were found to be macrophages (243). In vitro studies by Reiner and Malemud (244,245) have indicated that infection of murine macrophages with *L. donovani* amastigotes results in increased macrophage production of cyclooxygenase and 5-lipoxygenase metabolites of arachidonic acid. Both prostaglandin E_2 and leukotriene C_4 were produced in excess by *Leishmania*-infected cells and reduced the in vitro proliferative response of spleen cells (245). Others have attributed the reduced spleen cell response by phytohemagglutinin during murine leishmaniasis to decreased production of interleukin 2 as well as to a T-cell defect in interleukin 2 responsiveness (246).

It is noteworthy that concurrent *L. donovani* and *Toxoplasma gondii* infections in BALB/c mice did not result in decreased lymphoproliferative responses to *T. gondii* antigen (242), nor did BALB/c mice infected with *L. donovani* have reduced responses to several non-parasite-related antigens such as sperm whale myoglobin or pneumococcal polysaccharide (247). Conversely, in the case of *L. mexicana* infection, mice exhibited nonspecific immunosuppression in response to sheep erythrocytes at a time when they exhibited intense DTH

responses to leishmanial antigens (248). Overall, the data point to the importance of *Leishmania*-specific, rather than generalized, immune suppression in the
progression of leishmaniasis.

3. Human Cutaneous Leishmaniasis

It is not known whether immune responses in human leishmaniasis are analogous
to those among inbred mice. The typical cutaneous lesion in humans starts
as a papule, progressively enlarges, and eventually ulcerates. The ulcer may
persist for several months to a year before healing. Spontaneous cure of
naturally acquired disease is associated with the development of apparent
lifelong immunity against the infecting strain. For centuries, residents of the
Middle East exposed the bare bottoms of their infants to *Leismania*-infected
sandflies (249). The infants developed local lesions and after healing were
immune to reinfection. Likewise, iatrogenic infection with a live promastigote
"vaccine" administered at an inconspicuous site on the body has been effective
in preventing naturally acquired infection with the same leishmanial species in
Israel and Russia (250).

Clinical variants of cutaneous leishmaniasis provide potentially valuable
insights into the immunology of disease. Diffuse cutaneous leishmaniasis is
an anergic variant that is caused in the western hemisphere by members of
the *L. mexicana* complex and in Africa by *L. aethiopica*. The initial finding
is a nonulcerated papule at the site of the sandfly bite. Heavily parasitized
macrophages are present, but there is little in the way of a lymphocytic infiltrate. The disease is slowly progressive and persists for many years. Cutaneous
DTH and in vitro lymphoproliferative responses to leishmanial antigen are
absent.

To date, an antigen-specific, disease-enhancing T-cell population has not been
isolated from humans with cutaneous leishmaniasis. The best evidence for
immunosuppression comes from studies of patients with diffuse cutaneous
leishmaniasis acquired in the Dominican Republic (251,252). All of the patients
with diffuse cutaneous leishmaniasis who were studied lacked DTH and lympo-
proliferative responses to leishmanial antigens, in contrast to healthy residents
from the same region. Decreasing the number of glass-adherent cells (presumably
monocytes) or the addition of indomethacin, a prostaglandin inhibitor, to
patient mononuclear cells in vitro permitted expression of *Leishmania*-specific
lymphocyte proliferation. The findings suggested that mononuclear phagocytes,
rather than lymphocytes, were responsible for the failure of protective T-cell
populations to develop in patients with diffuse cutaneous leishmaniasis. Furthermore, cocultivation of lymphocytes and monocytes from HLA-identical leishmanin responders and nonresponders with diffuse cutaneous leishmaniasis also
identified the suppressor cells as monocytes.

4. Human Visceral Leishmaniasis

Relatively little is known about the control of cell-mediated immune responses during human infection with *L. donovani*. There is strong circumstantial evidence to suggest that *L. donovani* frequently produces self-resolving, asymptomatic infection. For example, the frequency of positive Leishmanin skin tests in an endemic area in East Africa was found to be greater than would have been predicted based on the incidence of disease (253). Second, during an outbreak of visceral leishmaniasis in northern Italy, 64% of asymptomatic household contacts and 40% of neighbors of persons with visceral leishmaniasis were found to have positive skin tests, whereas only 6% of controls from an area free of visceral leishmaniasis were positive (254). More recently, Badaro et al. (255,256) identified people with asymptomatic and oligosymptomatic *L. donovani chagasi* infection in a large prospective study in Brazil. Only a minority of those with serological or skin test evidence of infection went on to develop classical visceral leishmaniasis. Finally, a few humans have been experimentally inoculated with *L. donovani*. Visceral dissemination was reported in one person, while another developed a localized, spontaneously healing lesion at the site of cutaneous parasite inoculation (257).

Patients who suffer progressive visceral disease with *L. donovani* fail to develop cutaneous DTH and lymphocyte proliferative responses to leishmanial antigens (193,258,259). In addition, their lymphocytes fail to produce interleukin 2 and interferon-gamma in response to parasite antigens in vitro (193). Paradoxically, antileishmanial antibodies are produced in high titer (260-262), and there is evidence of polyclonal B-cell activation. To date no circulating suppressor T-cell population has been identified. Furthermore, depletion of CD8 cells and the addition of exogenous interleukin 2 have not reversed the leishmanial antigen-specific unresponsiveness of peripheral T cells in patients with Indian kala azar (263).

Leishmania donovani has been reported to suppress expression of class I and class II major histocompatibility gene products on infected murine macrophages (264). Parasite alterations in macrophage arachidonic acid metabolism may be responsible. In addition, neither *L. donovani* nor *L. major* elicit production of interleukin 1 by murine or human macrophages, respectively, infected in vitro (265,266). *Leishmania donovani* also reduced the secretion of interleukin 1 in response to *Listeria* or *Staphylococcus*. Interleukin 1 serves as a major signal for macrophage-dependent T-cell proliferation. Thus, *L. donovani* is capable of subverting in vitro two macrophage functions involved in the induction of T-cell-dependent antiparasitic immunity.

Some observers have reported more generalized immunodepression during visceral leishmaniasis, with decreased lymphoproliferative responses to lectins such as phytohemagglutinin (259,260) and, in a study from Kenya, anergy to purified protein derivative (PPD) and to streptokinase-streptodornase (259). This has not been a universal finding; in an Indian study, 72% of patients had DTH responses to PPD (260). The general immunodepression observed in some patients may be due to severe malnutrition, which often accompanies visceral leishmaniasis (267).

After clinically successful chemotherapy with drugs containing pentavalent antimony, the majority of patients develop lymphoproliferative and DTH responses to leishmanial antigens within 12-20 weeks. Although not well documented, these patients are thought to be relatively immune to reinfection. Whether immunity to *L. donovani* is acquired as a consequence of self-healing infection or after chemotherapy, visceral leishmaniasis can develop later if a patient becomes immunosuppressed. Badaro et al. (268) recently reported progressive visceral leishmaniasis in several immunocompromised Brazilian patients who were receiving steroids or other immunosuppressive agents. In one instance, a patient had moved away from areas of *L. donovani chagasi* transmission 20 years before progressive disease occurred. Fatal visceral leishmaniasis has been reported in a renal transplant recipient years after he has been moved from an endemic area (269). Visceral leishmaniasis has also been reported in persons with AIDS (270). These cases suggest the potential for long-term survival of *L. donovani*, even in normal hosts. Finally, Harrison et al. (267) found a correlation between the development of clinically apparent visceral leishmaniasis and malnutrition in residents living in an endemic area in northeastern Brazil. They hypothesized that the adverse effects of malnutrition on cell-mediated immune function predisposed to the development of progressive visceral disease.

The mechanisms by which potentially protective cell-mediated immune responses are blocked in patients with visceral leishmaniasis remain unknown. One possibility is the development of disease-enhancing *Leishmania*-specific T-cell populations. In addition, *Leishmania*-infected macrophages may play a suppressive role as suggested by findings discussed above. Finally, sera from patients with visceral leishmaniasis have been shown to suppress lymphocyte proliferative responses in a nonspecific manner in vitro (271,272). The relative contributions of lymphocyte, macrophage, and serum factors in mediating suppression of protective lymphocyte responses in vivo during human leishmaniasis remains uncertain.

In summary, the resolution of leishmanial infection and protection against reinfection appear to depend on complex interactions between helper/inducer and disease-enhancing mononuclear cell populations. The exact characteristics of the cell populations involved, the nature of their interactions, and the mechanisms that control them are not yet fully defined and provide exciting challenges for future investigation.

D. Consequences of Immune Responses

The degree to which the clinical manifestations of leishmaniasis are consequences of the host's immune responses is an area that has received relatively little attention. The ulceration of cutaneous lesions is in all likelihood due to host factors. Evidence for this hypothesis comes from clinical observations and animal studies. Cutaneous ulceration is a common feature of spontaneously resolving lesions, but it is not seen in the anergic variant, diffuse cutaneous leishmaniasis, even though the parasite burden is massive (3-6). Microscopically, necrosis of *Leishmania*-infected macrophages is prominent in self-healing animal and human lesions (131,149). Furthermore, induction of lymphocyte proliferation and interleukin 2 production in response to soluble *L. tropcia* antigen reached maximal levels coincident with ulceration of a lesion in one study (202).

More direct evidence for the role of immune responses in tissue destruction comes from Giannini's (273) studies in which the skin of mice was exposed to local, suberythematous levels of ultraviolet B irradiation. Inoculation of *L. major* into the irradiated skin was followed by parasite replication but not ulceration. In contrast, nonirradiated, control skin ulcerated as expected. The primary targets of UV-B radiation appeared to be host cells and not leishmanial parasites. UV-B irradiation of parasites in vitro did not affect their viability but did kill host cells. Furthermore, UV-B irradiation abrogated the induction of contact hypersensitivity to dinitrofluorobenzene and the induction of DTH responses to leishmanial antigens. These results suggest that local perturbations of skin-associated lymphoid tissue can influence the immunological responses and the subsequent development of clinical disease (273). In many instances the cost to the host of an effective immune response that eradicates *Leishmania* in the skin seems to be tissue destruction, ulceration, and scar formation. Finally, in the destructive, granulomatous lesions that characterize mucocutaneous leishmaniasis, the hyperergic response is detrimental to the host but is ineffective in eradicating parasites.

Even in visceral leishmaniasis, host immune responses probably have detrimental consequences. Humans and Syrian hamsters infected with *L. donovani* become profoundly cachectic (267). In contrast, genetically susceptible mice, which carry large parasite burdens, neither waste nor die. Parasite metabolism may contribute to wasting, but anorexia in humans and decreased food intake in hamsters are prominent. Patients with visceral leishmaniasis are reminiscent of those with the "consumption" of miliary tuberculosis or cachexia associated with AIDS or neoplasms. It has been hypothesized that the wasting observed during visceral leishmaniasis may be due to macrophage mediators such as tumor necrosis factor/cachectin or interleukin 1. The presence of fever during visceral leishmaniasis provides circumstantial evidence that interleukin 1 (274), cachectin

(275), or other yet to be identified endogenous pyrogens are produced. Recent evidence suggests that tumor necrosis factor/cachectin is elevated in the serum of patients with visceral leishmaniasis (276), and this cytokine has been shown to have catabolic effects (275). As noted earlier, monocytes infected with *L. major* or *L. donovani* in vitro do not produce interleukin 1 (265,266), but is is possible that circulating immune complexes (277-279), cachectin, or other factors stimulate interleukin 1 production in vivo. Further studies are needed to characterize the potentially detrimental consequences of these or other cytokines produced during visceral leishmaniasis.

VI. CONCLUSION

Leishmania species are prototypical intracellular parasites found solely in mononuclear phagocytes in mammals. Not only are the *Leishmania* important human pathogens in many areas of the developing world, but they have emerged as excellent model systems for the study of cell-mediated immunity. The *Leishmania* are easily propagated, each stage of parasite-phagocyte interactions can be easily studied in vitro, and excellent animal model systems of infection are available, including inbred strains of mice that vary dramatically in their susceptibility to infection. Investigations of leishmaniasis have been instrumental in defining (1) the steps involved in lymphocyte activation of macrophages to kill intracellular microbes, (2) the role of interferon-gamma as a macrophage-activating factor, (3) the genetic determinants of cell-mediated immune responses in mice, (4) the mechanisms that can mediate antigen-specific immunosuppression during intracellular infection, and (5) the potential contribution of immune responses to the clinical manifestations of disease. Ongoing studies of the mechanisms by which protective immunity is delayed or prevented in the various forms of leishmaniasis should provide further insight into the complex interactions between protective and disease-enhancing mononuclear cell populations. In summary, the study of leishmaniasis has provided important new information about general principles of cellular immunology.

REFERENCES

1. Walsh, J. A. Estimating the burden of illness in the tropics. In *Tropical Geographic Medicine* (K. S. Warren and A. A. F. Mahmoud, eds.). McGraw-Hill, New York, 1984, pp. 1073-1085.
2. Brown, H. W., and Neva, F. A. *Basic Clinical Parasitology*, 5th ed. Appleton-Century-Crofts, Norwalk, Conn., 1983.
3. Pearson, R. D., and de Sousa, A. Q. *Leishmania* species: kala-azar, cutaneous and mucocutaneous leishmaniasis. In *Principles and Practice of Infectious Diseases*, 2d ed. (G. L. Mandell, R. G. Douglas, Jr., and J. E. Bennett, eds.). John Wiley Medical, New York, 1985, Chap. 223, pp. 1522-1531.

4. Manson-Bahr, P. E. C., and Apted, F. I. C. Leishmaniasis. In *Manson's Tropical Diseases*, 18th ed. (P. E. C. Manson-Bahr, and F. I. C. Apted, eds.). Cassell, London, 1982, Chap. 7, pp. 93–115.

5. Chulay, J. D., and Manson-Bahr, P. E. C. Leishmaniasis. In *Hunter's Tropical Medicine* 36th ed. (G. T. Strickland, ed.). Saunders, Philadelphia, 1984, pp. 574–593.

6. Manson-Bahr, P. E. C., and Apted, F. I. C. Medical protozoology. In *Manson's Tropical Diseases*, 18th ed. (P. E. C. Manson-Bahr, and F. I. C. Apted, eds.). Cassell, London, 1982, pp. 637–686.

7. Jaffe, C. L., Grimaldi, G., and McMahon-Pratt, D. The cultivation and cloning of leishmania. In *Genes and Antigens of Parasites: A Laboratory Manual*, 2nd ed. (C. M. Morel, ed.) Fundaco Oswaldo Cruz, Rio de Janeiro, Brazil, 1984, pp. 47–91.

8. Sanyal, A. B., and Sen Gupta, P. C. Fine structure of *Leishmania* in dermal leishmanoid. *Trans. R. Soc. Trop. Med. Hyg. 61*:211–216 (1967).

9. Aleman, C. Finestructure of cultured *Leishmania brasiliensis*. *Exp. Parasitol. 24*:259–264 (1969).

10. Pham, T. D., Azar, H. A., Moscovic, E. A., and Kurban, A. K. The ultrastructure of *Leishmania tropica* in the oriental sore. *Ann. Trop. Med. Parasitol. 64*:1–4 (1970).

11. Gardener, P. J., Howells, R. E., and Molyneux, D. H. Ultrastructure of *Leishmania* amastigotes. *Trans. R. Soc. Trop. Med. Hyg. 67*:23 (1973).

12. Shaw, J. J., and Lainson, R. Leishmaniasis in Brazil. XI. Observations on the morphology of *Leishmania* of the *braziliensis* and *mexicana* complexes. *J. Trop. Med. Hyg. 79*:9–13 (1976).

13. Veress, B., Abdalla, R. E., and El Hassan, A. M. Electron microscope investigations on leishmaniasis in the Sudan. I. Morphometric studies on *Leishmania* amastigotes in various forms of human leishmaniasis. *Ann. Trop. Med. Parasitol. 74*:421–426 (1980).

14. Abdalla, R. E. Parasites in Sudanese cutaneous and mucosal leishmaniasis. *Ann. Trop. Med. Parasitol. 76*:299–307 (1982).

15. Ebert, F. Charakterisierung von *Leishmania donovani*-Stämmen mit der Disk-Elektrophorese. *Z. Tropenmed. Parasitol. 24*:517–524 (1973).

16. Gardener, P. F., Chance, M. L., and Peters, W. Biochemical taxonomy of *Leishmania*. II. Electrophoretic variation of malate dehydrogenase. *Ann. Trop. Med. Parasitol. 68*:317–325 (1974).

17. Brazil, R. P. Electrophoretic variation of the enzyme phosphoglucomutase in different strains of *Leishmania*. *Ann. Trop. Med. Parasitol. 72*:289–291 (1978).

18. Schnur, L. F., Chance, M. L. Ebert, F., Thomas, S. C., and Peters, W. The biochemical and serological taxonomy of visceralizing *Leishmania*. *Ann. Trop. Med. Parasitol. 75*:131–144 (1981).

19. Rassam, M. B., Al-Mudhaffar, S. A., and Chance, M. L. Isoenzyme characterization of *Leishmania* species from Iraq. *Ann. Trop. Med. Parasitol. 73*:527–534 (1979).

20. Chance, M. L., Peters, W., and Shchory, L. Biochemical taxonomy of *Leishmania*. I. Observations on DNA. *Ann. Trop. Med. Parasitol. 68*:307–316 (1974).

21. Decker, J. E., Schrot, J. R., and Levin, G. V. Identification of *Leishmania* spp. by radiorespirometry. *J. Protozool. 24*:463–470 (1977).

22. Schnur, L. F., and Zuckerman, A. Leishmanial excreted factor (EF) serotypes in Sudan, Kenya and Ethiopia. *Ann. Trop. Med. Parasitol. 71*:273–294 (1977).

23. Schnur, L. F., Zuckerman, A., and Greenblatt, C. L. Leishmanial serotypes as distinguished by the gel diffusion of factors excreted in vitro and in vivo. *Isr. J. Med. Sci. 8*:932–942 (1972).

24. Pratt, D. M., and David, J. R. Monoclonal antibodies that distinguish between New World species of *Leishmania*. *Nature 291*:581–583 (1981).

25. Arnot, D. E., and Barker, D. C. Biochemical identification of cutaneous leishmaniasis by analysis of kinetoplast DNA. II. Sequence homologies in *Leishmania* kDNA. *Mol. Biochem. Parasitol. 3*:47–56 (1981).

26. Wirth, D. F., and Pratt, D. M. Rapid identification of *Leishmania* species by specific hybridization of kinetoplast DNA in cutaneous lesions. *Proc. Natl. Acad. Sci. USA 79*:6999–7003 (1982).

27. Jackson, P. R., Wohlhieter, J. A., Jackson, J. E., Sayles, P., Diggs, C. L., and Hockmeyer, W. T. Restriction endonuclease analysis of *Leishmania* kinetoplast DNA characterizes parasites responsible for visceral and cutaneous disease. *Am. J. Trop. Med. Hyg. 33*:808–819 (1984).

28. Blackwell, J., Pratt, D. M., and Shaw, J. Molecular biology of *Leishmania*. *Parasitol. Today 2*:45–53 (1986).

29. Giannini, S. H., Schittini, M., Keithly, J. S., Warburton, P. W., Cantor, C. R., and Van der Ploeg, L. H. T. Karyotype analysis of *Leishmania* species and its use in classification and clinical diagnosis. *Science 232*:762–765 (1986).

30. Bradley, D. J., Taylor, B. A., Blackwell, J., Evans, E. P., and Freeman, J. Regulation of *Leishmania* populations within the host. III. Mapping of the locus controlling susceptibility to visceral leishmaniasis in the mouse. *Clin. Exp. Immunol. 37*:7–14 (1979).

31. Behin, R., Mauel, J., and Sordat, B. *Leishmania tropica*: pathogenicity and in vitro macrophage function in strains of inbred mice. *Exp. Parasitol. 48*: 81–91 (1979).

32. Gorczynski, R. M. Nature of resistance to leishmaniasis in experimental rodents. *Dev. Comp. Immunol. 6*:199–207 (1982).

33. Mock, B. A., Fortier, A. H., Potter, M., and Nacy, C. A. Genetic control of systemic *Leishmania major* infections: dissociation of intrahepatic amastigote replication from control by the *Lsh* gene. *Infect. Immun. 50*:588–591 (1985).

34. Blackwell, J. M. Genetic control of recovery from visceral leishmaniasis. *Trans. R. Soc. Trop. Med. Hyg. 76*:147–151 (1982).

35. Crocker, P. R., Blackwell, J. M., and Bradley, D. J. Expression of the natural resistance gene *Lsh* in resident liver macrophages. *Infect. Immun. 43*:1033–1040 (1984).

36. Nickol, A. D., and Bonventre, P. F. Visceral leishmaniasis in congenic mice of susceptible and resistant phenotypes: T-lymphocyte mediated immuno-suppression. *Infect. Immun. 50*:169–174 (1985).

37. Plant, J. E., Blackwell, J. M., O'Brien, A. D., Bradley, D. J., and Glynn, A. A. Are the *Lsh* and *Ity* disease resistance genes at one locus on mouse chromosome 1? *Nature 297*:510–511 (1982).

38. Cox, F. E. G. Leishmaniasis and mouse genetics. *Nature 291*:111–112 (1981).

39. Blackwell, J. M., Roberts, B., and Alexander, J. Response of BALB/c mice to leishmanial infection. *Curr. Trop. Microbiol. Immunol. 122*:97–106 (1985).

40. Howard, J. G., Hale, C., and Liew, F. Y. Genetically determined suscepti-bility to *Leishmania tropica* infection is expressed by haematopoietic donor cells in mouse radiation chimaeres. *Nature 288*:161–162 (1980).

41. Handman, E., Ceredig, R., and Mitchell, G. F. Murine cutaneous leish-maniasis: disease patterns in intact and nude mice of various genotypes and examination of some differences between normal and infected macrophages. *Aust. J. Exp. Biol. Med. Sci. 57*:9–29 (1979).

42. Nacy, C. A., Fortier, A. H., Pappas, M. G., and Henry, R. R. Susceptibility of inbred mice to *Leishmania tropica* infection: correlation of susceptibility with in vitro defective macrophage microbicidal activities. *Cell Immunol. 77*:298–307 (1983).

43. Howard, J. G., Hale, C., and Liew, F. Y. Immunological regulation of experimental cutaneous leishmaniasis. III. Nature and significance of spe-cific suppression of cell-mediated immunity in mice highly susceptible to *Leishmania tropica. J. Exp. Med. 152*:594–607 (1980).

44. Badaró, R., Jones, T. C., Lorenco, R., Cerf, B. J., Sampaio, D. Carvalho, E. M., Rocha, H., Teixeira, R., and Johnson, W. D., Jr. A prospective study of visceral leishmaniasis in an endemic area in Brazil. *J. Infect. Dis. 154*: 639–649 (1986).

45. Walton, B. C., and Valverde, L. Racial differences in espundia. *Ann. Trop. Med. Parasitol. 73*:23–29 (1979).

46. Sacks, D. L., and Perkins, P. V. Identification of an infective stage of *Leishmania* promastigotes. *Science 223*:1417–1419 (1984).

47. Sacks, D. L., Hieny, S., and Sher, A. Identification of cell surface carbohy-drate antigenic changes between noninfective and infective developmental stages of *Leishmania major* promastigotes. *J. Immunol. 135*:564–569 (1985).

48. Giannini, M. S. Effects of promastigote growth phase, frequency of subcul-ture, and host age on promastigote-initiated infections with *Leishmania donovani* in the golden hamster. *J. Protozool. 21*:521–527 (1974).

49. Wilson, M. E., Innes, D. J., de Sousa, A. Q., and Pearson, R. D. Early histo-pathology of experimental infection with *Leishmania donovani* in hamsters. *J. Parasitol. 73*:55–63 (1987).

50. Akiyama, H. J., and Haight, R. D. Interaction of *Leishmania donovani* and

hamster peritoneal macrophages. A phase-contrast microscopical study. *Am. J. Trop. Med. Hyg. 20*:539–545 (1971).

51. Williams, K. M., Sacci, J. B., and Anthony, R. L. Identification and recovery of leishmania antigen displayed on the surface membrane of mouse peritoneal macrophages in vitro. *J. Immunol. 136*:1853–1858 (1986).

52. Chang, K.-P. *Leishmania donovani*: promastigote-macrophage surface interactions in vitro. *Exp. Parasitol. 48*:175–189 (1979).

53. Zenian, A., Rowles, P., and Gingell, D. Scanning electron-microscopic study of the uptake of *Leishmania* parasites by macrophages. *J. Cell. Sci. 39*:187–199 (1979).

54. Chang, K.-P. Human cutaneous leishmania in a mouse macrophage line: propagation and isolation of intracellular parasites. *Science 209*:1240–1242 (1980).

55. Chang, K.-P. *Leishmania donovani*-macrophage binding mediated by surface glycoproteins/antigens: characterization in vitro by a radioisotopic assay. *Mol. Biochem. Parasitol. 4*:67–76 (1981).

56. Zenian, A. *Leishmania tropica*: biochemical aspects of promastigotes' attachment to macrophages in vitro. *Exp. Parasitol. 51*:175–187 (1981).

57. Pearson, R. D., Romito, R., Symes, P. H., and Harcus, J. L. Interaction of *Leishmania donovani* promastigotes with human monocyte-derived macrophages: parasite entry, intracellular conversion, and multiplication. *Infect. Immun. 32*:1249–1253 (1981).

58. Pearson, R. D., Harcus, J. L., Symes, P. H., Romito, R., and Donowitz, G. R. Failure of the phagocytic oxidative response to protect human monocyte-derived macrophages from infection by *Leishmania donovani*. *J. Immunol. 129*:1282–1286 (1982).

59. Pearson, R. D., Sullivan, J. A., Roberts, D., Romito, R., and Mandell, G. L. Interaction of *Leishmania donovani* promastigotes with human phagocytes. *Infect. Immun. 40*:411–416 (1983).

60. Pearson, R. D., Harcus, J. L., Roberts, D., and Donowitz, G. R. Differential survival of *Leishmania donovani* amastigotes in human monocytes. *J. Immunol. 131*:1994–1999 (1983).

61. Bray, R. S. *Leishmania mexicana*: attachment and uptake of promastigotes to and by macrophages in vitro. *J. Protozool. 30*:314–322 (1983).

62. Chang, K.-P. Cellular and molecular mechanisms of intracellular symbiosis in leishmaniasis. *Int. Rev. Cytol. (Suppl.) 14*:267–303 (1983).

63. Wyler, D. J. In vitro parasite–monocyte interactions in human leishmaniasis. Evidence for an active role of the parasite in attachment. *J. Clin. Invest. 70*:82–88 (1982).

64. Wyler, D. J., and Suzuki, K. In vitro parasite–monocyte interactions in human leishmaniasis: effect of enzyme treatments on attachment. *Infect. Immun. 42*:356–361 (1983).

65. Klempner, M. S., Cendron, M., and Wyler, D. J. Attachment of plasma membrane vesicles of human macrophages to *Leishmania tropica* promastigotes. *J. Infect. Dis. 148*:377–384 (1983).

66. Wilson, M. E., and Pearson, R. D. Evidence that *Leishmania donovani*

utilizes a mannose receptor on human mononuclear phagocytes to establish intracellular parasitism. *J. Immunol. 136*:4681–4688 (1986).

67. Dawidowicz, K., Hernandez, A. G., and Infante, R. B. The surface membrane of *Leishmania*. I. The effects of lectins on different stages of *Leishmania braziliensis*. *J. Parasitol. 61*:950–953 (1975).

68. Dwyer, D. M. Lectin binding saccharides on a parasitic protozoan. *Science 184*:471–473 (1974).

69. Dwyer, D. M. *Leishmania donovani*: surface membrane carbohydrates of promastigotes. *Exp. Parasitol. 41*:341–358 (1977).

70. Hernandez, A. G., Arguello, C., Ayesta, C., Dagger, F., Infante, R. B., Stojanovich, D., Dawidowicz, K., Riggione, F., and La Riva, G. The surface membrane of *Leishmania*. In *The Biochemistry of Parasites* (G. M. Slutzky, ed.). Pergamon, New York 1981, pp. 47–65.

71. Schottelius, J. Lectin typing of *Leishmania* strains from the New and Old World. In *Lectins–Biology, Biochemistry, Clinical Biochemistry*, Vol. II (T. C. Bog-Hansen, ed.). Walter de Gruyter, New York, 1982, pp. 531–541.

72. Jacobsen, R. L., Slutzky, G. M., Greenblatt, C. L., and Schnur, L. F. Surface reaction of *Leishmania*. I. Lectin-mediated agglutination. *Ann. Trop. Med. Parasitol. 76*:45–52 (1982).

73. Ebrahimzadeh, A., and Jones, T. C. A comparative study of different *Leishmania tropica* isolates from Iran: correlation between infectivity and cytochemical properties. *Am. J. Trop. Med. Hyg. 32*:694–702 (1983).

74. Wilson, M. E., and Pearson, R. D. Lectin binding to *Leishmania donovani*: stage-specific variations. *Infect. Immun. 46*:128–134 (1984).

75. Dwyer, D. M., and Gottlieb, M. The surface membrane chemistry of leishmania: its possible role in parasite sequestration and survival. *J. Cell Biochem. 23*:23–45 (1983).

76. Turco, S. J., Wilkerson, M. A., and Clawson, D. R. Expression of an unusual acid glycoconjugate in *Leishmania donovani*. *J. Biol. Chem. 259*:3883–3889 (1984).

77. Stahl, F., and Gordon, S. Expression of mannosyl-fucosyl receptor for endocytosis on cultured primary macrophages and their hybrids. *J. Cell. Biol. 93*:49–56 (1982).

78. Sung, S.-S. J., Nelson, R. S., and Silverstein, S. C. Yeast mannans inhibit binding and phagocytosis of zymosan by mouse peritoneal macrophages. *J. Cell. Biol. 96*:160–166 (1983).

79. Channon, J. Y., Roberts, M. B., and Blackwell, J. M. A study of the differential respiratory burst activity elicited by promastigotes and amastigotes of *Leishmania donovani* in murine resident peritoneal macrophages. *Immunology 53*:345–355 (1984).

80. Blackwell, J. M., Ezekowitz, R. A. B., Roberts, M. B., Channon, J. Y., Sim, R. B., and Gordon, S. Macrophage complement and lectin-like receptors bind *Leishmania* in the absence of serum. *J. Exp. Med. 162*:324–331 (1985).

81. Blackwell, J. M. Receptors and recognition mechanisms of *Leishmania* species. *Trans. R. Soc. Trop. Med. Hyg. 79*:606–612 (1985).

82. Colomer-Gould, V., Quintao, L. G., Keithly, J., and Nogueria, N. A common

major surface antigen on amastigotes and promastigotes of *Leishmania* species. *J. Exp. Med. 162*:902–916 (1985).

83. Etges, R., Bouvier, J., and Bordier, C. The major surface protein of *Leishmania* promastigotes is a protease. *J. Biol. Chem. 261*:9098–9101 (1986).

84. Russell, D. G., and Wilhelm, H. The involvement of the major surface glyco-protein (gp63) of *Leishmania* promastigotes in attachment to macrophages. *J. Immunol. 136*:2613–2620 (1986).

85. Chang, C. S., Inserra, T. J., Kink, J. A., Fong, D., and Chang, K.-P. Expres-sion and size heterogeneity of a 63 kilodalton membrane glycoprotein during growth and transformation of *Leishmania mexicana amazonensis. Mol. Biochem. Parasitol. 18*:197–210 (1986).

86. King, D. L., Chang, Y.-D., and Turco, S. J. Cell surface lipophosphoglycan of *Leishmania donovani. Mol. Biochem. Parasitol. 24*:47–53 (1987).

87. Turco, S. J., Hull, S. R., Orlandi, P. A., Jr., Shepherd, S. D., Homans, S. W., Dwek, R. A., and Rademaeker, T. W. Structure of the major fragment of the *Leishmania donovani* lipophosphoglycan. *Biochemistry 26*:6233–6238 (1987).

88. Orlandi, P. A., and Turco, S. J. Structure of the lipid moiety of the *Leish-mani donovani* lipophosphoglycan. *J. Biol. Chem. 262*:10384–10391 (1987).

89. Mosser, D. M., and Edelsons, P. J. Activation of the alternative complement pathway by leishmania promastigotes: parasite lysis and attachment to macrophages. *J. Immunol. 132*:1501–1505 (1984).

90. Wilson, M. E., and Pearson, R. D. Roles of CR3 and mannose receptors in the attachment and ingestion of *Leishmania donovani* by human mononu-clear phagocytes. *Infect. Immun. 56*:363–369 (1988).

91. Pearson, R. D., and Steigbigel, R. T. Mechanism of lethal effect of human serum upon *Leishmania donovani. J. Immunol. 125*:2195–2201 (1980).

92. Wozencraft, A. O., Sayers, G., and Blackwell, J. M. Macrophage type 3 complement receptors mediate serum-independent binding of *Leishmania donovani. J.Exp. Med. 164*:1332–1337 (1986).

93. Wyler, D. J., Sypek, J. P., and McDonald, J. A. In vitro parasite–monocyte interactions in human leishmaniasis: possible role of fibronectin in parasite attachment. *Infect. Immun. 49*:305–311 (1985).

94. Wright, S. D., Licht, M. R., Craigmyle, L. S., and Silverstein, S. C. Com-munication between receptors for different ligands on a single cell: ligation of fibronectin receptors induces a reversible alteration in the function of complement receptors on cultured human monocytes. *J. Cell. Biol. 99*:336–339 (1984).

95. Mesnick, S. R., and Eaton, J. W. Leishmanial superoxide dismutase: a possible target for chemotherapy. *Biochem. Biophys. Res. Commun. 102*: 970–976 (1981).

96. Murray, H. W. Susceptibility of *Leishmania* to oxygen intermediates and killing by normal macrophages. *J. Exp. Med. 153*:1302–1315 (1981).

97. Pearson, R. D., and Steigbigel, R. T. Phagocytosis and killing of the protozoan *Leishmania donovani* by human polymorphonuclear leukocytes. *J. Immunol. 127*:1438–1443 (1981).
98. Buchmüller, Y., and Mauel, J. Studies on the mechanisms of macrophage activation: possible involvement of oxygen metabolites in killing of *Leishmania enriettii* by activated mouse macrophages. *J. Reticuloendothel. Soc. 29*:181–192 (1981).
99. Avila, J. L., Convit, J., Pinardi, M. E., and Jacques, P. J. Loss of infectivity of mycobacterial and protozoal exoplasmic parasites after exposure in vitro to the polyenzymic cocktail "PIGO." *Biochem. Soc. Trans. 4*:680–681 (1976).
100. Reiner, N. E., and Kazura, J. W. Oxidant-mediated damage of *Leishmania donovani* promastigotes. *Infect. Immun. 36*:1023–1027 (1982).
101. Locksley, R. M., and Klebanoff, S. J. Oxygen-dependent microbicidal systems of phagocytes and host defense against intracellular protozoa. *J. Cell. Biochem. 22*:173–185 (1983).
102. Murray, H. W., and Cartelli, D. M. Killing of intracellular *Leishmania donovani* by human mononuclear phagocytes. Evidence of oxygen-dependent and -independent leishmanicidal activity. *J. Clin. Invest. 72*:32–44 (1983).
103. Murray, H. W. Interaction of *Leishmania* with a macrophage cell line: correlation between intracellular killing and the generation of oxygen intermediates. *J. Exp. Med. 153*:1690–1695 (1981).
104. Schmunis, G. A., and Herman, R. Characteristics of so-called natural antibodies in various normal sera against culture forms of *Leishmania*. *J. Parasitol. 56*:889–896 (1970).
105. Rezai, H. R., Sher, S., and Gettner, S. *Leishmania tropica, L. donovani* and *L. enriettii*: immune rabbit serum inhibitory in vitro. *Exp. Parasitol. 26*:257–263 (1969).
106. Ulrich, M., Ortiz, D. T., and Convit, J. The effect of fresh serum on the leptomonads of *Leishmania*. I. Preliminary report. *Trans. R. Soc. Trop. Med. Hyg. 62*:825–830 (1968).
107. Hindle, E., Hou, P. C., and Patton, W. S. Reports from the Royal Society's Kala Azar Commission in China. I. Serological studies on Chinese kala azar. *Proc. R. Soc. Lond. (Biol.) 100*:368–373 (1926).
108. Adler, S. Attempts to transmit visceral leishmaniasis to man. Remarks on the histopathology of leishmaniasis. *Trans. R. Soc. Trop. Med. Hyg. 33*:419–437 (1940).
109. Taub, J. The effect of normal serum on *Leishmania*. *Bull. Res. Counc. Isr. 6E*:55–57 (1956).
110. Lainson, R., and Strangways-Dixon, J. *Leishmania mexicana*: the epidemiology of dermal leishmaniasis in British Honduras. *Trans. R. Soc. Trop. Med. Hyg. 57*:242–265 (1963).
111. Ben Rachid, M. S. Action lytique du sérum humain normal vis-à-vis de *Leishmania infantum*. *Arch. Inst. Pasteur Tunis. 44*:155–161 (1967).

112. Franke, E. D., McGreevy, P. A., Katz, S. P., and Sacks, D. L. Growth cycle-dependent generation of complement-resistant *Leishmania* promastigotes. *J. Immunol. 134*:2713–2718 (1985).

113. Puentes, S. M., Sacks, D. L., da Silva, R. P., and Joiner, K. A. Complement binding by two developmental stages of *Leishmania major* promastigotes varying in expression of a surface lipophosphoglycan. *J. Exp. Med. 167*: 887–902 (1988).

114. Bray, R. S. *Leishmania*: chemotaxic responses of promastigotes and macrophages in vitro. *J. Protozool. 30*:322–329 (1983).

115. Handman, E., and Mitchell, G. F. Immunization with *Leishmania* receptor for macrophages protects mice against cutaneous leishmaniasis. *Proc. Natl. Acad. Sci. USA 82*:5910–5914 (1985).

116. Anderson, S., David, J. R., and Pratt, D. M. In vivo protection against *Leishmania mexicana* indicated by monoclonal antibodies. *J. Immunol. 131*:1616–1618 (1983).

117. Pearson, R. D., Wheeler, D. A., Harrison, L. H., and Kay, H. D. The immunobiology of leishmaniasis. *Rev. Infect. Dis. 5*:907–927 (1983).

118. Gorczynski, R. M., MacRae, S., Kuba, R., and Price, G. B. Macrophage heterogeneity and Ir-gene control as factors involved in the immune response of guinea pigs to infection with *Leishmania enriettii. Cell. Immunol. 60*:367–375 (1981).

119. Alexander, J., and Vickerman, K. Fusion of host cell secondary lysosomes with the parasitophorous vacuoles of *Leishmania mexicana*-infected macrophages. *J. Protozool. 22*:502–508 (1975).

120. Chang, K.-P., and Dwyer, D. M. Multiplication of a human parasite (*Leishmania donovani*) in phagolysosomes of hamster macrophages in vitro. *Science 193*:678–680 (1976).

121. Chang, K.-P., and Dwyer, D. M. *Leishmania donovani*-hamster macrophage interactions in vitro: cell entry, intracellular survival and multiplication of amastigotes. *J. Exp. Med. 147*:515–530 (1978).

122. Herman, R. Studies of the numbers and morphology of the intracellular form of *Leishmania donovani* grown in cell culture. *J. Protozool. 13*:408–418 (1966).

123. Bhattacharya, A., and Janovy, J., Jr. *Leishmania donovani*: autoradiographic evidence for molecular exchanges between parasites and host cells. *Exp. Parasitol. 37*:353–360 (1975).

124. Handman, E., and Spira, D. T. Growth of *Leishmania* amastigotes in macrophages from normal and immune mice. *Z. Parasitenkd. 53*:75–81 (1977).

125. Lewis, D. H., and Peters, W. The resistance of intracellular *Leishmania* parasites to digestion by lysosomal enzymes. *Ann. Trop. Med. Parasitol. 71*:295–312 (1977).

126. Berman, J. D., Fioretti, T. B., and Dwyer, D. M. In vivo and in vitro localization of *Leishmania* within macrophage phagolysosomes: use of colloidal gold as a lysosomal label. *J. Protozool. 28*:239–242 (1981).

127. Berman, J. D., Dwyer, D. M., and Wyler, D. J. Multiplication of *Leishmania* in human macrophages in vitro. *Infect. Immun. 26*:375–379 (1979).

128. Lewis, D. H. Infection of tissue culture cells of low phagocytic ability by *Leishmania mexicana mexicana. Ann. Trop. Med. Parasitol. 68*:327–336 (1974).

129. Mattock, N. M., and Peters, W. The experimental chemotherapy of leishmaniasis. I. Techniques for the study of drug action in tissue culture. *Ann. Trop. Med. Parasitol. 69*:349–357 (1975).

130. Berens, R. L., and Marr. J. J. Growth of *Leishmania donovani* amastigotes in a continuous macrophage-like cell culture. *J. Protozool. 26*:453–456 (1979).

131. Ridley, M. J.,and Ridley, D. S. Cutaneous leishmaniasis: immune complex formation and necrosis in the acute phase. *Br. J. Exp. Pathol. 65*:327–336 (1984).

132. Chang, K.-P. Antibody-mediated inhibition of phagocytosis in *Leishmania donovani*–human phagocyte interactions in vitro. *Am. J. Trop. Med. Hyg. 30*:334–339 (1981).

133. Herman, R. Cytophilic and opsonic antibodies in visceral leishmaniasis in mice. *Infect. Immun. 28*:585–593 (1980).

134. Gottlieb, M., and Dwyer, D. M. Protozoan parasite of humans: surface membrane with externally disposed acid phosphatase. *Science 212*:939–941 (1981).

135. Remaley, A. T., Glew, R. H., Kuhns, D. B., and Basford, R. E. *Leishmania donovani*: surface membrane acid phosphatase blocks neutrophil oxidative metabolite production. *Exp. Parasitol. 60*:331–341 (1985).

136. Haidaris, C. G., and Bonventre, P. F. A role for oxygen-dependent mechanisms in killing of *Leishmania donovani* tissue forms by activated macrophages. *J. Immunol. 129*:850–855 (1982).

137. Murray, H. W. Cell-mediated immune response in experimental leishmaniasis. II. Oxygen-dependent killing of intracellular *Leishmania donovani* amastigotes. *J. Immunol. 129*:351–357 (1982).

138. Brazil, R. P. In vivo fusion of lysosomes with parasitophorous vacuoles of *Leishmania*-infected macrophages. *Ann. Trop. Med. Parasitol. 78*:87–91 (1984).

139. Hart, P. D., Armstrong, J. A., Brown, C. A., and Draper, P. Ultrastructural study of the behavior of macrophages toward parasitic mycobacteria. *Infect. Immun. 5*:803–807 (1972).

140. Armstrong, J. A., and Hart, P. D. Response of cultured macrophages to *Mycobacterium tuberculosis*, with observations on fusion of lysosomes with phagosomes. *J. Exp. Med. 134*:713–740 (1971).

141. Jones, T. C., and Hirsch, J. G. The reaction between *Toxoplasma gondii* and mammalian cells. II. The absence of lysosomal fusion with phagocytic vacuoles containing living parasites. *J. Exp. Med. 136*:1173–1194 (1972).

142. Kress, Y., Tanowitz, H., Bloom, B., and Wittner, M. *Trypanosoma cruzi*:

infection of normal and activated mouse macrophages. *Exp. Parasitol. 41*: 385–396 (1977).

143. Rabinovitch, M., Dedet, J.-P. Ryter, A., Robineaux, R., Topper, G., and Brunet, E. Destruction of *Leishmania mexicana amazonensis* amastigotes within macrophages in culture by phenazine methsulfate and other electron carriers. *J. Exp. Med. 155*:415–431 (1982).

144. Mukkada, A. J., Meade, J. C., Glaser, T. A., and Bonventre, P. F. Enhanced metabolism of *Leishmania donovani* amastigotes at acid pH: an adaptation for intracellular growth. *Science 229*:1099–1101 (1985).

145. Zilberstein, D., and Dwyer, D. M. Antidepressants cause lethal disruption of membrane function in the human protozoan parasite *Leishmania*. *Science 226*:977–978 (1984).

146. Rabinovitch, M., Zilberfarb, V., and Ramazeilles, C. Destruction of *Leishmania mexicana amazonensis* amastigotes within macrophages by lysosomotropic amino acid esters. *J. Exp. Med. 163*:520–535 (1986).

147. Van der Ploeg, L. H. T., Giannini, S. H., and Cantor, C. R. Heat shock genes: regulatory role for differentiation in parasitic protozoa. *Science 228*:1443–1446 (1985).

148. Chang, K.-P. Leishmanicidal mechanisms of human polymorphonuclear phagocytes. *Am. J. Trop. Med. Hyg. 30*:322–333 (1981).

149. Ridley, D. S., and Ridley, M. J. The evolution of the lesion in cutaneous leishmaniasis. *J. Pathol. 141*:83–96 (1983).

150. Biozzi, G., Mouton, D., Sant´ Anna, O. A., Passos, H. C., Gennari, M., Reis, M. H. Ferreira, V. C. A., Heumann, A. M., Bouthillier, Y., Ibanez, O. M., Stiffel, C., and Sigueira, M. Genetics of immunoresponsiveness to natural antigens in the mouse. *Current Top. Microbiol. Immunol. 85*:31–98 (1979).

151. Hale, C., and Howard, J. G. Immunological regulation of experimental cutaneous leishmaniasis. 2. Studies with Biozzi high and low responder lines of mice. *Parasite Immunol. 3*:45–55 (1981).

152. Rezai, H. R., Farrell, J., and Soulsby, E. L. Immunological responses of *L. donovani* infection in mice and significance of T cell in resistance to experimental leishmaniasis. *Clin. Exp. Immunol. 40*:508–514 (1980).

153. Poulter, L. W. Mechanisms of immunity to leishmaniasis. I. Evidence for a changing basis of protection in self-limiting disease. *Clin. Exp. Immunol. 39*:14–26 (1980).

154. Hoover, D. L., Berger, M., Nacy, C. A., Hockmeyer, W. T., and Meltzer, M. S. Killing of *Leishmania tropica* amastigotes by factors in normal human serum. *J. Immunol. 132*:893–897 (1984).

155. Mosser, D. M., Wedgewood, J. S., and Edelson, P. J. Leishmania amastigotes: resistance to complement-mediated lysis is not due to a failure to fix C3. *J. Immunol. 134*:4128–4131 (1985).

156. Hoover, D. L., Berger, M., Hammer, C. H., and Meltzer, M. S. Complement-mediated serum cytotoxicity for *Leishmania major* amastigotes: killing by serum deficient in early components of the membrane attack complex. *J. Immunol. 135*:570–574 (1985).

157. Zuckerman, A. Parasitological review. Current status of the immunology of blood and tissue protozoa. I. *Leishmania. Exp. Parasitol. 38*:370–400 (1975).
158. Marsden, P. D. Current concepts in parasitology: leishmaniasis. *New Engl. J. Med. 300*:350–352 (1979).
159. Heyneman, D. Immunology of leishmaniasis. *Bull WHO 44*:499–514 (1971).
160. Bray, R. S. Leishmaniasis in the Old World. *Br. Med. Bull. 28*:39–43 (1972).
161. Bray, R. S. *Leishmania. Ann. Rev. Microbiol. 28*:189–217 (1974).
162. Jones, T. C. Interactions between murine macrophages and obligate intracellular protozoa. Am. J. Pathol. 102:127–132 (1981).
163. Preston, M. P., and Dumonde, D. C. Immunology of clinical and experimental leishmaniasis. In *Immunology of Parasitic Infections* (S. Cohen and E. H. Sadun, eds.). Blackwell Scientific Publications, Oxford, 1976.
164. Bray, R. S., and Bryceson, A. D. M. Cutaneous leishmaniasis of the guinea pig. Action of sensitized lymphocytes on infected macrophages. *Lancet ii*: 898–899 (1968).
165. Bryceson, A. D. M., Bray, R. S., Wolstencroft, R. A., and Dumonde, D. C. Immunity in cutaneous leishmaniasis of the guinea-pig. *Clin Exp. Immunol. 7*:301–341 (1970).
166. Blewett, T. M., Kadivar, D. M. H., and Soulsby, E. J. Cutaneous leishmaniasis in the guinea pig. Delayed-type hypersensitivity, lymphocyte stimulation, and inhibition of macrophage migration. *Am. J. Trop. Med. Hyg. 20*:546–551 (1971).
167. Bryceson, A. D. M., Bray, R. S., and Dumonde, D. C. Experimental cutaneous leishmaniasis. IV. Selective suppression of cell-mediated immunity during the response of guinea-pigs to infection with *Leishmania enriettii. Clin. Exp. Immunol. 16*:189–201 (1974).
168. Bryceson, A. D. M., and Turk, J. L. The effect of prolonged treatment with antilymphocyte serum on the course of infections with BCG and *Leishmania enriettii* in the guinea pig. *J. Pathol. 104*:153–165 (1971).
169. Bryceson, A. D. M., Preston, P. M., Bray, R. S., and Dumonde, D. C. Experimental cutaneous leishmaniasis. II. Effects of immune suppression and antigenic competition on the course of infection with *Leishmania enriettii* in the guinea-pig. *Clin. Exp. Immunol. 10*:305–335 (1972).
170. Preston, P. M., Carter, R. L., Leuchars, E., Davies, A. J. S., and Dumonde, D. C. Experimental cutaneous leishmaniasis. III. Effects of thymectomy on the course of infection of CBA mice with *Leishmania tropica. Clin. Exp. Immunol. 10*:337–357 (1972).
171. Preston, P. M., and Dumonde, D. C. Experimental cutaneous leishmaniasis. V. Protective immunity in subclinical and self-healing infection in the mouse. *Clin. Exp. Immunol. 23*:126–138 (1976).
172. Shov, C. B., and Twohy, D. W. Cellular immunity to *Leishmania donovani*. I. The effect of T cell depletion on resistance to *L. donovani* in mice. *J. Immunol. 113*:2004–2011 (1974).

173. Shov, C. B., and Twohy, D. W. Cellular immunity to *Leishmania donovani*. II. Evidence for synergy between thymocytes and lymph node cells in reconstitution of acquired resistance to *L. donovani* in mice. *J. Immunol. 113*:2012–2019 (1974).

174. Miller, H. C., and Twohy, D. W. Cellular immunity to *Leishmania donovani* in macrophages in culture. *J. Parasitol. 55*:200–207 (1969).

175. Mauel, J., Buchmüller, Y., and Behin, R. Studies on the mechanisms of macrophage activation. I. Destruction of intracellular *Leishmania enriettii* in macrophages activated by cocultivation with stimulated lymphocytes. *J. Exp. Med. 148*:393–407 (1978).

176. Mauel, J., Behin, R., and Louis, J. *Leishmania enriettii*: immune induction of macrophage activation in an experimental model of immunoprophylaxis in the mouse. *Exp. Parasitol. 52*:331–345 (1981).

177. Buchmüller, Y., and Mauel, J. Studies on the mechanisms of macrophage activation. II. Parasite destruction in macrophages activated by supernates from concanavalin A-stimulated lymphocytes. *J. Exp. Med. 150*:359–370 (1979).

178. Titus, R. G., Kelso, A., and Louis, J. A. Intracellular destruction of *Leishmania tropica* by macrophages activated with macrophage activating factor/interferon. *Clin. Exp. Immunol. 55*:157–165 (1984).

179. Nacy, C. A., Meltzer, M. S., Leonard, E. J., and Wyler, D. J. Intracellular replication and lymphokine-induced destruction of *Leishmania tropica* in C3H/HeN mouse macrophages. *J. Immunol. 127*:2381–2386 (1981).

180. Hoover, D. L., and Nacy, C. A. Macrophage activation to kill *Leishmania tropica*: defective intracellular killing of amastigotes by macrophages elicited with sterile inflammatory agents. *J. Immunol. 132*:1487–1493 (1984).

181. Hockmeyer, W. T., Walters, D., Gore, R. W., Williams, J. S., Fortier, A. H., and Nacy, C. A. Intracellular destruction of *Leishmania donovani* and *Leishmania tropica* amastigotes by activated macrophages: dissociation of these microbicidal effector activities in vitro. *J. Immunol. 132*:3120–3125 (1984).

182. Oster, C. N., and Nacy, C. A. Macrophage activation to kill *Leishmania tropica*: kinetics of macrophage response to lymphokines that induce antimicrobial activities against amastigotes. *J. Immunol. 132*:1494–1500 (1984).

183. Nacy, C. A. Macrophage activation to kill *Leishmania tropica*: characterization of a T cell-derived factor that suppresses lymphokine-induced intracellular destruction of amastigotes. *J. Immunol. 133*:448–453 (1984).

184. Haidaris, C. G., and Bonventre, P. F. Elimination of *Leishmania donovani* amastigotes by activated macrophages. *Infect. Immun. 33*:918–926 (1981).

185. Haidaris, C. G., and Bonventre, P. F. A role for oxygen-dependent mechanisms in killing of *Leishmania donovani* tissue forms by activated macrophages. *J. Immunol. 129*:850–855 (1982).

186. Chang, K.-P., and Chiao, J. W. Cellular immunity of mice to *Leishmania donovani* in vitro: lymphokine-mediated killing of intracellular parasites in macrophages. *Proc. Natl.Acad. Sci. USA 78*:7083–7087 (1981).

187. Murry, H. W., Rubin, B. Y., and Rothermel, C. D. Killing of intracellular *Leishmania donovani* by lymphokine-stimulated human mononuclear phagocytes. Evidence that interferon-γ is activating lymphokine. *J. Clin. Invest. 72*:1506–1510 (1983).

188. Hoover, D. L., Nacy, C. A., and Meltzer, M. S. Human monocyte activation for cytotoxicity against intracellular *Leishmania donovani* amastigotes: Induction of microbicidal activity by interferon-γ. *Cell. Immunol. 94*:500–511 (1985).

189. Douvas, G. S., Looker, D. L., Vatter, A. E., and Crowle, A. J. Gamma interferon activates human macrophages to become tumoricidal and leishmanicidal but enhances replication of macrophage-associated mycobacteria. *Infect. Immun. 50*:1–8 (1985).

190. Passwell, J. H., Shor, R., and Shoham, J. The enhancing effect of interferon-β and -γ on the killing of *Leishmania tropica major* in human mononuclear phagocytes in vitro. *J. Immunol. 136*:3062–3066 (1986).

191. Passwell, J. H., Shor, T., Gazit, E., and Shoham, J. The effects of Con A-induced lymphokines from the T-lymphocyte subpopulations on human monocyte leishmanicidal capacity and H_2O_2 production. *Immunology 59*:245–250 (1986).

192. Hoover, D. L., Finebloom, D. S., Crawford, R. M., Nacy, C. A., Gilbreath, M., and Meltzer, M. S. A lymphokine distinct from interferon-γ that activates human monocytes to kill *Leishmania donovani* in vitro. *J. Immunol. 136*:1329–1333 (1986).

193. Carvalho, E. M., Teixeira, R. A., Badaró, Reed, S. G., Jones, T. C., and Johnson, W. D., Jr. Absence of gamma interferon and interleukin 2 production during active visceral leishmaniasis. *J. Clin. Invest. 76*:2066–2069 (1985).

194. Scott, P., and Sher, A. A spectrum in the susceptibility of leishmanial strains to intracellular killing by murine macrophages. *J. Immunol. 136*:1461–1466 (1986).

195. Buchmüller, Y., and Mauel, J. Studies on the mechanisms of macrophage activation: possible involvement of oxygen metabolites in killing of *Leishmania enriettii* by activated mouse macrophages. *J. Reticuloendothel. Soc. 29*:181–192 (1981).

196. Scott, P., James, S., and Sher, A. The respiratory burst is not required for killing of intracellular and extracellular parasites by a lymphokine-activated macrophage cell line. *Eur. J. Immunol. 15*:553–558 (1985).

197. Pfefferkorn, E. R. Interferon-γ blocks the growth of *Toxoplasma gondii* in human fibroblasts by inducing the host cells to degrade tryptophan. *Proc. Natl. Acad. Sci. USA 81*:908–912 (1984).

198. Panosian, C. B., Sypek, J. P., and Wyler, D. J. Cell contact-mediated macrophage activation for antileishmanial defense. I. Lymphocyte effector

mechanism that is contact dependent and noncytotoxic. *J. Immunol. 133*: 3358–3365 (1984).

199. Sypek, J. P., Panosian, C. B., and Wyler, D. J. Cell contact-mediated macrophage activation for antileishmanial defense. II. Identification of effector cell phenotype and genetic restriction. *J. Immunol. 133*:3351–3357 (1984).

200. Sypek, J. P., Panosian, C. B., and Wyler, D. J. Antigen recognition by effector T cells in antileishmanial defense. *J. Infect. Dis. 152*:1057–1063 (1985).

201. Sypek, J. P., and Wyler, D. J. Cell contact-mediated macrophage activation for antileishmanial defence: mapping of the genetic restriction to the I region of the MHC. *Clin. Exp. Immunol. 62*:449–457 (1985).

202. Sadick, M. D., Locksley, R. M., and Raff, H. V. Development of cellular immunity in cutaneous leishmaniasis due to *Leishmania tropica. J. Infect. Dis. 150*:135–138 (1984).

203. Kirkpatrick, C. E., and Farrell, J. P. Leishmaniasis in beige mice. *Infect. Immun. 38*:1208–1216 (1982).

204. Merino, F., and Curz, I. Natural killer activity in experimental cutaneous leishmaniasis. *Int. Arch. Allergy Appl. Immunol. 73*:347–351 (1984).

205. Mauel, J., Behin, R., Biroum-Moerjasin, and Holle, B. Studies on protective cell-mediated mechanisms in experimental *Leishmania* infections. In *Mononuclear Phagocytes in Immunity, Infection and Pathology* (R. Van Furth, ed.). Blackwell Scientific, Oxford, 1975, pp. 663–672.

206. Handman, E., and Spira, D. T. Growth of *Leishmania* amastigotes in macrophages from normal and immune mice. *Z. Parasitenkd. 53*:75–81 (1977).

207. Handman, E., Ceredig, R., and Mitchell, G. F. Murine cutaneous leishmaniasis: disease patterns in intact and nude mice of various genotypes and examination of some differences between normal and infected macrophages. *Aust. J. Exp. Biol. Med. Sci. 57*:9–29 (1979).

208. Gorczynski, R. M., and MacRae, S. Analysis of subpopulations of glass-adherent mouse skin cells controlling resistance/susceptibility to infection with *Leishmania tropica*, and correlation with the development of independent proliferative signals to Lyt-1[+]/Lyt-2[+] lymphocytes. *Cell. Immunol. 67*:74–89 (1982).

209. Scott, P., Sacks, D., and Sher, A. Resistance to macrophage-mediated killing as a factor influencing the pathogenesis of chronic cutaneous leishmaniasis. *J. Immunol. 131*:966–971 (1983).

210. Scott, P. A. Impaired macrophage leishmanicidal activity at cutaneous temperature. *Parasite Immunol. 7*:277–288 (1985).

211. Howard, J. G. Immunological regulation and control of experimental leishmaniasis. *Int. Rev. Exp. Pathol. 28*:79–116 (1986).

212. Howard, J. G., Hale, C., and Chan-Liew, W. L. Immunological regulation of experimental cutaneous leishmaniasis. I. Immunogenetic aspects of susceptibility to *Leishmania tropica* in mice. *Parasite Immunol. 2*:303–314 (1980).

213. Howard, J. G., Hale, C., and Liew, F. Y. Immunological regulation of

experimental cutaneous leishmaniasis. III. Nature and significance of specific suppression of cell-mediated immunity in mice highly susceptible to *Leishmania tropica. J. Exp. Med. 152*:594–607 (1980).

214. Liew, F. Y., Howard, J. G., and Hale, C. Prophylactic immunization against experimental leishmaniasis. III. Protection against fatal *Leishmania tropica* infection induced by irradiated promastigotes involves Lyt-1$^+$2$^-$ T cells that do not mediate cutaneous DTH. *J. Immunol. 132*:456–461 (1984).

215. Liew, F. Y., Hale, C., and Howard, J. G. Prophylactic immunization against experimental leishmaniasis. IV. Subcutaneous immunization prevents the induction of protective immunity against fatal *Leishmania major* infection. *J. Immunol. 135*:2095–2101 (1985).

216. Liew, F. Y., Singleton, A., Cillari, E.,and Howard, J. G. Prophylactic immunization against experimental leishmaniasis. V. Mechanism of the anti-protective blocking effect induced by subcutaneous immunization against *Leishmania major* infection. *J. Immunol. 135*:2102–2107 (1985).

217. Liew, F. Y. Specific suppression of responses to *Leishmania tropica* by a cloned T cell line. *Nature 305*:630–632 (1983).

218. Mitchell, G. E., Curtis, J. M., Scollary, R. G., and Handman, E. Resistance and abrogation of resistance to cutaneous leishmaniasis in reconstituted BALB/c nude mice. *Aust. J. Exp. Biol. Med. Sci. 59*:539–554 (1981).

219. Behforouz, N. C., Wenger, C. D., and Mathison, B. A. Prophylactic treatment of BALB/c mice with cyclosporine A and its analog B-5-49 enhances resistance to *Leishmania major. J. Immunol. 136*:3067–3075 (1986).

220. Solbach, W., Forberg, K., and Rollinghoff, M. Effect of T-lymphocyte suppression on the parasite burden in *Leishmania major*-infected, genetically susceptible BALB/c mice. *Infect. Immun. 54*:909–912 (1986).

221. Solbach, W., Forberg, K., Kammerer, E., Bogdan, C., and Rollinghoff, M. Suppressive effect of cyclosporin A on the development of *Leishmania tropica*-induced lesions in genetically susceptible BALB/c mice. *J. Immunol. 137*:702–707 (1986).

222. Titus, R. G., Lima, G. C., Engers, H. D., and Louis, J. A. Exacerbation of murine cutaneous leishmaniasis by adoptive transfer of parasite-specific helper T cell populations capable of mediating *Leishmania major*-specific delayed-type hypersensitivity. *J. Immunol. 133*:1594–1600 (1984).

223. Titus, R. G., Ceredig, R., Cerottini, J.-C., and Louis, J. A. Therapeutic effect of anti-L3T4 monoclonal antibody GK1.5 on cutaneous leishmaniasis in genetically susceptible BALB/c mice. *J. Immunol. 135*:2108–2114 (1985).

224. Milon, G., Titus, R. G., Cerottini, J.-C., Marchal, G., and Louis, J. A. Higher frequency of *Leishmania major*-specific L3T4$^+$ T cells in susceptible BALB/c as compared with resistant CBA mice. *J. Immunol. 136*: 1467–1471 (1986).

225. Mossman, T. R., Cherwinski, H., Bond, M. W., Gledlin, M. A., and Coffman, R. L. Two types of murine helper T cell clone. I. Definition

according to profiles of lymphokine activities and secreted proteins. *J. Immunol. 136*:2348-2357 (1986).

226. Marvel, J., Mitchison, N. A., Oliveira, D. B. G., and O'Malley, C. The split within the CD4 (helper) T-cell subset, and its implications for immunopathology. *Mem. Inst. Oswaldo Cruz 82(Suppl.)*:260–273 (1987).

227. Handman, E., and Mitchell, G. F. Immunization with *Leishmania* receptor for macrophages protects mice against cutaneous leishmaniasis. *Proc. Natl. Acad. Sci. 82*:5910–5914 (1985).

228. Mitchell, G. F., and Handman, E. T-lymphocytes recognize *Leishmania* glycoconjugates. *Parasitol. Today 1*:61–63 (1985).

229. Handman, E., and Goding, J. W. The *Leishmania* receptor for macrophages is a lipid-containing glycoconjugate. *EMBO J. 4*:329–336 (1985).

230. Greenblatt, C. L., Kark, J. D., Schnur, L. F., and Slutzky, G. M. Do *Leishmania* serotypes mimic human blood group antigens? [letter] *Lancet 1*: 505–506 (1981).

231. Slutzky, G. M., and Greenblatt, C. L. Isolation of a carbohydrate-rich, immunologically active factor from cultures of *Leishmania tropica*. *FEBS Lett. 80*:401–404 (1977).

232. Handman, E., and Greenblatt, C. L. Promotion of leishmanial infections in non-permissive host macrophages by conditioned medium. *Z. Parasitenkd. 53*:143–147 (1977).

233. Slutzky, G. M., El-On, J., and Greenblatt, C. L. Leishmanial excreted factor: protein-bound and free forms from promastigote cultures of *Leishmania tropica* and *Leishmania donovani*. *Infect. Immun. 26*:916–924 (1979).

234. El-On, J., Schnur, L. F., and Greenblatt, C. L. *Leishmania donovani*: physiochemical, immunological, and biological characterization of excreted factor from promastigotes. *Exp. Parasitol. 47*:254–269 (1979).

235. Sacks, D. L., Scott, P. A., Asofsky, R., and Sher, F. A. Cutaneous leishmaniasis in anti-IgM-treated mice: enhanced resistance due to functional depletion of a B cell-dependent T cell involved in the suppressor pathway. *J. Immunol. 132*:2072–2077 (1984).

236. Scott, P., Natovitz, P., and Sher, A. B lymphocytes are required for the generation of T cells that mediate healing of cutaneous leishmaniasis. *J. Immunol. 137*:1017–1021 (1986).

237. Fahey, J. R., and Herman, R. Relationship between delayed hypersensitivity response and acquired cell-mediated immunity in C57BL/6J mice infected with *Leishmania donovani*. *Infect. Immun. 49*:447–451 (1985).

238. Dhaliwal, J. S., Liew, F. Y., and Cox, F. E. G. Specific suppressor T cells for delayed-type hypersensitivity in susceptible mice immunized against cutaneous leishmaniasis. *Infect. Immun. 49*:417–423 (1985).

239. Sheppard, H. W., Scott, P. A., and Dwyer, D. M. Recognition of *Leishmania donovani* antigens by murine T lymphocyte lines and clones. Species cross-reactivity, functional correlates of cell-mediated immunity, and antigen characterization. *J. Immunol. 131*:1496–1503 (1983).

240. Blackwell, J. M., and Ulczak, O. M. Immunoregulation of genetically controlled acquired responses to *Leishmania donovani* infection in mice: demonstration and characterization of suppressor T cells in non-cure mice. *Infect. Immun. 44*:97–102 (1984).
241. Scott, P. A., and Farrell, J. P. Experimental cutaneous leishmaniasis. I. Nonspecific immunodepression in BALB/c mice infected with *Leishmania tropica. J. Immunol. 127*:2395–2400 (1981).
242. Murray, H., Masur, H., and Keithly, J. S. Cell-mediated immune responses in experimental visceral leishmaniasis: I. Correlation between resistance to *Leishmania donovani* and lymphokine-generating capacity. *J. Immunol. 129*:344–350 (1982).
243. Murray, H. W., Carriero, S. M., and Donnelly, D. M. Presence of macrophage-mediated suppressor cell mechanism during cell-mediated immune response in experimental visceral leishmaniasis. *Infect. Immun. 54*:487–493 (1986).
244. Reiner, N. E., and Malemud, C. J. Arachidonic acid metabolism by murine peritoneal macrophages infected with *Leishmania donovani*: in vitro evidence for parasite-induced alterations in cyclooxygenase and lipoxygenase pathways. *J. Immunol. 134*:556–563 (1985).
245. Reiner, N. E., and Malemud, C. J. Arachidonic acid metabolism in murine leishmaniasis (donovani): ex-vivo evidence for increased cyclyooxygenase and 5-lipoxygenase activity in spleen cells. *Cell. Immunol. 88*:501–510 (1984).
246. Reiner, N. E., and Finke, J. H. Interleukin 2 deficiency in murine leishmaniasis donovani and its relationship to depressed spleen cell responses to phytohemagglutinin. *J. Immunol. 131*:1487–1491 (1983).
247. Reiner, N. E. Host–parasite relationship in murine leishmaniasis: pathophysiological and immunological changes. *Infect. Immun. 38*:1223–1230 (1982).
248. Perez, H., Pocino, M., and Malave, I. Nonspecific immunodepression and protective immunity in mice infected with *Leishmania mexicana. Infect. Immun. 32*:415–419 (1981).
249. Marinkelle, C. J. The control of leishmaniases. *Bull. WHO 58*:807–818 (1980).
250. Greenblatt, C. L. The present and future of vaccination for cutaneous leishmaniasis. In *Progress in Clinical and Biological Research*, Vol. 47. *New Developments with Human and Veterinary Vaccines* (A. Mizrahi, I. Hertman, M. A. Klingberg, and A. Kohn, eds). Alan R. Liss, New York, 1980, pp. 259–285.
251. Peterson, E. A., Neva, F. A., Oster, C. N., and Bogaret-Diaz, H. Specific inhibition of lymphocyte-proliferation responses by adherent suppressor cells in diffuse cutaneous leishmaniais. *New Engl. J. Med. 306*:387–392 (1982).
252. Peterson, E. A., and Neva, F. A., Barral, A., Correa-Coronas, R., Bogaert-Diaz, H., Martinez, D., and Ward, F. E. Monocyte suppression of antigen-

specific lymphocyte responses in diffuse cutaneous leishmaniasis patients from the Dominican Republic. *J. Immunol. 132*:2603–2606 (1984).

253. Southgate, B. A., and Manson-Bahr, P. E. C. Studies in the epidemiology of East African leishmaniasis. 4. The significance of the positive leishmanin test. *J. Trop. Med. Hyg. 70*:29–33 (1967).

254. Pampiglione, S., Manson-Bahr, P. E. C., La Placa, M., Borgatti, M. A., and Musumeci, S. Studies in Mediterranean leishmaniasis: 3. The leishmanin skin test in kala-azar. *Trans. R. Soc. Trop. Med. Hyg. 69*:60–68 (1975).

255. Badaró, R., Jones, T. C., Lorenco, R., Cerg, B. J., Sampaio, D., Carvalho, E. M., Rocha, H., Teixeira, R., and Johnson, W. D., Jr. A prospective study of visceral leishmaniasis in an endemic area in Brazil. *J. Infect. Dis. 154*: 639–649 (1986).

256. Badaró, R., Jones, T. C., Carvalho, E. M., Sampaio, D., Reed, S. G., Barral, A., Teixeira, R., and Johnson, W. D., Jr. New perspectives on a subclinical form of visceral leishmaniasis. *J. Infect. Dis. 154*:1003–1011 (1986).

257. Manson-Bahr, P. E. C. East African kala-azar with special reference to the pathology, prophylaxis and treatment. *Trans. R. Soc. Trop. Med. Hyg. 53*: 123–136 (1959).

258. Ho, M., Koech, D. K., Iha, D. W., and Bryceson, A. D. M. Immunosuppression in Kenyan visceral leishmaniasis. *Clin. Exp. Immunol. 51*:207–214 (1983).

259. Haldar, J. P., Ghose, S., Saha, K. C., and Ghose, A. C. Cell-mediated immune response in Indian kala azar and post-kala azar dermal leishmaniasis. *Infect. Immun. 42*:702–707 (1983).

260. Ghose, A. C., Haldar, J. P., Pal, S. C., Mishra, B. P., and Mishra, K. K. Serological investigations on Indian kala-azar. *Clin Exp. Immunol. 40*: 318–326 (1980).

261. Galvao-Castro, B., Sa Ferreira, J. A., Marzochi, K. F., Marzochi, M. C., Coutinho, S. G., and Lambert, P. H. Polyclonal B cell activation, circulating immune complexes and autoimmunity in human American visceral leishmaniasis. *Clin. Exp. Immunol. 56*:58–66 (1984).

262. Pearson, R. D., Evans, T., Naidu, T. G., Alencar, J. E., Wheeler, D., and Davis, J. S., IV. Humoral responses during South American visceral leishmaniasis. *Ann. Trop. Med. Parasitol. 80*:465–468 (1986).

263. Sacks, D. L., Lal, S. L., Shrivastava, S. N., Blackwell, J., and Neva, F. A. An analysis of T cell responsiveness in Indian kala-azar. *J. Immunol. 138*: 908–913 (1987).

264. Reiner, N. E., Ng, W., and McMaster, W. R. Parasite–accessory cell interactions in murine leishmaniasis. II. *Leishmania donovani* suppresses macropage expression for class I and class II major histocompatibility complex gene products. *J. Immunol. 138*:1926–1932 (1987).

265. Reiner, N. E. Parasite–accessory cell interactions in murine leishmaniasis. I. Evasion and stimulus-dependent suppression of the macrophage interleukin 1 response by *Leishmania donovani*. *J. Immunol. 138*:1919–1925 (1987).

266. Crawford, G. D., Wyler, D. J., and Dinarello, C. A. Parasite–monocyte interactions in human leishmaniasis: production of interleukin-1 in vitro. *J. Infect. Dis. 152*:315–322 (1985).
267. Harrison, L. H., Naidu, T. G., Drew, J. S., Alencar, J. E., and Pearson, R. D. Reciprocal relationships between undernutrition and the parasitic disease, visceral leishmaniasis. *Rev. Infect. Dis. 8*:447–453 (1986).
268. Badaró, R., Carvalho, E. M., Rocha, H., Queiroz, A. C., and Jones, T. C. *Leishmania donovani*: an opportunistic microbe associated with progressive disease in three immunocompromised patients. *Lancet 1*:647–648 (1986).
269. Ma, D. D. F., Concannon, A. J., and Hayes, J. Fatal leishmaniasis in renal transplant patient. *Lancet 2*:311–312 (1979).
270. Fernández-Guerrero, M. L., Aguado, J. M., Buzón, L., Barras, C., Montalbân, C., Martín, T., and Bouza, E. Visceral leishmaniasis in immunocompromised hosts. *Am. J. Med. 83*:1098–1102, 1987.
271. Barral, A., Carvalho, E. M., Badaró, R., and Barrel-Netto, N. Suppression of lymphocyte proliferative responses by sera from patients with American visceral leishmaniasis. *Am. J. Trop. Med. Hyg. 35*:735–742 (1986).
272. Wyler, D. J. Circulating factor from a kala-azar patient suppresses in vitro anti-leishmanial T cell proliferation. *Trans. R. Soc. Trop. Med. Hyg. 76*: 304–306 (1982).
273. Giannini, M. S. H. Suppression of pathogenesis in cutaneous leishmaniasis by UV irradiation. *Infect. Immun. 51*:838–843 (1986).
274. Dinarello, C. A. Interleukin-1. *Rev. Infect. Dis. 6*:51–95 (1984).
275. Beutler, B., and Cerami, A. Cachectin: more than a tumor necrosis factor. *New Engl. J. Med. 316*:379–385 (1987).
276. Scuderi, P., Lam, K. S., Ryan, K. J., Peterson, E., Salmon, S. E., Sterling, K. E., Finley, P. R., Ray, C. G., and Slymen, D. J. Raised serum levels of tumour necrosis factor in parasitic infections. *Lancet 2*:1364–1365 (1986).
277. Pearson, R. D., Alencar, J. E., Romito, R., Naidu, T. G., Young, A. C., and Davis, J. S. IV. Circulating immune complexes and rheumatoid factors in visceral leishmaniasis. *J. Infect. Dis. 147*:1102 (1983).
278. Carvalho, E. M., Andrews, B. S., Martinelli, R., Dutra, M., and Rocha, H. Circulating immune complexes and rheumatoid factor in schistosomiasis and visceral leishmaniasis. *Am. J. Trop. Med. Hyg. 32*:61–69 (1983).
279. Desjeux, P., Santoro, F., Afchain, D., Loyens, M., and Capron, A. Circulating immune complexes and anti-IgG antibodies in mucocutaneous leishmaniasis. *Am. J. Trop. Med. Hyg. 29*:195–198 (1980).

3
Pneumocystis carinii

PETER D. WALZER, C. KURTIS KIM, and MELANIE T. CUSHION
Cincinnati Veterans Administration Medical Center and University of Cincinnati College of Medicine, Cincinnati, Ohio

I. INTRODUCTION

Pneumocystis carinii was first described in 1909 by Chagas in the lungs of guinea pigs during his studies of experimental American trypanosomiasis (1). He thought the organism was a variant in the sexual life cycle of *Trypanosoma cruzi*. One year later, Carini found the organism in trypanosome-infected rats (2). The Delanöes then found identical forms in the lungs of rats that had not been infected with trypanosomes; they clearly established that these organisms represented a new genus and species and assigned the name *Pneumocystis carinii* in honor of Dr. Carini (3,4).

Although *P. carinii* was subsequently found in the lungs of humans and many other animals, the organism remained little more than a medical curiosity. The first association of *P. carinii* with human illness came in 1952 from the studies of Vanek and Jirovec, which implicated the organism as the cause of interstitial plasma cell pneumonia (5). This disease affected premature and debilitated infants in central and eastern Europe following World War II and had a high mortality rate; the histopathological picture was characterized by a prominent interstitial plasma cell infiltrate (6-8). Since the disease sometimes occurred in explosive outbreaks, it was known as the "epidemic" form of pneumocystosis. In the late 1950s, Ivady and Paldy reported on the successful treatment of interstitial plasma cell pneumonia with pentamidine (9,10), and the drug became generally accepted as the anti-*P. carinii* agent of choice. Interstitial plasma cell pneumonia gradually disappeared from Europe with improved socioeconomic conditions, but it still exists in many parts of the world where crowding, malnutrition, and poor health care abound (11-18).

Medical interest in *P. carinii* in the United States developed in the 1960s when the organism emerged as an important cause of pneumonia in the immuno-compromised host (7,8,12,19–36). Major targets included children with primary immunodeficiency diseases and patients of all ages receiving corticosteroids and other immunosuppressive drugs for the treatment of cancer, organ transplanta-tion, and other disorders. Cases of pneumocystosis were sporadic and were characterized histopathologically by the absence of any visible host inflamma-tory response, prompting some authors to call it the "hypoergic" form of *P. carinii* infection (37). The Centers for Disease Control (CDC), as the sole sup-plier of pentamidine in this country, maintained informal surveillance of *P. carinii*, which was helpful in delineating the epidemiological features of the disease (38–40). The experimental work of Sheldon, Frenkel, and other workers led to the establishment of animal models that have contributed much to our understanding of the pathogenesis of pneumocystosis (41–44).

In the 1970s, Hughes demonstrated that trimethoprim-sulfamethoxazole (TMP–SMX) was highly effective in both the therapy and prophylaxis of *P. carinii* pneumonia (45–47). Since TMP–SMX was less toxic than pentamidine, it became the drug of choice. The widespread use of TMP–SMX led to a marked decline in the number of cases of *P. carinii* pneumonia at most major medical centers (48).

With the emergence of the acquired immunodeficiency syndrome (AIDS) and other retroviral diseases in the 1980s, *P. carinii* regained medical attention (49, 49a,50). Pneumocystosis is the most common opportunistic infection in AIDS and a leading cause of morbidity and mortality (51–54). As the AIDS epidemic spreads, it can be expected that the number of cases of *P. carinii* pneumonia will continue to increase. The subtle clinical presentation, slow response to treat-ment, frequent relapses, and high rate of adverse reactions to TMP–SMX and pentamidine illustrate the new challenges posed by *P. carinii* pneumonia in AIDS patients (55–63).

Despite the rise in importance of *P. carinii*, our knowledge of the basic immunobiology of the organism remains at a rudimentary level. Until there is better understanding of *P. carinii's* growth, life cycle, metabolism, virulence factors, and structural and antigenic characteristics, it is unlikely that significant clinical progress in dealing with this organism can be made.

II. THE ORGANISM

A. Life Cycle and Epidemiology

1. Developmental Stages

Pneumocystis carinii exists as a pulmonary saprophyte in a wide variety of mammalian species in nature (64–72). Although the organisms in these different hosts are morphologically indistinguishable, it is likely that species or strain differences exist. The lack of a standard nomenclature system has led to different terms being used to describe the organism. Examples include *Pneumocystis sp* to refer to the organism in any host, *Pneumocystis carinii* for the organism in rats, and *Pneumocystis jiroveci* for the organism in humans (73). We have used *Pneumocystis carinii* in the present chapter to refer to the organism in any host because it is the most widely used term in the literature.

Studies of the life cycle of *P. carinii* have mainly relied on histochemical and ultrastructural analysis of organisms found in human and rat lung sections (74–96). Results of these studies differ in the number of identified stages and forms throughout the life cycle, the sequence of appearance of the stages within a life cycle, the existence of intracellular forms, and the taxonomic classification. Despite such differences, all investigators have consistently identified three major forms of *P. carinii*: trophic stage, precyst, and cyst (Fig. 1).

The *trophic stage* is the smallest of the stages and is also referred to as a trophozoite (74–76) or small thin-walled pneumocyst (83) (Fig. 1A, B). Depending on the specific subtype classification, investigators report a size range of 1–5 μm for this form. Few organelles populate the cytoplasm of the trophic stage. The most prominent feature is the nucleus, with an electron-dense area identified as a nucleolus sometimes present. The number of chromosomes has not yet been determined for any stage of *P. carinii*, but recent ultrastructural observations infer a haploid status for this form (80). Some investigators have observed electron-dense material in bell-shaped protrusions of the nucleus (83); however, the function of these "round bodies" has not been determined. Cytoplasmic organelles include one mitochondrion, rough endoplasmic reticulum, ribosomes, occasional vacuoles, and glycogen granules. Lipid globules have also been identified in some trophic forms (76,82). The rounded mitochondria of this and all forms of *P. carinii* have been interpreted as protozoan in nature. Although studies of the metabolic features of *P. carinii* are very limited, the presence of at least one mitochondrion means that the organism is capable of aerobic respiration with the oxidative metabolism of glucose and fatty acids for its energy source. The presence of glycogen granules within the cytoplasm of the organism has been thought to indicate glycogenesis, glyconeogenesis, or metabolism of low weight compounds by the organism (74,91).

The shape of the trophic form is quite pleomorphic and appears to be related to the method of fixation. In lung sections, *P. carinii* trophozoites have an irregular ameboid appearance, whereas in unfixed preparations examined under phase or Nomarski interference contrast microscopy, their shape becomes ellipsoidal and resembles a cluster of grapes (97). The boundaries of an individual organism in this developmental stage are defined by a cell wall that measures approximately 20–30 μm across and consists of three layers: an outer, electron-dense layer; a middle, electron-translucent layer; and an inner, trilaminar unit membrane characteristic of a plasmalemma (86). The term *cell wall* is

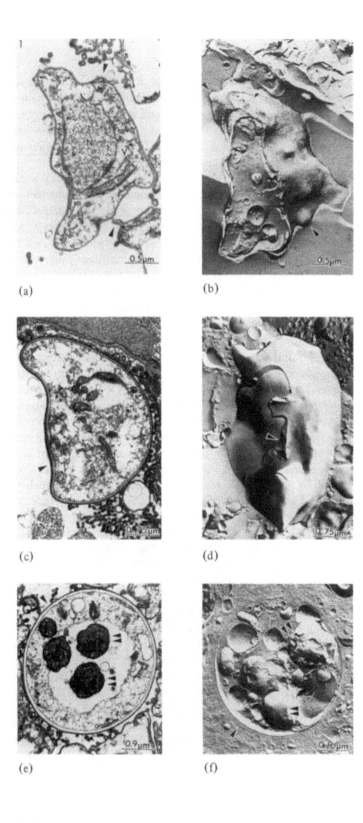

(a)

(b)

(c)

(d)

(e)

(f)

used here to describe the constraints of this form and all other stages of *P. carinii*, since "pellicle" denotes inclusion of supportive, flattened alveolar sacks, which have not been observed in any stage of *P. carinii*. Discontinuities on the cell wall surface are a characteristic feature; filopodia or tubular extensions are easily observed by ultrathin microscopy (75,82). The diameter of these projections varies, and the lumen is usually filled with dense granular material (83). It has been postulated that these expansions are used for nutritional uptake, attachment to host cells, or as a means of communication between organisms (80).

Freeze-fracture ultramicroscopy has revealed that the surface of the trophic form contains particles that may be randomly distributed, assume the conformation of rosettes, or encircle the base of tubular extensions (86). Rosettes are composed of circular arrangements of particles with a central depression measuring 60 nm in diameter. The function of such particles is not fully understood, but surface rosettes have been implicated in the process of endocytosis and exocytosis in other protozoan species. To date, these configurations have not been observed in yeast or mammalian cells.

Most investigators separate the uninuclear trophic stage into two subtypes: the small and large. Factors that differentiate the two include size, cytoplasmic inclusions, and composition of the cell wall.

The definition of the *precyst* stage of *P. carinii* varies considerably. In general, this form is considered an intermediate stage between the trophic and cystic stages with size dimensions of approximately 4-6 μm (Fig. 1C, D). The fairly consistent oval shape suggests a thickening and differentiation of the cell wall, which measures about 100 nm and is divided into three layers similar to those found in the trophic form. The cell surface of the precyst is smooth and

---

Figure 1 (a) Thin-section photograph of a trophic *P. carinii*. Note the irregular shape, a central nucleus (N) and mitochondira, and a few vacuoles (V); filopodia (arrows) are seen stretching from the cell body. Uranyl acetate and lead citrate stain. X28,000. (b) Freeze-fracture image of a trophic *P. carinii*. Note two layers of the pellicle. Filopodia (arrows) can be seen as bulges of cytoplasm. The smoothness of the vacuolar wall (V) is evident. X28,000. (c) Thin-section photograph of a precyst *P. carinii*. Note tightly packed outer layer of the cell wall (arrow). X19,000. (d) Freeze-fracture image of a precyst *P. carinii*. Note the smoothness of the surface and thickness of the wall (arrow). X19,000. (e) Thin-section photograph of a *P. carinii* cyst. Note the tightly packed wall and intracystic bodies (double arrows). Uranyl acetate and lead citrate strain. X16,000. (f) Freeze-fracture image of a *P. carinii* cyst. The fracture plane crossed the center of the cyst. Notice the tightly packed wall (arrow) and intracystic bodies (double arrows). X16,000 (Reprinted with permission from Ref. 82.)

completely devoid of any particles, but tubular extensions have been reported (73,82,86). Intracytoplasmically, the precyst contains one or more nuclei and mitochondria, which can be found singly or in clumps; these clumps have been observed frequently adjacent to the nucleus. Free ribosomes, endoplasmic reticulum, vacuoles, microtubules, and membranous structures have also been described for this stage.

Recent ultrastructural studies have identified three subtypes of the precyst stage (80). The early precyst is defined by an ovoid shape, a 40-50-nm cell wall, and a clump of mitochondria surrounding a single nucleus bound by an intact nuclear envelope with a nucleolus-like structure. Synaptonemal complexes have been found only in the early precyst stage. These structures represent the pairing of homologous chromosomes, a general indication of meiotic division (98). However, synaptonemal complexes have been reported to occur in haploid nuclei of higher plants and in the nonmeiotic nuclei of the ascomycete *Ascophanus* (99,100). Other indications of meiosis include observation of gamete fusion, cytological evidence of alternation of generation, and quantitation of DNA content of the various stages (98). Investigators have reported a reduction in nuclear size (2.0-0.5 μm) with a concomitant increase in the number of nuclei from one to eight in the precyst (80), and work in our laboratory has shown two uninuclear forms with a twofold nuclear size difference using light microscopic techniques (97). It therefore appears that *P. carinii* has a sexual phase, but further quantitation studies are required to document the process throughout the life cycle.

The intermediate precyst stage maintains a more spherical shape with an increase in thickness of the three-layer cell wall to 50-100 nm, due to a widening of the electron-lucent middle layer. Cytoplasmic inclusions unique to this intermediate stage include spindle microtubules, which appear to originate from a dense body termed the nucleus-associated organelle (NAO). Two to four nuclei associated with a clump of mitochondria are also found in this stage.

The late precyst is defined by its spherical shape and thickened three-layer cell wall (80-120 nm). Four or more rounded nuclei are usually found in association with NAOs. An interesting feature of this stage is the presence of parallel unit membranes, which appear to originate from the inner plasmalemma and function in the sequestration of cytoplasmic organelles into distinct units.

The *cyst* is the largest (5-8 μm) and the most recognizable stage of the organism (Fig. 1E, F). The cyst wall is composed of the three layers previously described and has a thickness of 70-120 nm. The three layers are uniform around the circumference of the spherical cyst, except at one pole, where a thickening of the electron-lucent layer imparts an irregularity. Freeze-fracture studies have shown the outer membrane surface to have dense fibrillar properties and the plasmalemma surface to contain many randomly scattered particles (88). The cyst commonly contains up to eight daughter forms, referred to as intracystic bodies or sporozoites. The intracystic bodies are spherical, about 1-2 μm in diameter, and contain a nucleus (0.5-1 μm) with nucleolus, rough endoplasmic reticulum, a mitochondrion, microtubules, and sometimes vacuoles and round bodies. Glycogen particles are rarely found within these daughter forms. The intracystic bodies have been reported to be attached to each other and/or the cyst wall by a stalklike or threadlike structure (80). The individual daughter forms are bounded by a double membrane wall (200-300 A). Besides these forms, glycogen granules, mitochondria, rough endoplasmic reticulum membranes, and ribosomes are found within the confines of the cyst wall. It is commonly accepted that the intracystic bodies excyst and transform into the trophic form.

In addition to the classic thick-walled cyst, a thin-walled cyst has been identified by some workers (83). This stage contains irregularly shaped daughter forms that comprise its entire internal contents. The nature of the thin-walled cyst is unclear, but it may represent the product of a cycle independent from the sexual, sporogenous thick-wall cyst cycle. For example, endopolygeny would be an alternative, asexual method of reproduction that would be initiated by serial mitotic divisions of the haploid trophic form. The resultant cyst would be thin-walled, since these mitoses would occur within the original trophic membrane. Other parasitic protozoans have cycles lending to autoinfection within the host (101,102), and it would not be unusual for *P. carinii* to possess this alternative developmental stage.

Other stages of *P. carinii* that have been identified include an empty or "ghost" cyst and crescent-shaped forms. Empty cysts are presumably the result of excystation and contain residual organelles and glycogen granules; at times a daughter form may remain. Controversy exists over whether the crescent form represents an intermediate stage in the maturation process or whether it represents a residual thick-walled cyst after excystation (73,76,80,86).

2. Proposed Life Cycles

A number of different life cycles for *P. carinii* have been proposed (75,76,80-83, 103,104). Earlier studies were characterized by identification of few developmental stages and simple life cycles; investigators defined development as a progression from the uninuclear form (most often called "trophozoite") directly to the cyst form by multiple nuclear divisions (Table 1). Most of these studies also recognized that the trophozoite could replicate itself by binary fission or a budding process.

More recent proposals have increased in complexity because of identification of additional developmental stages. One group of investigators proposed a life cycle that differs markedly from other cycles and includes a two-branch scheme (83). Both paths begin with the small trophic form, called a small thin-walled pneumocyst, which can enter an autoinfective cycle or stage designed for

Table 1 Summaries of Some Previously Proposed Life Cycles for *Pneumocystis carinii*

Investigator(s)	Source of *P. carinii*	Life-cycle stages	Life cycle
Vavra and Kucera, 1970 (82)	Rat	Small trophic form, large trophic form, precyst, cyst, intracystic bodies	1. Fission or budding of trophic form. 2. Large trophic state develops into precyst; development continues to mature cyst containing intracystic bodies; intracystic bodies grow and excyst.
Barton and Campbell, 1969 (75) Campbell, 1970 (76)	Rat Human	Small trophozoite, large trophozoite Precyst, thick-walled cyst, intracystic bodies	1. Budding and/or conjugation by trophozoites. 2. Trophozoite develops into precyst and continues development into mature cyst with intracystic bodies, which eventually excyst.
Bouton et al., 1977 (104)	Rat	Small trophozoite, large trophozoite, precyst (3 forms), mature cyst	1. Trophozoite develops to precyst to mature cyst.

Vossen et al., 1978 (83)	Rat	Thin-walled pneumocysts (subtypes A–C), thick-walled pneumocysts (subtypes A,B), intracellular pneumocysts (subtypes A,B)	1. Thin-walled cycle: Subtype A develops to subtype B pneumocyst, continues to multinucleated thin-walled pneumocyst to subtype C, to thin-walled pneumocyst with daughter cells; excystation. 2. Thick-walled cycle: subtype A develops to subtype B pneumocyst, development continues to precyst stage (subtype D), to thick-walled pneumocyst (subtype E) with rounded daughter forms; daughter forms continue to grow; some may become electron dense with excystation.
Matsumo and Yoshida, 1984, 1986 (80,81)	Rat	Trophozoites, early precyst, intermediate precyst, late precyst, cyst, intracystic bodies	1. Binary fission of trophozoites. 2. Sporogony (sexual cycle) mediated by conjugation of trophozoites; development to early, intermediate, late precyst; mature cyst with intracystic bodies followed by excystation. 3. Endogeny–asexual cyst cycle initiated by diploid or haploid trophozoite.

transmission. These authors also present micrographs that they have interpreted as illustrations of an intracellular phase of the *P. carinii* life cycle. Other workers have proposed a life cycle that includes a sexual phase of cyst development, on the basis of their ultrastructural observation of synaptonemal complexes (80, 81). They suggest that both conjugation and binary fission are mediated by the trophozoite stage.

The life-cycle studies conducted in our laboratory have focused on rat *P. carinii* obtained from infected lung homogenates or grown in tissue culture (103). Human *P. carinii* from bronchoalveolar lavage specimens has also been used. Most of these studies have used a combination of light microscopic and staining techniques to perform detailed examination of *P. carinii* stages in unfixed specimens. These procedures were chosen to avoid alterations induced by harsh reagents used in the fixation and embedding process. All developmental stages identified using these procedures were verified by examination of impression smears stained with Diff Quik, a variant of the Giemsa stain. From these data, we have proposed a life cycle for *P. carinii* that includes both an asexual and a sexual phase of development (Fig. 2). The predominant form of the organism in culture is the trophic form, which frequently occurs in large clusters together with other developmental stages. These forms appear to replicate by binary fission in the lung, and this replicatoon probably occurs in vitro as well. Initiation of the sexual cycle in other protozoans usually begins with gametic fusion and karyogamy (nuclear fusion). Since microgametic or macrogametic forms of *P. carinii* have not been identified, it may be possible that some forms identified as trophic stages function as isogametes (Fig. 2A, B) (105). Once nuclear fusion takes place, the diploid zygote is formed and is considered an early precyst (80). Subsequent meiosis and mitosis occur within the cyst wall, and the organism differentiates from the precyst to the mature cyst form. We have identified various cystic stages, based on the morphological changes of the intracystic bodies, ranging from ellipsoidal forms to very elongated thin forms (Fig. 2J-N). Presumably the crescent-shaped forms represent empty excysted cysts, although the actual process of excystment has not been adequately documented.

3. Taxonomy

Chagas' original misidentification of *P. carinii* as a schizogonic stage of the *Trypanosoma* species presaged the difficulties that would be encountered by investigators who attempted to assign taxonomy and define the life cycle of this organism. Almost 80 years later, the classification of *P. carinii* remains controversial and incompletely defined. Some authors have classified the organism as a fungus because it can be stained with fungal stains (e.g., methenamine silver) and because of certain ultrastructural characteristics (19,82,106). Most workers have classified *P. carinii* as a protozoan because of its similarities to *Toxoplasma*

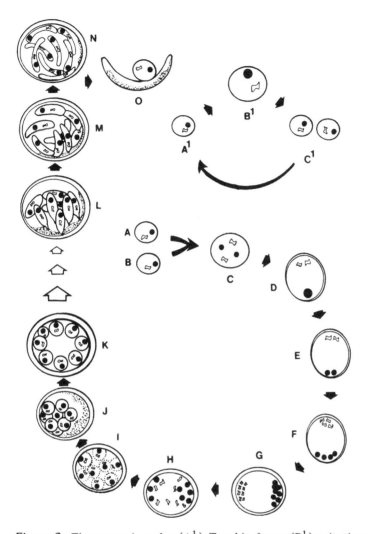

Figure 2 The asexual cycle: (A¹) Trophic form; (B¹) mitotic replication of trophic form; (C¹) trophic forms, products of binary fission. The sexual cycle: (A,B) Isogametic forms; (C) karyogamy; (D) early precyst, diploid zygote; (E) intermediate precyst, beginning of mitotic replication of nuclei; (F) intermediate precyst, four nuclei; (G) intermediate precyst, completion of nuclear replication, eight nuclei; (H) late precyst, migration of nuclei to periphery; (I) late precyst, initiation of compartmentalization of daughter forms; (J) early cyst, completed separation of daughter forms; (K) mature cyst, eight rounded daughter forms within a thick wall; (L) cyst containing ellipsoidal daughter forms; (M) cyst containing elongated daughter forms; (N) cyst containing thin, very elongated daughter forms; (O) collapsed, excysted cyst with trophic form. The progressive elongation of the daughter forms within the cyst (L–N) may represent the process required for excystation. These forms have been seen repeatedly in culture and in infected rat lung homogenates, although the actual process of excystment was not observed. (Reprinted with permission from Ref. 103.)

gondii, sensitivity to antiparasitic drugs, and specific ultrastructural properties. The words used to describe the developmental stages of *P. carinii* are based on terminology for protozoa. Arguments have been made that *P. carinii* belongs somewhere in the kingdom Protista, perhaps in the phylum Apicomplexa or Sarcomastigophora (subphylum Sarcodina, superclass Rhizopoda) (77,86). Classification of protozoans has been based primarily on morphological considerations. Since *P. carinii* lacks many basic organelles such as cytosomes or Golgi apparatus and specialized organelles associated with a parasitic existence such as rhoptries or micronemes, the assignment of a niche has been difficult. Recent application of molecular biology techniques to the taxonomy of *P. carinii* has revealed a close relationship with fungi (115).

4. Epidemiological Features

Infection with *P. carinii* appears to be acquired mainly by the respiratory route. Studies in athymic (nude) mice demonstrated that *P. carinii* could be transmitted by intrapulmonary injection of infected lung homogenates or prolonged exposure to other infected animals (107). Experiments in immunosuppressed, germ-free rats or rats raised in a protected environment implicated the airborne route as the major mode of spread; the infection could not be transmitted when soil, water, or food was used as the source of organism (108–110). One group of investigators has reported the successful transmission of *P. carinii* to nude mice or nude rats by intranasal inoculation (111–113), but other workers have been unable to confirm this finding (43,114,115). Although *P. carinii* is found in respiratory tract secretions (e.g., sputum) (116–118), it is unclear whether infection can be transmitted by direct contact with these substances.

Little is known about which developmental stage of *P. carinii* serves as the infective form. As with other protozoans, the thick-walled cyst is more resistant to adverse environmental conditions and would seem to be a logical candidate; however, the relatively large size of the cyst might make it more susceptible to upper airway defense mechanisms rather than being directly deposited in alveoli. Both cysts and trophozoites have been found in aerosols experimentally generated from infected lung homogenates (115), but a reproducible animal model of infection using this system has not yet been developed.

Environmental and ecological aspects of *P. carinii* infection have largely been overlooked (110). Studies of the soil, waterways, and air performed under natural conditions might reveal important information about sources of *P. carinii*, as have been found for fungi, mycobacteria, or environmental pollutants. Although histological stains could be used to identify *P. carinii* in the environment, more sophisticated and sensitive detection methods are needed.

Transmission of *P. carinii* by intrauterine or transplacental routes has been suggested by a few reports of pneumocystosis in newborn humans and rats

119–122). It is difficult to assess the validity of these claims because of their rarity and the lack of a suitable experimental model. Transmission of *P. carinii* by nonrespiratory routes implies the ability of the organism to travel beyond the lungs, something that has been documented rarely and only in severely immunocompromised patients (20,122). Nevertheless, the possibility of vertical transmission of *P. carinii* raises interesting questions and deserves further investigation.

Pneumocystis carinii infection in humans and in animals has a worldwide geographical distribution. Seroepidemiological surveys in humans have suggested that exposure to *P. carinii* occurs early in life, as evidenced by the fact that most (70–80%) healthy people have antibodies to the organism by age 3 or 4 (123, 124). A similar though less well defined age-related exposure to *P. carinii* also appears to occur in rodents (125). A few investigators have hypothesized that *P. carinii* infection is a zoonosis and have attempted to relate the incidence of pneumocystosis to occurrence of the disease in animals (68). However, the majority view holds that the organism is species- and host-specific; supporting evidence can be found from animal challenge experiments and antigenic studies (43,126,127).

B. Growth and Metabolism

1. In Vitro Culture Systems

Adaptation of protozoan parasites to the in vitro environment represents a unique scientific challenge. Factors that are not applicable to other microorganisms but that must be considered in parasite culture include the possibility of unknown vectors, assurance that the inoculum contains the infective stage, and unusual nutritive requirements, since parasite life-cycle stages often lack common organelles and have alternative metabolic cycles. It was not until 1976 that a system for the continuous culture of the human malarial parasite *Plasmodium falciparum* was established (128). Studies to enrich and optimize this system then followed (129,130). Recently, an in vitro cultivation system for *Cryptosporidium* was described that used a human fetal lung fibroblast line; although the organism underwent development in this system, quantitation has not yet been possible (131).

Tissue culture using anchor-dependent cell lines has been the principal in vitro method of growing *P. carinii*, with modest success achieved by only a few investigators (132–138) (Table 2). Three observations can be appreciated from this work: (1) few cell lines support replication of the parasite; (2) those cell lines that allow *P. carinii* growth have no obvious morphological, physiological, or donor specificity; and (3) the quantitation methods are not the same throughout the studies, and thus comparison is difficult. In addition, many other cell lines have been tried but not reported, as were solid and semisolid agar media preparations and chick embryo cultures (6,8,139).

Table 2 Studies of In Vitro Cultivation of *P. carinii*

Source of data	Cell lines supporting growth	Cell lines not supporting growth	Quantitation method		
			Form of PC	Stain	
Pifer et al. (132,133)	Chicken embryonic lung Vero	WI-38 L cells Rat lung	Cyst	Toluidine blue	
		Secondary chicken embryo fibroblast Owl monkey kidney Baby hamster kidney AV-3 WI38	Cyst	Toluidine blue	
Latorre et al. (134)	Vero Chang liver MRC-5	LLC–MK–2 FL McCoy	Microscopic observation of floating aggregates		
Bartlett et al. (135)	WI38 MRC-5		Trophozoite	Giemsa	
Cushion and Walzer (136,137); Cushion et al. (138)	A549 WI38 VA13	WI38 L2 4/4RM4 RFL-6	Nuclei Cyst	DQ CEV	

Our laboratory has used the A549 cell line as the primary support for growth studies of *P. carinii*, although we have found that a virally transformed WI-38 cell line also allows modest replication (137,138). The A549 line, which was derived from human lung carcinoma, has been presumptively identified as a type II pneumocyte but does not contain the functional capacities of the type II cell (e.g., does not secrete phosphatidylcholine) (140). Under optimal conditions a 10-fold replication of *P. carinii* occurs within a 7-day period, and up to three successive passages have been obtained by subculturing onto naive A549 monolayers.

Detailed studies have been performed analyzing a variety of factors affecting *P. carinii* growth in the A549 and WI-38VA13 cell lines (Table 3). The results indicated that the most favorable conditions include a temperature of 37°C, a stationary state of the culture flasks, and a 10-20% fetal bovine supplement to the culture media. Specific detrimental conditions included a temperature of 41°C, motion of the culture flasks, and addition of rat sera to the culture media.

Table 3 Effects of Environmental Conditions on *P. carinii* Growth

	Growth[a] of cell line	
Environmental condition	A549	VA13
Temperature		
Room temperature (25°C)	1.16	0.25
30°C	1.20	0.45
35°C	1.71	0.42
37°C	1.00	1.00
41°C	0.33	0.07
5% CO_2/motion		
Sealed flask/stationary	1.00	1.00
5% CO_2/stationary	0.92	1.30
Sealed/rocking	0.21	0.23
5% CO_2/rocking	0.19	0.27
NCTC vitamins 2 ✕		
Vitamins	1.77	1.02
No vitamins	1.00	1.00

[a]Expressed as the ratio of peak *P. carinii* counts obtained in experimental cultures to peak numbers in control cultures over a 7-10-day period. Control infected cultures have the value 1.00. Media in the controls contained 20% HyClone FBS and were stationary. Peak counts in control cultures ranged from 4.1×10^6 to 2.0×10^8/mL All data are a result of at least pooled triplicate flask counts.
Source: Reprinted with permission from Ref. 138.

Monitoring the system by phase contrast microscopy revealed that cultures on rocker platforms in constant motion did not permit attachment of the *P. carinii* to the monolayer. In other experiments the tissue culture medium from an infected culture was removed, the monolayer was thoroughly washed, and fresh medium was added. After several days, *P. carinii* organisms reappeared in the culture medium and increased in number. Thus, attachment to the cell monolayer appears to be an important requirement for *P. carinii* replication.

Important techniques that resulted from these studies have been the ability to quantitate the organism by assessment of nuclear replication and to monitor the culture dynamics by combined phase microscopic and staining methods (97). Through our in vitro studies we found that widely used stains that selectively stain the cyst wall (e.g., methenamine silver, toluidine blue, and cresyl echt violet) do not allow accurate assessment of organism growth, since these stains do not differentiate empty cysts from those that contain intracystic bodies (the actual replicating forms). Growth of *P. carinii* in our culture system is determined by enumerating organism nuclei in tissue culture supernates over time. The Diff Quik stain has been used successfully for this purpose and yields results identical to the more time-consuming Giemsa stain. Nuclei are stained reddish purple and cytoplasm blue; the cyst wall is not stained and presents itself as a halo around the intracystic bodies within (Fig. 3). No effort is made to differentiate stages of the organism, only to count the absolute number of nuclei. Therefore, this quantitation system includes both intracystic replication of daughter forms and extracystic replication of trophic forms. These techniques, in combination with physical separation modifications, have been applied to enumeration of *P. carinii* obtained from rat lung homogenates used for tissue culture inoculum. The ability to quantitate the inoculum has had important applications to studies of the life cycle, in vitro susceptibility to drugs, and characterization of growth kinetics of this organism.

2. In Vitro Drug Susceptibility Testing

Development of new anti-*P. carinii* drugs has rested primarily on the corticosteroid-treated rat model of pneumocystosis described later in this chapter. While this system has usually been a good predictor of drug activity in humans, it is time-consuming and expensive and permits evaluation of relatively few agents. In vitro systems of drug analysis offer potential advantages of speed and efficiency; several different approaches have been used to evaluate the effects of compounds on *P. carinii* (Table 4). Investigators who have been unable to grow the organism have analyzed drug effects by the use of lysosomotropic vital dyes and radiolabeled substrates and precursors (141,142). Workers who have succeeded in the culture of the organism have used cell monolayer systems to evaluate antimicrobial activity (143-146). These studies have provided valuable insights into susceptibility screening, but the results are difficult to compare; the

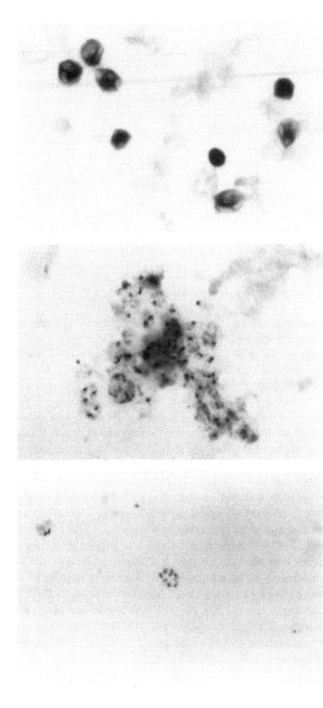

Figure 3 Rat lung homogenates. *Left*: Intracystic bodies in a single cyst. Cyst wall is not stained. Diff Quik stain. ×1350. *Middle*: Clusters of trophozoites and intracystic bodies in preparation of rat lung homogenates. Diff Quik stain. ×1700. *Right*: Cysts stained with cresyl echt violet. Wrinkled appearance is typical. ×1700.

Table 4 Methods Used to Assay the Effects of TMP–SMX and Pentamidine
Isethionate (PI) on *P. carinii* Growth In Vitro

| | | MIC (μg/ml) of: | |
| | | TMP–SMX | |
Investigators	Assay method	(ratio)	PI
Cushion et al. (146)	Nuclei per ml	1:19	0.1
Bartlett et al. (144)	Trophozoites per ml	50:200	0.5
Pifer et al. (143)	Cysts per ml	0.3:1.5	0.3
Pesanti (141)	Neutral red uptake	>200:200[a]	1.0
Pesanti and Cox (142)	$^{14}CO_2$ production from $[U-^{14}C]$ glucose	100:200[b]	1.0

[a]No inhibition was achieved with 200 μg of TMP and 200 μg of SMX per milliliter alone or
in combination.
[b]Decrease in viability only.
Source: Reprinted with permission from Ref. 146.

systems have differed in the cell line used, method of determining drug activity,
and amount of drug introduced.

In our laboratory, the A549 cell line is inoculated with rat *P. carinii* and
different concentrations of the antimicrobial drug to be tested (146). Efficacy
is evaluated by comparing *P. carinii* growth curves in the drug-treated and
control cultures over a 7-day period and calculating the ratio of the peak
organism counts achieved. As seen in Figure 4, TMP–SMX had dose-related
effects on *P. carinii* growth at concentrations achievable in serum. This system
has also been explored to study the mechanism of drug action, as illustrated in
Figure 5 with difluoromethyl ornithine (DFMO). This drug, which inhibits polyamine biosynthesis, has shown promising activity in the treatment of human
African trypanosomiasis and pneumocystosis (147). DFMO at concentrations
achievable in serum inhibited *P. carinii* growth in culture; this effect could be
overcome by the addition of the polyamine putrescine.

Unfortunately, in vitro drug sensitivity testing is plagued by the same technical problems that have made cultivation of *P. carinii* so difficult. In addition
to the factors discussed above, we have found a growing number of samples
where the in vitro effects of drugs on *P. carinii* do not correlate with their
activity in the rat model. DFMO, for example, has been ineffective in the treatment of pneumocystosis in immunosuppressed rats (148,149). Thus, considerably more experience is needed with both systems for proper assessment of their
role in the development of new anti-*P. carinii* drugs for human use.

3. Metabolism

Pneumocystis carinii has been the focus of only a few metabolic studies, owing to the difficulties encountered in in vitro cultivation. However, by using non-replicating organisms that were kept in tissue culture medium, some workers have been able to define certain metabolic activities using radiolabeled compounds (141,142). From these studies, it was reported that rat *P. carinii* was able to metabolize [^{14}C] glucose to CO_2, synthesize proteins from [^{3}H] amino acids, and incorporate [^{3}H] uridine into ribonucleic acid. Inhibitors of glucose

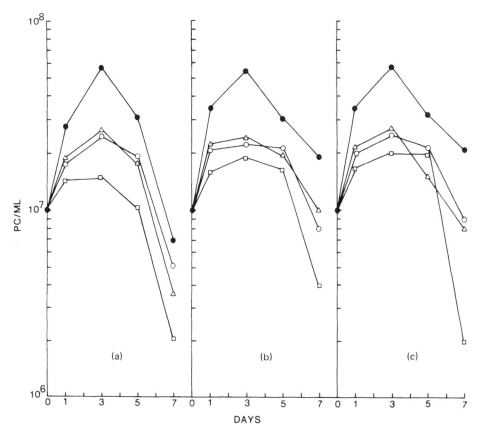

Figure 4 Effects of trimethoprim-sulfamethoxazole (TMP–SMX) on *P. carinii* growth in vitro. Rat *P. carinii* was cultured on A549 cell monolayers in (a) flasks or (b, c) multiwell plates with erythrocyte (a,b) lysed or (c) unlysed inocula. (●) control cultures; (△) TMP 1 µg/ml–SMX 19 µg/ml; (○), TMP 8 µg/ml–SMX 152 µg/ml; (□) TMP 16 µg/ml–SMX 304 µg/ml. Each data point represents the number of *P. carinii* nuclei of at least triplicate pooled samples.

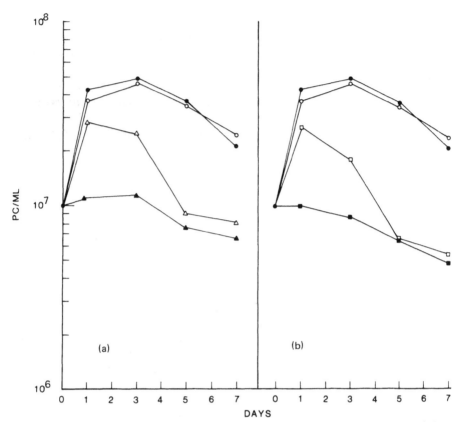

Figure 5 Effects of DFMO with and without putrescine on *P. carinii* growth in vitro. (a) (●) Control, no DFMO and no putrescine; (○) no DFMO, 0.1 mM putrescine; (△) 1 mM DFMO, 0.1 mM putrescine; (▲) 1 mM DFMO, no putrescine. (b) (●) Control, no DFMO and no putrescine; (○) no DFMO, 0.1 mM putrescine; (□) 10 mM DFMO, 0.1 mM putrescine; (■) 10 mM DFMO, no putrescine.

metabolism, protein synthesis, amino acid uptake, and uridine incorporation could effectively block these reactions, suggesting specificity of the pathways. A more recent report has suggested that *P. carinii* can synthesize phospholipids (but not disaturated phosphatidylcholine, a principal component of surfactant) from radiolabeled precursors (150). Although the system in these studies was contaminated by low numbers of bacteria and host cells, the investigators felt that these organisms did not contribute significantly to the activities measured.

In other work by the same investigators, *P. carinii* was found to utilize molecular oxygen by cyanide-sensitive, cytochrome-mediated pathways, a common system used by aerobic organisms (151). This finding is not surprising, since *P. carinii* does contain mitochondria and resides almost exclusively in the lung alveoli where it would have access to molecular oxygen. Low levels of antioxidant enzymes were detected in the same system, but superoxide dismutase was the only enzyme specifically associated with *P. carinii*. Lethal oxygen-mediated damage was effected against *P. carinii* by hydrogen peroxide and superoxide, but not by a hydroxyl-radical-generating system. The metabolism of *P. carinii* has been studied histochemically by the use of tetrazolium dye, which permits topographic localization of enzymatic activity within intact organisms (152). Lactic dehydrogenase, succinate dehydrogenase, and glutamate dehydrogenase produced strong reactions, suggesting that *P. carinii* has the potential for anaerobic glycolysis, Krebs cycle, and intermediary protein metabolism.

C. Immunology and Virulence

1. Antigenic Characteristics

The antigenic characteristics of *P. carinii* have mainly been evaluated by the direct (D) or indirect (I) fluorescent antibody (FA) technique (153–181). Organisms obtained from infected human or rat lungs or bronchoalveolar lavage fluid by enzyme digestion and/or density gradient centrifugation have been the primary source of study material; rat *P. carinii* grown in short-term culture has also been used. Sources of antibody have included sera from exposed subjects or immunized animals as well as monoclonal antibodies. *Pneumocystis carinii* organisms (cysts and trophozoites) stain brightly, with a typical rim pattern of fluorescence. Most attention has focused on the cyst form because it is more easily visualized as a discrete entity by light microscopy.

Overall, the data suggest that human and rat *P. carinii* have shared and species-specific antigenic determinants. The conflicting results of some studies presumably reflect differences in the preparation of the immunological reagents. The presence of most proteins on the surface of *P. carinii* is another potentially confounding variable. Some of these technical problems can be controlled when different sources of antibody are used in the same experiment (126). As seen in Table 5, serum specimens from rats with high antibody titers to rat *P. carinii* reacted well with mouse *P. carinii* but poorly with human *P. carinii*; mouse and human sera showed little reactivity with heterologous sources of the organism. By contrast, rabbits immunized with rat or human *P. carinii* showed good antibody titers to heterologous organisms. Some monoclonal antibodies bind *P. carinii* from different animal species by IFA, but other monoclonal antibodies do not (178–180).

The immunoperoxidase technique has been used to identify *P. carinii* in

Table 5 Comparison of Rat, Mouse, and Human *P. carinii* by Immunofluorescence

| Animal species | No. of specimens | Range of reciprocal IFA titer by source of *P. carinii*[a] | | |
		Rat	Mouse	Human
Rat	6	64–1 024 (6)	128–512 (6)	0–4 (3)
Mouse	6	0–4 (2)	64–256 (6)	0 (0)
Human	6	0–8 (4)	0–8	16–128 (6)
Rabbit A[b]	1	512	32	8
Rabbit B[c]	1	32	32	512

[a]The antigenic characteristics of rat, mouse, and human *P. carinii* were compared by the
indirect fluorescent antibody (IFA) technique. Data are ranges; the number of specimens
with a positive titer, that is, $\geqslant 4$, is given in parentheses.
[b]Immunized with rat *P. carinii*.
[c]Immunized with human *P. carinii*.
Source: Reprinted with permission from Ref. 126.

impression smears and tissue sections (122,182,183). By the use of rabbit antisera to rat and human *P. carinii*, differences in immunoreactivity have been
found in the specimens obtained from a small number of AIDS and non-AIDS
patients with pneumocystosis. A larger sample size as well as different sources of
antibody are needed to confirm and evaluate the significance of these findings.

The enzyme-linked immunosorbent assay (ELISA) has been used in several
serological studies of *P. carinii* infection (184–191). Crude soluble preparations
from *P. carinii*-infected rat lungs or organisms grown in short-term culture react
with human sera, suggesting shared antigenic determinants.

More recently, *P. carinii* antigens have been studied by the Western immunoblotting technique using polyclonal and monoclonal sources of antibody (127,
178,181,183,188,189). As seen in Figure 6, multiple bands were found with rat
P. carinii with rabbit antisera (127). The patterns of immunoreactivity of organisms derived from infected lungs or grown in culture were similar, suggesting that
P. carinii retains its antigenic characteristics with short-term cultivation. Bands
of 116, 50, and 45 kD were the principal immunoreactive moieties; these antigens appeared to be similar to antigens of 110–120 kD and 55–60 kD found in
other reports using somewhat different antigen preparations or electrophoretic
conditions.

The most prominent antigen in human *P. carinii* was a broad band of 40 kD
(Figure 6). Bands of 66 and 116 kD as well as other moieties were found with

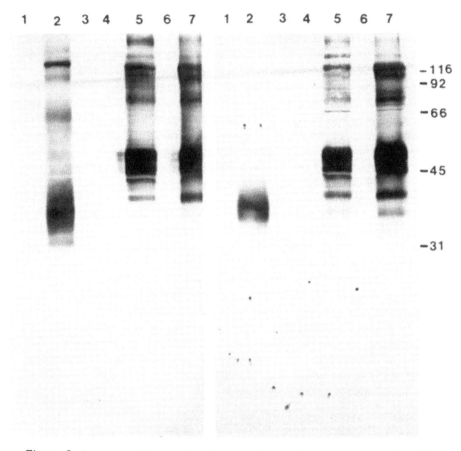

Figure 6 *Pneumocystis carinii* antigen and control preparations analyzed by immunoblotting using rabbit antisera to *P. carinii* diluted 1/100. *Left*: Rabbit antiserum to human *P. carinii* from an AIDS patient adsorbed with normal human lung. *Right*: Rabbit antiserum to tissue-culture-derived rat *P. carinii* adsorbed with A549 cells. Lanes of each panel are: 1, normal human lung; 2, lung-derived human *P. carinii* from an AIDS patient; 3, lung-derived human *P. carinii* from a non-AIDS patient; 4, normal rat lung; 5, lung-derived rat *P. carinii*; 6, A549 cells; 7, tissue-culture-derived rat *P. carinii*. Molecular weight markers on right. (Reprinted with permission from Ref. 127.)

some sources of antibody. The 40-kD band was present in six of seven lung specimens of AIDS patients with pneumocystosis but in only one of eight lung specimens from non-AIDS *P. carinii* patients. The reasons for this striking difference in immunoreactivity are unclear but may be related to such factors as age of the specimens, organism burden, or true antigenic differences.

Care must be used in interpreting the data obtained from immunoblotting studies because crude preparations have been used as antigens. The fact that the major immunoreactive bands were not found in a variety of control preparations suggests that they are specific for *P. carinii*. The clear-cut differences in antigens from rat and human *P. carinii* support the existence of species or strain differences in the organism. However, since these antigens were recognized by sera from rats and humans as well as from immunized rabbits, shared antigenic determinants also probably exist.

The biochemical and functional properties of the *P. carinii* antigens identified by immunoblotting have been the subject of considerable interest. When immunoblots of rat *P. carinii* were run in the absence of the reducing agent 2-mercaptoethanol, the prominent 110–120-kD band migrated with a molecular weight of more than 205 kD, suggesting that this larger moiety is composed of subunits held together by disulfide bands (189). However, different results were obtained with this procedure by another group of workers (178). The susceptibility of *P. carinii* antigens to treatment with proteases and sodium metaperiodate suggests the presence of protein and carbohydrate components. The presence of carbohydrates on the surface of *P. carinii* has recently been studied by the use of lectin probes, with glucosyl, galactosyl, and mannosyl residues being identified as prominent constituents (192).

2. Virulence Factors

Analysis of *P. carinii* virulence factors has been hampered by the low pathogenicity of the organism. Exposure to *P. carinii* in a variety of experimental settings initiates an immune response but results in no detectable tissue damage or clinical harm to the host (43,107,114,125,170). Thus, it has not been possible to calculate an infecting or lethal organism dose.

Within the alveolus, *P. carinii* attaches to a specific living cell, the type I pneumocyte (193). The interaction of *P. carinii* with this cell plays a central role in the host–parasite relationship in the infection and has been studied extensively in animal models by different electron microscopic techniques. Some workers have proposed that the tubular cytoplasmic extensions of *P. carinii* (filopodia) serve as the specialized organelle of adherence (75,77,82,194). Most other investigators have found that the surfaces of *P. carinii* and the type I pneumocyte are closely apposed without the fusion of cell membranes or changes in the intramembranous particles that have been typically observed with other microorganisms (85-91). It appears that *P. carinii* can change its shape to fit the countour of its immediate surroundings.

Whether the tight attachment of *P. carinii* to the type I pneumocyte is due solely to physical factors or also involves other mechanisms is unclear. It is possible that the tendency of *P. carinii* organisms to aggregate into clusters described above is related to its adherence properties. Histochemical stains have revealed the presence of carbodydrates on the surface of *P. carinii* and the type I pneumocyte (85,195), and, as mentioned earlier, the organism can bind to fluorescein-conjugated plant lectins (192). Perhaps *P. carinii* possesses a lectin that mediates attachment, as has been found with other protozoans (196-198).

Although the specific benefits *P. carinii* obtains from attachment to the type I pneumocyte are unknown, it is likely that this interaction contributes to organism growth and nutrition. Direct analysis of this adherence in vitro has not been feasible, because the type I pneumocyte does not replicate and no cell lines are available. However, as mentioned previously, attachment of *P. carinii* to the A549 cell monolayer is necessary for organism replication in tissue culture (137,138).

Pneumocystis carinii also interacts with other factors in the complex milieu of the alveolar microenvironment. Ultrastructural and in vitro studies have shown that *P. carinii* is covered by alveolar lung fluid and can bind surfactant (91,150); whether alveolar phospholipids provide nutrients or contribute to host defenses against the organism remains to be determined. It seems that *P. carinii* may not have direct contact with alveolar air but ordinarily needs molecular oxygen for growth and viability. In one report, organisms in an aerated portion of the lung exhibited typical staining characteristics and were attached to alveoli, whereas organisms in an atelectatic portion had lost their tinctorial properties, had become detached into the alveolar space, or had been phagocytosed (73). On the other hand, reports of the presence of *P. carinii* at extrapulmonary sites (e.g., intestine) and available in vitro data suggest the presence of metabolic pathways that would permit survival of the organism under reduced oxygenation (122,146,152).

3. Evasion Mechanisms

Little is known about the mechanisms employed by *P. carinii* to evade host defenses. Based on systems identified for other protozoans, the following areas might provide fertile ground for investigation.

1. Under appropriate conditions, stages in the life cycle of *P. carinii* may become activated that permit continued survival and replication within the host.
2. *Pneumocystis carinii* organisms attached to the type I pneumocyte may be protected from host immune effector responses.

3. *Pneumocystis carinii* may coat itself with surfactant or other host proteins and avoid antigenic recognition.
4. *Pneumocystis carinii* may elaborate substances that suppress host immune or inflammatory responses.

III. THE HOST

A. Host Defense Mechanisms

Exposure to *P. carinii* results in systemic and local immune responses in the host. Numerous data have been obtained about serum antibody levels, but little attention has been directed to cellular immune function.

1. Humoral Immunity

Although a variety of types of serological studies have been performed, attention has usually been focused on serum antibody responses to whole *P. carinii* organisms by the IFA and ELISA techniques. Population surveys have revealed that most healthy people have serum IgG antibodies by an early age (123,124,173, 185). In general, it has not been possible to distinguish, on the basis of single antibody titers, patients with pneumocystosis from other immunocompromised hosts or from healthy controls; however, some *P. carinii* patients have been able to develop a rise in serum antibody titers with paired specimens upon recovery from the disease (174). Hospital workers involved in the care of *P. carinii* patients may also experience a rise in serum IgG antibody levels (199). Limited serological studies suggest that serum antibodies to *P. carinii* can be found among AIDS patients but that this antibody response is impaired (127,189,191, 200–202).

Serum IgG antibody responses to *P. carinii* among rodents are similar to those in humans (125, 170, 171). Antibody titers are absent in young rats, are present in retired breeders, and develop in healthy rats with prolonged environmental exposure to the organism. Serum IgG antibodies develop in nu/+ mice but not in nu/nu mice inoculated with *P. carinii*, suggesting the importance of T cells in this response. Serum IgG antibody levels are suppressed in rats and mice administered corticosteroids to induce pneumocystosis; in general, there is an inverse relationship between antibody titer and extent of disease, which develops in the lungs. Antibody levels rise when corticosteroids are withdrawn and the infection is cleared.

Recent studies have examined serum IgG antibody responses to *P. carinii* by the Western blot technique (127,181,189). So far, IgG antibodies to the 116-, 50-, and 45-kD antigens of rat *P. carinii* and the 40-kD antigen of human *P. carinii* have been found among healthy human blood donors and among patients with pneumocystosis. Considerable variation has been found among individual subjects. IgG antibody responses by immunoblotting closely parallel the antibody responses by IFA in rats with experimental *P. carinii* infection; the 50-kD band is recognized slightly earlier than the 45- or 116-kD bands in some animals. Further serological studies are needed to determine if specific *P. carinii* antigens might have diagnostic value.

The development of serum IgM antibodies to *P. carinii* among healthy young children roughly parallels that of serum IgG antibodies (123,124). Serum IgM antibodies can be found in healthy adults, usually in low titer (199), but IgM antibody levels are low or absent in immunosuppressed patients even with recovery from pneumocystosis (174). Conflicting results have been obtained about serum IgM antibodies in AIDS patients (200,202).

The termporal formation of serum IgM antibodies to *P. carinii* in rats is very similar to that for IgG both in animals with active pneumocystosis and in animals with environmental exposure to the organism (181). Serum IgM antibodies to *P. carinii* measured by IFA are usually low in mice; however, in certain strains (e.g., C57BL/6N) or with a different serological technique (e.g., ELISA), IgM antibodies assume a more prominent component of the immune response (170,187). Studies of IgM antibody responses by the immunoblotting technique would be of interest, but problems have occurred in obtaining suitable reagents.

Serum IgA antibodies appear to be only a small part of the humoral immune response to *P. carinii* in humans or rodents (170,199), but detailed studies are lacking.

Only limited data are available about local antibody responses to *P. carinii*. IgG and IgM antibodies have been found in bronchoalveolar lavage fluid (BALF) of normal adults and a few AIDS patients with pneumocystosis (200). IgG antibodies are present in BALF of rats and correlate well with serum IgG antibody levels (125).

Despite their frequent presence, the role of serum and local antibodies in host defense against *P. carinii* is unclear. Antibodies with or without complement are not lethal for the organism and do not impair its growth in tissue culture (138,141). Since IgG, IgM, and IgA have been demonstrated on the surface of human and rat *P. carinii* by IFA (125,154), it is possible that these immunoglobulins function as opsonins; under certain in vitro conditions, antibodies enhance the phagocytes of *P. carinii* by alveolar macrophages (203). Defects in local IgA antibody and complement have been hypothesized as having a role in the pathogenesis of the interstitial plasma cell pneumonia form of pneumocystosis (11,155), but detailed evidence is not available.

Host defenses against *P. carinii* can also be studied by analyzing the immunological defects in patients with pneumocystosis. Children with primary immunodeficiency diseases are one of the major targets of the organism, with such diseases constituting the underlying illness in 13% of the cases of pneumocystosis reported to CDC before the discovery of AIDS (39,40). Patients with immune deficiency diseases provide the opportunity to examine host immune function without the influence of exogenous cytotoxic or immunosuppressive drugs. Early studies emphasized the role of antibody in the host defense against *P. carinii* because hypogammaglobulinemia was the only immune defect that could be detected (204); however, as testing of cellular immune function became more sophisticated, it became clear that children with pure B-cell defects constituted only a small fraction of the immunodeficient patients with pneumocystosis (12,39,205,206). By far the most common primary immune deficiency disease predisposing to *P. carinii* pneumonia is severe combined immune deficiency disease, a disorder with profound B- and T-cell defects.

2. Cellular Immunity

Cellular immune responses to *P. carinii* have been measured by a blastogenic assay in which proliferative responses were found in peripheral blood mononuclear cells (PBM) of healthy human adults but not among similar cells obtained from cord blood (207). Thus it appears that natural environmental exposure to *P. carinii* results in both humoral and cellular immune responses to the organism in the normal host.

It is generally considered that impaired cellular immunity is the principal host defect that predisposes to the development of pneymocystosis (208). Evidence for this conclusion is largely inferential (i.e., based on underlying illness) rather than based on direct experimental data. In the CDC study of 194 cases of *P. carinii* pneumonia, the major patient risk groups were leukemia, 47% of cases, of which acute lymphatic leukemia was the most common cell type (58 of 91 cases); Hodgkin's disease and other lymphomas, 18% of cases; and organ transplantation, 11% of cases (40). While some of these conditions may themselves depress host immune function, pneumocystosis almost never occurred in the absence of cytotoxic or immunosuppressive therapy. The occurrence of *P. carinii* pneumonia in such disparate underlying conditions as solid tumors or collagen vascular disease also reflected the effects of immunosuppressive therapy.

The risk of pneumocystosis in humans is related to the type and degree of immunosuppression. Corticosteroids, which have been by far the most commonly used drugs, cause lymphopenia characterized in peripheral blood primarily by a fall in T helper cells, with reversal of the T helper/T suppressor cell ratio (209,210). These agents also have other broad inhibitory effects on cellular immunity, the inflammatory response, and other host defense mechanisms (211).

The ability of corticosteroids to predispose to *P. carinii* can come from endogenous or exogenous sources. For example, a number of cases of pneumocystosis have occurred in patients with Cushing's syndrome, a disorder characterized by glucocorticoid overproduction; the risk of *P. carinii* appeared to correlate with serum cortisol levels (212–214). Corticosteroids administered as pharmacological agents can induce the development of pneumocystosis, and their effectiveness is enhanced when they are used in combination with other immunosuppressive drugs. The high frequency of *P. carinii* pneumonia in patients with acute lymphatic leukemia (ALL) compared with that in acute myelocytic leukemia (AML) probably reflects differences in chemotherapeutic regimens; corticosteroids are an integral part of most ALL but not AML protocols (215).

The relative importance of other agents in predisposing to pneumocystosis is less clear. A recent study of two multiple-drug (including prednisone) protocols used for the treatment of non-Hodgkin's lymphoma noted a much higher incidence of *P. carinii* pneumonia among patients who received the protocol containing bleomycin and cytarabine, drugs associated with pulmonary toxicity, than among patients who received the protocol containing mechlorethamine and procarbazine (216). Radiation therapy is commonly used with chemotherapy and has a variety of adverse effects on the host but has received little attention as a specific risk factor for *P. carinii* pneumonia. Although a few cases of pneumocystosis have been related to cyclophosphamide or methotrexate therapy (217,218), the effects of low-dose corticosteroids used concomitantly were not always ruled out. Recent interest has focused on the risk of *P. carinii* pneumonia in organ transplant patients administered immunosuppressive regimens containing cyclosporin (219–226). It appears that cyclosporin is generally associated with a lower frequency of opportunistic infections, including *P. carinii* pneumonia; however, since the specific drugs given with cyclosporin differ in these regimens, further data are needed to evaluate the specific effects of cyclosporin on *P. carinii*.

Protein malnutrition has become increasingly recognized as an important *P. carinii* predisposing risk factor. Although protein malnutrition may affect the host in a variety of ways, its major influence is on cell-mediated immunity (227). Infants who develop interstitial plasma cell pneumonia are frequently malnourished (6), and limited lymphocyte studies of such patients have demonstrated T-cell depression (228). *Pneumocystis carinii* was readily found in the lungs of children with kwashiorkor but not in children with normal nutrition from the same geographical area; conversely, children with cancer who developed pneumocystosis had poorer nutrition than did matched children without *P. carinii* pneumonia (28,229). Malnutrition may develop by itself or as a result of factors (e.g., anorexia, diarrhea) related to the underlying disease.

The most convincing evidence for the importance of impaired cell-mediated immunity in the development of *P. carinii* pneumonia comes from patients with AIDS. As mentioned elsewhere in this book, the prinicpal immunological defect in AIDS is a reduction in the number and function of T helper cells (230). Pneumocystosis is the most common opportunistic infection in AIDS, occurring in more than 60% of patients, as reported by CDC (51,52) and perhaps in up to

80–85% of patients during their lifetime (61). Autopsy surveys have revealed that *P. carinii* pneumonia is a leading cause of death in AIDS (53,54). Conversely, AIDS has become the most common underlying illness in patients who develop pneumocystosis. So strong is this association that *P. carinii* pneumonia has been used as a major epidemiological marker for AIDS and a principal indicator for entry into trials of aziothymidine (AZT) and other experimental drugs. It is highly likely that the continued spread of AIDS will be accompanied by a corresponding increase in the number of cases of pneumocystosis.

Recent studies have analyzed the proliferative responses of PBM to *P. carinii* at different stages of HIV infection (231). The antigen preparation was rat *P. carinii* grown in tissue culture that was similar to that used in an earlier study of healthy people (207). The results indicated that HIV class II (asymptomatic) and class III (lymphadenopathy) patients had a lower response to *P. carinii* and other antigens than did normal controls. Class IV patients (i.e., AIDS) had the lowest response, and this was not enhanced by AZT treatment. Thus, in the blastogenic assay, the host response to *P. carinii* appears to be similar to that to other antigens.

While *P. carinii* has been reported from a variety of other congenital or acquired immune deficiency states, the role of specific T-cell defects in the development of the infection has been obscured by the complex nature of these disorders (39). Pneumocystosis has been only rarely reported in patients with DiGeorge's syndrome (which is characterized by thymic hypoplasia and hence a pure T-cell defect) for reasons that are unclear (232). On the other hand, case reports of the occurrence of *P. carinii* pneumonia in obscure disorders (e.g., dyskeratosis congenita) characterized by impaired cellular immunity continue to emphasize the role of T cells in host defense against this organism (233).

Studies of *P. carinii* in experimental animals have generally supported data obtained in humans. In preliminary experiments, old rats with considerable environmental exposure to the organism exhibited spleen cell proliferative responses to *P. carinii* antigens, whereas very young rats did not (115). Rats and other animals administered corticosteroids and an antibiotic (usually tetracycline) in the drinking water to prevent bacterial infection for about 8 weeks spontaneously develop pneumocystosis with histopathological features identical to the disease in humans; this animal model, described in detail in Section III.B, has been extensively used to study *P. carinii* pneumonia (45). Cyclophosphamide and cyclosprorin alone induced pneumocystosis, but other immunosuppressive agents (e.g., drugs, irradiation) were successful only when combined with steroids (43,234). Severe protein malnutrition induced by a protein-free diet produced *P. carinii* pneumonia, and moderate malnutrition induced by a low (8%) protein diet enhanced pneumocystosis induced by corticosteroids (229,235).

The coricosteroid-treated rat model has permitted investigation of lymphocyte subsets by surface marker analysis at different stages of *P. carinii* pneumonia (236,237). Initially, there was some concern about this work because rats have been classified as "steroid-sensitive" and humans as "steroid-resistant" on the basis of susceptibility of their lymphoid tissues to the lytic properties of corticosteroids (238); however, this fear proved to be unwarranted. The corticosteroid regimen used to induce pneumocystosis in the rats resulted in profound general lymphocyte depletion. The lymphocytopenia in peripheral blood and lungs was characterized by a greater fall in T helper than in T suppressor cells with inversion of the T helper/T suppressor cell ratio, whereas such an imbalance in subsets was not found in thymus, spleen, or bone marrow. The data suggest that the greater sensitivity of pulmonary and systemic T helper cells to the effects of corticosteroids may be an important mechanism in the development of *P. carinii* pneumonia. Such effects appeared to be reversible upon withdrawal of the steroids.

Studies of spleen lymphoid cells have revealed impaired proliferative and plaque-forming responses in immunosuppressed rats (239,240); however, further investigation involving more purified antigen preparations and different body sites will be necessary to correlate functional studies with data obtained by analysis of lymphocyte surface markers. Such studies will also have to take into account the influence of other components (i.e., tetracycline and low-protein diet) of the immunosuppressive regimen. Tetracycline and protein malnutrition themselves did not alter the distribution of lymphocyte subsets but enhanced the magnitude of the effects of the corticosteroids (237).

Macrophages constitute an important component of the host pulmonary defense system against respiratory pathogens, but their specific role in *P. carinii* infection is poorly defined. No studies have been published with human alveolar macrophages, and techniques have not yet been developed to analyze the clearance of *P. carinii* in experimental animals after exogenous organism challenge. The principal investigative approach has been to conduct in vitro studies to examine the interaction of rat *P. carinii* with rat alveolar and mouse peritoneal macrophages (241). *Pneumocystis carinii* organisms added to freshly explanted macrophages were not engulfed but adhered readily to the surface of the cell. In one study, phagocytosis occurred promptly with the addition of rabbit antiserum to *P. carinii* but not with the addition of normal rabbit serum (203). In another study, alveolar macrophages grew in culture for 48 hr, and mouse peritoneal macrophages of any age were able to ingest *P. carinii* without the presence of antibody (242). Once taken up by the macrophage, *P. carinii* was rapidly digested. Macrophages from normal and corticosteroid-treated rats behaved in a similar manner, and their function was not altered by the presence of corticosteroids, complement, or anti-*P. carinii* drugs (e.g., pentamidine, trimethoprim-sulfamethoxazole) in the culture media.

These data demonstrate that alveolar macrophages can ingest and kill *P. carinii*. The susceptibility of the organism to acid pH and reactive oxygen moieties may contribute to the leth⊥ properties of macrophages (151). Thus, *P. carinii* resembles other extracellula respiratory pathogens (e.g., *Mycoplasma*) rather than true intracellular protozoans (e.g., *Toxoplasma*), which can resist macrophage killing. The enhancing effect of *P. carinii* antiserum on phagocytosis suggests a role for antibodies as opsonins, yet the ability of macrophages to engulf *P. carinii* in the absence of antibody under different experimental conditions illustrates the complex nature of this process.

The relevance of the in vitro studies to the development of pneumocystosis in the rat model in vivo is unclear. Although corticosteroids did not affect the interaction of macrophage monolayers with *P. carinii*, these drugs have a variety of effects on macrophages in other experimental systems and also impair the interaction of T lymphocytes with macrophages at the lymphokine level (243). Histopathologically, alveolar macrophages are not numerous in rat *P. carinii* pneumonia and do not appear to be very active in the phagocytosis of the organism (85,235). Thus, much more in vitro work is needed to better define the interaction of *P. carinii* with host macrophages.

Consideration of the role of polymorphonuclear leukocytes in the host defense against *P. carinii* reveals a paucity of clinical and experimental data. There have been a few case reports of pneumocystosis in patients with chronic granulomatous disease; in once instance, anti-*P. carinii* drugs were ineffective and cure of the infection occurred only after leukocyte transfusion (244,245). It has also been shown that production of polymorphonuclear leukocyte inflammatory response in the lungs of rats with gram-negative bacteria (*Pseudomonas*) protected against the subsequent development of *P. carinii* pneumonia induced by corticosteroids (246).

B. Pathogenesis

1. Human Studies

The pathogenic mechanisms involved in the development of human pneumocystosis have been most clearly defined in patients receiving immunosuppressive therapy. Here, the basic process appears to be reactivation of latent infection. Autopsy surveys have demonstrated asympotmatic pulmonary *P. carinii* infection only rarely in the normal population and in about 5% of patients with lymphoreticular malignancies (247–249). At some institutions the incidence of *P. carinii* pneumonia has been related to the intensity of cancer chemotherapy (250–252). "Outbreaks" of pneumocystosis have thus been related to such factors as changes in existing immunosuppressive regimens, more aggressive protocols, or greater clinical awareness of *P. carinii* rather than to contagion (253).

Evidence for person-to-person transmission of *P. carinii* having a role in the development of overt disease comes from the occurrence of pneumocystosis in individuals who had close contact with each other. Epidemics of *P. carinii* pneumonia have been well documented in orphanages and foundling homes (6,9). Outbreaks have occurred among immunosuppressed patients at major medical centers that could not be related to changes in chemotherapy (254, 255). Cases of pneumocystosis have been reported among persons who shared the same room or who were members of the same family (256–259). A rise in serum antibody titers to *P. carinii* has been found among some hospital personnel who cared for patients with pneumocystosis (199).

The process by which *P. carinii* pneumonia is initiated in patients with immune deficiency disorders in unclear. Perhaps organisms present in a latent state for long periods of time begin to propagate as the host's immune function becomes progressively impaired. Thus, the high frequency of pneumocystosis in immunodeficient siblings of children with primary immune deficiency diseases (39) or among patients with AIDS who have close or even sexual contact with each other may not be due to contagion. On the other hand, it is possible that exposure to sources of *P. carinii* at a critical point in the host's developing immunological dysfunction results in acquisition of infection and propagation of the organism.

2. Animal Models

The corticosteroid-treated rat has been the principal animal model for studies of pathogenesis of *P. carinii* pneumonia (260). As with humans receiving immuno-suppressive drugs, the mechanism of disease is reactivation of latent infection. Rats administered corticosteroids develop wasting and debilitation with loss of about 40% of their body weight; we routinely add a low-protein diet to this regimen because it enhances the intensity and uniformity of the pneumocystosis. *Pneumocystis carinii* organisms propagate slowly, gradually filling the alveolar spaces. A highly significant correlation has been found between the severity of *P. carinii* pneumonia, as judged by semiquantitative histopathological analysis of the extent of alveolar involvement, and the number of organisms in lung homogenates; at peak intensity of the disease, each lung may contain 10^9–10^{10} organisms (235,261). This system has been very valuable both in studies of pathogenesis and in the assessment of the efficacy of antimicrobial agents.

Development of pneumocystosis in the rat begins with attachment of the organism to the type I pneumocyte and is followed by a complex series of events in the alveolar microenvironment. The light and electron microscopic changes, whch are described in detail in Section III.C include alterations in the surface properties of alveolar lining cells and in alveolar-capillary permeability that culminate in damage to the type I pneumocyte (85,87,89,195,262). Physiological and biochemical events include altered respiratory mechanics, slight changes in arterial blood gases, and a fall in bronchoalveolar lavage surfactant phospholipids (263–266). Taken together, the data suggest diffuse alveolar injury, a process not specific for *P. carinii* but that can also be produced by a variety of infectious and noninfectious agents (267-269). The major difference in pneumocystosis is that these changes are slow to evolve and appear to be secondary to orgnism attachment.

When steroids are removed, the rat regains its weight and mounts a vigorous cellular and humoral immune response to clear *P. carinii* from the lung (43,125, 235,236). Yet, even after normal immune function has been restored, *P. carinii* can be found attached to the type I pneumocyte. Currently available anti-*P. carinii* drugs are not lethal and do not completely eliminate the organism from the lungs; reinstitution of corticosteroid treatment in the rat will induce *P. carinii* pneumonia even without exposure to exogenous sources of the organism (270). Similarly, in humans (particularly AIDS patients), relapses of pneumocystosis can occur once antimicrobial drugs have been stopped and the immunosuppressive conditions persist (56,57). It thus appears that the immune response developed by the host to *P. carinii* infection does not result in effective immunity, but the mechanisms by which this occurs require clarification.

Pneumocystosis has been studied in corticosteroid-treated mice (114,170, 171,271). The steroid dose on a mg/kg basis is usually about one-half that used in rats because at slightly higher doses the mice can die within a few weeks of presumed overwhelming bacterial sepsis. *Pneumocystis carinii* pneumonia in the mice is not as extensive as that achieved in rats, but otherwise the histopathological features are very similar to those in rats and humans. Mouse strains differ in their susceptibility to corticosteroid-induced pneumocystosis, with C3H being among the most sensitive and DBA/2N and DBA/1J being among the most resistant strains. In one study, C3H/HeJ mice, which are resistant to the effects of endotoxin and have defects in macrophage function, had more extensive pneumocystosis and higher serum antibody levels to *P. carinii* than did C3HeB/FeJ mice, which are immunologically normal (171).

Pneumocystosis has been induced by corticosteroids in rabbits, ferrets, and guinea pigs with histological features similar to the disease in humans (272,273), but there has been only modest interest in using these animals as experimental models. Attempts to produce pneumocystosis in hamsters by corticosteroid administration have been unsuccessful (42,273). Perhaps exploration of the pulmonary defense mechanisms in the hamster might reveal important insights about the host-parasite relationship in *P. carinii* infection.

Experimental transmission studies of *P. carinii* performed in corticosteroid-treated animals raised under conventional conditions have been inconclusive because of the development of pneumocystosis in steroid-treated controls (44). Thus, investigators have had to turn to animals raised in a germ-free environment.

Attempts to develop congenitally immunodeficient animals as experimental models of *P. carinii* infection have produced conflicting results. Our early studies demonstrated that human and rat *P. carinii* could be transmitted to outbred Swiss nude mice (107), but our later transmission experiments performed with a different outbred strain of nude mice at another institution were unsuccessful (114). Our limited attempts to establish *P. carinii* infection in nude rats have also been unsuccessful (115). In contrast, another group of investigators have been able to transmit *P. carinii* to both nude mice and nude rats and to examine the effects of various immunological manipulations (e.g., lymphocyte transfer) on the course of the infection (111–113).

The reasons for the divergent results of experimental *P. carinii* infection in nude mice and rats are unclear but may be related to factors in the organism or in the animal host. It is possible that some strains of *P. carinii* differ in virulence or host specificity. Investigators who have had the most success with nude mice have used mouse *P. carinii* as the major source of organisms (113), and previous attempts to transmit *P. carinii* from one normal immunosuppressed animal species to another have been unsuccessful (19,43,274). Perhaps there are strain differences among nude mice in susceptibility to exogenous *P. carinii* infection. An additional possibility is that environmental factors, which can influence immune function of nude mice (44), might influence their susceptibility to *P. carinii*.

Spontaneous outbreaks of pneumocystosis have occurred in colonies of nude mice and mice with severe combined immunodeficiency (275–277). The infection is usually mild or asymptomatic in young animals, similar to the picture achieved in experimental transmission studies. However, in older mice, pneumocystosis develops as a chronic illness that results in wasting and, ultimately, death. These outbreaks, which appear to be becoming more common, are of both theoretical and practical importance. They clearly demonstrate that naturally acquired *P. carinii* infection can result in devastating illness in the appropriate immunodeficient animal host. If the outbreaks could be developed into an experimental model system, they might reveal important data about human *P. carinii* infection.

Mice with pneumocystosis pose serious technical and economic problems for breeding facilities and are of little value to investigators who wish to work with disease-free animals. Control measures have involved identifying the source of *P. carinii* and efforts to eliminate the organism from the colony. Preliminary studies using IFA have suggested mouse *P. carinii* as the organism involved in some of the outbreaks (277); this information is important because preventive efforts might be different if another source of the organisms (e.g., humans) had been implicated. The principal control measure has been depopulation of the animal colony with redevelopment under more stringent barrier conditions, but this has not always been successful. While antimicrobial drugs have not yet been explored, it is unlikely that currently available agents could eradicate *P. carinii* from the animal colony because they are not lethal to the organism. Special filtered cages might help prevent the spread of *P. carinii* to uninfected mice, but they also appear to enhance the severity of pneumocystosis in mice already infected with the organism (115).

Cases of naturally acquired *P. carinii* pneumonia have been reported in animals in whom an immunodeficiency disease was proven (e.g., hairless guinea pig) or strongly suspected (e.g., dogs, goats, swine, horses, primates) (69,274, 278–282). The emergence of AIDS has stimulated interest in retrovirus infection in animals; however, so far, *P. carinii* has not been the dominant opportunistic infection as in humans. A recent autopsy survey of cats with feline leukemia virus infection failed to reveal *P. carinii* (283).

C. Pathology

1. Human Pneumocystosis

Gross features of human *P. carinii* pneumonia depend on whether the disease is diffuse, focal, or nodular and whether there is concomitant infection with other organisms. When pathological specimens are available for gross evaluation, *P. carinii* pneumonia usually has been well established because early infection may not be detected by chest X-ray.

In the advanced diffuse form of pneumocystosis, all lobes of the lungs are involved by the disease process. The lungs are bulky and densely consolidated with a rubbery consistency. The cut surfaces are yellowish grey to reddish grey, granular, and dry with obliteration of the air spaces. Overall, the changes are similar to those found with diffuse alveolar damage caused by a variety of etiologies, which are manifested clinically as the adult respiratory distress syndrome. In less severely infected areas, foci of consolidation, atelectasis, and compensatory hyperinflation are intermixed. In the epidemic infantile form of pneumocystosis (interstitial plasma cell pneumonia), dark red liverlike lungs are seen in those who died rapidly (11).

The focal form of pneymocystosis seen by chest X-ray may represent an earlier stage of the disease, since patients may develop diffuse changes later. Except for the extent of involvement, the gross features in the focal form are similar to those of the diffuse form.

The nodular form is rare, with only a few cases having been reported (284–289). Both solitary and multiple nodules as well as cavitation have been found.

On histopathological examination, *P. carinii* pneumonia typically shows both alveolar interstitial thickening and frothy honeycombed material in the lumens (Fig. 7). The interstitial thickening is attributed to hyperplasia and hypertrophy of type II pneumocytes, interstitial edema, cellular infiltrates composed of lymphocytes with a few macrophages or plasma cells, and sometimes mild fibrosis. However, the cellular infilatrates are usually scanty and are sometimes lacking in the alveolar septa, whereas perivascular and peribronchial

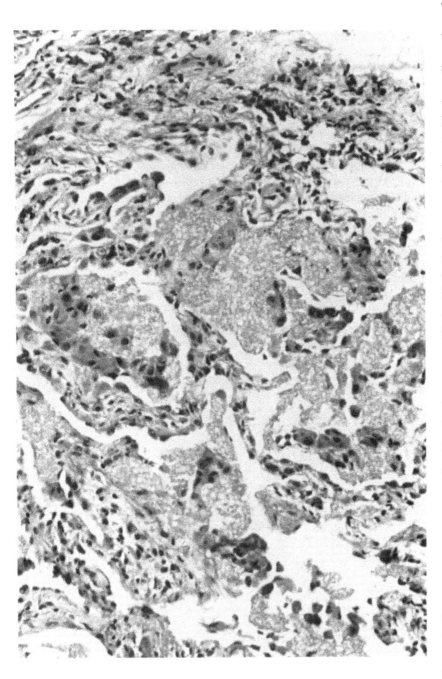

Figure 7 Human *P. carinii* pneumonia. Alveolar lumens are filled with frothy honeycombed material. A small number of pulmonary macrophages are intermixed. Alveolar septa reveal features of interstitial pneumonia with hyperplasia and hypertrophy of Type II pneumocytes, edema, mononuclear cell infiltrates, and mild fibrosis. Hematoxylin-eosin stain. X250.

infiltrates may be more noticeable. The lymphocytes are mainly small mature lymphocytes, but transformed lymphocytes and plasma cells are occasionally seen. The alveolar lumens are filled with frothy honeycombed material that contains numerous cysts (Fig. 8). Inflammatory cells are generally inconspicuous, but, when present, a few macrophages and rarely neutrophils can be seen.

In contrast to immunosuppressed patients, infants with the epidemic form of pneumocystosis show a heavy interstitial plasma cell infiltrate (6,8,37). The reasons for this difference are unclear but are probably more related to factors in the host (e.g., immature immune system) than to factors in the organism (e.g., antigenic differences). Although cases of interstitial plasma cell pneumonia still occur, there has been little apparent interest in performing detailed studies of the histological features or pathogenesis of this form of pneumocystosis.

One of the problems in histological studies of pneumocystosis is that typical features of well-established disease may not always be present in the pathological specimen (284,286,290-292). For example, in one study the frothy honeycombed alveolar material was absent in 47% of the cases (293). We have found that autopsy or open lung biopsy specimens, which are of sufficient size to permit detailed examination, will reveal typical histological features of *P. carinii* pneumonia in at least a few loci even though atypical features may be more prominent. Such atypical changes include hyaline membrane formation, prominent interstitial fibrosis, necrotizing and nonnecrotizing granulomas, focal multinucleated giant cells, organizing pneumonia, dense interstitial or intraalveolar

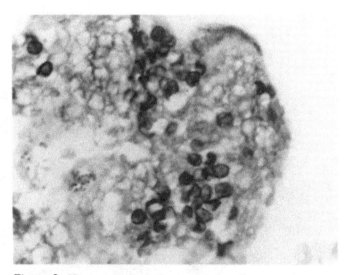

Figure 8   Human *P. carinii* pneumonia. Clusters of cysts are seen in frothy honeycombed material. Grocott's methenamine silver stain. ×900.

inflammatory cell infiltrates, and focal calcification (Fig. 9). Since pneumocystosis patients frequently have a hsitory of other conditions (e.g., chemotherapy, radiation therapy, oxygen toxicity, other pulmonary infections) that can cause lung damage, it is often impossible to determine to what extent these atypical changes are due to *P. carinii*. We have usually found far fewer organisms in areas of atypical histological features than in areas with typical histological features; the one exception is the presence of hyaline membranes where compact aggregates of *P. carinii* are frequently seen. It is imperative for pathologists to examine the specimen meticulously to identify the organisms, since small biopsy material may contain only a few organisms and crush artifacts in such material may alter the histopathological changes.

In cases of pneumocystosis presenting as a solitary nodule, necrotizing or nonnecrotizing granulomas containing *P. carinii* or frothy honeycombed material may be found (284–289).

2. Experimental Pneumocystosis

Histopathologically, *P. carinii* pneumonia in corticosteroid-treated rats develops slowly over time (43,235). Although the intensity of the infection varies somewhat among individual rats sacrificed at any given time, it is light to moderate in most rats by week 4, moderate to severe at week 6, and reaches peak intensity at weeks 7 and 8. In rats with light infection (defined as less than 25% alveolar involvement with *P. carinii*), organisms are first detected sporadically along the alveolar septa, especially in the subpleural region. The alveolar septa are normal. Typically, there is multifocal involvement of the lung with *P. carinii*. As the infection progresses, organisms are found mostly in the alveolar lumens where the intralveolar frothy material starts accumulating. The classic honeycombed appearance of this exudate does not develop until extensive disease is established. The alveolar septa reveal thickening with hyperplasia and hypertrophy of type II pneumocytes. This change is present focally in moderate (25–50% alveoli involved) infection and becomes more apparent in heavy (50–75% alveoli involved) and very heavy (>75% alveoli involved) infection. Other changes include interstitial edema and mild mononuclear cell infiltrates in the alveolar septa and in the peribronchial and perivascular regions. These infiltrates, which are not conspicuous, are composed mainly of small lymphocytes and varying admixtures of macrophages and plasma cells (Fig. 10).

With discontinuation of the corticosteroids, alveolar macrophages become very prominent in phagocytosis of *P. carinii*, and multinucleated cells can be found (235). Hypertrophy of type II pneumocytes continues. A heavy mononuclear cell infiltrate develops, particularly in the peribronchial and perivascular areas. This is accompanied systemically by a rise in the lymphocyte count and return of the T-cell subsets toward normal (236). There is also the progressive development of pulmonary interstitial fibrosis. This finding is important because

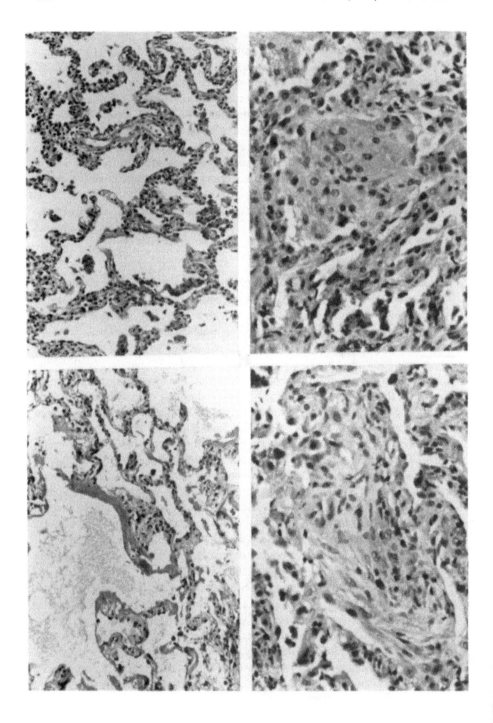

it demonstrates in an experimental system that recovery of pneumocystosis can be associated with long-lasting histological changes in the lung.

3. Ultrastructural Studies

Electron microscopic studies have been performed on lung biopsy and autopsy specimens of humans and animals with pneumocystosis. The available data suggest that the ultrastructural features of *P. carinii* pneumonia in humans are similar to those in corticosteroid-treated rats; since many more detailed studies have been performed in rats, the analysis here is confined to this animal model.

The ultrastructural changes parallel the growth of *P. carinii* and light microscopic changes. After several weeks of corticosteroid administration, there is a decrease in the cell surface glycocalyx of the type I pneumocyte demonstrable by histochemical stains (e.g., ruthenium red) (195). There are also alterations in alveolar-capillary permeability, as noted by the leakage of the marker, horseradish peroxidase, from the vascular space into the alveolar space (262). This is followed at the peak intensity of *P. carinii* pneumonia by degenerative changes in the type I pneumocyte, which begin with subepithelial bleb formation and are followed by denudation of the basement membrane (85,88,89). This membrane appears to be the site of exudation of fibrin and serum proteins into the alveolar space, which contribute to the formation of the foamy material. Other components of this material include degenerative membranes of *P. carinii* and the host and myelin figures presumed to represent pulmonary surfactant.

Along with these findings, the type II pneumocytes exhibit a progressive increase in size and in labellar bodies. These hypertrophic changes are a host reparative response to alveolar injury regardless of cause. The type I cell does not replicate and is thought to develop through differentiation of the type II cell (267–269). However, interpretation of the significance of these findings in *P. carinii* infection is complicated by the fact that similar changes can be produced in type II pneumocytes by the administration of tetracycline drugs alone (294).

Figure 9 Atypical histological features of human *P. carinii* pneumonia. *Upper left*: Prominent hyaline membranes along the alveolar septa. Clusters of cysts are usually found by Grocott's methenamine silver stain. Hematoxylin-eosin stain. X140. *Upper right*: Lack of alveolar honeycombed material. The alveolar septa reveal interstitial inflammation identical to usual interstitial pneumonia. Organisms are rarely found in this histological picture. Hematoxylin-eosin stain. X140. *Lower left*: Organizing exudate obliterating the alveolar lumen, resulting in features of organizing pneumonia. Hematoxylin-eosin stain. X250. *Lower right*: Changes resembling noncaseating epithelioid granuloma. Hematoxylin-eosin stain. X250.

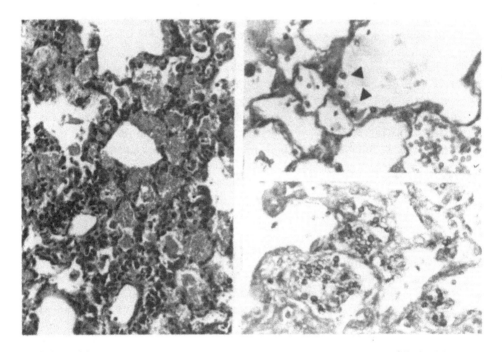

Figure 10 Rat *P. carinii* pneumonia. *Left*: Alveolar lumens are filled with frothy honeycombed material. The features are essentially identical to human *P. carinii* pneumonia. Hematoxylin-eosin stain. X200. *Upper right*: In early infection, cysts (arrowheads) are found mainly along the alveolar septa. Note the absence of honeycombed material in alveolar lumens. Grocott's methenamine silver stain. X500. *Lower right*: In severe infection, typical honeycombed material containing cysts and trophozoites is present. Grocott's methenamine silver stain. X500.

4. Staining of Histological and Cytological Material

Two basic types of stains have been used to identify *P. carinii*. Stains such as Grocott's or Gomori's methenamine silver, which selectively stain the wall of *P. carinii* cysts, have been the most popular. The silver stain can be applied to tissue sections, imprint smears, and respiratory secretions; organisms appear black against a light green background.We use the silver stain for all histopathological sections in both clinical and experimental work. The silver stain is time-consuming and requires a high degree of technical expertise, although simpler, more rapid modifications of the basic procedure are now in use (295-301).

At times, combinations of methenamine silver with other stains have been used to examine the interaction of *P. carinii* with host tissues. One example has been the use of hematoxylin-eosin counterstain to analyze the inflammatory cellular response. Periodic acid Schiff (PAS) and sodium bisulfite resorcinol stains have been used to identify basement membranes (302).

Several other selective cell-wall stains have been used to identify *P. carinii* in imprint smears or respiratory secretions. The popularity of these stains stems from the fact that they are simple, rapid, and easy to perform. We have favored cresyl echt violet (CEV) for routine use in our laboratory; *P. carinii* cysts stain pink while tissues assume a yellow background (235,261,303). Toluidine blue O, which stains the organism pink against a blue background, has been favored by other authors (304-306). Gram-Weigert appears to stain both the cell wall and some of the internal contents of the cyst (307,308).

Various forms of *P. carinii* cysts can be demonstrated with cell-wall stains: round, wrinkled, crescentic, round with targeted appearance, and comma-shaped dark staining in rounded cysts (Fig. 11). They measure 4-6 μm in diameter in tissue sections but are slightly larger in cytology preparations. The comma-shaped structures or dark bodies within cysts on silver stain appear to represent focal thickening of the cyst wall and not sporozoites or other intracytoplasmic organelles (309). The round cyst forms of *P. carinii* can sometimes mimic fungi (e.g., *Histoplasma, Candida, Cryptoccus*), especially when only a few organisms are present in a specimen; the presence of wrinkled and crescentic forms of *P. carinii* and the lack of budding are distinguishing morphological features.

The major advantages or cyst-wall stains are that they can be analyzed rapidly and do not require a great deal of expertise for proper interpretation. Thus, unless there are major errors in staining technique, even a relatively inexperienced observer can make the diagnosis of *P. carinii* in most clinical situations. The major disadvantage of cyst-wall stains is that they do not stain the internal contents of the organism, and hence empty cysts, live cysts, and dead cysts all share the same tinctorial characteristics. While this may not be important in histological sections, it has been a major drawback in working with *P. carinii* in tissue culture or fresh clinical specimens.

The second type of *P. carinii* stains stain trophozoites, intracystic bodies, and

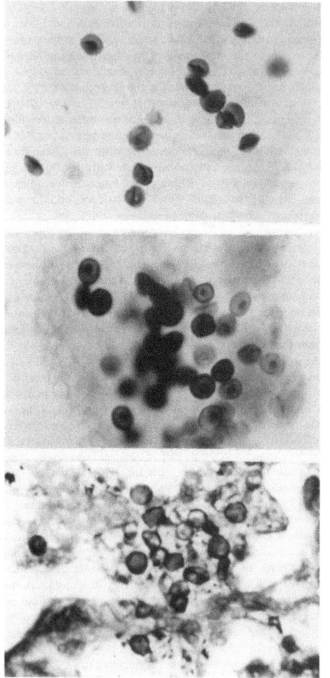

Figure 11 *Pneumocystis carinii* cysts stained with Grocott's methenamine silver. X1300. *Left*: Cysts in honeycombed material in tissue preparation. *Middle*: Cysts in honeycombed material in cytology smear. Note prominent targetoid appearance. *Right*: Wrinkled and crescentic forms are seen.

all intermediate forms. Giemsa stain is the prototype, but similar results can be obtained with Wright-Giemsa and polychrome methylene blue (305,310, 311). We favor Diff Quik, a variant of the Wright-Giemsa stain, because it is very rapid (can be accomplished in less than 1 min) and gives staining results similar to those achieved with the standard Giemsa stain (137,261). Recent studies indicate that *P. carinii* can also be seen with Wright's and Gram's stains in lung imprint smears and bronchoalveolar lavage fluid (311–316), but it is unclear what specific role these stains will have in diagnosis of this infection.

The major advantage of stains such as Diff Quik or Giemsa is that they provide important information about the biology of *P. carinii*. Trophozoites appear as single or clustered dark bluish-red nuclei surrounded by faint blue cytoplasm; intracystic bodies have similar staining characteristics (Fig. 3). As mentioned previously, we have used the Diff Quik stain to monitor the growth and life cycle stages of *P. carinii* in tissue culture. The number of organisms identified with these stains is 5–10 times greater than the number of organisms identified by selective cell-wall stains.

In our experience, Diff Quik types of stains work well in imprint smears and respiratory secretions but are not suitable for tissue sections. The major limitation to these stains is that they also stain host cells. It takes a longer period of time and a greater degree of experience to properly examine a slide for the presence of *P. carinii*; care must be taken not to confuse platelets or debris with organisms. We have also found that this type of stain does not work well on tissues that have been previously frozen.

In recent years, there has been increased interest in the use of cytology in the diagnosis of pneumocystosis (317–321). Specimens include touch preparations, bronchoalveolar lavage, bronchial washings and brushings, needle aspiration, concentration smears, suspension smears, and sputum. Although identification of the organisms is needed to make the diagnosis, the smears from bronchoalveolar lavage and needle aspiration often show frothy honeycombed material (Fig. 12). Examination of Papanicolaou stained slides under fluorescence microscopy has revealed *P. carinii* nuclei (177). Other stains (e.g., acridine orange, ethidium bromide, propidium iodide) as well as monoclonal and polyclonal antibodies have been used to identify the organism by fluorescence microscopy (192,322) but have not yet gained widespread clinical application.

Specialized light microscopic techniques are also helpful in examining *P. carinii* in fresh specimens. In our laboratory, phase contrast, Nomarski interference contrast, and bright field microscopy with oblique illumination all provide excellent views of the organism (97). These techniques can be combined with erythrosin B dye to examine organism viability, and with Triton X–Giemsa stain to study life-cycle stages. As clinical experience with *P. carinii* continues to grow, these microscopic techniques should assume an increasingly important role

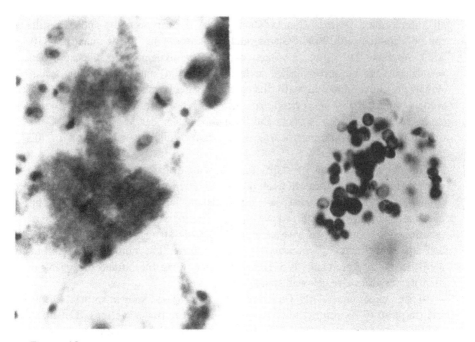

Figure 12 *Left*: Honeycombed material of a bronchoalveolar lavage smear from an AIDS patient. Papanicolaou stain. X530. *Right*: *P. carinii* cysts in honeycombed material. Grocott's methenamine silver stain. X680.

in detection of the organism in respiratory secretions, lung homegenates, or other fresh specimens.

IV. THE DISEASE

A. Clinical Manifestations

1. Immunocompromised Host

The clinical manifestations of pneumocystosis include asymptomatic infection in the normal host and life-threatening pneumonia in the immunocompromised host; however, a spectrum of disease between these two extremes has not yet been established. In other words, it is unknown whether *P. carinii* causes a self-limited bronchitis, pneumonitis, or other forms of respiratory disease in healthy or immunosuppressed people. This situation has resulted from a lack of sensitive, noninvasive diagnostic techniques.

The clinical features of pneumocystosis are compared in three large series in Table 6 and 7. Two of these studies were conducted prior to the onset of AIDS.

Table 6 Signs and Symptoms of Pneumocystosis

	Series			
			NIH–NYC	
Sign/symptom	CDC (168 pts)	St. Jude (80 pts)	Non-AIDS (38 pts)	AIDS (48 pts)
Dyspnea	91%	90%[a]	66%	68%
Fever	66%	98%	87%	81%
Cough	47%	80%	71%	81%
Sputum	7%	0%	21%	23%
Chest pain	7%	–	24%	23%
Cyanosis	39%	65%	–	–
Rales	33%	0%	34%	30%
Duration (median)	14 days	–	5 days	28 days

[a]Expressed as tachypnea in children.

Table 7 Laboratory Values in Pneumocystosis[a]

	Series			
			NIH–NYC	
Value	CDC	St. Jude	Non-AIDS	AIDS
pH	7.46	7.47	–	–
pO_2 (mmHg)	46	49	52	69
pCO_2 (mmHg)	34	29	–	–
A–A gradient	–	–	59	41
Total WBC/mm^3	11,800	–	4,600	4,900
Neutrophils/mm^3	–	4086	3,562	3,315
Lymphocytes/mm^3	–	–	396	643
Total protein (g/100 ml)	5.6	–	–	–
Albumin (g/100 ml)	–	<3.0[b]	3.1	3.25

[a]Mean or median values.
[b]62% of the patients had a serum albumin <3.0 g/100 ml.

The CDC series, which is based on analysis of patients treated with pentamidine isethionate before the introduction of trimethoprim-sulfamethoxazole (TMP-SMX), includes patients from all regions of the country and a variety of underlying illnesses (40). The St. Jude's Children's Hospital study is concerned with pediatric cancer patients treated at a single institution (27,28). The third study is a comparison of the features of pneumocystosis in AIDS and non-AIDS patients treated at the National Institutes of Health (NIH) and at the Memorial Sloan-Kettering Cancer Center and the New York Hospital in New York City (NYC) during the period 1970–1983 (57).

The cardinal features of pneumocystosis are shortness of breath, fever, and a dry, nonproductive cough (Table 6). These symptoms, whether individually or in varying combinations, are present in almost all patients during the course of their disease. In some instances, one of these manifestations (e.g., high fever) may be the predominant clinical problem, which could cause confusion in a diagnostic workup. The cough in pneumocystosis is occasionally productive of small amounts of sputum; hemoptysis has (rarely) been reported, but it is unclear whether it was due to *P. carinii* or to other causes. Chest pain can also occur.

Pneumocystosis in the compromised host varies from an acute illness with abrupt onset to a chronic, insidious process. Although this variation in symptomatology occurs in virtually all underlying illnesses, certain patterns of reactivity have emerged that can help focus diagnostic thinking. Typically, in patients with cancer or other diseases requiring immunosuppressive therapy, symptoms are present 1–2 weeks before diagnosis of *P. carinii* is established. The symptoms frequently begin after corticosteroids have been tapered or discontinued. Some children with primary immune deficiency diseases may be sick for weeks to months; it may be difficult to separate *P. carinii* from other causes of respiratory illness and chronic debilitation. Pneumocystosis in patients with AIDS follows a similar, more protracted clinical course. As noted in the NIH/NYC series, the median duration of symptoms in AIDS patients was 28 days versus 5 days in non-AIDS patients investigated at the same institutions. Symptoms of *P. carinii* in AIDS patients seem to occur with the same frequency as in non-AIDS patients but are typically more subtle; thus, the clinician needs to perform a careful and more detailed history in order for *P. carinii* to get adequate consideration in the differential diagnosis.

On physical examination, tachypnea and tachycardia are frequently present in the acutely ill patient but may be absent in the more chronically ill individual. Physical findings are generally mild in comparison with the degree of symptomatic respiratory impairment. Rales occur in about one-third of the adult patients, but other findings on lung auscultation are unusual. Cyanosis is more frequent in children than in adults. Children may also exhibit flaring of the nasal alae and intercostal retractions.

Laboratory tests exhibit a variety of abnormalities in pulmonary function (Table 7). Blood gases typically show hypoxemia, increased alveolar-arterial oxygen gradient, and respiratory alkalosis. These abnormalities tend to be less severe in AIDS patients than in other immunosuppressed hosts. In the late stages of pneumocystosis, a respiratory acidosis may develop. Other tests reveal impaired diffusing capacity, vital capacity, and total lung capacity, and an elevated ratio of forced expiratory volume in 1 sec (FEV1) to forced vital capacity (FVC) (63,323). Nuclear medicine studies show increased lung uptake on gallium scan and increased clearance of inhaled 99m-technetium diethylenetriamine penta-acetate (tcDTPA) (182,324–329). This latter substance has been used as a marker for alveolar-capillary membrane permeability.

Radiographic changes classically show bilateral diffuse alveolar infiltrates emanating from the perihilar region (28,40,57,330) (Fig. 13). Frequently, there is apical sparing. Early in the infection the infiltrates may be patchy, but with progression, dense consolidation and air bronchograms develop. Although pneumocystosis has frequently been described as causing an "interstitial pneumonia," the disease process actually represents a combination of alveolar or air-space consolidation with variable interstitial infiltrate (331).

A variety of atypical radiographic manifestations of pneumocystosis have been reported, including unilateral predominance of infiltrate, lobar consolidation, nodular lesions, cavitation, pneumatocele, pneumothorax, pneumomediastinum, and pleural effusion (215,284–289,331–337). The occurrence of pneumocystosis with normal chest X-ray has also been well documented (215, 327,337,338); this appears to be more common in AIDS patients, particularly since the development of more aggressive diagnostic approaches. In such cases the gallium scan, blood gases, or other pulmonary function tests are usually abnormal.

Few other laboratory alterations consistently occur in *P. carinii* pneumonia. The patient's white blood cell count is usually governed by his underlying disease or immunosuppressive therapy. Leukopenia and/or lymphopenia are not uncommon. Serum albumin levels vary considerably, but overall are below normal; this supports the role of protein malnutrition in the pathogenesis of pneumocystosis.

2. Interstitial Plasma Cell Pneumonia

Since interstital plasma cell pneumonia has virtually disappeared from Western industrialized countries, physicians have tended to consider the disease to be of historical rather than of practical importance. However, this form of pneumocystosis has continued to be found in other parts of the world; with modern international travel, the disease could present difficult diagnostic problems for physicians unfamiliar with it. Such a situation is illustrated by the occurrence of *P. carinii* pneumonia in Vietnam refugees in the United States (15–18).

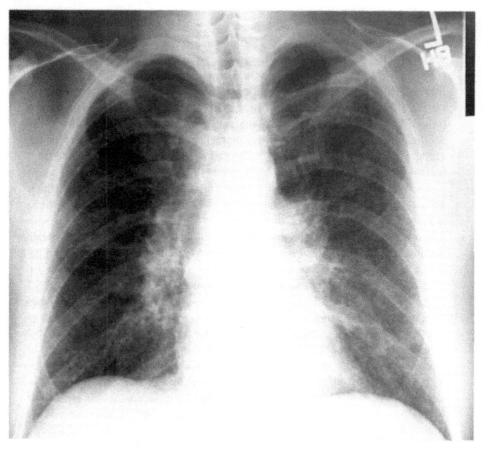

Figure 13   Chest radiograph of an AIDS patient with *P. carinii* pneumonia. Note typical bilateral infiltrates.

The classical clinical setting for interstitial plasma cell pneumonia is the orphanage or related institution that houses chronically debilitated infants, often born prematurely, under crowded conditions. The disease occurs throughout the first year of life, with a peak age incidence of 6 weeks to 4 months (6–8). The clinical manifestations are nonspecific and begin insidiously with restlessness, lethargy, or poor feeding. Respiratory difficulties develop gradually and are characterized by tachypnea, facial cyanosis, and mild cough; fever is frequently absent. As the disease worsens, there may be flaring of nasal alae, sternal retraction, and use of the accessory muscles of respiration. Physical findings are unusual and may include fine rales or focal areas of decreased resonance and bronchial breathing. Chest X-ray shows diffuse pulmonary infiltrates.

B. Diagnosis

Pneumocystis carinii pneumonia should be considered in any compromised host who develops fever, respiratory symptoms, or infiltrates on chest X-ray. These clinical features can be mimicked by a long list of other infectious agents including gram-positive and gram-negative bacteria, legionella, mycobacteria, fungi, viruses, parasites, mycoplasmas, and chlamydia. A similar clinical picture can be caused by noninfectious etiologies including tumor, hemorrhage, edema, fibrosis, oxygen, radiation, and drugs. The frequence of occurrence of *P. carinii* in AIDS and its subtle and varied presentation have raised medical interest in the clinical manifestations of this organism. Patients with HIV infection frequently develop fever and a variety of other prodromal symptoms for weeks to months before developing pneumocystosis as the first manifestation of AIDS. Whether these clinical symptoms are all due to *P. carinii* is as yet unclear.

Optimal patient management depends on establishment of a specific diagnosis, since it is not possible to cover all of the above causes of pulmonary infiltrates with empirical therapy. At the present time the definitive diagnosis of *P. carinii* can only be made by morphological or histopathological demonstration of the organism. *Pneumocystis carinii* is only rarely present in sputum or gastric secretions or non-AIDS patients (40,116–118,339–342), and thus an invasive procedure is usually necessary to establish diagnosis. Transtracheal aspiration has occasionally revealed *P. carinii*; since this procedure bypasses mouth flora, it may be more useful in identifying fastidious bacterial or fungal pathogens (117). Enthusiasm for performing transtracheal aspiration varies considerably among medical centers, and caution should be used with patients who are severely hypoxemic or thrombocytopenic or who have bleeding disorders. Percutaneous needle aspiration/biopsy of the lung has been frequently performed in children (343–352). Enthusiasm for this procedure among adults has waned because of the small amount of tissue obtained and the high frequency of complications.

Open-lung biopsy has traditionally given the greatest diagnostic yield and hence has served as the "gold standard" for other procedures (307,353–364). With open biopsy, the tissue sample, which is obtained under direct visualization and controlled conditions, is of sufficient quantity to permit both culture and adequate histological examination. Clinical and experimental studies have been performed comparing lung homogenates with tissue sections in detecting light *P. carinii* infection (261,363,364). The biopsy usually requires the use of operating room facilities and general anesthesia. When performed early in the course of the patient's illness by experienced personnel, serious complications are uncommon; however, morbidity rises precipitously when lung biopsy is performed in the late stages of the disease as a last ditch measure.

Over the past decade fiber-optic bronchoscopy has emerged as the most commonly used procedure in the diagnostic workup of pulmonary infiltrates in immunosuppressed adults (365-388). In early studies, fiber-optic bronchoscopy was combined with washings and brushings; in later studies, bronchoalveolar lavage and transbronchial biopsy were added to the regimen. Although a large number of studies have been performed, it is difficult to make meaningful comparisons because of differences in patient populations, study design, specific procedures employed, and methods of handling and evaluating specimens. Despite these limitations, several general conclusions appear warranted: first, fiber-optic bronchoscopy with bronchoalveolar lavage and/or transbronchial biopsy makes the diagnosis of pneumocystosis at least 90% of the time in AIDS patients. Such a high diagnostic yield reflects, at least in part, a higher organism burden in AIDS patients than in other compromised hosts. Bronchoalveolar lavage is more efficacious than washings or brushings, carries little morbidity, and hence has emerged as the procedure of choice. Transbronchial biopsy can make the diagnosis of *P. carinii* in some patients in whom lavage has been unrevealing; however, this procedure is considerably more invasive and has a higher rate of complications. Opinion varies at different medical centers about the need for transbronchial biopsy in the diagnostic workup of these patients.

Second, the yield from bronchoscopy with lavage and/or biopsy is generally lower in non-AIDS patients, although exceptions to this statement have occurred at selected institutions (381). Since non-AIDS patients constitute a heterogeneous population, it is difficult to extrapolate from one group to another. For example, the type of immunosuppression and opportunistic pulmonary infections encountered by granulocytopenic patients with acute myelogenous leukemia are different from those encountered by renal transplant recipients. In addition, experience with AIDS patients has increased the technical expertise both in performing diagnostic procedures and in the laboratory's ability to diagnose *P. carinii* and other oportunistic pathogens. Histological staining procedures used to identify the organism, which were formerly performed only in specialized facilities, can now be routinely performed in cytology or microbiology laboratories.

The continued increase in the number of cases of pneumocystosis associated with AIDS has put a strain on the medical care system and has led to efforts to develop less invasive procedures and control medical costs. Performance of bronchosocopy at the bedside and in the outpatient setting, and the use of control-tipped reusable catheters are examples of this trend (397). Recently, studies at two medical centers demonstrated that *P. carinii* can be diagnosed in about 50% of AIDS patients by the use of induced sputum (389-391). The procedure involves inhalation of a mist of hypertonic saline generated by an ultrasonic nebulizer. Whether induced sputum will achieve widespread use in diagnosis of *P. carinii* is as yet unclear; nevertheless, this approach represents a simple, noninvasive, and inexpensive technique.

The diagnosis of pneumocystosis in patients with compatible clinical features should be pursued aggressively and requires close cooperation between the patient's primary physician, subspecialty consultants, and the laboratory. Algorithms have now been developed to help in this evaluation (392). Induced sputum can serve as a first step in assessing AIDS patients but should not delay other procedures. If sputum is unrewarding, fiber-optic bronchoscopy with lavage and perhaps biopsy should then be performed. The patient is usually started on therapy on the basis of initial analysis of this specimen and pending results of further studies.

The major dilemma facing the clinician occurs when the diagnosis is not established or the patient is not responding to therapy. While it is possible that *P. carinii* is resistant to the antimicrobial agents being used, it is also possible that there are other treatable conditions that could only be revealed by more invasive procedures. Concomitant infection with other organisms is not uncommon in AIDS patients or other immunosuppressed hosts. The clinician is then faced with three alternative courses of action: more broad-spectrum (and empirical) therapy, repeat bronchoscopy, or open-lung biopsy. We favor open-lung biopsy because it offers the highest diagnostic yield. In a study of a small series of bone marrow transplant recipients, open-lung biopsy clearly had a higher diagnostic yield than did transbronchial biopsy in patients who had both procedures performed simultaneously (378). Open-lung biopsy has also been favored over transbronchial biopsy for the diagnosis of Kaposi's sarcoma of the lung (393). Open-lung biopsy is currently performed less often than in the past, and controversy still exists in the realm of risk–benefit analysis over the precise role of open biopsy in the evaluation of pulmonary infiltrates in the compromised host (394,395). Perhaps the most important determining factor in the success of open-lung biopsy or other invasive diagnostic procedures is the amount of delay encountered before they are performed; none of these techniques will do much good if they are considered only as a last resort option when the patient's condition has deteriorated to near death. Unfortunately, the specific cause of pulmonary infiltrates in some patients cannot be established even with open-lung biopsy or at autopsy (355,396).

Immunological techniques are of potential value in the diagnosis of pneumocystosis. As mentioned previously, the organism has been identified both by immunofluorescence and immunoperoxidase staining in lungs and respiratory tract secretions (118,179,182); however, the lack of commercially available reagents has limited this approach. Serum antibody detection systems have had considerable application in infants with interstitial plasma cell pneumonia but have been of little value in the diagnosis of pneumocystosis in the compromised host (123,124,154,157,174,185,201). The high prevalence of serum antibodies in the normal population has been a major contributory factor to this problem; while a rise in serum antibody titers has occurred in some *P. carinii* patients over time, serology has usually not been able to distinguish active disease from prior exposure to the organism. Serum antigen detection methods have used counter-immunoelectrophoresis (CIE) and, to a lesser extent, latex agglutination. Initial experience with CIE was promising (124), and attempts were made to apply the test to the diagnosis of pneumocystosis in a variety of clinical and experimental settings (121,397–403). However, because of problems of sensitivity, specificity, and reproducibility, the consensus of most investigators is that the test is unreliable as a diagnostic tool (168,185,201,260,404–407).

Up to the present time, immunodiagnostic techniques of *P. carinii* have used whole organisms or crude extracts as the source of antigenic material. With the recent progress made in identifying specific *P. carinii* antigens by Western blotting, it is hoped that immunological techniques will find greater application in the diagnosis of this infection.

C. Treatment and Prevention

1. Natural History of *P. carinii* Infection

Pneumocystis carinii infection in the normal host causes no apparent symptoms or tissue damage. Pneumocystosis in the form of interstitial plasma cell pneumonia had a mortality rate of 25–60% in different series; however, spontaneous recovery from even severe disease was felt to occur (6–8). By contrast, *P. carinii* pneumonia in the immunocompromised host is almost always fatal once clinical signs and symptoms develop. There is progressive hypoxemia and respiratory insufficiency, usually leading to ventilator support. Whether or not *P. carinii* can cause mild or self-limited symptomatic respiratory disease is unknown.

Spread of *P. carinii* beyond the lungs appears to be quite uncommon. The organism was found in the spleen of 1 of 19 children with cancer who died from pneumocystosis, but not in the spleen or lymph modes of 200 institutionalized infants who succumbed to the disease (79,408). At least 20 cases of disseminated pneumocystosis have been reported in the literature (122). The 14 non-AIDS patients had a variety of underlying diseases, particularly primary immune deficiency disorders (12,29,408–415). Major sites of extrapulmonary involvement were lymph node, bone marrow, spleen, and liver; multiorgan involvement also occurred. The six cases of documented pneumocystosis in AIDS patients have been reported only recently (415–420). The precise frequency of extrapulmonary spread of *P. carinii* in AIDS is unclear, but the sites of involvement may be different. For example, the organism has been associated with auditory polyps and an intestinal mass presenting as an acute abdomen. In some locations (e.g., retina, brain) there has been controversy as to whether the organisms found actually represent *P. carinii* (418,419,421,422).

Pneumocystis carinii probably spreads from the lungs by hematogenous and/or lymphatic routes. The presence of the organism in extrapulmonary sites has been suspected from the demonstration of the typical foamy, honeycombed eosinophilic material on hematoxylin and eosin stain in the affected organ. The host inflammatory response is variable and nonspecific. The diagnosis is confirmed by methenamine silver stain, but organisms have also been demonstrated by electron microscopy and immunoperoxidase staining (122). Systematic and in-depth studies are needed to obtain reliable data about the frequency and clinical significance of the extrapulmonary spread of *P. carinii*. This effect will be greatly helped by the availability of specific and well-characterized immunological reagents. It should be possible to survey autopsy or surgical specimens by immunohistology. Alternatively, soluble antigen detection systems might be employed if current technical problems can be overcome.

2. Treatment

Treatment of pneumocystosis has largely been empirical because little is known about the organism's metabolism. The corticosteroid-treated rat model has been the principal tool of drug development (423). Since it takes about 3 months to complete each experiment, relatively few agents have been tested. Drugs that are active against rat *P. carinii* have also been found to be effective against human pneumocystosis (43,45,148,424,425); in general, drugs that have shown no activity against rat *P. carinii* have usually been ineffective against human *P. carinii*, but some exceptions (e.g., DFMO) have occurred (147). Tissue culture represents another system of drug evaluation and offers promise for studies of mechanism of action and drug interaction (143-146).

Over the past 10-15 years, two major drugs have been used in the treatment of human pneumocystosis: TMP-SMX and pentamide isethionate. Prospective controlled trials as well as a variety of other studies have shown that these two drugs are equally effective in the treatment of *P. carinii* pneumonia in AIDS and non-AIDS patients, with an overall success rate of about 75% (40,46,55-58,62, 384,426,427).

TMP-SMX is administered orally or intravenously in a dose of 20 mg/kg per day TMP and 100 mg/kg per day SMX in four divided doses for 14 days in non-AIDS patients. The parenteral route is preferred in patients who are acutely ill or who have gastrointestinal problems that may interfere with absorption of the drug. Adjustments in dose should be made according to serum concentrations; optimal levels of TMP are 3-5 μg/ml in children and $\geqslant 5$ μg/ml in adults, and those for SMX are 100-150 μg/ml (428,429). In general, sulfonamide levels are more widely available than TMP levels in hospital laboratories. It is not uncommon that the dosage of TMP-SMX can be reduced downward following this procedure. The fact that TMP–SMX is well tolerated has made it the treatment of choice for pneumocystosis in non-AIDS patients. Adverse reactions occur in about 10–15% of patients and usually consist of mild gastrointestinal complaints or skin rash. More serious problems (e.g., hematological or hepatic toxicity) are uncommon.

Pentamidine is an old drug used in the treatment of African trypanosomiasis and was the first agent to be found effective in the treatment of pneumocystosis (9,10,38,39,430,431). Pentamidine was formerly available only to physicians in the United States as an investigational drug through the Centers for Disease Control but recently has been licensed (Pentam, Lyphomed, Inc.). Pentamidine is administered parenterally in a single dose of 4 mg/kg per day for 14 days in non-AIDS patients. Although the intramuscular route was formerly preferred, the intravenous route is now widely used and is not associated with any greater degree of toxicity (432,433). To be given intravenously, pentamidine must be diluted in 50–250 ml of a 5% dextrose solution (because of poor solubility in saline) and infused over a period of at least 60 min.

Pentamidine has considerable toxicity, with about 50% of non-AIDS patients experiencing adverse effects. Local reactions (pain, swelling, sterile abscess) frequently occur at the site of intramuscular injection. A variety of systemic reactions (dizziness, flushing, cardiac arrhythmias) have been reported with intramuscular and intravenous administration. Perhaps the most notable of these reactions is hypotension, which may persist for several hours and require vigorous supportive therapy. Nephrotoxicity (azotemia) is frequent but usually reversible in the absence of other drugs or conditions that impair renal function. Alterations in glucose metabolism are also quite prominent (434–436). Hypoglycemia, sometimes associated with elevated insulin levels, may occur during or following the completion of therapy and appears to be enhanced by the presence of renal insufficiency. The manifestations of hypoglycemia vary in severity from an asymptomatic laboratory value to a life-threatening condition. Hyperglycemia, sometimes progressing to frank diabetes mellitus and requiring insulin therapy, is usually a later event. Abnormal liver function tests, hypocalcemia, and a variety of other adverse reactions to pentamidine have also been reported (437–440).

Response to TMP–SMX or pentamidine is variable but has occurred on the average after about 4 days of treatment in non-AIDS patients (427). Clinically, this response is characterized by improvement in fever, shortness of breath, and arterial blood gases followed later by changes in the chest X-ray. The major question that arises in clinical decision making is what to do when there is no response to therapy. If, as indicated previously, infection with another organism or another cause of pulmonary infiltrates is suspected, a more vigorous diagnostic approach is indicated. If drug failure is suspected, it seems reasonable to continue with initial anti-*P. carinii* drug as long as the patient's condition has stabilized. However, if there has been no improvement after 5-6 days of treatment, consideration should be given to substituting the other drug. The use of TMP-SMX and pentamidine in combination does not enhance treatment efficacy and may well increase the risk of adverse reactions (425,441).

Pneumocystosis in patients with AIDS has presented new therapeutic challenges. A recently completed prospective study and several retrospective reports indicate that TMP-SMX and pentamidine are equally effective in the treatment of the first episode of *P. carinii* pneumonia in AIDS, with response rates similar to those achieved in other immunocpmpromised hosts (55-45,62). However, AIDS patients tend to respond more slowly to treatment, and hence it is usually prudent to wait longer (at least 7 days) before considering drug failure. Despite clinical improvement, the majority of AIDS patients have persisting *P. carinii* on repeat bronchoscopy following treatment; in some cases organisms can be found even after the patient has been given the drug for many weeks (442-444). This finding presumably reflects the high *P. carinii* burden in AIDS patients, but the viability of the remaining organisms is unknown. Another distressing problem is the high rate of recurrence of pneumocystosis in AIDS; the published literature suggests that this occurs in 20-30% of patients, but more recent evidence suggests that the frequency is considerably higher (50%). Such a recurrence rate contrasts with a general rate of 1-2% in non-AIDS patients and a rate of 10-15% at selected pediatric hospitals (56). Whether this recurrence represents relapse due to persisting organisms or reinfection is as yet unclear. Treatment of these recurrent episodes is usually more difficult than treatment of the primary episodes, but controlled studies are lacking.

The features of pneumocystosis in AIDS have led to the practice of longer duration of therapy (at least 3 weeks). A more difficult question is whether or not to perform repeat bronchoscopy. This procedure might become important if it could be shown that persistence of *P. carinii* was associated with a higher frequency of relapses or treatment failures. Perhaps an even more prolonged course of therapy would be necessary to achieve organism eradication, but studies to answer this question have not yet been performed.

AIDS patients have a very high frequency (50-80%) of adverse reactions to TMP-SMX, including fever, rash, leukopenia, thrombocytopenia, and hepatic disturbances (55-62). These effects usually appear during the second week of therapy and are often severe enough to necessitate discontinuation of the drug. It is unknown whether these adverse reactions represent some form of hypersensitivity or direct drug toxicity. The sulfonamide component has been implicated as the etiological agent, although it has been suggested that TMP may be responsible for some cases of rash (63). Unfortunately, there are few firm guidelines in management. In some cases TMP-SMX may be continued at the same or reduced dose without further problems, whereas in other instances continuation of the drug results in severe and sometimes life-threatening toxic reactions. We believe it is reasonable to continue TMP-SMX as long as the side effects are mild, but the drug should be stopped if the effects become more pronounced.

The problems of TMP-SMX therapy in AIDS patients have stimulated renewed interest in the pharmacological properties of the drug. One area of concern is the relationship of TMP-SMX to folinic acid. In the therapy of toxoplasmosis, the administration of folinic acid ameliorates the bone marrow toxicity of pyrimethamine and sulfadiazine but does not interfere with their activity against the organism. While anecdotal reports have suggested that folinic acid might interfere with the effectiveness of TMP-SMX against *P. carinii* (445), data from the rat model as well as clinical experience indicate that this is not the case (427,446). Folinic acid does not prevent the adverse reactions of TMP-SMX in AIDS patients but might be helpful in preventing bone marrow toxicity, which can occur in patients with poor marrow reserve (e.g., renal or bone transplant recipients). In such patient populations the administration of 5-10 mg/day of folinic acid seems to be a prudent measure.

Another area of interest has been in the hypersensitivity properties of TMP-SMX. Some AIDS patients who have suffered adverse reactions to sulfonamides or TMP-SMX have experienced no toxic effects upon rechallenge; however, it is unknown which subset of patients might have this procedure safely applied. Some authors have proposed a scheme for drug desensitization (447). Conflicting results have been noted when other sulfonamides such as the fixed combination of pyrimethamine and sulfadoxine (Fansidar) or sulfones (dapsone) have been administered to AIDS patients with a history of sulfonamide allergy or adverse reactions to TMP-SMX (447-452). Recent case reports of unusual adverse reactions have increased awareness of the potential spectrum of toxicity that might be encountered with this family of drugs (453-455). Thus, at the present time considerable caution must be used in considering the administration of any sulfonamide or sulfone to an AIDS patient who has had an adverse reaction to TMP-SMX.

The occurrence of pneumocystosis in AIDS has resulted in a marked increase in the use of pentamidine. AIDS patients experience a high frequency of adverse reactions to pentamidine; the toxic effects are similar to those seen in other immunocompromised hosts, but the frequency of neutropenia and possibly hypoglycemia is considerably higher. The mechanism of these effects is unknown. The increased clinical demand for pentamidine has rekindled investigatory interest in the drug. New assays for measuring pentamidine levels have been developed (456,457). On the basis of data obtained in those studies as well as in earlier reports (458-461), it appears that pentamidine levels in serum are low even in experimentally induced renal failure (462); the drug is bound to tissues and released slowly over time (weeks to months). It is hoped that this renewed interest in pentamidine will lead to better knowledge of the drug's pharmaco-kinetics and a more rational dosing schedule.

Attention is also being devoted to alternative delivery systems. Aerosol administration of pentamidine results in much higher administration of the drug in the lung than in other body sites and appears to be an effective form of therapy and prophylaxis of pneumocystosis in the rat model (461,463–465). Published results of the use of aerosolized pentamidine in a small number of patients appear to be promising (466).

Several alternative drugs are available for the treatment of pneumocystosis. Pyrimethamine and sulfadiazine in doses used to treat toxoplasmosis have been successful in the therapy of a small number of cases of *P. carinii* pneumonia (467–469) but have never received widespread clinical attention or been used in controlled trials. More recently, dapsone in a dose of 100 mg/day combined with trimethoprim in a dose of 20 mg/kg per day was evaluated in an open trial in the treatment of pneumocystosis in AIDS patients; the therapeutic response was similar to that observed with TMP–SMX (63). This same group of investigators in another uncontrolled study found dapsone alone to be less effective than when used in combination with TMP (61).

One of the most promising new drugs in trimetrexate, a lipid-soluble deriva-tive of methotrexate that is a much more potent inhibitor of rat *P. carinii* dihyrdrofolate reductase (DHFR) than TMP or pyrimethamine (470). Tri-metrexate has been successful in the treatment of rat and human pneumocys-tosis when used alone or combined with a sulfonamide; bone marrow toxicity is minimized by the administration of large doses of folinic acid (471,472). Trimetrexate may be an important drug in patients who fail or cannot tolerate conventional anti–*P. carinii* therapy.

There is accumulating evidence that DFMO represents a new type of thera-peutic approach to *P. carinii* pneumonia (147,473,474). This drug inhibits orni-thinc decarboxylase, a necessary step in the synthesis of polyamines, which play an important role in the replication of eukaryotic cells. While DFMO has inhib-itory effects on a variety of protozoans, its main clinical use has been in the treatment of African trypanosomiasis. The use of DFMO in the treatment of *P. carinii* pneumonia has mainly been on a compassionate basis in patients who have failed or have experienced serious adverse reactions to TMP–SMX or pentamidine. The clinical experience with DFMO in more than 100 patients with pneumocystosis has been briefly summarized in a recent symposium (147). Of 53 persons who received the drug for more than 2 weeks, 70% achieved a good clinical response; 12 of these responders had begun therapy on ventilator sup-port. DFMO was usually well tolerated, with adverse reactions (e.g., thrombo-cytopenia, leukopenia, high-frequency hearing loss, patchy alopecia, diarhhea) being reversible upon reduction in dose or cessation of therapy.

Drug development research efforts in the rat model and in vitro have focused on two broad areas: inhibitors of folic acid synthesis and analogues of pentamidine. A variety of antifol combinations have been effective in therapy of experimental pneumocystosis (43,45,475-477). With few exceptions (e.g., trimetrexate), DHFR inhibitors used alone have shown little anti-*P. carinii* activity, whereas sulfonamides, sulfones, or sulfonylureas used as single agents have been highly effective against the organism (148,478-480). Interesting structure-activity relationships have been discovered: anti-*P. carinii* activity has been found with carbutamide, which possesses a terminal amino group, but not with tolbutamide, which has a terminal methyl group. Further studies with closer attention to drug dosing schedules are needed to determine which folic acid inhbitors, used alone or in combination, are the most effective form of therapy.

An earlier report noted that hydroxystilbamidine, a diamidine related to pentamidine, showed activity against rat *P. carinii* (43). A more recent study explored a variety of cationic compounds with similar structural properties (149). These drugs have been used for many years in the therapy of veterinary African trypanosomiasis, but for reasons of toxicity or lack of potential clinical demand had never been developed for human use. Several of these agents (e.g., diminazene, imidocarb, amicarbalide, quinapyramine, isometamidium) were at least as effective as pentamidine in the treatment of rat pneumocystosis. Further exploration of these compounds or their analogues should be a fruitful area of investigation.

Other promising areas of drug development include purine nucleosides (e.g., 9-deazainosine) (145) and unusual combinations (e.g., clindamycin and primaquine). A long list of compounds has been tried in the treatment of clinical or experimental pneumocystosis without success. Claims for efficacy of some agents (e.g., rifampin) have been made without histological documentation of the presence of *P. carinii* (481,482).

At the present time, treatment of pneumocystosis in AIDS patients is in a stage of flux. Since TMP-SMX and pentamidine have similar rates of therapeutic response and adverse reactions, neither agent has emerged as the clear-cut drug of choice. TMP-SMX is favored by many clinicians because it has well-defined pharmacology and activity against other infectious agents. Pentamidine might be favored on the basis of more rapid clinical improvement and lower (but not statistically significant) early mortality in the only published comparative controlled clinical trial (62). There is a pressing need for large, randomized, controlled multiinstitutional trials so that the role of newer agents such as trimetrexate and other folic acid inhibitors, DFMO, and aerosolized pentamidine can be properly assessed. AIDS patients are desperate for any signs of hope, and physicians are frequently tempted to embark on treatment regimens before their efficacy, toxicity, and cost have been established.

A variety of factors may affect a patient's ability to respond to anti-*P. carinii* therapy, including status of underlying disease, nutrition, degree of respiratory impairment, prior lung damage, concomitant infection with other opportunistic pathogens, and total leukocyte and lymphocyte counts (40,57,60). The role of specific factors in relation to the prognosis of pneumocystosis is sometimes difficult to evaluate. Cytomegalovirus infection, for example, is frequently present in *P. carinii* patients, but a definite relationship between these organisms has not yet been shown in clinical or experimental systems (483). Vigorous supportive measures such as the maintenance of adequate oxygenation and nutrition as well as careful fluid and electrolyte balance are an important part of medical management. Since the need for ventilator support is usually associated with poor prognosis, the decision as to whether to institute such a measure in AIDS patients has posed difficult medical and ethical questions (60,484). Even more heroic measures (e.g., the use of mebrane lung support or continuous negative chest wall pressure) have been advocated in severe cases of respiratory distress in the past (485–488). The need for cytotoxic or immunosuppressive therapy to treat a malignancy or prevent transplant rejection must be carefully balanced against the suppression of host defenses, which promotes the development of pneumocystosis. Immunotherapy offers a potentially important adjunct to anti-*P. carinii* drugs, but, so far, few studies have been done.

A major controversial area involves the use of corticosteroids (427,489–493). One side of this argument is based on the hypothesis that the pathogenesis of pneumocystosis in some patients is related at least in part to the host inflammatory response. Evidence for this comes from the following sources: Many patients receiving immunosuppressive therapy develop clinical evidence of *P. carinii* pneumonia after the corticosteroid dose has been tapered; clinical improvement in the treatment of pneumocystosis in a few AIDS patients was associated with the institution of corticosteroid therapy; the development of corticosteroid-induced pneumocystosis in the rat model can be delayed by bacterial infection, which evokes pyogenic response. However, strong arguments can been made against the use of corticosteroids: These agents are by far the most commonly used drugs that predispose to the development of *P. carinii* pneumonia in humans; several cases of pneumocystosis in AIDS patients have been related to corticosteroid administration; pneumocystosis spontaneously develops in rats with corticosteroid administration and clears when these agents are withdrawn. In addition, when corticosteroids have been studied in other serious infections (e.g., bacterial sepsis) in rigorously controlled trials, these agents have been shown to have no therapeutic benefit.

Potential indications for the adjunctive use of corticosteroids in the treatment of pneumocystosis might be as a short-term measure to reduce host inflammatory response or as a last ditch effort when other therapeutic modalities have failed. Traditionally, great caution has been advised in contemplating the use of corticosteroids not only because of their effects on *P. carinii*, but also because they might promote infection with other opportunistic pathogens. At the present time, we see no reason to change this recommendation. Patients receiving corticosteroids or other immunosuppressive drugs who develop pneumocystosis should have the dose tapered to as low a level as necessary to control the underlying disease. A recent preliminary report has suggested that corticosteroids might improve the therapeutic response of AIDS *P. carinii* patients with respiratory insufficiency (493); however, until large well-controlled studies are performed, we feel that corticosteroids should not be used in the treatment of *P. carinii* pneumonia in AIDS.

3. Long-Term Prognosis

The long-term prognosis and follow-up of patients who survive pneumocystosis are receiving increasing attention. This information is important because of the studies in the rat model that have noted the development of pulmonary fibrosis (235). Infants and children who have recovered from *P. carinii* pneumonia do not show any abnormalities on follow-up pulmonary function testing (494,495), but the picture is more complex in adults. One study of renal transplant patients showed mild residual pulmonary function abnormalities 15–20 months after recovery from the disease; these alterations correlated with radiological and pathological features of the acute illness (496). A case report in an adult documented the development of interstitial fibrosis (497). Pulmonary fibrosis can be found occasionally at autopsy in patients who have recovered from pneumocystosis, but the relationship of *P. carinii* to these changes is not clear. These patients frequently have been subjected to a variety of other insults (e.g., radiation, chemotherapy, oxygen toxicity, infectious agents) that may have contributed to the pathological changes. Long-term follow-up studies of AIDS patients who have recovered from pneumocystosis would be of interest.

4. Prevention

Pneumocystis carinii pneumonia can be prevented by the daily administration of TMP-SMX in a dose of 5 mg/kg TMP and 25 mg/kg SMX per day (47,498-501). Chemoprophylaxis is indicated for anyone who has recovered from pneumocystosis but continues in an immunocompromised state, and certain high-risk patient groups including children with acute leukemia (original group for whom chemoprophylaxis was developed); infants with primary immune deficiency disorders, particularly severe combined immune deficiency; bone marrow, heart, and liver transplant recipients; and patients with AIDS. The need for chemoprophylaxis can be related to frequency of pneumocystosis at different institutions. An outbreak of *P. carinii* pneumonia among renal transplant recipients at one hospital and increased incidence of the disease among patients on a particular oncology protocol at another hospital led to the use of prophylactic

TMP-SMX (216-219). A case for the use of chemoprophylaxis might be made in adults with acute lymphatic leukemia whose cytotoxic therapy is similar to that for children, whereas chemoprophylaxis is usually not needed in adults with acute myelogenous leukemia who have different cytotoxic therapy and a low incidence of pneumocystosis. TMP-SMX requires care because severe adverse reactions may occur not only in AIDS patients but also in persons with impaired renal function (e.g., renal transplant recipients) who are receiving immunosuppressive drugs (azathioprine) (502).

TMP-SMX is given daily, but animal and clinical studies have shown that intermittent dosage is also effective (424,501). The important thing is not to discontinue the drug for a long period of time because the chemoprophylactic effect of TMP-SMX exists only as long as the drug is being given; cases of delayed development of pneumocystosis have been documented after chemoprophylactic TMP-SMX had been discontinued (498). TMP-SMX and other anti-*P. carinii* drugs exert a static rather than cidal effect on the organism (270, 503). In vitro and microscopic studies suggest that these drugs act mainly on the trophozoite form, whereas the cyst seems to be impermeable (146,241). There is a great need in *P. carinii* drug development for agents that can kill the cyst form of the organism.

Prophylactic TMP-SMX is well tolerated in non-AIDS patients but has found little application in persons with AIDS. The fixed combination of pyrimethamine and sulfadoxine (Fansidar), which was first used in prophylaxis in the epidemic form of pneumocystosis (504), has been used in limited numbers of AIDS patients with mixed results (448-452). Toxicity considerations with this drug and other sulfonamides or sulfones are the same as those discussed under treatment. Pentamidine, administered intravenously or via aerosol, is currently receiving a lot of attention, but controlled studies have not yet been performed. Immunological approaches to *P. carinii* prophylaxis have attracted little interest. The results of active immunization in the rat model or the administration of immune plasma or serum globulin preparations in small numbers of humans have been discouraging (27,505,506).

In considering environmental preventive measures, there is solid clinical and experimental evidence to support the communicability of *P. carinii*; however, the exact risk of specific patient populations in hospital settings is a matter of debate. While official CDC guidelines indicate that isolation of *P. carinii* patients is not necessary, we and other workers feel that these patients should not be directly exposed to other immunocompromised hosts (199,254). The use of respiratory isolation precautions or a private room have been the most commonly used techniques for isolating *P. carinii* patients. The duration of isolation is arbitrary, but commonly 5-10 days of therapy has been used (427).

REFERENCES

1. Chagas, C. Nova tripanozomiaza humana. *Mem. Inst. Oswaldo Cruz 1*:159–218 (1909).
2. Carini, A. Formas de eschizogonia do *Trypanozoma lewisi. Comm. Soc. Med. Sao Paolo* Aug. 16, p. 204 (1910).
3. Delanöe, P., and Delanöe, M. Sur les rapporte des kystos de carinii le *Trypanosoma lewisi. Compt. Rend. Acad. Sci. 155*:658–660 (1912).
4. Delanöe, P., and Delanöe, M. De la rarete de *Pneumocystis carinii* chez cobayes de la region de Paris; absense de kysts chez d'autres animaus lapin, grenouille, zanguilles. *Bull. Soc. Pathol. Exot. 7*:271–274 (1914).
5. Vanek, J., and Jirovec, O. Parasitaere Pneumonie. Interstitielle plasmazellen Pneumonie der Fruehgeborenen verursacht durch *Pneumocystis carinii. Abl. Bakt. 158*:120–127 (1952).
6. Gajdusek, D. C. *Pneumocystis carinii*—etiologic agent of interstitial plasma cell pneumonia of premature and young infants. *Pediatrics 19*:543–565 (1957).
7. Sheldon, W. H. Pulmonary *Pneumocystis carinii* infection. *J. Pediatr. 61*:780–791 (1962).
8. Robbins, J. B. *Pneumocystis carinii* pneumonitis: a review. *Pediatr. Res. 1*:131–158 (1967).
9. Ivady, G., Paldy, L., Koltay, M., et al. *Pneumocystis carinii* pneumonia. *Lancet 1*:616–617 (1967).
10. Ivady, G., and Paldy, L. Treatment of *Pneumocystis carinii* pneumonia in infancy. *Natl. Cancer Inst. Monogr. 43*:201–208 (1976).
11. Dutz, W., Post, C., Vessal, K., and Kohut, E. Endemic infantile *Pneumocystis carinii* infection: the Shiraz study. *Natl. Cancer Inst. Monogr. 43*:31–38 (1976).
12. Burke, B. A., and Good, R. A. *Pneumocystis carinii* infection. *Medicine 52*:23–51 (1973).
13. Vigneault, M., and Planneton, A. Occurrence of pneumocystosis. *Can. Med. Assn. J. 101*:586–590 (1969).
14. Hyun, B. H., Varga, C. F., and Thalheimer, L. J. *Pneumocystis carinii* pneumonitis occurring in an adopted Korean infant. *JAMA 195*:784–786 (1966).
15. Redman, J. *Pneumocystis carinii* pneumonia in an adopted Vietnamese infant. *JAMA 320*:1561–1563 (1974).
16. Gleason, W. A., Roden, V. J., and DeCastro, F. *Pneumocystis carinii* in Vietnamese infants. *J. Pediatr. 87*:1001–1002 (1975).
17. Nordin, J., and Myers, M. G. *Pneumocystis carinii* in Vietnamese foundling. *Am. J. Dis. Child. 129*:1361 (1975).
18. Giebink, G. S., Sholler, L., and Keenan, T. P. *Pneumocystis carinii* pneumonia in two Vietnamese refugee infants. *Pediatrics 58*:115–118 (1976).
19. Minielly, J. A., Mills, S. D., and Holley, K. E. *Pneumocystis carinii* pneumonia. *Can. Med. Assoc. J. 100*:846–854 (1969).

20. Walzer, P. D. *Pneumocystis carinii* infection: a review. *South Med. J. 70*(11):1330–1337 (1977).
21. Easterly, J. A., and Warner, N. E. *Pneumocystis carinii* pneumonia. *Arch. Pathol. 80*:433–441 (1965).
22. Rifkind, D., Faris, T. D., and Hill, R. D. *Pneumocystis carinii* pneumonia. *Ann. Intern. Med. 65*:943–956 (1966).
23. Vogel, C. V., Cohen, M. H., Powell, R. D., et al. *Pneumocystis carinii* pneumonia. *Ann. Intern. Med. 68*:97–108 (1968).
23a. DeVita, V. T., Jr., Goodell, B., Hubbard, S., Geelhoed, G. W., and Young, R. C. Pneumocystis pneumonia in patients with cancer: clinical setting. *Natl. Cancer Inst. Monogr. 43*:41–46 (1976).
24. Gentry, L. O., Ruskin, J., and Remington, J. S. *Pneumocystis carinii* pneumonia. *Calif. Med. 116*:6–14 (1972).
25. Geelhoed, G. W., Levin, B. J., Adkins, P. C., et al. The diagnosis and management of *Pneumocystis carinii* pneumonia. *Ann. Thoracic Surg. 14*:335–346 (1972).
26. Rosen, P., Armstrong, D., and Ramos, C. *Pneumocystis carinii* pneumonia. *Am. J. Med. 53*:428–436 (1972).
27. Hughes, W. T., Prince, R. A., Kim, H. Y., Koburn, T. P., Grigsby, D., and Feldman, S. *Pneumocystsi carinii* pneumonitis in children with malignancies. *J. Pediatr. 82*:404–415 (1973).
28. Hughes, W. T., Sanyal, S. K., and Price, R. A. Signs, symptoms, and pathophysiology of *Pneumocystis carinii* pneumonitis. *Natl. Cancer. Inst. Monogr. 43*:77–84 (1976).
29. LeClair, R. A. Descriptive epidemiology of interstitial pneumocystic pneumonia. *Am. Rev. Resp. Dis. 99*:542–547 (1969).
30. LeClair, R. A. Transplantation pneumonia, associated with *Pneumocystis carinii*, among recipients of cardiac transplants. *Am. Rev. Resp. Dis. 100*: 874–875 (1969).
31. Sedaghatian, M. R., and Singer, D. B. *Pneumocystis carinii* in children with malignant disease. *Cancer 29*:772–776 (1972).
32. Stinson, E. B., Bieber, C. P., Griepp, R. B., et al. Infectious complications after cardiac transplantation in man. *Ann. Intern. Med. 74*:22–36 (1971).
33. Solberg, C. O., Meuwissen, J. H., Needham, R. N., Good, R. A., and Matsen, J. M. Infectious complications in bone marrow transplant patients. *Br. Med. J. 1*:18–23 (1971).
34. Goodell, B., Jacobs, J. B., and Powell, R. D. *Pneumocystis carinii*: the spectrum of diffuse interstitial pneumonia in patients with neoplastic diseases. *Ann. Intern. Med. 72*:337–340 (1970).
35. Rosen, P., Armstrong, D., and Ramos, C. *Pneumocystis carinii* pneumonia. *Am. J. Med. 53*:428–436 (1972).
36. DeVita, V. T., Goodell, B., Hubbard, S., Geelhoed, G. W., and Young, R. C. Pneumocystis pneumonia in patients with cancer: clinical setting. *Natl. Cancer Inst. Monogr. 43*:41–47 (1976).
37. Dutz, W. *Pneumocystis carinii* pneumonia. *Pathol. Ann. 5*:309–341 (1970).

38. Western, K. A., Perera, D. R., and Schultz, M. G. Pentamidine isethionate in the treatment of *Pneumocystis carinii* pneumonia. *Ann. Intern. Med. 73*: 695–702 (1970).

39. Walzer, P. D., Schultz, M. G., Western, K. A., and Robbins, J. B. *Pneumocystis carinii* pneumonia and primary immune deficiency diseases of infancy and childhood. *J. Pediatr. 82*:416–422 (1973).

40. Walzer, P. D., Perl, D. P., Krogstad, D. J., Rawson, P. G., and Schultz, M. G. *Pneumocystsis carinii* pneumonia in the United States: epidemiologic, clinial and diagnostic features. *Ann. Intern. Med. 80*:83–93 (1974).

41. Sheldon, W. H. Experimental pulmonary *Pneumocystis carinii* infection in rabbits. *J. Exp. Med. 110*:147–160 (1959).

42. Frenkel, J. K., and Havenhill, M. A. The corticoid sensitivity of golden hamsters, rats, and mice. *Lab Invest. 12*:1204–1220 (1963).

43. Frenkel, J. K., Good, J. T., and Schultz, J. A. Latent *Pneumocystis* infection of rats, relapse, and chemotherapy. *Lab. Invest. 15*:1559–1577 (1966).

44. Walzer, P. D. Experimental models for *Pneumocystis carinii* infection. In *Pneumocystis carinii Infections*. (L. S. Young, ed.). Marcel Dekker, New York, 1984, pp. 7–75.

45. Hughest, W. T., McNabb, P. C., and Makres, T. D. Efficacy of trimethoprim and sulfamethoxazole in the prevention and treatment of *Pneumocystis carinii* pneumonitis. *Antimicrob. Agents Chemother. 5*:289–293 (1974).

46. Hughes, W. T., Feldman, S., Chaudhary, C. C., Ossi, M. J., Cox, F., and Sanyal, S. K. Comparison of pentamidine isethionate and trimethoprim-sulfamethoxazole in treatment of *Pneumocystis carinii* pneumonia. *J. Pediatr. 92*:285–291 (1978).

47. Hughes, W. T., Kuhn, S., and Chaudhary, S. Successful chemoprophylaxis for *Pneumocystis carinii* pneumonitis. *New Engl. J. Med. 297*:1419–1426 (1977).

48. Hughes, W. T. Five-year absence of *Pneumocystis carinii* pneumonitis in a pediatric oncology center. (letter) *J. Infect. Dis. 150*:305–306 (1984).

49. Gottlieb, M. S., Schroff, R., Schanker, H. M., Weisman, J. D., Fan, P. T., Wolf, R. A., and Saxon, A. *Pneumocystis carinii* pneumonia and mucosal candidiasis in previously healthy homosexual men: evidence of a new acquired cellular immunodeficiency. *New Engl. J. Med. 305*:1425–1431 (1981).

49a. Ueda, N., Iwata, K., Tokuoka, H., Akagi, T., Ito, J., and Muzushima, M. Adult T-cell leukemia with generalized cytomegalic inclusion disease and *Pneumocystis carinii* pneumonia. *Acta Pathol. Jap. 29*:221–232 (1979).

50. Masur, H., Michelis, M. A., Greene, J. B., Onorato, I., Stouwe, R. A., Holzman, R. S., Wormser, G., Brettman, L., Lange, M., Murray, H. W., and Cunningham-Rundles, S. An outbreak of community-acquired *Pneumocystis carinii* pneumonia: initial manifestations of cellular immune dysfunction. *New Engl. J. Med. 305*:1431–1438 (1981).

51. Fauci, A. S., Macher, A. M., Lingo, D. M., Lane, H. C., Rook, A. H., Masur, H., and Gelman, E. P. Acquired immunodeficiency syndrome:

epidemiologic, clinical, immunologic, and therapeutic considerations. *Ann. Intern. Med. 100*:92–106 (1984).

52. DeVita, V. T., Broder, S., Fauci, A. S., Kovacs, J. A., and Chabner, B. A. Developmental therapeutics in the acquired immunodeficiency syndrome. *Ann. Intern. Med. 106*:568–581 (1987).

53. Niedt, G. W., and Schinella, R. A. Acquired immunodeficiency syndrome: a clinicopathologic study of 56 autopsies. *Arch. Pathol. Lab. Med. 109*:724–734 (1985).

54. Moskowitz, L., Hensley, G. T., Chan, J. C., and Adams, K. Immediate cause of death in the acquired immunodeficiency syndrome. *Arch. Pathol. Lab. Med. 109*:735–738 (1985).

55. Engelberg, L. A., Lerner, C. W., and Tapper, M. L. Clinical features of *Pneumocystis* pneumonia in the acquired immune deficiency syndrome. *Am. Rev. Resp. Dis. 130*:689–694 (1984).

56. Haverkos, H. W. Assessment of therapy for *Pneumocystis carinii* pneumonia. *Am. J. Med. 76*:501–508 (1984).

57. Kovacs, J. A., Hiemenz, J. W., Macher, A. M., Stover, D., Murray, H. W., Shelhamer, J., Lane, H. C., Urmacher, C., Honig, C., Longo, D. L., Parker, M. M., Natanson, C., Parrillo, J. E., Fauci, A. S., Pizzo, P. A., and Masur, H. *Pneumocystis carinii* pneumonia: a comparison between patients with the acquired immunodeficiency syndrome and patients with other immunodeficiencies. *Ann. Intern. Med. 100*:663–671 (1984).

58. Small, C. B., Harris, C. A., Friedland, G. H., and Klein, R. S. The treatment of *Pneumocystis carinii* pneumonia in the acquired immunodeficiency syndrome. *Arch. Intern. Med. 145*:837–840 (1985).

59. Gordin, F. M., Simon, G. L., Wofsy, C. B., et al. Adverse reactions to trimethoprim-sulfamethoxazole in patients with the acquired immunodeficiency syndrome. *Ann. Intern. Med. 100*:495–499 (1984).

60. Wachter, R. M., Luce, J. M., Turner, J. Intensive care of patients with the acquired immunodeficiency syndrome—outcome and changing patterns of utilization. *Am. Rev. Resp. Dis. 134*:891–896 (1986).

60a. Catteral, J. R., Potasman, I., and Remington, J. S. *Pneumocystis carinii* pneumonia in the patient with AIDS. *Chest 88*:758–762 (1985).

60b. Farthing, C. F., Shanson, D. C., Gazzard, B. G. The acquired immune deficiency syndrome: problems associated with the management of *Pneumocystis carinii* pneumonia. *J. Infect. 11*:103–108 (1987).

61. Mills, J. *Pneumocystis carinii* and *Toxoplasma gondii* infections in patients with AIDS. *Rev. Infect. Dis. 8*:1001–1011 (1986).

62. Wharton, J. M., Coleman, D. L., Wofsy, C. B., Luce, J. M., Blumenfeld, W., Hadley, W.K., Ingram-Drake, L., Volberding, P. A., and Hopewell, P. C. Trimethoprim-sulfamethoxazole or pentamidine for *Pneumocystis carinii* pneumonia in the acquired immunodeficiency syndrome. *Ann. Intern. Med. 105*:37–44 (1986).

63. Leoung, G. S., Mills, J., Hopewell, P. C., Hughes, W., and Wofsy, C. Dapsone-trimethoprim for *Pneumocystis carinii* pneumonia in the acquired immunodeficiency syndrome. *Ann. Intern. Med. 105*:45–48 (1986).

64. Sheldon, W. H. Subclinical pneumocystis pneumonitis. *Am. J. Dis. Child 97*: 287-297 (1959).
65. Lainson, R., and Shaw, J. J. Pneumocystis and histoplasma infections in wild animals from the Amazon region of Brazil. *Trans. R. Soc. Trop. Med. Hyg. 69*:505-508 (1975).
66. Poelma, F. G. *Pneumocystis carinii* infections in zoo animals. *Z. Parasitenkd. 46*:61-68 (1975).
67. Poelma, F. G., and Broekhuizen, S. *Pneumocystis carinii* in hares, *Lepus europaeus* Pallas, in the Netherlands. *Z. Parasitenkd. 40*:195-202 (1972).
68. Kucera, K. Exact correlation in epidemics of *Pneumocystis* pneumonia. *Folia Parasitol. 13*:343-360 (1966).
68a. Kucera, K. Le pneumocystose en tant quanthropozoonose. *Ann. Parasitol. 42*:565-581 (1967).
69. Juranek, D. D. *Pneumocystosis* (CRC Handbook Series in Zoonoses, Vol. I.) (J. S. Steele, ed.). CRC Press, Boca Raton, Fla., 1982, pp. 197-205.
70. Settnes, O. P., and Lodal, J. Prevalence of *Pneumocystis carinii* Delanoe and Delanoe 1912 in rodents in Denmark. *Nord. Vet. Med. 32*:17-27 (1980).
71. Shista, T., Kurimoto, H., and Yoshida, Y. Prevalence of *Pneumocystis carinii* in wild rodents in Japan. *Zentralbl. Bakt. Hyg. A. 261*:381-389 (1986).
71a. Matsumoto, Y. M., Yamata, T., Tegoshi, T., Yoshida, Y., Gotoh, S., Suzuki, J., and Matsubayashi, K. Pneumocystis infection in macaque monkeys. *Parasitol. Res. 73*:324-327 (1987).
72. Goyot, P., Mojon, M., and Petavy, A. F. *Arvicola ternestris*, Linnaeus 1758, a reservoir of *Pneumocystis* sp. Delanoe and Delanoe 1912. *Z. Parasitenkd. 72*:685-687 (1986).
73. Frenkel, J. K. *Pneumocystis jiroveci* n sp from man: morphology, physiology, and immunology in relation to pathology. *Natl. Cancer Inst. Monogr. 43*:13-30 (1976).
74. Barton, E. G., and Campbell, W. G. Further observations on the ultrastructure of pneumocystosis. *Arch. Pathol. 83*:527-534 (1967).
75. Barton, E. G., Jr., and Campbell, W. G., Jr. *Pneumocystis carinii* in the lungs of rats treated with cortisone acetate. Ultrastructural observations relating to the life cycle. *Am. J. Pathol. 54*:209-236 (1969).
76. Campbell, W. G. Ultrastructure of pneumocystis in human lungs: life cycle of human pneumocystosis. *Arch. Pathol. 93*:312-324 (1972).
77. Ham, E. H., Greenberg, S. D., Reynolds, R. C., and Singer, D. B. Ultrastructure of *Pneumocystis carinii* *Exp. Mol. Pathol. 14*:362-372 (1971).
78. Wang, N. S., Huang, S. W., and Thurlbeck, W. M. Combined *Pneumocystis carinii* and cytomegalovirus infection. *Arch. Pathol. 90*:529-535 (1970).
79. Price, R. A., and Hughes, W. T. Histopathology of *Pneumocystis carinii* infestation and infection in malignant disease in childhood. *Human Pathol. 5*:737-752 (1974).
80. Matsumoto, Y., and Yoshida, Y. Sporogony in *Pneumocystis carinii*: synaptonemal complexes and meiotic nuclear divisions observed in precysts. *J. Protozool. 31*:420-428 (1984).

81. Matsumoto, Y., and Yoshida, Y. Advances in *Pneumocystis* biology. *Parasitol. Today 2*:137–142 (1986).
82. Vavra, J. and Kucera, K. *Pneumocystis carinii* Delanoe, its ultrastructures and ultrastructural affinities. *J. Protozool. 17*:463–483 (1970).
83. Vossen, M. E. M. H., Beckers, P.J. A., Meuwissen, J. H. E., and Stadboulders, A. M. Developmental biology of *Pneumocystis carinii*: an alternative view on the life cycle of the parasite. *Z. Parasitenkd. 55*:101–118 (1978).
84. Haselton, P. S. A., Curry, Rankin, E. H. *Pneumocystis carinii* pneumonia: a light microscopal and ultrastructural study. *J. Clin. Pathol. 34*:1138–1146 (1981).
85. Yoneda, K., and Walzer, P. D. The interaction of *Pneumocystis carinii* with host cells: an ultrastructural study. *Infect. Immun. 29*:692–703 (1980).
86. Yoneda, K., Walzer, P. D., Richey, C. S., et al. *Pneumocystis carinii*: freeze fracture study of various stages of the organism. *Exper. Parasitol. 53*:68–76 (1982).
87. Yoneda, K., and Walzer, P. D. Attachment of *Pneumocystis carinii* to type I alveolar cells: study by freeze fracture electron microscopy. *Infect. Immun. 40*:812–815 (1983).
88. Henshaw, N. G., Carson, J. L., and Collier, A. M. Ultrastructural observations in *Pneumocystis carinii* attachment to rat lung. *J. Infect. Dis. 151*: 181–186 (1985).
89. Lanken, P. N., Minda, M., Pietra, G. G., and Fishman, A. P. Alveolar response to experimental *Pneumocystis carinii* pneumonia in the rat. *Am. J. Pathol. 99*:561–578 (1980).
90. Long, E. C., Smith, J. S., and Meier, J. L. Attachment of *Pneumocystis carinii* to rat pneumocytes. *Lab Invest. 54*:609–614 (1986).
91. Yoshida, Y., Matsumoto, Y., Yamada, M., Okabayashi, K., Yoshikawa, H., and Nakazawa, M. *Pneumocystis carinii*: electron microscopic investigation of the interation of trophozoite and alveolar lining cell. *Zbl. Bakt. Microbiol. Hyg. A 256*:390–399 (1984).
92. Takeuchi, S. Electron microscopic observation of *Pneumocystis carinii. Jap. J. Parasitol. 29*:427–453 (1980).
93. Yamada, M. Transmission-electron microscopic observations of *Pneumocystis carinii* pneumonia in nude mice. *Jap. J. Parasitol. 35*:339–353 (1986).
94. Yoshikawa, H., and Yoshida, Y. Freeze fracture studies on *Pneumocystis carinii*. I. Structural alteration of the pellicle during the development from trophozoite to cyst. *Z. Parasitenkd. 72*:463–477 (1986).
95. Yoshikawa, H., Morioka, H., and Yoshida, Y. Freeze-fracture localization of filipin-sterol complexes in plasma- and cyto-membranes of *Pneumocystis carinii. J. Protozool. 34*:131–137 (1987).
96. Yoshikawa, H., Morioka, H., and Yoshida, Y. Freeze fracture studies on *Pneumocystis carinii*. II. Fine structure of the trophozoite. *Parasitol. Res. 73*:132–139 (1987).
97. Ruffolo, J. J., Cushion, M. T., and Walzer, P. D. Microscopic techniques for studying *Pneumocystis carinii* in fresh specimens. *J. Clin. Microbiol. 23*: 17–21 (1986).

98. Heywood, P., and Magee, P. T. Meiosis in protists. Some structural and physiological aspects of meiosis in algae, fungi and protozoa. *Bacteriol. Rev. 40*:190–240 (1976).

99. Sen, S. K. Synaptonemal complexes in haploid petunia and antirrhinom sp. *Naturwissenschaften 57*:550 (1970).

100. Zickler, D. Fine structure of chromosome pairing in ten ascomycetes: meiotic and premeiotic (oritotic) synaptonemal complexes. *Chromosoma 40*:401–416 (1973).

101. Current, W. L. *Cryptosporidium* and cryptosporidiosis. In *Acquired Immune Deficiency Syndrome* (M. S. Gottleib and J. B. Groupman, eds.) Liss, New York, 1984, pp. 355–373.

102. Navin, T. R., and Juranek, D. D. Cryptosporidiosis—clinical, epidemiologic, and parasitologic review. *Rev. Infect. Dis. 6*:315–327 (1984).

103. Cushion, M. T., Ruffolo, J. M., and Walzer, P. D. Analysis of the developmental stages of *Pneumocystis carinii* in vitro. *Lab Invest. 58*:324–331 (1988).

104. Bouton, C., Kernbaum, S., Christol, D., Dinh, H. T., Vezinet, F., Gutman, L., Seman, M., and Bastin, R. Diagnostic morphologique du *Pneumocystis carinii. Pathol. Biol. 25*:153–160 (1977).

105. Lee, J. J., Hotner, S. H., and Bouee, E. C. An illustrated guide to the protozoa. Society of Protozoologists, Lawrence, Kan., 1985, p. 359.

106. Csillag, A. Contributions to the taxonomical classification of the so-called *Pneumocystis carinii. Acta Microbiol. Acad. Sci. Hung. 4*:1–8 (1957).

107. Walzer, P. D., Schnelle, V., Armstrong, D., and Rosen, P. P. The nude mouse: a new experimental model for *Pneumocystis carinii* infection. *Science 197*:177–179 (1977).

108. Hendley, J. O., and Weller, T. H. Activation and transmission in rats of infection with *Pneumocystis carinii. Proc. Soc. Exp. Biol. Med. 137*:1401–1404 (1971).

109. Hughes, W. T. Natural mode of acquisition for de novo infection with *Pneumocystis carinii. J. Infect. Dis. 145*:842–848 (1982).

110. Hughes, W. T., Bartley, D. L., and Smith, B. M. A natural source of infection due to *Pneumocystis carinii. J. Infect. Dis. 147*:595 (1983).

111. Furuta, T., Ueda, K., and Fujiwara, K. Experimental *Pneumocystis carinii* infection in nude rats. *Jap. J. Exp. Med. 54*:65–72 (1984).

112. Furuta, T., Ueda, K., Fujiwara, K., and Yamanouchi, K. Cellular and humoral immune responses of mice subclinically infected with *Pneumocystis carinii. Infect. Immun. 47*:544–548 (1985).

113. Furuta, T., Uedo, K., Kyuwa, S., and Fujiwara, K. Effect of T-cell transfer on *Pneumocystis carinii* in nude mice. *Jap. J. Exp. Med. 54*:57–64 (1984).

114. Walzer, P. D., and Powell, R. D. *Pneumocystis carinii* infection in nude and steroid treated normal mice. In *Proceedings of the Third International Workshop on Nude Mice.* (N. D. Reed, ed.). Gustav Fisher, New York, 1982, pp. 123–132.

115. Walzer, P. D. Unpublished observations.
116. Erschul, J. W., Williams, L. P., and Meighan, P. P. *Pneumocystis carinii* in hypopharyngeal material. *New Engl. J. Med. 267*:926–927 (1962).
117. Lau, W. K., Young, L. S., and Remington, J. S. *Pneumocystis carinii* pneumonia: diagnosis by examination of pulmonary secretions. *JAMA 236*:2399–2402 (1976).
118. Lim, S. K., Eveland, W. C., and Porter, R. J. Development and evaluation of a direct fluorescent antibody method for the diagnosis of *Pneumocystis carinii* pneumonitis from sputa or tracheal aspirates from humans. *Appl. Microbiol. 27*:144–149 (1974).
119. Bazaz, G. R., Manfredi, O. L., Howard, R. G., and Claps, A. S. *Pneumocystis carinii* pneumonia in three full-term siblings. *J. Pediatr. 76*:767–769 (1970).
120. Pavlica, F. The first observation of congenital pneumocystic pneumonia in a fully developed stillborn child. *Ann. Paediatr. 198*:177–184 (1962).
121. Pifer, L. L., Lattuada, C. P., Edwards, C. C., et al. *Pneumocystis carinii* in germ-free rats: implications for human patients. *Diagn. Microbiol. Infect. Dis. 2*:23 (1984).
122. Carter, T. R., Cooper, P. H., Petri, W. A., Kim, C. K., Walzer, P. D., and Guerrant, R. L. *Pneumocystis carinii* infection of the small intestine in a patient with the acquired immunodeficiency syndrome. *Am. J. Clin. Pathol.* (in press).
123. Meuwissen, J. H. E., Tauber, I., Leewenberg, A. D. E. M., Beckers, P. J. A., and Siehen, J. Parasitologic and serologic observations of infection with *Pneumocystis* in humans. *J. Infect. Dis. 136*:43–49 (1977).
124. Pifer, L. L., Hughes, W. T., Stagno, S., and Woods, D. *Pneumocystis carinii* infection: evidence for high prevalence in normal and immunosuppressed children. *Pediatrics 62*:35–41 (1978).
125. Walzer, P. D., and Rutledge, M. E. Humoral immunity in experimental *Pneumocystis carinii* pneumonia. I. Systemic and local antibody responses in rats. *J. Lab. Clin. Med. 97*:820–833 (1981).
126. Walzer, P. D., and Rutledge, M. E. Comparison of rat, mouse, and human *Pneumocystis carinii* by immunofluorescence. *J. Infect. Dis. 142*:449 (1980).
127. Walzer, P. D., and Linke, M. J. A comparison of the antigenic characteristics of rat and human *Pneumocystis carinii* by immunoblotting. *J. Immunol. 138*:2257–2265 (1987).
128. Trager, W., and Jensen, J. B. Human malaria parasites in continuous cultures. *Science 193*:673–675 (1976).
129. Divo, A. A., and Jensen, J. B. Studies on serum requirements for the cultivation of *Plasmodium falciparum*. 2. Medium enrichment. *Bull. WHO 60*(4):571–575 (1982).
130. Jensen, J. B., and Trager, W. *Plasmodium falciparum* in culture: use of outdated erythrocytes and description of the candle jar method. *J. Parasitol. 63*:883–886 (1977).

131. Current, W. L., and Haynes, T. B. Complete development of *Cryptosporidium* in cell culture. *Science 224*:603–605 (1984).
132. Pifer, L. L., Hughes, W. T., and Murphy, M. J. Propagation of *Pneumocystis carinii* in vitro. *Pediatr. Res. 11*:305–316 (1977).
133. Pifer, L. L., Woods, D., and Hughes, W. T. Propagation of *Pneumocystis carinii* in Vero cell cultures. *Infect. Immun. 20*:66–68 (1978).
134. Latorre, C. R., Sulzer , A. T., and Norman, L. G. Serial propagation of *Pneumocystis carinii* in cell line cultures. *Appl. Environ. Microbiol. 33*: 1204–1206 (1977).
135. Bartlett, M. S., Vervanac, P. A., and Smith, J. W. Cultivation of *Pneumocystis carinii* with WI-38 cells. *J. Clin. Microbiol. 10*:796–799 (1979).
136. Cushion, M. T., and Walzer, P. D. Cultivation of *Pneumocystis carinii* in lung-derived cell lines. *J. Infect. Dis. 149*:644 (1984).
137. Cushion, M. T., and Walzer, P. D. Growth and serial passage of *Pneumocystis carinii* in the A549 cell line. *Infect. Immun. 44*:245–251 (1984).
138. Cushion, M. T., Ruffolo, J. J., Linke, M. J., and Walzer, P. D. *Pneumocystis carinii*: growth variables and estimates in the A549 and WI-38 VA 13 human cell lines. *Exper. Parasitol. 60*:43–54 (1985).
139. Smith, J. W., and Bartlett, M. S. In vitro cultivation of *Pneumocystis*. In *Pneumocystis carinii Pneumonia* (L. S. Young, ed.). Marcel Dekker, New York, 1984, pp. 107–137.
140. Hay, R. J., Williams, C. D., Macy, M., and Lavappa, K. S. Cultured cell lines for research on pulmonary physiology available through the American Type Tissue Culture Collection. *Am. Rev. Resp. Dis. 125*:222–232 (1982).
141. Pesanti, E. L. IN vitro effects of antiprotozoan drugs and immune serum on *Pneumocystis carinii*. *J. Infect. Dis. 141*:755–759 (1980).
142. Pesanti, E. L., and Cox, C. Metabolic and synthetic activities of *Pneumocystis carinii* in vitro. *Infect. Immun. 34*:908–914 (1981).
143. Pifer, L. L., Pifer, D. D., and Woods, D. R. Biological profile and response to anti-pneumocystis agents of *Pneumocystis carinii* in cell culture. *Antimicrob. Agents Chemother. 24*:674–678 (1983).
144. Bartlett, M. S., Eichholtz, R., and Smith, J. W. Antimicrobial susceptibility of *Pneumocystis carinii* in culture. *Diagn. Microbiol. Infect. Dis. 3*:381–387 (1985).
145. Bartlett, M. S., Marr, J. J., Queener, S. F., Klein, R. S., and Smith, J. W. Activity of inosine analogues against *Pneumocystis carinii* in culture. *Antimicrob. Agents Chemother. 30*:181–183 (1986).
146. Cushion, M. T., Stanforth, D., Ruffolo, J. J., Linke, M. J. and Walzer, P. D. An in vitro system of testing the susceptibility of *Pneumocystis carinii* to antimicrobial agents. *Antimicrob. Agents Chemother. 28*:796–801 (1985).
147. McCann, P. P., Bacchi, C., Clarkson, A. B., Bey, P., Sjoersdma, A., Schecter, P. J., Walzer, P. D., and Barlow, J. R. Inhibition of polyamine biosynthesis by a-difluoromethylornithine in African trypanosomiasis and

Pneumocystis carinii as a basis of chemotherapy: biochemical and clinical aspects. *Am. J. Trop. Med. Hyg. 35*:1153–1156 (1986).

148. Hughes, W. T., and Smith, B. L. Efficacy of diaminodiphenylsulfone and other drugs in murine *Pneumocystis carinii* pneumonitis. *Antimicrob. Agents Chemother. 26*:436–440 (1984).

149. Walzer, P. D., Kim, C. K., Joy, J. M., Linke, M. J., and Cushion, M. T. Cationic antitrypanosomal and other antimicrobial drugs in the threatment of experimental *Pneumocystis carinii* pneumonia. *Antimicrob. Agents Chemother* (in press).

150. Pesanti, E. L. Phospholipid profile of *Pneumocystis carinii* and its interaction with alveolar type II epithelial cells. *Infect. Immun. 55*:736–74 (1987).

151. Pesanti, E. L. *Pneumocystis carinii*: oxygen uptake, antioxidant enzymes, and susceptibility to oxygen-mediated damage. *Infect. Immun. 44*:7–11 (1984).

152. Mazer, M. A., Kovacs, J. A., Swann, J. C., Parrillo, J. E., and Masur, H. Histoenzymological study of selected dehydrogenase enzymes in *Pneumocystis carinii. Infect. Immun. 55*:727–730 (1987).

153. Brzosko, W. J., Mandalinski, K., and Neweslawski, A. Fluorescent antibody and immunoelectrophoretic evaluation of the immune reaction in children with pneumonia induced by *Pneumocystis carinii. Exp. Med. Microbiol. 19*:397–405 (1967).

154. Brzosko, W. J., Madalinski, K., Crawczynski, K., and Nowoslawski, A. Immunohistochemistry in studies on the pathogenesis of pneumocystis pneumonia in infants. *Ann. NY Acad. Sci. 177*:156–170 (1971).

155. Brzosko, W. J., Krawczynski, K., Madalinski, K., and Nowoslawski, A. Immunopathologic aspects of *Pneumocystis carinii* pneumonia in infants as revealed by immunofluorescence and electron microscopy. *Natl. Cancer Inst. Monogr. 43*:163–169 (1976).

156. Ikai, T. *Pneumocystis carinii*: production of antibody either specific to trophozoite or cyst wall. *Jap. J. Parasitol. 29*:115–126 (1980).

157. Kagan, I. G., and Norman, L. N. Serology of pneumocystosis. *Natl. Cancer Inst. Monogr. 43*:121–125 (1976).

158. Kim, H. K., Hughes, W. T., and Feldman, S. Studies of morphology and immunofluorescence of *Pneumocystis carinii. Proc. Soc. Exp. Biol. Med. 141*:304–309 (1972).

159. Libertin, C. R., Woloschak, G. E., Wilson, W. R., and Smith, T. F. Analysis of *Pneumocystis carinii* cysts with a fluorescence-activated cell sorter. *J. Clin. Microbiol. 20*:877–880 (1984).

160. Lim, S. K., Eveland, W. C., and Porter, R. J. Development and evaluation of a direct fluorescent antibody method for the diagnosis of *Pneumocystis carinii* infections in experimental animals. *Appl. Microbiol. 26*:666–671 (1973).

161. Lim, S. K., Jones, R. H., and Eveland, W. C. Fluorescent antibody studies in experimental *Pneumocystis. Proc. Soc. Exp. Biol. Med. 136*:675–679 (1971).

162. Meuwissen, J., Leeuwenberg, A., and Heeren, J. New method for study of infections with *Pneumocystis carinii*. *J. Infect. Dis. 127*:209–210 (1973).

163. Meuwissen, J. H. Infections with *Pneumocystis carinii*. *Natl. Cancer Inst. Monogr. 43*:133–136 (1976).

164. Minielly, J. A., McDuffie, F. C., and Holley, K. E. Immunofluorescent identification of *Pneumocystis carinii*. *Arch. Pathol. 90*:561–566 (1979).

165. Norman, L., and Kagan, I. G. A preliminary report of an indirect fluorescent antibody test for detecting antibodies to cysts of *Pneumocystis carinii* in human sera. *Am. J. Clin. Pathol. 58*:170–176 (1972).

166. Norman, L., and Kagan, I. G. Some observations on the serology of *Pneumocystis carinii* infections in the United States. *Infect. Immun. 8*:317–321 (1973).

167. Walzer, P. D., Rutledge, M. E., and Yoneda, K. A new method of separating *Pneumocystic carinii* from infected lung tissue. *Exp. Parasitol. 47*:356–368 (1979).

168. Milder, J. E., Walzer, P. D., Coonrod, J. D., and Rutledge, M. E. Comparison of histological and immunological techniques for detection of *Pneumocystis carinii* in rat bronchial lavage fluid. *J. Clin. Microbiol. 11*:409–417 (1980).

169. Stahr, B., Walzer, P. D., and Yoneda, K. Effect of proteolytic enzymes on *Pneumocystis carinii* in rat lung tissue. *J. Parasitol. 67*:196–203 (1981).

170. Walzer, P. D., and Rutledge, M. E. Serum antibody responses to *Pneumocystis carinii* among different strains of normal and athymic (nude) mice. *Infect. Immun. 35*:620–626 (1982).

171. Walzer, P. D., Rutledge, M. E., and Yoneda, K. Experimental *Pneumocystis carinii* pneumonia in C3H/HeJ and C3HeB/FeJ mice. *J. Reitculoendothel. Sox. 33*:1–9 (1983).

172. Reinhardt, D., Kaplan, W., and Chandler, F. W. Morphologic resemblance of zygomycete spores to *Pneumocystis carinii* cysts in tissue. *Am. Rev. Resp. Dis. 115*:170–172 (1977).

173. Shepherd, V. B., Jameson, B., and Knowles, G. K. *Pneumocystis carinii* pneumonitis: a serological study. *J. Clin. Pathol. 32*:773–777 (1979).

174. Jameson, B. Serology of *Pneumocystis carinii*. In *Pneumocystis carinii Pneumonia* (L. S. Young, ed.). Marcel Dekker, New York, 1984, pp. 97–106.

175. Gradus, M. S., and Ivey, M. H. An improved method of isolating *Pneumocystis carinii* from infected rat lungs. *J. Parasitol. 72*:690–698 (1986).

176. Trull, A. K., Warren, R. E., and Thiru, S. Novel immunofluorescent test for *Pneumocystis carinii*. *Lancet 1*:271 (1986).

177. Ghali, V. S., Garcia, R. L., and Skolom, J. Fluorescence of *Pneumocystis carinii* in Papanicolaou smears. *Hum. Pathol. 15*:907–909 (1984).

178. Gigliotti, F., Stokes, D. D., Cheatham, A. B., Davis, D. S., and Hughes, W. T. Development of monoclonal antibodies to *Pneumocystis carinii*. *J. Infect. Dis. 154*:315–322 (1986).

179. Kovacs, J. A., Swann, J. C., Shelhamer, J., Gill, V., Ognibene, F., Parillo, J. E., and Masur, H. Prospective evaluation of a monoclonal antibody in diagnosis of *Pneumocystis carinii* pneumonia. *Lancet 2*:1-3 (1986).
180. Matsumoto, Y., Amayai, T., Yamada, M., Imanishi, J., and Yoshida, Y. Production of a monoclonal antibody with specificity for the pellicle of *Pneumocystis carinii* by hybridoma. *Parasitol. Res. 73*:228-233 (1987).
181. Walzer, P. D., Stanforth, D., Linke, M. J., and Cushion, M. T. *Pneumocystis carinii*: immunoblotting and immunofluorescent analysis of serum antibodies during rat infection and recovery. *Exper. Parasitol. 6*:319-328 (1987).
182. Levin, M., McLeod, R., Young, Q., Abrahams, C., Chambliss, M., Walzer, P. D., and Kabins, S. A. Pneumocystis pneumonia: importance of a gallium scan for early diagnosis and description of a new peroxidase techniques to demonstrate *Pneumocystis carinii. Am. Rev. Resp. Dis. 128*:182-185 (1983).
183. Lee, C. H., Bolinger, C. D., Bartlett, M. S., Kohler, R. B., Wilde, C. E., and Smith, J. W. Production of monoclonal antibody against *Pneumocystis carinii* by using a hybrid of rat spleen and mouse myeloma cells. *J. Clin. Microbiol, 23*:505-508 (1986).
184. Maddison, S. E., Hayes, G. W., Ivey, M. H., et al. Fractionation of *Pneumocystis carinii* antigens used in an enzyme-linked immunosorbent assay for antibodies and in the production of antiserum for detecting *Pneumocystis carinii* antigenemia. *J. Clin. Microbiol. 15*:1029-1035 (1982).
185. Maddison, S. E., Hayes, G. V., Slemenda, S. B., Norman, L. G., and Ivey, M. H. Detection of specific antibody by enzyme-linked immunsorbent assay and antigenemia by counterimmunoelectrophoresis in humans infected with *Pneumocystis carinii. J. Clin. Microbiol. 15*:1036-1043 (1982).
186. Leggiadro, R. J., Yolken, R. H., Simkins, J. H., and Hughes, W. T. Measurement of *Pneumocystis carinii* antigen by enzyme immunoassay. *J. Infect. Dis. 144*:484 (1981).
187. Furuta, T., Fujiwara, K., and Yamanouchi, K. Detection of antibodies to *Pneumocystis carinii* by enzyme-linked immunosorbent in experimentally infected mice. *J. Parasitol. 71*:522-523 (1985).
188. Graves, D. C., McNabb, S. J., Ivey, M. H., and Worley, M. A. Development and characterization of monoclonal antibodies to *Pneumocystis carinii. Infect. Immun. 51*:125-133 (1986).
189. Graves, D. C., McNabb, S. J., Whorley, M. A., Downs, J. D., and Ivey, M. H. Analysis of rat *Pneumocystis carinii* antigens recognized using Western immunoblotting. *Infect. Immun. 54*:96-103 (1986).
190. Radulescu, S., Niculeseu, D., Petrasincu, D., Lazar, L., Butnariu, J., Baciu, M. C., Buttucea, L. V., and Maneseu, V. Evaluation of enzyme linked immunosorbent assay as a serodiagnostic tool–clinical and epidemiological aspects of pneumocystosis in young infants. *Arch. Roun. Path. Exp. Microbiol. 45*:117-128 (1986).

191. Pifer, L. L., Neill, H. B., Langdon, S., Baltz, S., Clark, S. F., and Edwards, C. C. Evidence for depressed humoral immunity to *Pneumocystis carinii* antigens in homosexual males, commercial plasma donors, and in patients with the acquired immunodeficiency syndrome. *J. Clin. Microbiol. 25*: 991–995 (1987).

192. Cushion, M. T., DeStefano, J., and Walzer, P. D. Surface carbohydrates of *Pneumocystis carinii* detected by fluoresceinated lectin probes. *Exp. Parasitol.* (in press).

193. Walzer, P. D. Attachment of microorganisms to host cells: relevance of *Pneumocystis carinii. Lab. Invest. 54*:589–592 (1986).

194. Murphy, M. J., Pifer, L. L., and Hughes, W. T. *Pneumocystis carinii* in vitro. *Am. J. Pathol. 88*:387–402 (1977).

195. Yoneda, K., and Walzer, P. D. The effect of corticosteroid treatment on the cell surface glycocalyx of the rat pulmonary alveolus: relevance to the host–parasite relationship in *Pneumocystis carinii* infection. *Br. J. Exper. Pathol. 65*:347–354 (1984).

196. Farthing, M. J. G., Pereira, M. E. A., and Keusch, G. T. Description and characterization of a surface lectin from *Giardia lamblia. Infect. Immun. 51*:661–667 (1986).

197. Ravdin, J. I., Murphy, C. F., Salata, R. A., Guerrant, R. L., and Hewlett, E. L. The *N*-acetyl-*D*galactosamine inhibitable adherence lectin of *Entamoeba histolytica*. I. Partial purification and relationships to amebic *in vitro* virulence. *J. Infect. Dis. 151*:804–815 (1985).

198. Barondes, S. H. Lectins in cellular slime molds. In *The Lectins. Properties, Functions and Applications in Biology and Medicine.* (I. E. Liener, N. Sharon, and I. J. Goldstein, eds.). Academic Press, New York, 1986, pp. 467–491.

199. Giron, J. A., Martinez, S., and Walzer, P. D. Should inpatients with *Pneumocystis carinii* be isolated? *Lancet, 2*:46 (1982).

200. Rankin, J. A., Walzer, P. D., Dwyer, J. M., Schraeder, C. E., Enriquez, R., and Merrill, W. W. Immunologic alterations in bronchoalveolar lavage fluid in the acquired immune deficiency syndrome (AIDS). *Am. Rev. Resp. Dis. 128*:189–194 (1983).

201. Maddison, S. E., Walls, K. W., Haverkos, H. W., and Juranek, D. D. Evaluation of serologic tests for *Pneumocystis carinii* antibody and antigenemia in patients with acquired immunodeficiency syndrome. *Diagn. Microbiol. Infect. Dis. 2*:69 (1984).

202. Hofmann, B., Odum, N., Platz, P., Ryder, L. P., Svejgaard, A., Nielsen, P. B., Holten-Adnersen, W., Gerstoft, J., Nielsen, J. O., and Mojon, M. Humoral responses to *Pneumocystis carinii* in patients with acquired immunodeficeincy syndrome and in immunocompromised homosexual men. *J. Infect. Dis. 152*:838–840 (1985).

203. Masur, H., and Jones, T. C. The interaction in vitro of *Pneumocystis carinii* with macrophages and L cells. *J. Exp. Med. 147*:157–170 (1978).

204. Burke, B. A., Krovetz, L. J., and Good, R. A. Occurrence of *Pneumocystis*

carinii pneumonia in children with agammaglobulinemia. *Pediatrics 28*: 196–205 (1961).

205. Leggiardro, R. J., Winkelstein, J. A., and Hughes, W. T. Prevalence of *Pneumocystis carinii* pneumonitis in severe combined immunodeficiency. *J. Pediatr. 99*:96–98 (1981).
206. Saulsbury, F. T., Bernstein, M. T., and Winkelstein, J. A. *Pneumocystis carinii* pneumonia as the presenting infection in congenital hypogammaglobulinemia. *J. Pediatr. 95*:559–561 (1979).
207. Herrod, H. G., Valenski, W. R., Woods, D. R., and Pifer, L. L. The in vitro response of human lymphocytes to *Pneumocystis carinii* antigen. *J. Immunol. 126*:59–61 (1981).
208. Walzer, P. D. Pneumocystosis. In *Tropical and Geographic Medicine* (K. S. Warren and A. A. F. Mahmoud, eds.). McGraw-Hill, New York, 1983, pp. 293–298.
209. Slade, J. D., and Hepburn, B. Prednisone-induced alterations of circulating human lymphocyte subsets. *J. Lab. Clin. Med. 101*:479–487 (1983).
210. Ten Berge, R. J. M., Sauerwein, H. P., Young, S. L., and Schellekens, P. T. L. A. Administration of presdisolone in vivo affects the ratio of OKT4/OKT8 and the LDH-isoenzyme pattern of human T lymphocytes. *Clin. Immunol. Immunopathol. 30*:91–103 (1984).
211. Fauci, A. S., Dale, D. C., and Balow, J. E. Corticosteroid therapy: mechanisms of action and clinical consideration. *Ann. Intern. Med. 84*:304–315 (1976).
212. Anthony, L. B., and Greco, F. A. *Pneumocystis carinii* pneumonia: complication of Cushing's syndrome. *Ann. Intern. Med. 94*:488–489 (1981).
213. Fulkerson, W. J., and Newman, J. H. Endogenous Cushing's syndrome complicated by *Pneumocystis carinii* pneumonia. *Am. Rev. Resp. Dis. 129*:188–189 (1984).
214. Graham, B. S., and Tucker, W. S. Opportunistic infections in endogenous Cushing's syndrome. *Ann. Intern. Med. 101*:334–338 (1984).
215. Young, L. S. Clinical aspects of pneymocystosis in man: epidemiology, Clinical manifestations, diagnostic approaches, and sequelae. In *Pneumocystis carinii Pneumonia* (L. S. Young, ed.). Marcel Dekker, New York, 1984, pp. 139–174.
216. Browne, M. T., Hubbard, S. M., Longo, D. L., Fisher, R., Wesley, R., Ihde, D. H., and Pizzo, P. A. Excess prevalence of *Pneumocystis carinii* pneumonia in patients treated for lymphoma with combination chemotherapy. *Ann. Intern. Med. 104*:338–344 (1986).
217. Miller, J. J., Williams, G. F., and Leissring, J. D. Multiple late complications of therapy with cyclophosphamide, including ovarian destruction. *Am. J. Med. 50*:530–535 (1971).
218. Perruquet, J. L., Harrington, T. M., and Davis, D. E. *Pneumocystis carinii* pneumonia following methotrexate therapy for rheumatoid arthritis. *Arthritis Rheum. 26*:1291–1292 (1983).
219. Hardy, A. M., Wajszcuk, C. P., Suffredini, A. F., Hakala, T. R., and Ho, M.

Pneumocystis carinii pneumonia in renal transplant patients. *J. Infect. Dis. 149*:143–147 (1984).

220. Ballardie, F. W., Winearls, C., Cohen, J., Carr, D. H., Rees, A. J., and Williams, G. *Pneumocystis carinii* pneumonia in renal transplant recipients–clinical and radiologic features, diagnosis and treatment. *Quart. J. Med. 57*:729–747 (1986).

221. The Canadian Multicentre Transplant Study Group. A randomized clinical trial of cyclosporine in cadaveric renal transplantation: analysis at three years. *New Engl. J. Med. 314*:1219–1225 (1986).

222. Ballardie, F. W., Winearls, C. G., and Williams, G. Cyclosoprin and steroids in renal transplantation: risk of *Pneumocystis carinii* pneumonia. *Lancet 2*:638–639 (1984).

223. Dutz, W., and Burke, B. A. Cytologic diagnosis of *Pneumocystis carinii. Natl. Cancer Inst. Monogr. 43*:157–161 (1976).

224. Kay, H. E., Watson, J. G., Jameson, B., Morgenstern, G. R., and Powles, R. L. Infections in bone marrow transplantation using cyclosporine. *Transplantation 36*:491–495 (1983).

225. Busuttil, R. W., Goldstein, L. I., Danovitch, G. M., Ament, M. E., and Memsic, L. D. Liver transplantation today. *Ann. Intern. Med. 104*:377–389 (1986).

226. Hofflin, J. M., Potasman, I., Baldwin, J. C., Oyer, P. E., Stinson, E. B., and Remington, J. M. Infectious complications in heat transplant recipients receiving cyclosporine and corticosteroids. *Ann. Intern. Med. 106*:209–216 (1987).

227. Chandra, R. K. Cell-mediated immunity in nutritional imbalance. *Fed. Proc. 39*:3088–3092 (1980).

228. Gleason, W. A., Jr., and Roodman, S. T. Reversible T cell depression in malnourished infants with *Pneumocystis* pneumonia. *J. Pediatr. 90*:1032–1033 (1977).

229. Hughes, W. T., Price, R. A., Sisko, F., Havron, W. S., Kefatos, A. G., Schonland, M., and Smythe, P. M. Protein calorie malnutrition: a host determinant for *Pneumocystis carinii* infection. *Am. J. Dis. Child. 128*:44–52 (1974).

230. Masur, H. The compromised host: AIDS and other diseases. This volume, Chap. 1.

231. Hagler, D. N., Deepe, G. S., and Walzer, P. D. Blastogenic responses to *Pneumocystis carinii* among HIV patients. (submitted)

232. Di George, A. M. Congenital absence of the thymus and its immunological consequences: occurrence with congenital hypoparathyroidism. *Birth Defects 4*:116–123 (1968).

233. Wiedemann, H. P., McGuire, J., Dwyer, J. M., Sabetta, J., Gee, J. B. L., Smith, G. J. W., and Loke, J. Progressive immune failure in dyskeratosis congenita. Report of an adult in whom *Pneumocystis carinii* and fatal disseminated candidiasis developed. *Arch. Intern. Med. 144*:397–399 (1984).

234. Hughes, W. T., and Smith, B. Provocation of infection due to *Pneumocystis carinii* by cyclosporin A. *J. Infect. Dis. 145*:767 (1982).
235. Walzer, P. D., Powell, R. D., Yoneda, K., Rutledge, M. E., and Milder, J. E. Growth characteristics and pathogenesis of experimental *Pneumocystis carinii* pneumonia. *Infect. Immun. 27*:929–937 (1980).
236. Walzer, P. D., LaBine, M., Redington, T. J., and Cushion, M. T. Lymphocyte changes during chronic administration and withdrawal of corticosteroids: relevance to *Pneumocystis carinii* pneumonia. *J. Immunol. 133*: 2502–2508 (1984).
237. Walzer, P. D., LaBine, M., Redington, T. J., and Cushion, M. T. Predisposing factors in *Pneumocystis carinii* pneumonia: effects of tetracycline, protein malnutrition, and corticosteroids on the host. *Infect. Immun. 46*: 747–753 (1984).
238. Claman, H. N. Corticosteroids and lymphoid cells. *New Engl. J. Med. 287*: 388–397 (1972).
239. Vohra, H., Mahajan, R. C., Ganguly, N. K., and Sharma, B. K. Assay of plaque forming cells during infection with *Pneumocystis carinii. Indian J. Med. Res. 79*:604–609 (1984).
240. Vohra, H., Mahajan, R. C., Ganguly, N. K., and Sharma, B. K. Profile of lymphocyte number and function during experimental *Pneumocystis carinii* infection in rats. *Indian J. Med. Microbiol. 4*:181–189 (1986).
241. Masur, H. Inreraction between *Pneumocystis carinii* and phagocytic cells. In *Pneumocystis carinii Pneumonia* (L. S. Young, ed.). Marcel Dekker, New York, 1984, pp. 77–95.
242. Von Behren, L. A., and Pesanti, E. L. Uptake and degradation of *Pneumocystis carinii* by macrophages in vitro. *Am. Rev. Resp. Dis. 118*:1051–1059 (1978).
243. Masur, H., Murray, H. W., and Jones, T. C. Effect of hydrocortisone on macrophage response to lymphokine. *Infect. Immun. 35*:709 (1982).
244. Adinoff, A. D., Johnston, R. B., Dolen, S., and South, M. A. Chronic granulomatous disease and *Pneumocystis carinii* pneumonia. *Pediatrics 69*: 133 (1982).
245. Pedersen, F. K., Johansen, K. S., Rosenkvist, J., Tygstrup, I., and Valerius, N. H. Refractory *Pneumocystis carinii* infection in chronic granulomatous disease: successful treatment with granulocytes. *Pediatrics 64*:935–938 (1979).
246. Pesanti, E. L. Effects of bacterial pneumonitis on development of pneumocystosis in rats. *Am. Rev. Resp. Dis. 125*:723–726 (1982).
247. Easterly, J. A. *Pneumocystis carinii* in lungs of adults at autopsy. *Am. Rev. Resp. Dis. 94*:935–937 (1968).
248. Hamlin, W. A. *Pneumocystis carinii. JAMA 204*:173–174 (1968).
249. Sedaghatian, M. R., and Singer, D. B. *Pneumocystis carinii* in children with malignant disease. *Cancer 29*:772–776 (1972).
250. Perera, D. R., Western, K. A., Johnson, H. D., et al. *Pneumocysis carinii* pneumonia in a hospital for children. *JAMA 214*:1074–1078 (1970).

251. Hughes, W. T., Feldman, S., Aur, R. J. A., et al. Intensity of immunosuppressive therapy and the incidence of *Pneumocystis carinii* pneumonitis. *Cancer 36*:2004–2009 (1975).

252. Chusid, M. J., and Heyrman, K. A. An outbreak of *Pneumocystis carinii* pneumonia at a pediatric hospital. *Pediatrics 62*:1031–1035 (1978).

253. Cox, F., Allen, R., and Long, W., Jr. Pneumocystis pneumonia in hospitals: outbreaks or improved recognition? *South. Med. J. 73*:1566–1567 (1980).

254. Singer, C., Armstrong, D., Rosen, P. P., and Schottenfeld, D. *Pneumocystis carinii* pneumonia: a cluster of eleven cases. *Ann. Intern. Med. 82*:772–777 (1975).

255. Ruebush, T. K., Weinstein, R. A., Bachner, R. L., Wolff, D., Bartlett, M., Gonzales-Crussi, F., Silzer, A. J., and Schultz, M. G. An outbreak of pneumocystis pneumonia in children with acute leukemia. *Am. J. Dis. Child. 132*:143–148 (1978).

256. Ruskin, J., and Remington, J. S. The compromised host and infection. *JAMA 202*:1070–1074 (1967).

257. Brazinsky, J. H., and Phillips, J. E. Pneumocystis pneumonia transmission between patients with lymphoma. *JAMA 209*:1527 (1969).

258. Watanabe, J. M., Chinchinian, H., and Weitz, C. *Pneumocystis carinii* pneumonia in a family. *JAMA 193*:685–686 (1965).

259. Yates, J. W., Ellison, R. R., and Plager, J. *Pneumocystis carinii* in a husband and wife. *Lancet 2*:610 (1975).

260. Walzer, P. D., and Young, L. S. The clinical relevance of animal models of *Pneumocystis carinii* pneumonia. *Diag. Microbiol. Infect. Dis. 2*:1–6 (1984).

261. Kim, C. K., Foy, J. M., Cushion, M. T., Stanforth, D., Linke, M. J., Hendrix, H. L., and Walzer, P. D. A comparison of histologic and quantitative techniques in the evaluation of experimental *Pneumocystis carinii* pneumonia. *Antimicrob. Agents Chemother. 31*:197–201 (1987).

262. Yoneda, K., and Walzer, P. D. Mechanism of alveolar injury in experimental *Pneumocystis carinii* pneumonia in the rat. *Br. J. Exp. Pathol. 62*: 339–346 (1981).

263. Kernbaum, S., Masliah, J., Alcindor, L. G., Bouton, C., and Christol, D. Phospholipase activities of bronchoalveolar lavage fluid in rat *Pneumocystis carinii* pneumonia. *Br. J. Exp. Pathol. 64*:75–80 (1983).

264. Brun-Pascaud, M., Pocidalo, J. J., and Kernbaum, S. Respiratory and pulmonary alterations in experimental *Pneumocystis carinii* pneumonia in rats. *Bull. Eur. Physiopathol. Resp. 21*37–41 (1985).

265. Stokes, D. C., Hughes, W. T., Alderson, P. O., King, R. E., and Garfinkel, D. J. Lung mechanisms, radiography and ^{67}Ga scintigraphy in experimental *Pneumocystis carinii* pneumonia. *Br. J. Exp. Pathol. 67*:383–393 (1986).

266. Sheehan, P. M., Stokes, D. C., Yeh, Y., and Hughes, W. T. Surfactant phospholipids and lavage phospholipase A^2 in experimental *Pneumocystis carinii* pneumonia. *Am. Rev. Resp. Dis. 134*:526–531 (1986).

267. Adamson, I. Y. R., and Bowden, P. H. The pathogenesis of bleomycin induced pulmonary fibrosis in mice. *Am. J. Pathol. 77*:85 (1974).
268. Evans, M. J., Cabla, L. J., Stephens, R. J., and Freeman, G. Renewal of alveolar epithelium in the rat following exposure to NO₂. *Am. J. Pathol. 70*:175–190 (1973).
269. Gail, D. B., and Lenfant, C. J. M. Cells of the lung: biology and clinical implications. *Am. Rev. Resp. Dis. 127*:366–387 (1983).
270. Hughes, W. T. Limited effect of trimethoprim sulfamethoxazole prophylaxis on *Pneumocystis carinii. Antimicrob. Agents Chemother. 16*: 333–335 (1979).
271. Walzer, P. D., Powell, R. D., and Yoneda, K. *Pneumocystis carinii* pneumonia in different strains of cortisonized mice. *Infect. Immun. 24*:939–947 (1979).
272. Sheldon, W. H. Experimental pulmonary *Pneumocystis carinii* infection in rabbits. *J. Exp. Med. 110*:147–160 (1959).
273. Yoshida, Y., Yamada, M., Shiota, T., et al. Provocation experiment: *Pneumocystis carinii* in several kinds of animals. *Zbl. Bakt. Microbiol. Hyg., I. Abt. Orig. A 250*:206–212 (1981).
274. Farrow, B. R. H., Watson, A. D. J., and Hartley, W. J. Pneumocystis pneumonia in the dog. *J. Comp. Pathol. 82*:447–453 (1972).
275. Ueda, K., Goto, Y., Yamazaki, S., and Fujiwara, K. Chronic fatal pneumocystosis in nude mice. *Jap. J. Exp. Med. 47*:475–482 (1977).
276. Weir, E., Brownstein, D. G., and Barthold, S. W. Spontaenous wasting disease in nude mice associated with *Pneumocystis carinii* infection. *Lab. Animal Sci. 36*:140–144 (1986).
277. Walzer, P. D., Kim, C. K., Linke, M. J., Pogue, C., Chrisp, C., Huerkamp, W. J., Wixson, S. K., Levro, A. V., and Shultz, L. D. Outbreaks of *Pneumocystis carinii* pneumonia in colonies of immunodeficient mice (submitted).
278. McConnel, E. E., Basson, P. A., and Pienaar, J. C. Pneumocystosis in a domestic goat. *Onderstepoort J. Vet. Res. 38*:117–126 (1971).
279. Shively, J. N., Dellers, R. W., Buergelt, C. D., Hsu, F. S., Kabelac, L. P., Moe, K. K., Tennant, B., and Vaughn, J. T. *Pneumocystis carinii* pneumonia in two foals. *J. Am. Vet. Med. 162*:648–652 (1973).
280. Shivley, J. N., Moe, K. K., and Dellers, R. W. Fine structure of spontaneous *Pneumocystis carinii* pulmonary infection in foals. *Cornell Vet. 64*: 72–88 (1974).
281. Long, G. G., White, J. D., and Stookey, J. L. *Pneumocystis carinii* infection in splenectomized owl monkeys. *J. Am. Vet. Med. Assoc. 167*:651–654 (1975).
282. Chandler, F. W., McClure, H. M., and Campbell, W. G. Pulmonary *Pneumocystis* in nonhuman primates. *Arch. Pathol. Lab. Med. 100*:163–167 (1976).
283. Hagler, D. N., Kim, C. K., and Walzer, P. D. Feline leukemia virus and *Pneumocystis carinii* infection. *J. Parasitol. 73*:1284–1286 (1987).

284. LeGolvan, D. P., and Heidelberger, K. Disseminated granulomatous *Pneumocystis carinii* pneumonia. *Arch. Pathol. 95*:344–348 (1973).

285. Cross, A. S., and Steigbiegel, R. T. *Pneumocystis carinii* pneumonia presenting as localized nodular densities. *New Engl. J. Med. 291*:831–832 (1974).

286. Hartz, J. W., Geisinger, K. R., Scharyj, M., and Muss, H. B. Granulomatous pneumocystosis presenting as solitary pulmonary nodule. *Arch. Pathol. Lab. Med. 109*:466–469 (1985).

287. Bier, S. *Pneumocystis carinii* presenting as a single pulmonary nodule. *Pediatr. Radiol. 15*:59–60 (1986).

288. Barrio, J. L., Manuel, S., Rodriguez, J. L., Saldana, M. J., and Pitchenik, A. E. *Pneumocystis carinii* pneumonia presenting as cavitating and noncavitating solitary pulmonary nodules in patients with the acquired immunodeficiency syndrome. *Am Rev. Resp. Dis. 134*:1094–1096 (1986).

289. Eng., R. H., Bishburg, E., and Smith, S. M. Evidence for destruction of lung tissues during *Pneumocystis carinii* infection. *Arch. Intern. Med. 147*: 746–749 (1987).

290. Cruickshank, B. Pulmonary granulomatous pneumocystosis following renal transplantation. *Am. J. Clin. Pathol. 63*:384–390 (1975).

291. Burke, B. A., and Good, R. A. *Pneumocystis carinii* infection. *Medicine 52*:23–51 (1973).

292. Askin, F. B., and Katzenstein, A. L. Pneumocystis infection masquerading as diffuse alveolar damage: a potential source of diagnostic error. *Chest 79*:420–422 (1981).

293. Weber, W. R., Askin, F. B., and Dehner, L. P. Lung biopsy in *Pneumocystis carinii* pneumonia: a study of typical and atypical features. *Am. J. Clin. Pathol. 67*:11–19 (1977).

294. Gottschall, J. I., Walzer, P. D., and Yoneda, K. Morphological changes in the rat type II pneumocytes induced by oxytetracycline. *Lab Invest. 41*: 5–12 (1979).

295. Churukian, C. J., and Schenk, E. A. Rapid Grocott's methenamine-silver nitrate method for fungi and *Pneumocystis carinii*. *Am. J. Clin. Pathol. 68*: 428–428 (1977).

296. Musto, L., Flanigan, M., and Elbadawi, A. Ten-minute silver stain for *Pneumocystis carinii* and fungi in tissue sections. *Arch. Pathol. Lab. Med. 106*:292–294 (1982).

297. Pintozzi, R. L. Technical methods—modified Grocott's methenamine–silver nitrate method for quick staining of *Pneumocystis carinii*. *J. Clin. Pathol. 31*:803–805 (1978).

298. Smith, J. W., and Hughes, W. T. A rapid staining technique for *Pneumocystis carinii*. *J. Clin. Pathol. 25*:269–271 (1972).

299. Senba, M. A reliable silver staining method for identification of *Pneumocystis carinii* in histologic sections. *Tohoku J. Exp. Med. 143*:397–404 (1984).

300. Shimono, L. H., and Hartman, B. A simple and reliable rapid methenamine

silver stain for *Pneumocystis carinii* and fungi. *Arch. Pathol. Lab. Med. 100*:855–856 (1986).
301. Bush, J. B., and Markus, M. B. Diagnosis of *Pneumocystis carinii* pneumonia by various staining methods. *S. Afr. J. Sci. 82*:577–579 (1986).
302. Waldrop. F. S., Younker, T. D., and Puchtler, H. Histochemical observations on *Pneumocystis carinii*: selective demonstration of honeycomb forms. *Histochemistry 63*:1–6 (1979).
303. Bowling, M. C., Smith, I. M., and Wescott, S. L. A rapid staining procedure for *Pneumocystis carinii. Am. J. Med. Technol. 39*:267–268 (1973).
304. Charlvardjian, A. M., and Grawe, L. A. A new procedure for the identification of *Pneumocystis carinii* in tissue sections and smears. *J. Clin. Pathol. 16*:383–385 (1963).
305. Kim, H. K., and Hughes, W. Comparison of methods for identification of *Pneumocystis carinii* in pulmonary aspirates. *Am. J. Clin. Pathol. 60*:462–466 (1973).
306. Gosey, L. L., Howard, R. M., Witebsky, F. G., Ognibene, F. P., Wu, T. C., Gill, V. J., and MacLowry, J. D. Advantages of a modified toluidine blue O stain and bronchoalveolar lavage for the diagnosis of *Pneumocystis carinii* pneumonia. *J. Clin. Microbiol. 22*:803–807 (1985).
307. Rosen, P. P., Martini, N., and Armstrong, D. *Pneumocystis carinii* pneumonia: diagnosis by lung biopsy. *Am. J. Med. 58*:794–801 (1975).
308. Bouton, C., Kernbaum, S., Christol, D., Dinh, H. T., Vezinet, F., Gutman, L., Seman, M., and Bastin, R. Diagnostic morphologique du *Pneumocystis carinii. Pathol. Biol. 25*:153–160 (1977).
309. Watts, J. C., and Chandler, F. W. *Pneumocystis carinii* pneumonitis. *Am. J. Surg. Pathol. 10*:744–751 (1985).
310. Hughes, W. T. Current status of laboratory diagnosis of *Pneumocystis carinii. Crit. Rev. Clin. Lab. Sci. 6*:145–170 (1975).
311. Pintozzi, R. L., Blecka, L. J., and Nanos, S. The morphologic identification of *Pneumocystis carinii. Acta. Cytol. (Baltimore) 23*:35–39 (1979).
312. Smith, J. W., and Bartlett, M. S. Laboratory diagnosis of *Pneumocystis carinii* infection. *Clin. Lab. Med. 2*:393–406 (1982).
313. Macher, A. M., Shelhamer, J., Maclowry, J., Parker, M., and Masur, H. *Pneumocystis carinii* identified by gram stain of lung imprints. *Ann. Intern. Med. 99*:484–485 (1983).
314. Felegie, T. P., Pasculle, A. W., and Dekker, A. Recognition of *Pneumocystis carinii* by gram stain in impression smears of lung tissue. *J. Clin. Microbiol. 20*:1190–1191 (1984).
315. Domingo, J., and Waksa, H. W. Wright's stain in rapid diagnosis of *Pneumocystis carinii. Am. J. Clin. Pathol. 81*:511–514 (1984).
316. Rankin, J. A., and Young, K. R. Gram staining of *Pneumocystis* sporozoites. *Ann. Intern. Med. ?*:919 (1985).
317. Greaves, T. S., and Strigle, S. M. The recognition of *Pneumocystis carinii* in routine Papanicolaou-stained smears. *Acta Cytol. 29*:714–20 (1985).
318. Fleury, J., Escudier, E., Pocholle, M. J., Carre, C., and Bernaudin, J. F. Cell

population obtained by bronchoalveolar lavage in *Pneumocystis carinii* pneumonitis. *Acta Cytol. 29*:721–726 (1985).

319. Orenstein, M., Webber, C. A., and Heurich, A. E. Cytologic diagnosis of *Pneumocystis carinii* infection by bronchoalveolar lavage in acquired immune deficiency dysndrome. *Acta Cytol. 29*:727–731 (1985).

320. Sun, T., Chess, Q., and Tanenbaum, B. Morphologic criteria for the identification of *Pneumocystis carinii* in Papanicolaou-stained preparations. (letter) *Acta Cytol. 30*:80–82 (1986).

321. Rorat, E., Garcia, R. L., and Skolom, J. Diagnosis of *Pneumocystis carinii* pneumonia by cytologic examination of bronchial washings. *JAMA 254*: 1950–1951 (1985).

322. Thomson, R. B., Jr., and Smith, T. F. Acridine orange staining of *Pneumocystis carinii. J. Clin. Microbiol. 16*:191–192 (1982).

323. Coleman, D. L., Dodek, P. M., Golden, J. A., Luce, J. M., Golden, E., Gold, W. M., and Murray, J. F. Correlation between serial pulmonary function tests and fiberoptic bronchoscopy in patients with *Pneumocystis carinii* pneumonia and the acquired immune deficiency syndrome. *Am. Rev. Resp. Dis. 129*:491–493 (1984).

324. Levenson, S. M., Warren, R. D., Richman, S. D., Johnston, G. S., and Chabner, B. A. Abnormal pulmonary gallium accumulation in *P. carinii* pneumonia. *Radiology 119*:395–398 (1976).

325. Turbiner, E. H., Yeh, S. J., Rosen, P. P., Manjlt, S. B., and Benua, R. S. Abnormal gallium scintigraphy in *Pneumocystis carinii* pneumonia with a normal chest radiograph. *Radiology 127*:437–438 (1978).

326. Barron, T. F., Birnbaum, N. S., Shane, L. B., Goldsmith, S. J., and Rosen, M. J. *Pneumocystis carinii* pneumonia studied by gallium scan. *Radiology 154*:791–793 (1985).

327. Coleman, D. L., Hattner, R. S., Luce, J. M., Dodek, P. M., Golden, J. A., and Murray, J. F. Correlation between gallium lung scans and fiberoptic bronchoscopy in patients with suspected *Pneumocystis carinii* pneumonia and the acquired immune deficiency syndrome. *Am. Rev. Resp. Dis. 130*: 1166–1169 (1984).

328. Jones, D. K., and Higenbottam, T. W. *Pneumocystis* pneumonia increases the clearance rate of inhaled ^{99m}Tc DTPA from lung to blood. *Chest 88*: 631–632 (1985).

329. Mason, G. R., Duane, G. B., Mena, I., and Effros, R. M. Accelerated solute clearance in *Pneumocystis carinii* pneumonia. *Am. Rev. Resp. Dis. 135*: 864–868 (1987).

330. Paldy, L., and Ivady, G. Roentgenologic diagnosis of interstitial plasma cell pneumonia in infancy. *Natl. Cancer Inst. Monogr. 43*:99–118 (1976).

331. Doppman, J. L., and Geelhoed, G. W. Atypical radiographic features in *Pneumocystis carinii* pneumonia. *Natl. Cancer Inst. monogr. 43*:89–95 (1976).

332. Friedman, B. A., Wenglin, B. D., Hyland, R. W., et al. Roentgenographically atypical *Pneumocystis carinii* pneumonia. *Am. Rev. Resp. Dis. 111*: 89–96 (1975).

333. Byrd, R. B., and Horn, B. R. Infection due to *Pneumocystis carinii* simulating lobar bacterial pneumonia. *Chest 70*:91–92 (1976).
334. Forrest, J. V. Radiographic findings in *Pneumocystis carinii* pneumonia. *Radiology 103*:539–544 (1972).
335. Reed, J. C., and Madewell, J. E. The air bronchogram in interstitial disease of the lung. *Radiology 116*:1–9 (1975).
336. Luddy, R. E., Champion, L. A., and Schwartz, A. D. *Pneumocystis carinii* pneumonia with pneumatocele formation. *Am. J. Dis. Child. 131*:470 (1977).
337. Dee, P., Winn, W., and McKee, K. *Pneumocystis carinii* infection: radiologic and pathologic correlation. *Am. J. Radiol. 132*:741 (1979).
338. Mones, J. M., Saldana, M. J., and Oldham, S. A. Diagnosis of *Pneumocystis carinii* pneumonia. *Chest 89*:522–526 (1986).
339. Fortuny, I. E., Tempero, K. F., and Amsden, T. W. *Pneumocystis carinii* pneumonia diagnosed from sputum and successfully treated with pentamidine isethionate. *Cancer 26*:911–913 (1970).
340. Mreiden, T., Rao, G., Philipp, F., et al. *Pneumocystis carinii* penumonia. *JAMA 236*:2392–2393 (1976).
341. Chan, H., Pifer, L., Hughes, W. T., Feldman, S., Pearson, T. A., and Woods, D. Comparison of gastric contents to pulmonary aspirates for the cytologic diagnosis of *Pneumocystis carinii* pneumonia. *J. Pediatr. 90*:243–244 (1977).
342. Kagan, I. G., and Norman, L. The laboratory diagnosis of *Pneumocystis carinii* pneumonia. *Health Lab. Sci. 14*:155–163 (1977).
343. Krumholz, R. A., Manfredi, F., Weg, J. G., et al. Needle biopsy of the lung. *Ann. Intern. Med. 65*:293–307 (1966).
344. Jacobs, J. B., Vogel, C., Powell, R. D., et al. Needle biopsy in *Pneumocystis carinii* pneumonia. *Radiology 93*:525–530 (1969).
345. Mimica, I., Donoso, E., Howard, J. E., et al. Lung puncture in the etiologic diagnosis of pneumonia. *Am. J. Dis. Child. 122*:278–282 (1971).
346. Cohen, M. L., and Weiss, E. B. *Pneumocystis carinii* pneumonia: percutaneous lung biopsy and review of the literature. *Chest 60*:195–199 (1971).
347. Chaudhary, S., Hughes, W. T., Feldman, S., Sanyal, S. K., Coburn, T., Ossi, M., and Cox, F. Percutaneous transthoracic needle aspiration of lung. Diagnosing *Pneumocystis carinii* pneumonitis. *Am. J. Dis. Child. 131*: 902–907 (1977).
348. Youmans, C. R., Middleton, J. M., Derrick, J. R., et al Percutaneous needle biopsy of the lung for diffuse parenchymal disease. *Dis. Chest 54*:105–111 (1968).
349. Bandt, P., Blank, N., and Castellino, R. A. Needle diagnosis of pneumonitis. *JAMA 220*:1578–1580 (1972).
350. Palmer, D. L., and Lusk, R. Needle aspiration of the lung in complex pneumonias. *Chest 78*:16–21 (1980).
351. Linnemann, C. C., Jr. Lung punctures. *Chest 78*:1–2 (1980).
352. Castellino, R. A. Percutaneous pulmonary needle diagnosis of *Pneumocystis carinii* pneumonitis. *Natl. Cancer Inst. Monogr. 43*:137–140 (1976).

353. Gaensler, E. A., Moister, M. V., and Hamm, J. Open lung biopsy in diffuse pulmonary disease. *New Engl. J. Med. 270*:1319–1331 (1964).

354. Klassen, K. P., and Andrews, N. C. Biopsy of diffuse pulmonary lesions. *Ann. Thorac. Surg. 4*:117–124 (1967).

355. Singer, C., Armstrong, D., Rosen, P. P., Walzer, P. D., et al. Diffuse pulmonary infiltrates in immunosuppressed patients: a prospective study of 80 cases. *Am. J. Med. 66*:110–120 (1979).

356. Greenman, R. L., Goodall, P. T., and King, D. Lung biopsy in immunocompromised hosts. *Am. J. Med. 59*:488 (1975).

357. Geelhoed, G. W., Levin, B. J., Adkins, P. C., et al. The diagnosis and management of *Pneumocystis carinii* pneumonia. *Ann. Thoracic Surg. 14*: 335–346 (1972).

358. Geelhoed, G. W. Open lung biopsy in the diagnosis of *Pneumocystis carinii* pneumonia. *Natl. Cancer. Inst. Monogr. 43*:141–147 (1976).

359. Burt, M. E. Prospective evaluation of aspiration needle, cutting needle, transbronchial, and open lung biopsy in patients with pulmonary infiltrates. *Ann. Thorac. Surg. 32*:146–161 (1981).

360. Wolff, L. J., Bartlett, M. S., Baehner, R. L., Grosfeld, J. L., and Smith, J. W., The causes of interstitial pneumonitis in immunocompromised children: an aggressive, systematic approach to diagnosis. *Pediatrics 60*: 41–45 (1977).

360a. Prober, C. G., Whyte, H., and Smith, C. R. Open lung biospy in immunocompromised children with pulmonary infiltrates. *Am. J. Dis. Child. 138*: 60–63 (1984).

360b. Rossiter, S. J., Miller, C., Churg, A. M., et al. Open lung biopsy in the immunosuppressed patient: is it really beneficial? *J. Thorac. Cardiovasc. Surg. 77*:338–345 (1979).

361. Michaelis, L. L., Leight, G. S., Jr., Powell, R. D., Jr., et al. Pneumocystis pneumonia: the importance of early open lung biopsy. *Ann. Surg. 183*: 301–306 (1976).

362. Tyras, D. H., Campbell, W., Corley, C., et al. The role of early open lung biopsy in the diagnosis and treatment of *Pneumocystis carinii* pneumonia. *Ann. Thorac. Surg. 18*:571–577 (1974).

363. Thomson, R. B., Jr., Smith, T. F., and Wilson, W. R. Comparison of two methods used to prepare smears of mouse lung tissue for detection of *Pneumocystis carinii. J. Clin. Microbiol. 16*:303–306 (1982).

364. Gay, J. D., Smith, T. F., and Ilstrup, D. M. Comparison of processing techniques for detection of *Pneumocystis carinii* in open-lung biopsy specimens. *J. Clin. Microbiol. 21*:150–151 (1985).

365. Repsher, L. H., Schroter, G., and Hammond, W. S. Diagnosis of *Pneumocystis carinii* pneumonitis by means of endobronchial brush biopsy. *New Engl. J. Med. 287*:340–341 (1972).

366. Repsher, L. H., Levin, D. C., Matthay, R. A., and Stamford, R. E. Transbronchial lung biopsy via the fiberoptic bronchoscope in the diagnosis of diffuse pulmonary infiltrates in the immunosuppressed host. *Natl. Cancer Inst. Monogr. 43*:127–132 (1976).

367. Levin, D. C., Wicks, A. B., and Ellis, J. H. Transbronchial lung biopsy via the fiberoptic bronchoscope. *Am. Rev. Resp. Dis. 110*:4–12 (1974).

368. Scheinhorn, D. J., Joyner, L. R., and Whitcomb, M. E. Transbronchial forceps lung biopsy through the fiberoptic bronchoscope in *Pneumocystis carinii* pneumonia. *Chest 66*:294–295 (1974).

369. Finley, R., Kieff, E., Thomsen, S., et al. Bronchial brushing in the diagnosis of pulmonary disease in patients at risk for opportunistic infection. *Am. Rev. Resp. Dis. 100*:379–387 (1974).

370. Drew, W. L., Finley, T. N., Mintz, L., and Klein, H. Z. Diagnosis of *Pneumocystis carinii* pneumonia by bronchopulmonary lavage. *JAMA 230*:713–715 (1974).

371. Chopra, S. K., and Ben-Isaac, F. Transbronchial lung biopsy using fiberoptic bronchoscope. *South Med. J. 77*:302–304 (1977).

372. Pennington, J. E., and Feldman, N. T. Pulmonary infiltrates and fever in patients with hematologic malignancy: assessment of transbronchial biopsy. *Am. J. Med. 62*:581–587 (1977).

373. Cunningham, J. H., et al. Trephine air drill, bronchial brush, and fiberoptic transbronchial lung biopsies in immunosuppressed patients. *Am. Rev. Resp. Dis. 115*:213–220 (1977).

374. Kelley, J., Landis, J. N., Davis, G., Trainer, T. D., Jakab, G., and Green, G. W. Diagnosis of pneumonia due to *Pneumocystis* by segmental pulmonary lavage via the fiberoptic bronchoscope. *Chest 74*:24–28 (1978).

375. Wilson, R. K., Fechner, R. E., Greenberg, S. D., Estrada, R., and Stevens, P. M. Clinical implications of a "nonspecific" transbronchial biopsy. *Am. J. Med. 65*:252–256 (1978).

376. Lauver, G. L., Hasan, F. M., Morgan, R. B., and Campbell, S. C. The usefulness of fiberoptic bronchoscopy in evaluating new pulmonary lesions in the immunocompromised host. *Am. J. Med. 66*:580–585 (1979).

377. Nishio, J. W. Fiberoptic bronchoscopy in the immunocompromised host: the significance of a "nonspecific" transbronchial biopsy. *Am. Rev. Resp. Dis. 121*:307–312 (1980).

378. Springmeyer, S. C., Silvestri, R. C., Sale, G. E., et al. The role of transbronchial biopsy for the diagnosis of diffuse pneumonias in immunocompromised marrow transplant recipients. *Am. Rev. Resp. Dis. 126*:736–765 (1982).

379. Hedemark, L. L., Kronenberg, R. S., Rasp, F. L., et al. The value of bronchoscopy in establishing the etiology of pneumonia in renal transplant recipients. *Am. Rev. Resp. Dis. 126*:981–985 (1982).

380. Hopkin, J. M., Young, J. A., Turney, J. H., Adu, D., and Michael, J. Rapid diagnosis of obscure pneumonia in immunosuppressed renal patients by cytology of alveolar lavage fluid. *Lancet 2*:299–301 (1983).

381. Stover, D. E., Zaman, M. B., Hajdu, S. I., Lange, M., Gold, J., and Armstrong, D. Bronchoalveolar lavage in the diagnosis of diffuse pulmonary infiltrates in the immunosuppressed host. *Ann. Intern. Med. 101*: 1–7 (1984).

382. Coleman, D. L., Dodek, P. M., Luce, J. M., Golden, J. A., Gold, W. M., and

Murray, J. F. Diagnostic utility of fiberoptic bronchoscopy in patients with *Pneumocystis carinii* pneumonia and the acquired immune deficiency syndrome. *Am. Rev. Resp. Dis. 128*:795–799 (1983).

383. Ognibene, F. P., Shelhamer, J., Gill, V., Macher, A. M., Loew, D., Parker, M. M., Gelmann, E., Fauci, A. S., Parrillo, J. E., and Masur, H. The diagnosis of *Pneumocystis carinii* pneumonia in patients with the acquired immunodeficiency syndrome using subsegmental bronchoalveolar lavage. *Am. Rev. Resp. Dis. 129*:929–932 (1984).

384. Murray, J. F., Felton, C. P., Garay, G. M., Gottlieb, M. S., Hopewell, P. C., Stover, D. E., and Teirstein, A. S. Pulmonary complications of the acquired immunodeficiency syndrome. *New Engl. J. Med. 310*:1682–1688 (1984).

385. Hartman, B., Koss, M., Hui, A., Baumann, W., Athos, L., and Boylen, T. *Pneumocystis carinii* pneumonia in the acquired immunodeficiency syndrome (AIDS). Diagnosis with bronchial brushings, biopsy, and bronchoalveolar lavage. *Chest 87*:603–607 (1985).

386. Glassroth, J. The pulmonary complcations of AIDS. *Chest 87*:562–563 (1985).

387. Caughey, G., Wong, H., Gamsu, G., and Golden, J. Nonbronchoscopic bronchoalveolar lavage for the diagnosis of *Pneumocystis carinii* pneumonia in the acquired immunodeficiency syndrome. *Chest 88*:659–662 (1985).

388. Barrio, J. L., Harcup, C., Baier, H. J., and Pitchenik, A. E. Value of repeat fiberoptic bronchoscopies and significance of nondiagnostic results in patients with the acquired immunodeficiency syndrome. *Am. Rev. Resp. Dis. 135*:422–425 (1987).

389. Pitchenik, A. E., Ganjei, P., Torres, A., Evans, D. A., Rubin, E. and Baier, H. Sputum examination for the diagnosis of *Pneumocystis carinii* pneumonia in the acquired immunodeficiency syndrome. *Am. Rev. Resp. Dis. 133*:226–229 (1986).

390. Bigby, T. D., Margolskee, D., Curtis, J. L., Micheael, P. F., Sheppard, D., Hadley, W. K., and Hopewell, P. C. In usefulness of induced sputum in the diagnosis of *Pneumocystis carinii* pneumonia in patients with the acquired immunodeficiency syndrome. *Am. Rev. Resp. Dis. 133*:515–518 (1986).

391. Luce, J. M. Sputum induction in the acquired immunodeficiency syndrome. *Am. Rev. Resp. Dis. 133*:513–514 (1986).

392. Murray, J. F., Garay, S. M., Hopewell, P. C., Mills, J., Snider, G. L., and Stover, D. E. Pulmonary complications of the acquired immunodeficiency syndrome: an update. *Am. Rev. Resp. Dis. 135*:504–509 (1987).

393. Ognibene, F. P., Steis, R. G., and Macher, A. M. Kaposi's sarcoma causing pulmonary infiltrates and respiratory failure in the acquired immunodeficiency syndrome. *Ann. Intern. Med. 102*:471–475 (1985).

394. Aelony, Y. The role of transbronchial biopsy for the diagnosis of diffuse pneumonia in immunocompromised marrow transplant recipients. *Am. Rev. Resp. Dis. 127*:329–330 (1983).

395. Robin, E. D., and Burke, C. M. Lung biopsy in immunosuppressed patients. *Chest 89*:276–278 (1986).
396. Suffredini, A. F., Ognibene, F. P., Lack, E. E., Simmons, J. T., Brenner, M., Gill, V. J., Lane, H. C., Fauci, A. S., Parrillo, J. E., Masur, H., and Shelhamer, J. H. Nonspecific interstitial pneumonitis: a common cause of pulmonary disease in the acquired immunodeficiency syndrome. *Ann. Intern. Med. 107*:7–13 (1987).
397. Meyers, J. D., Pifer, L. L., Sale, G. E., and Thomas, E. D. The value of *Pneumocystis carinii* antibody and antigen detection for diagnosis of *Pneumocystis carinii* pneumonia after marrow transplantation. *Am. Rev. Resp. Dis. 120*:1283–1287 (1979).
398. Stagno, S., Pifer, L. L., Hughes, W. T., Brasfield, D. M., and Tiller, R. E. *Pneumocystis carinii* in young immunocompetent infants. *Pediatrics 66*: 56–62 (1980).
399. Stagno, S., Brasfield, D., Brown, M., et al. Infant pneumonitis associated with cytomegalovirus, chlamydia, *Pneumocystis* and ureaplasma: a prospective study. *Pediatrics 68*:322 (1981).
400. Robert, N. J., Pifer, L. L., Niell, H. B., Woods, D. R., Neely, C. L., Miller, J. H., and Churchill, H. Incidence of *Pneumocystis carinii* antigenemia in ambulatory cancer patients. *Cancer 53*:1878–1881 (1984).
400a. Pifer, L. L., Niell, H. B., Morrison, B. J., Counce, J. D., Jr., Freeman, J. M., Woods, D. R., and Neely, C. L. *Pneumocystis carinii* antigenemia in adults with malignancy, infection, or pulmonary disease. *J. Clin. Microbiol. 20*: 887–890 (1984).
401. Shann, F., Walters, S., Pifer, L. L., Graham, D. M., Jack, I., Uren, E., Birch, D., and Stallman, N. D. Pneumonia associated with infection with pneumocystis, respiratory syncytial virus, chlamydia, mycoplasma, and cytomegalovirus in children in Papua New Guinea. *Br. Med. J. 292*:314–317 (1986).
402. Jarowenko, M., Pifer, L., Kerman, R., and Kahn, B. D. Serologic methods for the early diagnosis of *Pneumocystis carinii* infection in renal allograft recipients. *Transplantation 41*:436–442 (1986).
403. Pifer, L. L. Serodiagnosis of *Pneumocystis carinii*. *Chest 87*:698–700 (1985).
404. Tanabe, K., Furuta, T., Ueda, K., Tanaka, H., and Shimada, K. Serological observations of *Pneumocystis carinii* infection in humans. *J. Clin. Microbiol. 22*:1058–1060 (1985).
405. Hughes, W. T. Serodiagnosis of *Pneumocystis carinii*. *Chest 87*:700 (1985).
406. Walzer, P. D., Cushion, M. T., Juranek, D. J., Walls, K., Smith, J. W., Bartlett, M. W., Armstrong, D., Gold, J., Young, L. S., Pesanti, E., Graves, D. C., Ivey, M. B., Masur, H., and Kovacs, J. Serodiagnosis of *Pneumocystis carinii*. *Chest 9*:935 (1987).
407. Young, L. S. Antigen detection in *Pneumocystis carinii* pneumonia. *Serodiagn. Immunotherapy 1*:163–167 (1987).

408. Barnett, R. N., Hull, J. G., Vortel, V., and Schwarz, J. *Pneumocystis carinii* in lymph nodes and spleens. *Arch. Pathol.* 88:175–180 (1969).

409. Anderson, C. D., and Barrie, B. J. Fatal *Pneumocystis* pneumonia in an adult. *Am. J. Clin. Pathol.* 34:365–370 (1960).

410. Asen, C. F., and Baltzan, M. A. Systemic dissemination of *Pneumocystis carinii* pneumonia. *Can. Med. Assoc. J.* 104:809–812 (1971).

411. Barnett, R. N., Hull, J. G., Vortel, V., and Schwarz, J. *Pneumocystis carinii* in lymph nodes and spleens. *Arch. Pathol.* 88:175–180 (1969).

412. Henderson, D. W., Humeniuk, V., Meadows, R., et al. *Pneumocystis carinii* pneumonia with vascular and lymph nodal involvement. *Pathology* 6:235–241 (1974).

413. Jarnum, S., Rasmussen, E. F., Ohlsen, A. S., et al. Generalized *Pneumocystis carinii* infection with severe idiopathic hypoproteinemia. *Ann. Int. Med.* 68:138–145 (1968).

414. Livingstone, C. S. Pneumocystis pneumonia occurring in a family with agammaglobulinemia. *Can. Med. Assoc. J.* 90:1223–1225 (1964).

415. Rahimi, S. A. Disseminated *Pneumocystis carinii* in thymic alymphoplasia. *Arch. Pathol.* 97:162–165 (1974).

416. Coulman, C. U., Greene, I., and Archibald, R. W. R. Cutaneous pneumocystosis. *Ann. Intern. Med.* 106:396–398 (1987).

417. Grimes, M. M., LaPook, J. D., Bar, M. H., Wasserman, H. S., and Dwork, A. Disseminated *Pneumocystis carinii* infection in a patient with acquired immunodeficiency syndrome. *Hum. Pathol.* 18:307–308 (1987).

418. Kwok, S., O'Donnell, J. J., and Wood, I. S. Retinal cotton-wool spots in a patient with *Pneumocystis carinii* infection. *New Engl. J. Med.* 307:184–185 (1982).

419. Macher, A. M., Bardenstein, D. S., Zimmerman, L. E., et al. *Pneumocystis carinii* choroiditis in a male homosexual with AIDS and disseminated pulmonary and extrapulmonary *P. carinii* infection. *New Engl. J. Med.* 316:1092 (1987).

420. Schinella, R. A., Breda, S. D., and Hammerschlag, P. E. Otic infection due to *Pneumocystis carinii* in an apparently healthy man with antibody to the human immunodeficiency virus. *Ann. Intern. Med.* 106:399–400 (1987).

421. Holland, G. N., Gottlieb, M. S., and Foos, R. Y. Retinal cotton-wool patches in acquired immunodeficiency syndrome. *New Engl. J. Med.* 307:1704 (1982).

422. Follansbee, S. E., Busch, D. F., Wofsy, C. B., Coleman, D. L., Gullet, J., Aurigemma, G. P., Ross, T., Hadley, W. K., and Drew, W. L. An outbreak of *Pneumocystic carinii* pneumonia in homosexual men. *Ann. Intern. Med.* 96:705–713 (1982).

423. Walzer, P. D. Experimental *Pneumocystis carinii* infection. In *Experimental Models in Antimicrobial Chemotherapy*, Vol. 3 (O. Zak and M. A. Sande, eds.). Academic Press, Orlando, Fla., 1986, pp. 185–201.

424. Hughes, W. T., and Smith, B. L. Intermittent chemoprophylaxis for *Pneumocystis carinii* pneumonia. *Antimicrob. Agents Chemother.* 24:300–301 (1983).

425. Kluge, R. M., Spaulding, D. M., and Spain, J. A. Combination of pentamidine and trimethoprim-sulfamethoxazole in the therapy of *Pneumocystis carinii* pneumonia in rats. *Antimicrob. Agents Chemother. 13*:975–978 (1978).

426. Siegel, S. E., Wolff, L. J., Baehner, R. L., and Hammond, D. Treatment of *Pneumocystis carinii* pneumonia. *Am. J. Dis. Child. 138*:1051–1054 (1984).

427. Young, L. S. Treatment and prevention of *Pneumocystis carinii* infection. In *Pneumocystis carinii Pneumonia* (L. S. Young, ed.). Marcel Dekker, New York, 1984, pp. 175–194.

428. Hughes, W. T. Trimethoprim-sulfamethoxazole therapy for *Pneumocystis carinii* pneumonitis in children. *Rev. Infect. Dis. 4*:602–607 (1982).

429. Young, L. S. Trimethoprim-sulfamethoxazole in the treatment of adults with pneumonia due to *Pneumocystis carinii*. *Rev. Infect. Dis. 4*:608–613 (1982).

430. Pearson, R. D., and Hewlett, E. L. Pentamidine for the treatment of *Pneumocystis carinii* pneumonia and other protozoal diseases. *Ann. Intern. Med. 103*:782–786 (1985).

431. Drake, S., Lampasona, V., Nicks, H. L., and Schwarzmann, S. W. Pentamidine isethionate in the treatment of *Pneumocystis carinii* pneumonia. *Clin. Pharm. 4*:507–516 (1985).

432. Navin, T. R., and Fontaine, R. E. Intravenous versus intramuscular pentamidine. *New Engl. J. Med. 311*:1701–1702 (1984).

433. Mallory, D. L., Parrillo, J. E., Bailey, K. R., Akin, G. L., Brenner, M., Lane, H. C., Fauci, A. S., and Masur, H. Cardiovascular effects and safety of intravenous and intramuscular pentamidine isethionate. *Crit. Care Med. 15*:503–505 (1987).

434. Stahl-Bayliss, C. M., Kalman, C. M., and Laskin, O. L. Pentamidine-induced hypoglycemia in patients with the acquired immune deficiency syndrome. *Clin. Pharmacol. Ther. 39*:271–275 (1986).

435. Bouchard, P., Sai, P., and Reach, G. Diabetes mellitus following pentamidine-induced hypoglycemia in humans. *Diabetes 31*:40–45 (1982).

436. Osei, K., Falko, J. M., Nelson, K. P., and Stephens, R. Diabetogenic effect of pentamidine. *Am. J. Med. 77*:41–46 (1984).

437. Murphey, S. A., and Josephs, A. S. Acute pancreatitis associated with pentamidine therapy. *Arch. Intern. Med. 141*:56–58 (1981).

438. Salmeron, S., Petitpretz, P., Katlama, C., Herve, P., Brivet, F., Simonneau, G., Duroux, P., and Regnier, B. Pentamidine and pancreatitis. *Ann. Intern. Med. 105*:140–141 (1986).

438a. Sensakovic, J. W., Suarez, M., Perez, G., Johnson, E. S., and Smith, L. G. Pentamidine treatment of *Pneumocystis carinii* pneumonia in the acquired immunodeficiency syndrome. *Arch. Intern. Med. 145*:2247 (1985).

439. Kempin, S. J., Jackson, C. W., and Edwards, C. C. In vitro inhibition of platelet function and coagulation by pentamidine isethionate. *Antimicrob. Agents Chemother. 12*:451–454 (1977).

440. Levy, M. A., Senior, R. M., and Sneider, R. E. Severe Thrombocytopenic

purpura complicating pentamidine therapy for *Pneumocystis carinii* pneumonia. *Cancer 34*:441–443 (1974).

441. Milder, J. E., Walzer, P. D., and Powell, R. D. Treatment of *Pneumocystis carinii* pneumonia with trimethoprim-sulfamethoxazole and pentamidine: problems of efficacy and toxicity. *South Med. J. 72*:1626-1628 (1979).

442. Shelhamer, J. H., Ognibene, F. P.. Macher, A. M., Tuazon, C., Steiss, R., Longo, D., Kovacs, J. A., Parker, M. M., Natanson, C., Lane, H. C., Fauci, A. S., Parrillo, J. E., and Masur, H. Persistence of *Pneumocystis carinii* in lung tissue of acquired immunodeficiency syndrome patients treated for *Pneumocystis* pneumonia. *Am. Rev. Resp. Dis. 130*:1161–1165 (1984).

443. DeLorenzo, L. J., Maguire, G. P., Wormser, G. P., Davidian, M. M., and Stone, D. J. Persistence of *Pneumocystis carinii* pneumonia in the acquired immunodeficiency syndrome. Evaluation of therapy by follow-up trans-bronchial lung biopsy. *Chest 88*:79–83 (1985).

443a. El-Sadr. W., and Sidhu, G. Persistence of trophozoites after successful treatment of *Pneumocystis carinii* pneumonia. *Ann. Intern. Med. 105*: 889–890 (1986).

444. Hughes, W. T. Persistence of pneumocystis. *Chest 88*:4–5 (1985).

445. Nunn, P., and Allistone, J. Resistance to trimethoprim-sulfamethoxazole in the treatment of *Pneumocystis carinii* pneumonia—implication of folinic acid. *Chest 86*:149–150 (1984).

446. D'Antonio, R. G., Johnson, D. B., Winn, R. E., Van Dellen, A. F., and Evans, M. E. Effect of folinic acid on the capacity of trimethoprim-sulfamethoxazole to prevent and treat *Pneumocystis carinii* pneumonia in rats. *Antimicrob. Agents Chemother. 29*:327–329 (1986).

447. Hughes, T. E., Almgren, J. D., McGuffin, R. W., and Omoto, R. J. Co-trimoxazole desensitization in bone marrow transplantation. *Ann. Intern. Med. 105*:148 (1986).

448. Gottlieb, M. S., Knight, S., Mitsuyasu, R., Weisman, J., Roth, M., and Young, L. S. Prophylaxis of *Pneumocystis carinii* infection in AIDS with pyrimethamine-sulfadoxine. *Lancet 2*:398-399 (1984).

449. Navin, T. R., Miller, K. D., Striale, R. F., and Lobel, H. O. Adverse reactions associated with pyrimethamine-sulfadoxine prophylaxis for *Pneumocystis carinii* infections in AIDS. *Lancet 1*:1332 (1985).

450. Edelson, P. J., Metroka, C. E., and Friedman-Kien, A. Dapsone. Trimethoprim-sulfamethoxazole, and the acquired immunodeficiency syndrome. *Ann. Intern. Med. 103*:963 (1985).

451. Pearson, R. D., and Hewlett, E. L. Use of pyrimethamine-sulfadoxine (Fansidar) in prophylaxis against chloroquine-resistant *Plasmodium falciparum* and *Pneumocystis carinii. Ann. Intern. Med. 106*:714–718 (1987).

452. Fischl, M. A., and Dickinson, G. M. Fansidar prophylaxis of *Pneumocystis* pneumonia in the acquired immunodeficiency syndrome. *Ann. Intern. Med. 105*:629 (1986).

453. Antonow, D. R. Acute pancreatitis associated with trimethoprim-sulfamethoxazole. *Ann. Intern. Med. 104*:363–365 (1986).

454. Liu, L. X., Seward, S. J., and Crumpacker, C. S. Intravenous trimethoprim-sulfamethoxazole and ataxia. *Ann. Intern. Med. 104*:448–450 (1986).
455. Zitelli, B. J., Alexander, J., Taylor, S., Miller, K. D., Howrie, D. L., Kuritsky, J. N., Perez, T. H., and Van Thiel, D. H. Fatal hepatic necrosis due to pyrimethamine-sulfadoxine (Fansidar). *Ann. Intern. Med. 106*:393–395 (1987).
456. Bernard, E. M., Donnelly, H. J., Maher, M. P., and Armstrong, D. Use of a new bioassay to study pentamidine pharmacokinetics. *J. Infect. Dis. 152*: 750–754 (1985).
457. Conte, J. E., Upton, R. A., Phelps, R. T., Wofsy, C. B., Zurlinden, E., and Lin, E. T. Use of a specific and sensitive assay to determine pentamidine pharmacokinetics in patients with AIDS. *J. Infect. Dis. 154*:923–929 (1986).
458. Waalkes, P. T., Denham, C., and DeVita, V. T. Pentamidine: clinical pharmacologic correlations in man and mice. *Clin. Pharm. Therap. 11*: 505–512 (1970).
459. Waalkes, T. P., and DeVita, V. T. The determination of pentamidine (4,4'-diamidinophenoxypentane) in plasma, urine, and tissues. *J. Lab. Clin. Med. 75*:871–878 (1970).
460. Waalkes, T. P., and Makulu, D. R. Pharmacologic aspects of pentamidine. *Natl. Cancer Inst. Monogr. 43*:171–176 (1976).
461. Waldman, R. H., Pearce, D. E., and Martin, R. A. Pentamidine isethionate levels in lungs, livers, and kidneys of rats after aerosol or intramuscular administration. *Am. Rev. Resp.Dis. 108*:1004–1006 (1973).
462. Navin, T. R., Dickinson, C. M., Adams, S. R., Mayersohn, M., and Juranek, D. D. Effect of azotemia in dogs on the pharmacokinetics of pentamidine. *J. Infect. Dis. 155*:1020–1026 (1987).
463. Debs, R. J., Straubinger, R. M., Brunette, E. N., Lin, J. M., Lin, E. J., Montgomery, A. B., Friend, D. S., and Papahadjopoulos, D. P. Selective enhancement of pentamidine uptake in the lung by aerosoloization and delivery in liposomes. *Am. Rev. Resp. Dis. 135*:731–737 (1987).
464. Debs, R. J., Blumenfeld, W., Brunette, E. N., Straubinger, R. M., Montgomery, A. B., Lin, E., Agabian, N., and Papahadjopoulos, D. Successful treatment with aerosolized pentamidine of *Pneumocystis carinii* pneumonia in rats. *Antimicrob. Agents Chemother. 31*:37–41 (1987).
465. Girard, P.-M., Brun-Pascaud, M., Farinotti, R., Tamisier, L., and Kernbaum, S. Pentamidine aerosol in prophylaxis and treatment of murine *Pneumocystis carinii* pneumonia. *Antimicrob. Agents Chemother. 31*: 978–981 (1987).
466. Montgomery, A. B., Debs, R. J., Luce, J. M., Corkery, K. J., Turner, J., Brunette, E. N., Lin, E. T., and Hopewell, P. C. Aerosolised pentamidine as sole therapy for *Pneumocystis carinii* pneumonia in patients with acquired immunodeficiency syndrome. *Lancet* Aug. 29:480–483 (1987).
467. Kirby, H. B., Kenamore, B., and Guckian, J. C. *Pneumocystis carinii* pneumonia treated with pyrimethamine and sulfadiazine. *Ann. Intern. Med. 75*:505–509 (1971).

468. Whisnant, J. K., and Buckley, R. H. Successful pyrimethamine-sulfadiazine therapy and *Pneumocystis* pneumonia in infants with x-linked immunodeficiency with hyper-IgM. *Natl. Cancer Inst. Monogr.* 43:211–216 (1976).

469. Young, R. C., and DeVita, V. T., Jr. Treatment of *Pneumocystis carinii* pneumonia: current status of the regimens of pentamidine isethionate and pyrimethamine-sulfadiazine. *Natl. Cancer Inst. Monogr.* 43:193–198 (1976).

470. Allegra, C. J., Kovacs, J. A., Drake, J. C., Swan, J. C., Chabner, B. A., and Masur, H. Activity of antifolates against *Pneumocystis carinii* dihydrofolate reductase and identification of a potent new agent. *J. Exp. Med.* 165:926–931 (1987).

471. Queener, S. F., Bartlett, M. S., Jay, M. A., Durkin, M. M., and Smith, J. W. Activity of lipid-soluble inhibitors of dihydrofolate reductase against *Pneumocystis carinii* in culture and in a rat model of infection. *Antimicrob. Agents Chemother.* 31:1323–1327 (1987).

472. Allegra, C. J., Chabner, B. A., Tuazon, C. U., Ogata-Arakaki, D., Baird, B., Drake, J. C., Simmons, J. T., Lack, E. E., Shelhamer, J. H., Balis, F., Walker, R., Kovacs, J. A., Lane, C., and Masur, H. Trimetrexate for the treatment of *Pneumocystis carinii* pneumonia in patients with the acquired immunodeficiency syndrome. *New Engl. J. Med.* 317:978–985 (1987).

473. Golden, J. A., Sjoerdsma, A., and Santi, D. V. *Pneumocystis carinii* pneumonia treated with alpha-difluoromethylornithine. A prospective study among patients with the acquired immunodeficiency syndrome. *West. J. Med.* 141:613–623 (1984).

474. Sjoerdsma, A., Golden, J. A., Schechter, P. J., Barlow, J. L. R., and Santi, D. V. Successful treatment of lethal protozoal infections with the ornithine decarboxylase inhibitor alpha-difluoromethylornithine. *Trans. Assoc. Am. Phys.* 98:70–79 (1984).

475. Hussain, Z., Carlson, M. L., Craig, I. D., and Lannigan, R. Efficacy of tetroxoprim/sulfadizone in the treatment of *Pneumocystis carinii* in rats. *J. Antimicrob. Chemother.* 15:575–578 (1985).

476. Yoshida, Y., Takeuchi, S., Ogino, K., Ikai, T., and Yamada, M. Studies on *Pneumocystis carinii* and *Pneumocystis carinii* pneumonia. III. Therapeutic experiment of the pneumonia with pyrimethamine + sulfamonomethoxine and trimethoprim + sulfamethoxozole. *Jap. J. Parasitol.* 26:367–375 (1977).

477. Yamada, M., Takeuchi, S., Shiota, T., Matsumoto, Y., Yoshikawa, H., Okabayashi, K., Tegoshi, T., Yoshikawa, T., and Yoshida, Y. Experimental studies on the chemoprophylaxis for *Pneumocystis carinii* pneumonia with intermittent administration of trimethoprim-sulfamethoxazole and pyrimethamine-sulfamonomethoxine. *Jap. J. Parasitol.* 35:287–294 (1985).

478. Hughes, W. T., Smith, B. L., and Jacobus, D. P. Successful treatment and prevention of murine *Pneumocystis carinii* pneumonitis with 4,4'-sulfonylbisformanilide. *Antimicrob. Agents. Chemother.* 29:509–510 (1986).

479. Hughes, W. T., and Smith-McCain, B. L. Effects of sulfonylurea compounds on *Pneumocystis carinii*. *J. Infect. Dis.* 153:944–947 (1986).

480. Walzer, P. D., Kim, C. K., Foy, J. M., Linke, M. J., and Cushion, M. T. Inhibitors of folic acid synthesis in the treatment of experimental *Pneumocystis carinii* pneumonia. *Antimicrob. Agents Chemother. 32*: 96–103 (1988).
481. Szychowska, Z., Prandota-Schoepp, A., and Chabydzinska, S. Rifampin for *Pneumocystis carinii* pneumonia. *Lancet 1*:935 (1983).
482. Hughes, W. T., Rifampin for *Pneumocystis carinii* pneumonia. *Lancet 2*: 162 (1983).
483. Pesanti, E. L., and Shanley, J. D. Murine cytomegalovirus and *Pneumocystis carinii. J. Infect. Dis. 149*:643 (1984).
484. Steinbrook, R., Lo, B., Moulton,J., Saika, G., Hollander, H., and Volberding, P. A. Preferences of homosexual men with AIDS for life-sustaining treatment. *New Engl. J. Med. 314*:457–460 (1986).
485. Geelhoed, G. W. Pulmonary and extrapulmonary support for patients with *Pneumocystis carinii* pneumonia. *Natl. Cancer Inst. Monogr. 43*: 187–191 (1976).
486. Geelhoed, G. W., Corso, P., and Joseph, W. L. The role of membrane lung support in transient acute respiratory insufficiency of *Pneumocystis carinii* pneumonia. *J. Thorac. Cardiovasc. Surg. 68*:802–809 (1974).
487. Sanyal, S. K., McGaw, D., Hughes, W. T., Harris, K. S., and Rogers, R. W. Continuous negative chest wall pressure as therapy of severe respiratory distress in the older child. *J. Pediatr. 85*:230 (1974).
488. Sanyal, S. K., Avery, T. L., Hughes, W. T., Kumar, M. A. P., and Harris, K. S. Management of severe respiratory insufficiency due to *Pneumocystis carinii* pneumonia in immunosuppressed hosts. *Am. Rev. Resp. Dis. 116*: 223 (1977).
489. MacFadden, D. K., Edelson, J. D., and Rebuck, A. S. *Pneumocystis carinii* pneumonia in the acquired immune deficiency syndrome: response to inadvertent steroid therapy. *Can. Med. Assoc. J. 132*:1161–1163 (1985).
490. Begin, P. Steroid use in *Pneumocystis carinii* pneumonia. *Can. Med. Assoc. J. 133*:640–641 (1985).
491. Shafer, R. W., Offit, K., Macris, N. T., Horbar, G. M., Ancona, L., and Hoffman, I. R. Possible risk of steroid administration in patients at risk for AIDS. *Lancet 1*:934–395 (1985).
492. El-Sadr, W., Sidhu, G., Diamond, G., Zuger, A., Berman, D., Simberkoff, M. S., and Rahal, J. J. High dose corticosteroids as adjunct therapy in severe *Pneumocystis carinii* pneumonia. *AIDS Res. 2*:349–355 (1986).
493. MacFadden, D. K., Hyland, R. H., Inouye, T., Edelson, J. D., Rodriguez, C. H., and Rebuck, A. S. Corticosteroids as adjunctive therapy in treatment of *Pneumocystis carinii* pneumonia in patients with acquired immunodeficiency syndrome. *Lancet 1*:1477–1479 (1987).
494. Foltanska, H., Przyblska, H., and Winnicki, S. Assessment of respiratory system in children after *Pneumocystis carinii* pneumonia. *Pediatr. Pol. 51*: 1417–1420 (1976).
495. Sanyal, S. K., Mariencheck, W. C., Hughes, W. T., Parvey, L. S., Tsiatis, A. A., and Mackert, P. W. Course of pulmonary dysfunction in children

surviving *Pneumocystis carinii* pneumonitis. *Am. Rev. Resp. Dis. 124*: 161–166 (1981).

496. Suffredini, A. F., Owens, G. R., Tobin, M. J., Slasky, B. S., Peel, R. L., and Costa, F. Long-term prognosis of survivors of *Pneumocystis carinii* pneumonia. *Chest 89*:229–233 (1986).

497. Whitcomb, M. E., Schwartz, M. I., Charles, M. A., and Larson, P. H. Interstitial fibrosis after *Pneumocystis carinii* pneumonia. *Ann. Intern. Med. 73*:761–765 (1970).

498. Wolff, L. J., and Baehner, R. L. Delayed development of *Pneumocystis* pneumonia following administration of short-term high-dose trimethoprim-sulfamethoxazole. *Am. J. Dis. Child. 132*:525–526 (1978).

499. Harris, R. E., McCallister, J. A., Allen, S. A., Barton, A. S., and Baehner, R. L. Prevention of *Pneumocystis* pneumonia. *Am. J. Dis. Child. 134*: 35–38 (1980).

500. Wilber, R. B., Feldman, S., Malone, W. J., Ryan, M., Aur, R. J. A., and Hughes, W. T. Chemoprophylaxis for *Pneumocystis carinii* pneumonitis. *Am. J. Dis. Child. 134*:643–648 (1980).

501. Hughes, W. T., Rivera, G. K., Schell, M. J., Thornton, D., and Lott, L. Successful intermittent chemoprophylaxis for *Pneumocystis carinii* pneumonitis. *New Engl. J. Med. 316*:1627–1632 (1987).

502. Bradley, P. P., Warden, G. D., Maxwell, J. G., and Rothstein, G. Neutropenia and thrombocytopenia in renal allograft recipients treated with trimethoprim-sulfamethoxazole. *Ann. Intern. Med. 93*:560–562 (1980).

503. Western, K. A., Norman, L., and Kaufmann, A. F. Failure of pentamidine isethionate to provide chemoprophylaxis against *Pneumocystis carinii* infection in rats. *J. Infect. Dis. 131*:273–276 (1975).

504. Dutz, W. T., Post, C., Jennings-Khodadad, E., Fakouhi, T., Kohut, E., and Bandarizadeh, B. Therapy and prophylaxis of *Pneumocystis carinii* pneumonia. *Natl. Cancer Inst. Monogr. 43*:179–185 (1976).

505. Hughes, W. T., Kim, H. K., and Price R. A. Attempts at prophylaxis for murine *Pneumocystis carinii* pneumonitis. *Curr. Ther. Res. Clin. Exp. 15*: 581–587 (1973).

506. Burke, B. A. *Pneumocystis carinii* infection: diagnosis and pathogenesis. *Natl. Cancer Inst. Monogr. 43*:151–154 (1976).

ADDITIONAL REFERENCES

Conte, J. E., Upton, R. A., and Lin, E. T. Pantamidine pharmacokinetics in patients with AIDS with impaired renal function. *J. Infect. Dis. 156*:885–890 (1987).

Kovacs, J. A., Ng, V., Masur, H., Leoung, G., Hardley, W. K., Evans, G., Lane, H. C., Ognibene, F. P., Shelhamer, J., Parrillo, J., and Gill, V. J. Diagnosis of *Pneumocystis carinii* pneumonia: Improved detection in sputum with use of monoclonal antibodies. *N. Engl. J. Med. 318*:589–593 (1988).

Stokes, D. C., Gigliotti, F., Rehg, J. E., Snellgrove, R. L., and Hughes, W. T. Experimental *Pneumocystis carinii* pneumonia in the ferret. *Br. J. Exp. Pathol. 68*:267–276 (1987).

4
Toxoplasma gondii

BENJAMIN J. LUFT
State University of New York at Stony Brook, Stony Brook, New York

I. INTRODUCTION

Toxoplasma gondii is an obligate intracellular protozoan that causes significant morbidity and mortality in both humans and animals. In 1908 the parasite was first described as the causative agent of a significant zoonosis (1,2), and in 1928 the organism was first isolated from a human (3). However, its life cycle was not established until 1969, when it was shown that *T. gondii* was a coccidian and the definitive host was found to be the cat (4).

In 1937 Wolf and Cowen (5) and Sabin and Olitski (6) established *Toxoplasma* as a cause of neonatal encephalitis in humans, and it was subsequently found that the infection can be congenitally acquired (7). With the development in 1948 of a reliable serological test to detect anti-*Toxoplasma* antibody, the Sabin-Feldman dye test (8), the wide spectrum of clinical manifestations and ubiquitous nature of the infection throughout the world could first be fully appreciated. It is currently estimated that 3300 infants born in the United States are congenitally infected with *T. gondii* at an average lifetime cost per child of over $67,000 (9). Although *Toxoplasma* has long been recognized as a significant problem in the immunocompromised host (10–13), with the advent of the acquired immune deficiency syndrome (AIDS), toxoplasmic encephalitis is being recognized in epidemic proportions. (14). Therefore, now more than ever, the need to control this disease is clearly evident for both humanitarian and economic reasons.

The purpose of this chapter is to place the clinical manifestations of toxoplasma infection in the compromised host into perspective, with particular attention to the host-parasite immunological interaction. Knowledge of the host's ability to develop a protective response and of the parasite's capacity to suppress or evade these responses will give us insight into the pathogenesis of this disease as well as into the development of new rational therapeutic and diagnostic modalities.

II. EPIDEMIOLOGY

A. Sources of Infection

Toxoplasma gondii is a coccidian that is classified among the sporozoa in the suborder Eimeria. Human infection with *Toxoplasma* is found throughout the world. The prevalence of infection is generally less at high altitudes, in cold regions, and in hot and arid climates. In the United States, between 10 and 60% of adults are seropositive for *Toxoplasma* depending on the geographical location. The incidence of infection increases with age and does not vary between sexes. Common-source outbreaks of acute toxoplasma infection within families are common, although there is no evidence of human-to-human transmission (15).

The organism infects all orders of mammals and some birds. It has been isolated from herbivorous, carnivorous, and omnivorous animals. However, only in the cat can the organism complete its life cycle and produce oocysts. The presence of cats seems to be of prime importance in the transmission of infection (16,17). Several outbreaks of toxoplasmosis have been directly linked to food or water contaminated with oocysts (18,19). An increased prevalence of toxoplasma infection is not always directly correlated with the presence of cats, and a high prevalence of toxoplasmosis among humans have been found in areas without cats (20). The infection can also be transmitted (and thereby perpetuated) by eating meat of animals previously infected with *Toxoplasma* (21-23) as well as via the placenta (24).

Besides food contaminated with oocysts or meat from animals previously infected with *Toxoplasma*, milk (particularly goat's milk) has been implicated as a source of *Toxoplasma* (25). Infection with *T. gondii* may be acquired through blood product transfusions as a result of persistent parasitemia in normal asymptomatic blood donors or leukocytes from patients with chronic myelogenous leukemia (26). Transmission may also occur in laboratory workers by self-inoculation of tachyozoites, tissue cysts, or oocysts (27). Infection has also been transmitted by the transplantation of organs containing *Toxoplasma* tissue cysts (28-30).

B. Immunocompromised Hosts

In immunocompromised hosts, severe infection is more commonly recognized, most often manifesting itself as a necrotizing encephalitis. However, even so, toxoplasmosis compromises a very small minority, less than 5%, of significant cerebral infections in patients with immunocompromising conditions (31,32).

The most common neoplasm associated with *Toxoplasma* is Hodgkin's disease; however, *Toxoplasma* causes significant disease in only a small minority of such patients. Similarly, significant toxoplasma infection has been reported only sporadically in cardiac (28-30,33-36), kidney (37-43), bone marrow (44-47), and liver transplant recipients (48). It has been noted to occur with inordinate frequency in cardiac transplant recipients compared with other organ transplant recipients. Britt (34) noted that significant toxoplasma infection occurred in 3% of cardiac transplant recipients and comprised 15% of the central nervous system infections. At Papworth Hospital, 5% of cardiac transplant recipients developed clinically significant toxoplasma infection, and two died as a result of the infection (36). In contrast, in large series of other types of transplant recipients including renal (32,49), liver (50), and bone marrow (51) recipients, clinically significant toxoplasma infection has occurred in 1% or less of patients.

The most striking predilection for the development of significant toxoplasma infection has been in patients with the acquired immune deficiency syndrome (AIDS) (14,52). Depending on the risk group associated with the development of AIDS, clinically apparent *T. gondii* infection has been reported in as many as 40% of patients. For instance, in studies from Miami (53) and New York (54), toxoplasmic encephalitis was present in over 40% of Haitian patients with AIDS. In a review of autopsies at Jackson Memorial Hospital in Miami between 1979 and 1982, toxoplasmic encephalitis was the leading cause of death among Haitian patients who came to autopsy (55). Similarly, toxoplasmic encephalitis was noted with very high frequency in Africans with AIDS (56). Toxoplasmic encephalitis occurred in 5% of homosexual patients with AIDS or generalized lymphadenopathy seen at the University of California at San Francisco (57) and in 2.6% of homosexual patients in New York with AIDS (52). In the review of the clinical experience of neurological disease in AIDS patients at New York Hospital Memorial Sloan-Kettering Cancer Center (58-60), *Toxoplasma* accounted for 38% of known central nervous system infections and 36% of focal intracerebral lesions. It has been estimated that toxoplasmic encephalitis may eventually afflict 10-15% of AIDS patients (60). These studies emphasize the pervasiveness and importance of toxoplasma infection as a significant cause of morbidity and mortality in AIDS patients.

III. LIFE CYCLE

There are two cycles in the development of *Toxoplasma* that can be linked into a life cycle (17) (Fig. 1). In the cat, which is the definitive host for *Toxoplasma*, the organism undergoes the complete life cycle, including both an enteroepithelial cycle and an extraintestinal cycle. The enteroepithelial cycle of development is similar to that of other coccidians. In other mammalian and avian hosts, which are incidental hosts, the organism only has an extraintestinal phase of

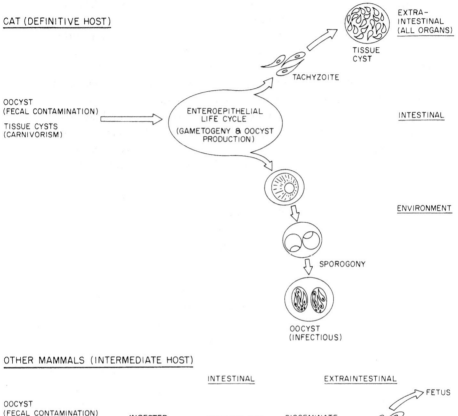

Figure 1   Life cycle of *Toxoplasma gondii*.

development. The enteroepithelial cycle results in the productions of oocysts, whereas in the extraintestinal cycle the tachyzoite form and tissue cysts are found.

A. Oocysts

Ovoid in shape and 10-12 μm in diameter, oocysts have been found only in members of the cat family. After the cat ingests either tissue cysts or oocysts, *T. gondii* is released and invades the epithelial cells of the small intestine, where it undergoes an enteroepithelial cycle (17,61). The organism undergoes sequential stages of development and multiplication, finally resulting in the formation of oocysts. During the multiplicative part of the cycle, the organism appears to asexually divide by endodyogeny, by schizogony, and by splitting of single merozoites from the main nucelated mass. This occurs 3-15 days after infection.

Gametocytes are found throughout the entire small intestine and, in particular, the ileum. Each male gametocyte produces approximately 12 microgametes, which escape and fertilize macrogametes. After fertilization the zygote becomes surrounded by an oocystic wall, and the oocysts are discharged into the lumen, leaving the host with the feces. Sporogony occurs outside the body and requires 2-21 days. The zygote further develops by dividing into two sporoblasts. Each sporoblast develops a wall and thereby becomes a sporocyst. Within the sporocyst there are two further divisions, producing four sporozoites. Therefore, each oocyst contains eight sporozoites. The prepatent period to oocyst production varies between 3 and 24 days depending on the form of organism ingested. The sporulated oocysts are infectious (61). Millions of oocysts are excreted in the feces each day for approximately 2-3 weeks (17).

Under favorable conditions (e.g., warm, moist soil), oocyts may remain infectious for more than a year. Oocysts have been demonstrated in between 0 and 23% of the cats in a given geographical location at a given time (24). The importance of oocysts in the transmission of toxoplasma infection is beginning to be documented both by careful epidemiological studies (18,19,62) and by serological tests developed to detect antibody to sporozoite antigens (63). Ingestion of food contaminated with oocysts is probably how herbivorous animals and humans become infected. It would also account for the equal prevalence of infection among vegetarians and meat-eating subjects in a given geographical area (64).

B. Tachyzoites

Crescent to ovoid in shape (approximately 3 μm X 7 μm), the tachyzoite is seen in the acute stage of the infection or the recrudescence of a chronic infection. In all mammals, including cats, infected by ingestion of food contaminated with cysts or oocysts, tachyzoites can be found in the lamina propria, mesenteric nodes, and distant organs. The tachyzoite is an obligate intracellular parasite that can infect every kind of mammalian cell. The tachyzoite's ability to invade cells is discussed in more detail in Section VI. The organism multiplies by endodyogeny, a process in which two daughter cells develop within a mother cell. Within each daughter cell, a Golgi apparatus, ribosomes, and mitochondria develop (17). As the daughter cells grow within the parent cell, the inner membrane of the latter disappears and its outer membrane joins the daughter cell to form the pellicle. The tachyzoites proliferate within vacuoles in the host cell and continue to proliferate until 8-16 organisms accumulate within the host cell, which then lyses. Tachyzoites, also called pseudocysts, may accumulate in host cells for a prolonged time without forming a true cyst. The tachyzoite cannot survive the digestive juices of the stomach (65); however, it may be involved in the transmission of infection in laboratory accidents. *Toxoplasma* has been isolated from blood donated by an asymptomatic person for transfusion (66) and has also been transmitted through blood product transfusions (26). Prolonged parasitemia has been demonstrated in asymptomatic patients (67) as well as in chronically infected mice (68), indicating that transfused blood products may be vehicles for transmission of infection.

C. Tissue Cysts

Tissue cysts vary in size (10-100 μm in diameter) and contain up to 3000 bradyzoites (Fig. 2). The bradyzoites slowly divide by endodyogeny. The outer membrane of the tissue cysts is probably a combination of host and parasite origin. The cyst is characteristic of chronic infection but can be found as early as 6-12 days after infection. The tissue cyst is found most commonly in heart, striated muscle, and brain; however, any organ can be chronically infected. Cysts have been found in experimental infection of guinea pigs 5 years after infection (69) and probably persist in host tissue for the life of the host. The mechanisms involved in the transformation of actively dividing tachyzoites to slowly dividing bradyzoites have not yet been delineated. With immunosuppression, the tissue cyst ruptures and the organism proliferates as a tachyzoite. The presence of cysts in tissue culture systems devoid of antibody indicates that other factors such as gamma interferon may be involved in cyst formation (70). However, further immunohistological studies must be performed to determine whether the tissue cyst found in vivo is antigenically the same as that seen in tissue culture models (see Section V). The tissue cyst begins to form a membrane that is of parasitic origin in the vacuole of an infected cell. Ultimately, the wall of the mature cyst is believed to represent a combination of host and/or parasitic components (71-73). Immunohistochemical staining has revealed that the surface of the mature cysts contains antigens of parasitic origin (74).

The tissue cyst is associated with transmission because it persists in tissues of

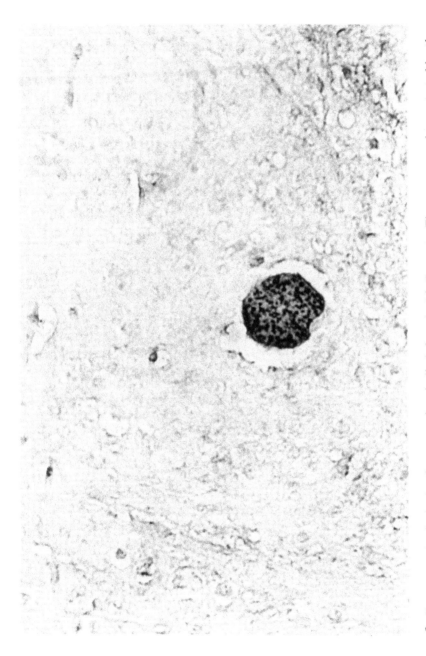

Figure 2 Tissue cyst in the brain of a mouse chronically infected with *T. gondii*. Tissue cyst was demonstrated by the use of and avidon-biotin-based immunohistochemical procedure.

chronically infected animals, which may be ingested by carnivores, including humans. Undercooked meat has been implicated as the source of several common-source outbreaks of toxoplasmosis (21-23). In various surveys, as much as 25% of the mutton and pork in butcher shops contains *Toxoplasma* (24). However, it is rare for beef to contain *Toxoplasma* except for those occasions on which it is contaminated with pork (22,23). After ingestion, the cyst wall is disrupted by peptic or tryptic digestion, which liberates viable *T. gondii* bradyzoites. The bradyzoites resist peptic and tryptic digestion and survive several hours after exposure to these digestive enzymes and are capable of invading the host through the digestive tract. The cyst may also be important in the transmission of infection in organ transplantation (28-30). It has been demonstrated that heart transplant patients who are seronegative for *Toxoplasma* antibody and receive a heart from a seropositive donor have a high incidence of developing disseminated toxoplasmosis. This mode of transmission has also been demonstrated in other organ transplant recipients (75).

IV. GROWTH AND METABOLISM

Toxoplasma gondii is an obligate intracellular parasite. Although it is capable of limited nucleic acid synthesis and respiration in a host-cell-free environment (76), active replication of tachyzoites occurs only with host cells. The reasons for the parasite's dependence on the host cell for growth are not entirely clear. *Toxoplasma* has all the organelles necessary for independent existence including mitochondria, Golgi apparatus, ribosomes, and endoplasmic reticulum (77).

Jones (78) and Sethi et al. (79) found that the growth of *T. gondii* did not require the presence of the host cell nucleus, since *Toxoplasma* was able to proliferate in enucleated fibroblasts. Schwartzman and Pfefferkorn (80) used a mutant host cell line that was defective in pyrimidine synthesis to demonstrate that *T. gondii* is capable of de novo pyrimidine synthesis. In addition, they provided circumstantial evidence that *Toxoplasma* was capable of pyrimidine salvage from the host cell under certain circumstances. Subsequently, the enzymatic pathways in *T. gondii* leading to the synthesis of uridine monophosphate have been characterized (81). In contrast to these findings, there is some evidence to indicate that *Toxoplasma* lacks the ability of de novo purine synthesis. This was suggested by the experiments of Perotto et al. (76), in which extracellular *Toxoplasma* incorporated radiolabeled adenine and guanine into its own nucleic acid but did not utilize formate or glycine. Pfefferkorn and Pfefferkorn (82) utilized fibroblasts from patients with Lesch-Nyhan disease, which are genetically defective in purine salvage, to show that the parasite has the capability of incorporating these precursors into their nucleic acids. Radiolabeled hypoxanthine in the medium was readily incorporated into the parasite, which indicated the presence of a parasite-specific hypoxanthine phosphoribosyl transferase that converts these purines into their corresponding 5' nucleotides. These studies support the contention that although de novo synthesis of purines may be impaired in *Toxoplasma*, the organism has the enzymes necessary for the conversion of one nucleotide to another. Furthermore, purine salvage pathways may prove to be ideal targets for the development of new chemotherapeutic agents (83).

Pfefferkorn and Pfefferkorn (84) showed that host cell protein synthesis was not necessary for the growth of the organism. In these experiments, host cell protein synthesis was blocked either by muconomycin A or by using a temperature-sensitive Chinese hamster ovary cell mutant that had a thermolabile positive RNA synthetase. In both circumstances, host cell protein synthesis was inhibited while *T. gondii* infected and grew normally in the infected cells. However, these studies did not eliminate the possibility that host cell mitochondrial biosynthesis is important to the growth of *T. gondii*, since cells treated with various inhibitors or mutant cells did not have abnormal mitochondrial function.

Another hypothesis about the obligate intracellular parasitism of *T. gondii* relates to the possibility that potassium concentrations may have a profound role in its metabolism. Takeuchi et al. (85) found that sodium- or potassium-dependent ATPase was negligible in the parasite, indicating that *T. gondii* lacks a sodium pump and is probably freely permeable to potassium and sodium ions. Furthermore, they found that protein synthesis and NAD pyrophosphatase of *T. gondii* was activated by 150 millimolar KCl. These findings support the hypothesis that high concentrations of potassium are ncessary for *T. gondii* metabolism. This may account for the fact that various ionophores have had such potent anti-*Toxoplasma* effects in vitro (86–88).

V. ANTIGENIC STRUCTURE

A. Tachyzoites

The characterization and purification of *Toxoplasma* antigens would be useful for the development of more sensitive serological tests. Knowledge of the biochemical constituents of the cell membrane and their functional significance may help to explain how the organism evades host cell killing. Recently, certain antigens have been identified and purified that may be important in the development of a protective immune response or in the parasite's ability to suppress and thereby subvert the host's immune response. The recent application of gene cloning in the production of *Toxoplasma* antigen (89) in an extracellular environment offers the possibility to produce large amounts of a well-characterized antigen that will be useful in diagnostic tests and possibly for vaccine development.

A major obstacle to the biochemical characterization of *T. gondii* is the difficulty of obtaining large quantities of purified preparations of organisms. Because *Toxoplasma* is an obligate intracellular parasite, it can be cultivated only in vivo or in vitro in tissue culture. This has caused most crude antigen preparations to be contaminated with host cell debris (90). In addition, antigen preparations from organisms prepared from the peritoneal cavities of mice are coated with murine antibody within 1–2 days after infection (91). In order to circumvent or reduce these problems, investigators have compared the various biochemical moieties identified in polyacrylamide gelelectrophoresis (PAGE) to host cell controls or have utilized antisera specific to *Toxoplasma* to immunoprecipitate antigens for PAGE or to identify antigens by the Western blot technique (92).

Handman et al. (91) determined the antigenic structure of *Toxoplasma* tachyzoites. The proteins of *Toxoplasma* tachyzoites of the RH strain were biosynthetically labeled with [^{35}S]methionine and solubilized with the detergent Nonidet P-40. The antigens were precipitated with antiserum *Toxoplasma* collected from mice chronically infected with *Toxoplasma*. Thirty-two bands were identified in one-dimensional PAGE gels, and approximately 70 spots were seen on autoradiographs of two-dimensional PAGE gels. When solubilized surface antigens from radioiodinated tachyzoites were immunoprecipitated with the polyvalent serum and one-dimensional PAGE was performed, a remarkably simple pattern was revealed that consisted of four major proteins. Using similar methodology, Johnson et al. (93) studied antigenic components of the soluble and insoluble fractions of RH strain tachyzoites fractionated by ultracentrifugation. In these studies, they identified seven antigenic polypeptides in the insoluble fraction. These investigators also found 10 antigenic polypeptides in the solbule fraction. Four of the polypeptides in the soluble fraction had molecular weights identical to those of polypeptides found in the insoluble fraction of the organism. Three of these common polypeptides have molecular weights identical to those of the three peptides found on the membrane of the tachyzoite found by Handman et al. (91). Further characterization of one of the insoluble antigens (mol. wt. 43,000) was performed by Ogata et al. (94). In their study, they prepared three monoclonal antibodies that reacted with the 43,000 molecular weight antigen in the insoluble portion of the organism. Each monoclonal antibody localized to the tachyzoite in a specific and unique manner. The antigen specific to these monoclonal antibodies was purified. Two of the three monoclonal antibodies bound only to the purified antigen for which they had specific affinity, whereas the third cross-reacted.

The 30,000 molecular weight membrane protein of *Toxoplasma* has been isolated (95) and it has been calculated that it comprises between 3 and 5% of the total protein of *T. gondii*. Apparently the 30,000 molecular weight membrane protein is a major multivalent antigen with a single immunodominant region with two or more identical epitopes (96). It was also demonstrated that single monoclonal antibodies directed against the 30,000 molecular weight antigen inhibit 25–50% of the specific binding of antibodies of patients with toxoplasmosis to the antigenic extract of tachyzoites (96). IgM antibody to this purified antigen has been found in patients with acute toxoplasmosis, and IgG antibodies to this antigen have been found in patients with latent infection (96, 97,98a). It is noteworthy that subjects without clinical or serological evidence of toxoplasma infection may have naturally occurring antibodies against various *Toxoplasma* antigens including those with 30,000 molecular weight (98).

The presence of antigens of similar molecular weights in both the membrane and soluble fraction of the organism raises the possibility that certain cytoplasmic antigens may be secreted onto the surface of the tachyzoite. Brzosko et al. (99) demonstrated immunoelectromicroscopically that antigenic material found on the surface of the tachyzoite was of cytoplasmic origin. However, these investigators could not discern whether this material may have come from other disrupted tachyzoites, whether it leaked through a damaged cell membrane, or whether it was secreted onto membrane. Johnson et al. (100) demonstrated that a monoclonal antibody that reacted to an antigen in the soluble fraction of the tachyzoite also bound to the cell membrane of the organism. This was felt to be consistent with the hypothesis that some cytoplasmic antigens are secreted onto the parasite membrane. Further support for this hypothesis comes from the development of monoclonal antibodies that react to both membrane and cytoplasmic antigens (100-102).

Polysaccharides are present on the membrane of *T. gondii* tachyzoites and are antigenic (103). Mauras et al. (104) found that *Toxoplasma* binds [^{125}I] concanavalin A but does not signfiicantly bind wheat germ agglutinin, indicating the presence of glycopeptides on the surface of the organism. In addition, they determined that the parasite's receptor affinity for concanavalin A was on the same order of magnitude as for other cell systems, but the number of sites per parsasite was low. Further characteristics of the glycosylated peptides were delineated by Johnson et al. (93). In these studies, RH strain tachyzoites were disrupted and fractionated into a soluble and an insoluble fraction by ultracentriugation. Polypeptide analysis of the two fractions by sodium dodecyl sulfate (SDS) PAGE revealed nine and eight parasite-derived polypeptides in the soluble and insoluble fractions, respectively. The soluble fraction contained no polypeptides that would bind to ^{125}I-Con A; however, three polypeptides from the insoluble fraction bound ^{125}I-Con A. Subsequently, Johnson et al. (100) developed a monoclonal antibody that reacted to a parasite cell membrane antigen whose binding was markedly diminished when the tachyzoites were pretreated with periodate, suggesting that this antigenic epitope was composed mainly of carboyhydrate. Further evidence that polysaccharides are antigenically important is derived from studies that used polysaccharides isolated from *Toxoplasma* of the antigen preparation in enzyme-linked immunosorbent assays (105-107). Mineo et al. (106) observed a reaction between polysaccharides extracted from *Toxoplasma* tachyzoites and IgM antibody from humans acutely infected with *T. gondii*. The IgG antibody response to polysaccharides was low or absent. In their polysaccharide preparations, no protein components were found. In contrast, Naot et al. (108) found that both IgG and IgM antibodies recognize *T. gondii* polysaccharides.

Further characterization of the antigenic moieties of the tachyzoites recognized by various classes of antibodies has been possible utilizing the sensitive Western blot analysis. Partanan et al. (109) found that the IgG in humans naturally infected with *T. gondii* recognizes polypeptides that ranged in molecular weight from 27,000 to 67,000 and that the pattern of antigens recognized by IgG antibody was similar. In contrast, sera of two patients that contained *Toxoplasma*-specific IgM antibody, only 35,000- and 60,000-D polypeptides were recognized. In a study by Ehrlich et al. (110), the authors noted the heterogeneity of the humoral response, with the number of antigenic determinants recognized varying from individual to individual. This may have been due to different lengths of time after initial infection, antigenic differences in the infecting strain, stage (oocyst or cyst) of the infecting organism, and genetic variability of the host. In this study five major antigens and approximately 15 minor antigens with molecular weights ranging from 110,000 to 6000 were identified. A 6000 molecular weight antigen reacted uniquely with the serum sample of acutely infected individuals. IgM and/or IgG antibodies specific for the 6000 molecular weight antigen were present in acutely infected individuals; however, in five of nine chronically infected subjects, IgG antibody against this antigen was also present. These data indicated that the presence of IgM antibody directed against the 6000 molecular weight antigen correlated with acute infection. The authors hypothesized that the IgM antibody response to this low molecular weight antigen represents the initial immune response to the infection, followed by an IgM response to other antigens and an IgG response directed against the 6000 antigen and higher molecular weight antigens.

Sharma et al. (111) further delineated the antigenic moieties recognized by IgM and IgG antibodies. In these studies they found that *Toxoplasma*-antigen-specific IgM antibody from acutely infected individuals recognized between two and seven antigens, whereas IgG antibody from these individuals recognized at least 20 different polypeptides. Most of the major bands recognized by IgM antibodies were also present in the patterns attained with IgG antibodies. In addition, these investigators found that the periodation of the antigen abolished or reduced the IgM and IgG reactivity to certain antigenic moieties. Sharma et al. (111) also found that periodic acid Schiff reagent stain detected three antigenic moieties recognized by *Toxoplasma*-specific antibody. This study further delineates the importance of glycoproteins in the humoral response to *T. gondii*. Subsequently, Partanan (112) had the opportunity to study sequential serum specimens from a patient who developed acute glandular toxoplasmosis as a result of a laboratory accident. In this study, Partanan confirmed the findings of

Ehrlich et al. (110) and Sharma et al. (111) that only a few antigen bands were detectable by IgM antibody whereas IgG antibody detected a complex antigen pattern. In addition, in contrast to their previous study (109), they also detected intense staining of a 6000-D band when they used 15% instead of 10% polyacrylamide gel. These authors also found that the IgA response to *Toxoplasma* closely paralleled the IgM response

B. Strain-Specific Antigens

Toxoplasma is considered to be one species of organism. Strains of organisms have been differentiated by their varying degree of virulence and their propensity for tissue cyst formation. In an attempt to define differences in the protein constituency of three strains of *T. gondii*, Bloomfield and Remington (90) compared the electrophoretic patterns of the proteins by tube PAGE. They were not able to discern any differences. Subsequently, Handman et al. (91) used two-dimensional PAGE to discern differences. Immune precipitation of the membrane antigens of three strains of *Toxoplasma* (C37 strain, avirulent; C56 strain, moderately virulent; RH strain, virulent) revealed the same pattern of antigens. The patterns of antigens did not vary whether antisera from mice chronically infected with RH, C56, or C37 strains were used. In another study by Kasper and Ware (63), three strains of *Toxoplasma* (RH, P, and C strains) were compared by PAGE of whole antigen preparations. In these studies, eight major proteins were shared among the various strains. However, there appeared to be several minor staining proteins that were present in the C and P strains but not in the RH strain preparation. When a Western blot analysis was performed using the three different tachyzoite strains as antigen and pooled human antisera, four major and seven to ten minor antigens were detected in all three strains. In addition, various minor strain-specific antigens unique to each strain appeared. Thus, by using the exquisitely sensitive Western blot anlaysis, it was demonstrated that major tachyzoite antigens and proteins are shared by different strains of *Toxoplasma*; however, there are unique minor strain-specific proteins that are able to elicit a humoral response.

C. Stage-Specific Antigens

Toxoplasma has five stages of development. In the cat, the organism undergoes an enteroepithelial cycle with schizogonic and gametogenic stages found in the epithelium of the small intestine; oocysts, each containing two sporocysts, are excreted in the feces. Two additional stages are found in the extraintestinal cycle: the tachyzoites, which occur during acute infection, and bradyzoites within tissue cysts, which are found during subacute and chronic infection. In nonfeline hosts, these latter two stages compose the entire life cycle of the organism. Differences between the various stages of the organism have been inferred by differences in histopathological staining patterns. For instance, the bradyzoites have large granules that stain with periodic acid Schiff (PAS). During the enteroepithelial stages, the organism again is found to have increased amounts of PAS-positive material (17).

Lunde and Jacobs (113) first demonstrated antigenic differences between bradyzoites and tachyzoites using fluorescein conjugated antibradyzoite and antitachyzoite antisera. Antiserum directed against the tachyzoites reacted to the tachyzoites and partially to the bradyzoites, whereas antiserum directed against the bradyzoites reacted to the bradyzoites but not to the tachyzoites. Furthermore, absorption of tachyzoite and bradyzoite antisera by bradyzoites ablated the positive reaction of the antitachyzoite serum with tachyzoites but did not affect the positive reaction between the antibradyzoite serum and the bradyzoites. Subsequently, Kasper et al. (114) demonstrated that two monoclonal antibodies specific to two membrane antigens found on the tachyzoite failed to recognize membrane antigens on the bradyzoite.

Toxoplasma sporozoites have been shown to express stage-specific antigens. Sporozoite-specific monoclonal antibodies have shown minimal activity against tachyzoites in both enzyme-linked and immunofluorescent assays (114). This indicates that there may be immunogens common to both stages but present in unequal amounts. When the surface membrane proteins of tachyzoites and sporozoites from two strains of *T. gondii* (RH and C strains) were compared by one- and two-dimensional PAGE, marked differences were seen (63,114). In the sporozoite preparation, five proteins were present that could not be found in the radioiodinated tachyzoite preparations. In contrast, two proteins identified on the tachyzoite surface could not be found on the sporozoite (63,114). When whole tachyzoite and oocyst preparations were compared, there were 10–12 protein bands in the oocyst preparation not seen in the tachyzoites. A carbohydrate stain (periodic acid Schiff) revealed 9–10 bands in the oocyst/sporozoite preparation that were not present in the tachyzoite preparation.

When the differences in the antigenic determinants were compared between sporozoites and tachyzoites by Western blot analysis, further differences were determined. These analyses were performed with sera obtained from subjects who were involved in an epidemiologically well documented common-source outbreak due to ingestion of water contaminated with oocysts (62). Control sera were obtained from the same cohort of subjects who did not demonstrate clinical symptoms or signs of infection and had a nominally elevated antibody titer. When sera from individuals acutely infected with *Toxoplasma* oocysts were used, at least five unique stage-specific oocyst/sporozoite antigens and three stage-specific tachyzoite antigens were recognized by IgG antibody. The acute IgM anibody also showed sporozoite/oocyst stage specificity. Serum from acutely infected convalescent individuals was also able to distinguish certain antigens unique to the oocysts or tachyzoites. Interestingly, although the oocyts stained strongly with PAS, periodate treatment resulted in no significant change in the antigenicity of any major unique stage-specific antigen of the oocyst. This information may be useful in epidemiological studies that may be capable of determining not only whether the patient was infected but also the actual stage of organism involved in the infection. In addition, vaccine strategies may have to consider antigenic differences in the different stages of the organism in order to abort the infection before it reaches the intracellular environment.

D. Protective Antigens

The antigenic determinants of *Toxoplasma* have a diverse and not well understood impact on the host's immune response. When purified antigens have been used to vaccinate animals, some antigen preparations have been found to have a protective effect (115,116), whereas others have had a deleterious effect on host resistance to infection (117). The passive transfer of monoclonal antibodies directed against specific antigenic determinants has been useful in further delineating the relative roles of humoral and cell-mediated immunity in host resistance to *Toxoplasma*.

Both Hauser and Remington (118) and Sethi et al. (119) have determined that when tachyzoites of the highly virulent RH strain are preincubated with various monoclonal antibodies directed against antigenic moieties found on the parasite's membrane, unelicited peritoneal macrophages either effectively reduced the proliferation of these tachyzoites or killed them, whereas tachyzoites not treated with monoclonal antibodies proliferated. Hauser and Remington (118) found that pretreatment with the monoclonal antibodies also enhanced phagocytosis. Monoclonal antibodies that have activity in vitro systems have not been uniformly effective in passively transferring immunity. On the contrary, the monoclonal antibody directed against the 30,000 molecular weight antigen was found to be parasiticidal in vitro with the addition of complement, but passive immunization aggravated the infection. Passively immunized mice had a greater mortality and greater numbers of brain cysts than nonimmunized controls when challenged with a relatively avirulent strain of *T. gondii* (117). Johnson et al. (120) tested seven monoclonal antibodies specific to membrane antigens for their ability to passively immunize mice. Three of the seven monoclonal antibodies were able to afford the mice significant protection against a moderately virulent strain of *T. gondii*. Interestingly, one of the protective monoclonal antibodies was directed against an antigenic fraction with a molecular weight of 35,000 and slight reactivity was noted with a 14,000 molecular weight antigen. The other protective monoclonal antibodies were directed against an antigen with molecular weight of 14,000. Two monoclonal antibodies that were not found to be protective recognized the 21,000 and/or 14,000 molecular weight surface antigens. It is not clear whether the monoclonal antibodies directed against the 35,000 molecular weight antigen described by Handman et al. (91) and Johnson et al. (120), which has a protective effect in acute infection with *Toxoplasma*, are directed against the same 30,000 molecular weight antigen described by Kasper (117), which exacerbated infection. Active immunization with partially purified antigens that included the 35,000 and 14,000 molecular weight antigens conferred partial immunity to infection with *Toxoplasma* (116), whereas active immunization with the 30,000 molecular weight antigen exacerbated acute infection with *T. gondii* (117). If these antigens are the same, the reasons for the discrepancies in the protective effect of monoclonal antibodies directed against the same antigens is not clear; perhaps they are due to differences in isotypes among the monoclonal antibodies or reflect the fact that various monoclonal antibodies recognize different epitopes on the same antigen and therefore confer varying degrees of immunity or serve as blocking antibodies. The reasons why a purified antigen preparation induces protective immunity or immunosuppression may be related to the methods used in antigen preparation and antigen presentation to the host.

Sharma et al. (115) demonstrated that a monoclonal antibody directed against a cytoplasmic antigen conferred passive immunity to mice infected with a moderately virulent strain of *T. gondii*. This study indicated that monoclonal antibodies directed against cytoplasmic antigens or membrane antigens can confer resistance to infection with *T. gondii*. Further studies need to be performed to determine whether or not the antigen recognized by the monoclonal antibody described by Sharma et al. (115) is a cytoplasmic antigen that is secreted to the surface of the organism and therefore available to binding by the antibody. Another possibility is that the membrane structure of the tachyzoite changes during the course of the infection, thereby making this antigen available for binding during the infection.

Various preparations of killed organisms or fractions of the organism have been employed as vaccines. Studies in guinea pigs using lysed or formalin-killed organisms protected the animals from lethal infection with the virulent RH strain of *T. gondii* (121). However, in each of these studies, the organism could be recovered from the tissues of surviving guinea pigs (122). Krahenbuhl et al. (122) demonstrated that injection of killed *Toxoplasma* organisms protected mice against a lethal infection with an avirulent strain. By using differential centrifugation, Araujo and Remington (123) showed that various fractions of disrupted tachyzoites protected against lethal infection with an avirulent strain of *T. gondii*. The antigen preparations were found to be equally effective whether administered with or without Freund's incomplete adjuvant. Furthermore, administration of *Toxoplasma* RNA was able to significantly protect mice against infection with an avirulent strain of *Toxoplasma*, especially when the RNA was administered with Freund's incomplete adjuvant. It is important to note that in these experiments the protective effects of the various preparations of *Toxoplasma* may be eliciting nonspecific immunity. In addition to the protection against *Toxoplasma* infection afforded by vaccination with *Toxoplasma* RNA, similarly treated mice also resisted infection with a phylogenetically unrelated organism, *Listeria monocytogenes*. Similarly, fractions of *Toxoplasma* antigens injected with Freund's incomplete adjuvant also protected mice from infection with other intracellular pathogens. Fractions of *Toxoplasma* have been shown to nonspecifically potentiate natural killer cell activity in mice that had been previously uninfected with *T. gondii* (124) and to augment natural killer cell activity of peripheral blood lymphocytes of humans in vitro (125).

VI. EVASION OF HOST DEFENSE

Toxoplasma gondii is able to evade the host's immune system by numerous strategies; it has the ability to (1) invade, persist, and grow in numerous types of cells including the nonactivated macrophage; (2) suppress host defenses; and (3) shed immunoglobulins bound to its surface. Each of these mechanisms of evasion of the host's immune response will be considered in turn.

A. Host Cell Invasion

Toxoplasma is able to infect all mammalians except perhaps the nonnucleated red blood cell. This ability to infect all cell types distinguishes *Toxoplasma* from other intracellular pathogens that infect phagocytic cells (e.g., *Listeria monocytogenes, Leishmania*) exclusively. The intracellular habitat of the organism may play a role in protecting it from the host's immune response. The mechanism

Table 1 Proposed Mechanisms of Evasion of Host Defense

Intracellular habitat

Active invasion of all mammalian cells

Evasion of killing by professional phagocytes

   Avoids triggering oxidative burst

   Organism-derived scavengers of oxygen-derived products

   Prevention of phagosome–lysosome fusion

   Prevention of phagosome acidification

Antibody shedding

Induction of immunosuppression

   Depressed primary antibody response

   Depressed cellular immunity

of host cell infection is controversial, with some reports demonstrating an active method of parasite penetration into the host cell while others present evidence supporting *Toxoplasma* induction of phagocytosis by professional phagocytic and nonphagocytic cells (126).

Knowledge of the precise biochemical mechanisms for specific attachment and invasion of tachyzoites into host cells may lead to a molecular definition of these important tachyzoite proteins and new rational therapeutic modalities. Jones et al. (127) presented light and electron microscopic evidence that *Toxoplasma* gains entry into both phagocytic and nonprofessional phagocytic cells because of its ability to induce phagocytosis. In their studies, phagocytosis was the mechanism of entry into macrophages, fibroblasts, and HeLa cells. They postulated that *Toxoplasma* stimulated phagocytosis by secretion of an enzyme or other factor onto the surface of the host cell. Ryning and Remington (128) showed that cytochalasin D, a compound that blocks phagocytosis by preventing microfilament formation, dramatically inhibited entry of *T. gondii* into macrophages or bladder tumor cells. These results indicated the active participation of the host cell in *Toxoplasma*'s entry. In contrast to these findings, Silva et al. (129) found that cytochalasin B inhibited entry of *Toxoplasma* into macrophages or LA-9 cells by 50%, whereas similar concentrations of cytochalasin B inhibited the incorporation of epimastigotes of *T. cruzi* or yeast cells into macrophages by 98%. These authors suggested that there are at least two mechanisms used by *T. gondii* for invasion of host cells: active invasion by the parasite and active participation (perhaps phagocytosis) by the host cell. The reason for the discrepancy between Ryning and Remington (128) and Silva et al. (129) may be the possibility that the cytochalasin D interfered with the active myosin system of the parasite as well as the microfilament formation of the host cell. It has been recently demonstrated that myosin has been localized to the anterior pole of the organism (130).

Phagocytosis occurring simultaneously or concurrently with active invasion of the host cell has been propsoed by several other investigators. Studies by Nichols and O'Connor (131) demonstrated by electron microscopy that within 15-30 sec after inoculation of *Toxoplasma* into the host, the organism invades several kinds of leukocytes. Using electron microscopy, they distinguished invasion from phagocytosis by demonstrating that the host cell membrane is disrupted as the parasite penetrates it. These investigators showed electron microscopic evidence that although invasion appeared to be the predominant means of cellular entry of *Toxoplasma*, some phagocytosis also occurs.

B. Evasion of Oxidative and Nonoxidative Killing

Besides purportedly having the ability to actively invade mononuclear phagocytes in order to circumvent killing, *Toxoplasma* avoids triggering the oxidative burst upon ingestion by nonactivated macrophages (132,133). In addition, it contains scavengers of oxygen-derived products (134) that may be detrimental to the mononuclear phagocyte's ability to kill or restrict the intracellular growth of *T. gondii* by an oxidative burst. *Toxoplasma gondii* tachyzoites have been found to be more resistant to the toxic effects of hydrogen peroxide than either *Leishmania* or *Trypanosoma cruzi*. This greater resistance of *T. gondii* to H_2O_2 is probably due to high levels of two H_2O_2 scavengers found within the organism—catalase and glutathione. Furthermore, *Toxoplasma* also contains levels of superoxide dismutase that may be protective against oxygen radicals (134). Inhibition of *T. gondii* catalase by preincubation with aminotraizole enhanced the susceptibility of the organism to killing by H_2O_2 or by nonactivated mouse peritoneal macrophages (134), indicating that this protective mechanism of the organism may be important in evading the immune response. In addition, *Toxoplasma* is able to subvert the nonoxidative lysosome-dependent toxicity by preventing phagosome–lysosome fusion (135,135a) and phagosome acidification (135b). These abnormalities in phagosome-lysosome function may be due to *Toxoplasma*-induced alterations of the phagosome, including elaborate structural modification of phagosomes by *Toxoplasma* surface proteins (135c).

C. Antibody Shedding

One mechanism by which *Toxoplasma* may evade the host's humoral immune system is by shedding membrane-bound immunoglobulins or by releasing soluble antigens, which could serve as a "sink" by complexing specific antibodies in vivo and thereby preventing antibody from binding to the organism surface. Dzbenski and Zielinska (136) showed that when *Toxoplasma* antiserum was used to coat tachyzoites, 5-20% of the organisms were able to remove antibody from their surface by forming a cap to the medium. Dubremetz et al. (137,138) also found that *Toxoplasma* was able to shed membrane-specific antibody in a unique manner. By using a monoclonal antibody specific for the 30,000 molecular weight membrane antigen, they showed that preincubation of the tachyzoites with this antibody had no effect on the tachyzoite's ability to invade HeLa cells. However, immunofluorescence studies of the bound monoclonal antibody revealed much smaller amounts of antibody in the intracellular tachyzoite than were found in similarly treated tachyzoites that did not invade the HeLa cell. Electron microscopic studies of parasites fixed during the process of invasion showed the monoclonal antibody to be present on the surface of the tachyzoite that was still outside the cell, whereas the portion of the parasite within the cell was almost devoid of antibody. These investigators felt that during host cell invasion tachyzoites shed the antibody and they hypothesized that the antigen was shed along with the antibody.

The presence of soluble *Toxoplasma* antigens has been demonstrated in the serum of both animals and humans acutely infected with *Toxoplasma* (139,140). In addition, *Toxoplasma* antigens have been detected in the ocular fluids of rabbits with experimental toxoplasmic chorioretinitis (141). In addition, using monoclonal antibodies, Araujo et al. (142) showed that the soluble antigen found in the serum of acute infected humans is also present on the membrane of tachyzoites. In the in vivo situation, these soluble antigens may prevent the antibodies' access to the tachyzoite's surface. The shedding of the antigen-antibody complex may be responsible for the immune complexes detected in the serum of patients with acute toxoplasmosis (143–145).

D. Organism-Induced Immunosuppression

1. Animal Models

Acute and chronic infection with *Toxoplasma* have paradoxical effects on the cell-mediated immune system. Chronic infection with *Toxoplasma* confers upon mice nonspecific resistance to a variety of intracellular pathogens and to transplantable and autochthonous tumors. However, acute and chronic infection with *Toxoplasma* also appear to have a profound immunosuppressive effect on other immunological functions. Strickland et al. (146) and Huldt (147) demonstrated that the primary humoral response to immunization with sheep red blood cells in mice chronically infected with *Toxoplasma* was depressed compared with uninfected controls. In addition, Huldt et al. noted severe atrophy of the thymus associated with acute infection (148). Hibbs et al. (149) also showed that chronically infected mice that were reinfected with the same strain of *Toxoplasma* had a suppressed primary antibody response to sheep red blood cells and to tetanus toxoid; however, the secondary antibody response to both sheep red blood cells and tetanus toxoid remained intact. In addition, primary humoral response in mice to *Clostridium welchii typhii* vaccine, louping ill virus vaccine, bovine serum albumin, and live louping ill virus has been depressed in mice with *Toxoplasma* (150). Buxton et al. (151) demonstrated that the antibody response to enzootic abortion vaccine and louping ill vaccine was significantly depressed in sheep infected for 7 or 28 days with *Toxoplasma* compared with uninfected controls.

The immunosuppression associated with *Toxoplasma* has not been limited to depressed antibody response to primary immunization. Hibbs et al. (152) observed a prolongation of allograft survival in mice that were chronically infected and received a skin graft from mice that differed at the H-2 histocompatibility locus. Strickland et al. (146) and Chan et al. (153) showed markedly depressed blastogenic response of splenocytes of the T-cell mitogens concanavalin A and phytohemagglutinin as well as the B-cell mitogen lipopolysaccharide. This immunosuppression was found in mice acutely and chronically infected with *T. gondii*. McLeod et al. (154) were not able to confirm this finding when they studied mice infected either intravenously or intraperitoneally with *T. gondii*. However, McLeod et al. (155) demonstrated that mice infected periorally with an avirulent strain of *T. gondii* had marked suppression in lymphocyte proliferation to concanavalin A.

The mechanisms involved in the immunodepression that occurs with murine toxoplasmosis are dynamic, with different lymphocyte subpopulations being involved at different times during the infection. The immunosuppression evoked by the parasitic infection may allow the parasite the ability to survive within the host by not permitting a protective response to develop. As mentioned above, depression in the primary antibody response to sheep red blood cells (SRBC) has been demonstrated in mice chronically infected with *T. gondii*. Suzuki et al. (156) confirmed these observations and also demonstrated that the humoral response to the T-independent antigen dinitrophenylated Ficoll (DNP-Ficoll) was also suppressed by toxoplasma infection. However, this suppression occurred when mice were primed after infection. Once the priming was established prior to infection, the suppressive effect did not occur (157). These data suggested that both T and B lymphocytes may be suppressed independently of of each other during toxoplasma infection and that this suppression of B-lymphocyte function can occur independently of the T cell. Also, the immuno-suppression demonstrated pertained only to the initiation and not to the expression of memory cells (157). In vitro studies revealed that splenocytes from infected mice had a diminished capacity to mount an SRBC DNP-Ficoll-specific plaque-forming cell response. Furthermore, Suzuki and Kobayashi found that a plastic adherent (158–160), radioresistant (159) spleen cell had a suppressive effect on the ability of normal mouse spleen cells to mount an SRBC-specific plaque-forming cell response in vitro (157).

Lymphocyte proliferation to the T-cell mitogen concanavalin A has been shown to be markedly depressed in mice acutely and chronically infected with *T. gondii*. Chan et al. (153) studied the mechanisms involved in the depression of lymphocyte proliferation to concanavalin A in C57 black mice acutely infected with either the virulent RH or less virulent C56 strain of *Toxoplasma*. In these studies, the proliferative response and interleukin 2 production of splenocytes and T-enriched cells from infected mice were significantly depressed compared to uninfected controls. Removal of macrophages or addition of indomethacin improved the proliferative response of splenocytes from mice infected with the less virulent strain of *T. gondii* but had no effect on the proliferative response of splenocytes of mice infected with the RH strain of *T. gondii*. These data indicated that there was a defect in T-lymphocyte function in infected mice that was independent of the macrophage. In addition, lymphocyte proliferation of the splenocytes and T lymphocytes of mice infected with the less virulent strain of *Toxoplasma* could be reconstituted with the addition of exogenous interleukin 2, but their peak response never reached the control group. Subsequent studies by Luft et al. (161) revealed that during acute infection with tachyzoites of the RH strain, Thy 1.2^+, Lyt 2.2^+, Lyt 1.2^- and Thy 1.2, Lyt, 1.2^+, Lyt 2.2^-, are generated that suppress the proliferative response of normal splenocytes to concanavalin A. Jones et al. (161a) demonstrated that during acute toxoplasma infection there is a striking increase in the absolute and relative number of Lyt 2^+ T cells in both the spleens and lymph nodes of infected mice. The nonspecific suppressor cells thus demonstrated may play a role in the pathogenesis of persistent toxoplasma infection.

In a study performed by Kasper (117), vaccination with a purified membrane antigen (mol. wt. 30,000) of the tachyzoite decreased resistance to infection to an avirulent strain of *T. gondii*. Vaccinated mice had an increased mortality to infection, and surviving mice had significantly greater numbers of intracerebral tissue cysts. The mechanisms involved in the increased susceptibility due to vaccination have not been defined, but it may be that this particular antigen preparation may preferentially induce suppressor cell activity.

Depression of Natural Killer Cell Activity. Natural killer cell activity has been shown to be augmented during the early phase of acute toxoplasma infection (162,163). However, Kamiyama and Hagiwara (163) also showed that this augmentation of natural killer cell activity early in infection was followed by suppression of activity 2 weeks postinfection. During the early period of infection when there was augmentation of natural killer cell activity, interferon could not be detected in the serum; however, when NK activity was depressed, significant titers of interferon could be detected in the serum. This suppression of natural killer activity during the latter part of infection could not be reversed by administration of interferon or interferon inducers. In cell-mixing experiments, these authors found no direct suppressor effect on natural killer cell function by splenocytes of infected mice. Kamiyama and Tatsumi (164) also reconfirmed the findings of Huldt et al. (148) and Beverly and Henry (165) that infection with *Toxoplasma* is associated with marked changes in the thymus, in particular the loss of cortical lymphocytes in rabbits (165) and congenitally infected mice (148). Furthermore, Kamiyama and Tatsumi (164) showed that thymocytes from uninfected mice showed significant sensitivity to cytolytic activity of natural killer cells, whereas thymocytes from mice infected with *T. gondii* did not. They speculated that during the course of *T. gondii* infection, thymocytes expressing the natural killer target antigen were eliminated from the thymus. This would explain the significant cortical atrophy in the thymus during acute infection. However, in earlier experiments (162,163), investigators were not able to demonstrate the presence of natural killer cell activity in the thymus during the course of acute toxoplasma infection. Therefore, the direct cytolytic effect of natural killer cells on thymocytes during acute *T. gondii* infections is still speculative.

2. Human Studies

The cell-mediated immune response plays an important role in host resistance to *Toxoplasma* in both animals and humans. However, early studies revealed that the ability to elicit delayed hypersensitivity reaction to intradermally injected *Toxoplasma* antigen showed may require months to develop after infection (166–170). Luft et al. (171) studied the kinetics of the lymphoproliferative response to *Toxoplasma* antigen and mitogens of patients acutely infected with *T. gondii* compared with chronically infected controls. In these studies, there was no significant difference in lymphocyte proliferation to phytohemmagglutinin or pokeweed mitogen. The peak proliferative response to *Toxoplasma* antigen was significantly depressed in acutely infected compared with chronically infected control patients. When the kinetics of the proliferative response of mononuclear cells or helper T cells (Leu 3 positive) alone were studied, it was determined that there was a significant depression in the peak proliferative response. This depression was due not to the presence of a Leu 2 positive suppressor T cell but to the induction of an adherent suppressor cell (171a). Luft et al. (171) also showed that there were marked alterations in the T-cell subpopulations during acute infection with *T. gondii*. In particular, patients with prolonged illness due to *Toxoplasma* had significantly increased numbers of suppressor/cytotoxic (leu 2 positive) T cells and an inverted helper/inducer to suppressor/cytotoxic T-cell ratio. Abnormalities in the relative and absolute numbers of T-lymphocyte subpopulations were also noted in patients with asymptomatic lymphadenopathy. In these patients, T-cell abnormalities were found to be due to either increased numbers of suppressor/cytotoxic T cells or decreased numbers of helper/inducer T cells. Abnormalities in T-cell subpopulations were found to persist for as long as 7 months after the onset of infection and to be associated with a severe reduction in the number of helper/inducer T cells. Further studies of the functional activity of the elevated numbers of suppressor/cytotoxic T cells (CD8 positive) demonstrated that these cells could be activated to suppress *Toxoplasma*-specific immune response by preincubation with *Toxoplasma* antigen (172). Both the induction and suppressive activity of the suppressor T cells were found to be antigen-specific. Subsequently, Yano et al. (173) also demonstrated in a patient with acute toxoplasmosis the presence of a Leu 2-positive suppressor T cell that was induced by *Toxoplasma* antigen to suppress both *Toxoplasma*-specific and tuberculin-specific responses (173). DeWaele et al. (174,174a) also noted increased numbers of suppressor/cytotoxic T cells that also expressed the activation of antigens OKT10 and OKIa (174,

174a) in patients with acute toxoplasmic lymphadenopathy. Subsequently it
was demonstrated that clonal expansion of *Toxoplasma*-antigen-specific suppres-
sor/cytotoxic cells are induced preferentially in patients with acute symptomatic
T. gondii infection (172,175).

E. Virulence Factors

As mentioned in Section V, there has been no demonstration of signficiant
differences in antigenic moieties between the various strains of *Toxoplasma*.
However, Kaufman et al. (176,177) were able to correlate the in vivo virulence
of strains of *Toxoplasma* in mice to their invasiveness and their rate of multiplication in tissue culture. Furthermore, it has been shown that an avirulent strain
of *Toxoplasma* can become more virulent by repeated passage in a host (178,
179). The relationship of an organism's tendency to transform from the tachyzoite stage to the tissue cyst to its virulence or ability to recrudesce with
immunosuppression has not been studied. However, the limiting membrane of
the cyst wall is thicker in the less virulent strains of *T. gondii* (180).

Penetration enhancing factor (PEF) is a protein that was isolated from *Toxoplasma* tachyzoites. This factor seems to alter the host cell membrane in such a
way as to facilitate parasite invasion of the host cell (181-185). In a study by
Lycke et al. (184) it was demonstrated that in addition to enhancing the penetration of *Toxoplasma* into host cells in tissue culture, this factor can increase the
virulence of *Toxoplasma* for mice if it is injected concomitantly with the organisms. This increase in virulence was measured by time to death or percent mortality and was demonstrable with either the extremely virulent RH strain or the
relatively avirulent C56 or C5 strains of organisms. Although PEF would seem to
be an important virulence factor, there have been no studies to determine
whether there are differences in the amounts of PEF present in organisms of
varying virulence. However, with the development of a monoclonal antibody to
PEF (186), it may be possible to quantitate differences in PEF between strains
of *Toxoplasma* of varying virulence and decipher its physiochemical properties.

VII. DEVELOPMENT OF PROTECTIVE IMMUNITY

Infection with *T. gondii* induces changes in a variety of host immune responses.
These include potentiation of nonspecific resistance to a variety of phylogenetically distinct intracellular pathogens and autochthonous and transplanted
tumors (187-191) as well as the acquisition of *Toxoplasma*-specific protective
humoral and cellular immunity (192-196). Paradoxically, as discussed earlier,
certain aspects of antigen-specific and nonspecific immune function are depressed. It becomes evident that infection with *Toxoplasma* involves a tenuous
balance between a protective immune response and the down regulation or

suppression of the immune response. This tenuous balance may be upset as a result of aging, pregnancy, or iatrogenic immunosuppression. The role and relative importance of each of the arms of the protective immune system to resistance to toxoplasma infection or chronic persistence of infection has not been fully defined, but there is evidence that natural, cell-mediated and humoral immunity play important roles in resistance to infection. Therefore, each of these aspects of the immune response in regard to toxoplasma infection will be discussed in turn.

A. Cellular Immunity

Thymus-dependent immunity to *Toxoplasma* plays a prominent role in the protective immune response. Evidence that T cells are involved in the early response to infection comes from studies indicating that T-cell-deficient mice are unable to develop protective immunity and thereby control the infection. Even if infections in the T-cell-deficient mice are controlled temporarily by chemotherapy, protective immunity fails to develop (197), and the mice die after the cessation of antimicrobial chemotherapy. Injection of thymocytes into homologous athymic mice reconstitutes the ability of the mice to develop resistance to *Toxoplasma*. In a series of experiments that Frenkel and Taylor (198) performed with athymic and B-cell-depleted mice, all athymic mice infected with *T. gondii* died within 7 days after infection, whereas 42% of heterozygous (nu/+) controls and the B-cell-depleted mice died at an average of 30 days postinfection. Because congenitally acquired athymic mice are known to have high endogenous natural killer and macrophage activity despite abnormal cell-mediated immunity, it would seem evident that the T cell plays an important role in early resistance to infection. Furthermore, passive transfer of antibody to nude mice did not alter the outcome or prolong time to death. Passive transfer of T cells immunized to *T. gondii* also confers partial protection to guinea pigs infected with the virulent RH strain of *T. gondii* (199). Recently, Suzuki and Remington (199a) demonstrated that both Lyt 2^+ and Lyt 1^+ cells from immunized mice can confer resistance to the naive animal. Chinchilla and Frenkel (200,201) showed that lymphocytes from immune donors can produce a lymphokine that confers specific strain-restricted immunity to nonphagocytic cells in vitro. This specific mediator was found to have a molecular weight between 3000 and 5000 (202). Administration of γ-interferon has been shown to confer remarkable resistance to mice in vivo (202a), and treatment of mice with monoclonal antibodies directed against γ-interferon causes these animals to be highly susceptible to *T. gondii* infection (202b). These studies provide further evidence of the primacy of cell-mediated immunity in acquired resistance to *Toxoplasma* and the possible presence of multiple mediators that confer immunity. Because the activated macrophage can effectively kill *T. gondii* in vitro, these cells are the primary effector cells (203). However, both natural killer cells (229) and cytotoxic T cells (203a) are capable of killing *T. gondii* in vitro.

1. Phagocytic Cells

It has long been suggested that the activated macrophage plays a preeminent role in the resistance to toxoplasma infection. Peritoneal macrophages from mice acutely and chronically infected with *Toxoplasma* have a remarkable ability to kill not only intracellular *Toxoplasma* (203) but also other unrelated phylogenetically distinct facultative and obligate intracellular pathogens (204) as well as tumor target cells (205). Macrophages and human monocyte-derived macrophages become activated after being exposed to lymphokines produced by sensitized lymphocytes cocultured with *Toxoplasma* antigen (206–209). The ability of lympohcytes from acutely infected mice to activate macrophages in vitro correlated temporarily with the in vivo acquisition of activated macrophages (194). The major mediator of macrophage activation is gamma-interferon (210,211). As discussed earlier, the induction of increased microbial activity is associated with increased oxygen-dependent and independent mechanisms of microbial activity.

The ability of *Toxoplasma* to infect and proliferate within mononuclear phagocytes had been felt to facilitate the dissemination of infection by serving as a haven from antibody-dependent cytotoxicity. However, the ability of mononuclear phagocytes to kill or inhibit the protection of *T. gondii* in vitro is dependent on the length of time that the monocytes are cultured prior to challenge. It was shown by McLeod et al. (212) that in monocytes cultured in vitro for less than 4 hr prior to challenge with *Toxoplasma*, greater than 80% of human peripheral blood monocytes that phagocytosed also killed and eliminated the organism. Similarly, Wilson and Remington (213) demonstrated that both human peripheral blood moncytes and polymorphonuclear leukocytes challenged within 1 hr of isolation were able to eliminate or retard the multiplication of the organism. Elimination of *Toxoplasma* from the granulocyte proceeded more slowly than from the cultured monocyte, but both cell types inhibited replication of *Toxoplasma* to an equivalent extent. Interestingly, Sklenar et al. (175) demonstrated that during acute infection with *T. gondii* there is an increase in the absolute numbers of monocytes. These data suggest that the circulating monocyte or polymorphonuclear leukocyte may be a first-line defense mechanism against *T. gondii* infection prior to the development of acquired immunity.

The ability of phagocytes to kill *T. gondii* is dependent on oxygen-dependent and independent microbicidal activity. In cell-free systems it has been determined that *Toxoplasma* is fairly resistant to exposure to hydrogen peroxide (214). However, the presence of peroxidase and halide synergistically augments the activity of hydrogen peroxide (214,215). Hydroxyl radicals and singlet oxygen have been implicated as being potently toxoplasmacidal in a series of experiments utilizing the xanthine–xanthine oxidase system and the intermediate oxygen metabolite scavengers superoxide dismutase and catalase (214,216).

Murine peritoneal macrophages and human monocyte-derived macrophages failed to mount a respiratory burst upon phagocytosis with *T. gondii* (132,133). In contrast, phagocytosis and killing of *T. gondii* by freshly isolated monocytes was accompanied by a remarkable oxidative burst (212,213,215). The ability of the murine macrophage to kill or inhibit the intracellular multiplication of *Toxoplasma* has been directly correlated to the amount of oxygen metabolites released after stimulation with phorbol myristate acetate (133). Macrophages activated either in vivo or in vitro were found to have an increased capacity to mount an oxidative burst upon phagocytosis of *T. gondii*. In addition, the addition of lymphokines after phagocytosis can activate the macrophage to kill or inhibit the multiplication of *Toxoplasma* (217). Resident peritoneal macrophages also acquired the ability to kill *Toxoplasma* when cocultured with xanthine–xanthine oxidase, which produced the needed oxygen metabolites (214). In contrast to murine peritoneal macrophages, resident rat peritoneal and alveolar macrophages kill *T. gondii* without involvement of toxic metabolites of oxygen (217a,217b).

The capacity of monocytes or monocyte-derived macrophages to kill or inhibit the multiplication of *T. gondii* has been correlated with the level of myeloperoxidase within the phagocytes. Freshly isolated monocytes that have been demonstrated to kill *T. gondii* contain myeloperoxidase and undergo a respiratory burst as measured by O_2^-, H_2O_2, and O_2 consumption in response to PMA. At 72 hr, the respiratory burst in response to PMA is more vigorous; however, myleoperoxidase levels are diminished, as is the ability to kill *T. gondii* (218,219). Murine resident peritoneal macrophages and 5–10-day cultured human monocyte-derived macrophages, which have no myeloperoxidase and a markedly diminished respiratory burst, also have no effect on intracellular proliferation of the organism (219a). However, coating *Toxoplasma* tachyzoites with eosinophil peroxidase prior to ingestion by murine resident peritoneal macrophages gives the phagocyte substantial toxoplasmacidal activity (215). It should be noted that lymphokine activation of macrophages or 3-day-old monocytes, which enables these cells to kill *T. gondii*, does not enhance the production of myeloperoxidase, indicating the multiplicity of mechanisms involved in intracellular killing. McLeod and Remington (220) first suggested that oxygen-independent mechanisms may be involved in the microbicidal activity of mononuclear phagocytes. In a series of experiments involving the use of inhibitors of various metabolic pathways or cell function, they showed that the serine esterase inhibitor toxyllysine chloromethyl ketone (TLCK) abrogated killing or inhibition of growth of *T. gondii* by activated macrophages. Unfortunately, TLCK may also decrease the levels of intracellular reduced glutathione and thereby affect the peroxidative processes and toxic oxygen radicals within mouse macrophages. Aminophylline, which increases concentration of cyclic AMP by inhibition of phosphodiesterase, also diminished the microbicidal capacity of the activated macrophages. Although these studies were not definitive, they suggested that serine esterases and cyclic AMP levels may play a role in the killing of these intracellular pathogens.

The relative contribution of oxygen-independent mechanisms involved in the killing of *T. gondii* may depend on the population of mononuclear phagocytic cells being studied. For instance, antioxidative manipulations were more detrimental to the activated macrophage's ability to inhibit the intracellular growth of *T. gondii* than they were to the ability of the 1-day-old monocyte (221). This difference was interpreted by Murray et al. (221) to mean that oxygen-independent mechanisms might play a more substantial role in the 1-day-old monocyte's activity or may reflect increased amounts of intracellular oxygen metabolites that are inaccessible to the actions of the inhibitors. Wilson and Haas (217) found monocyte-derived macrophages activated by concanavalin A-induced lymphokines had enhanced toxoplasmacidal activity but did not increase O_2^- release in response to phorbol myristate acetate or zymosan, two potent inducers of the oxidative burst; nor did the activated phagocyte have increased nitroblue tetrazolium reduction around the ingested parasite. Antioxidants did not reverse the anti-*Toxoplasma* activity of these activated macrophages. Furthermore, phagosome-lysosome fusion of *T. gondii*-infected cells was not significantly enhanced in lymphokine-stimulated monocyte-derived macrophages. These results suggested that lymphokine-activated monocyte derived macrophages exhibit anti-*Toxoplasma* activity independently of oxidative metabolism.

Further evidence that nonoxidative mechanisms are involved in anti-*Toxoplasma* activity is derived from studies that employed monocytes from patients with chronic granulomatous disease (CGD) (221). In these studies, 1-day-old monocytes from CGD patients displayed microbistatic effects. Treatment of CGD monocytes with mitogen- or antigen-stimulated lymphokines enhanced toxoplasmastatic activity and induced toxoplasmacidal activity as well. However, there was no reversal in the low to absent levels of H_2O_2 or nitroblue tetrazolium reduction. In addition, parasitized endothelial and mouse kidney cells cocultured with lymphokine inhibited the intracellular proliferation of *T. gondii* (222,223). Gamma-interferon appears to be the lymphokine necessary for induction of the nonoxidative anti-*Toxoplasma* activity (224–226).

2. Natural Killer Cells

Natural killer (NK) cells are lymphocytes that are distinct from T cells, B cells, and macrophages and have cytotoxic activity against various tumor target cells to which the host has not been previously sensitized. Natural killer cells have also been found to have cytotoxic activity against various protozoans, including *T. gondii* (227) and fungal targets (228). Hauser et al. (162) demonstrated that increased natural killer cell activity is augmented during acute infection with *T. gondii*.

This increase in NK activity was paralleled by a concomitant rise in interferon activity in the serum of the infected mice. Kamiyama and Hagiwara (163) similarly found augmented levels of NK activity in the splenocytes of mice infected for 3 days with tachyzoites of the Beverly strain; however, in contrast to Hauser et al. (162), NK cytotoxicity was markedly and significantly diminished between 12 and 47 days after infection. Sklener et al. (175) showed that during acute infection with *T. gondii* in humans there is an increase in the absolute number of lymphocytes bearing the cell membrane marker (leu 7) for NK cells.

Subsequently, Hauser et al. (124) demonstrated that both the soluble and particulate fractions of *Toxoplasma* tachyzoites enhanced NK activity. Treatment of the fraction with heat, protease, or periodate diminished the ability to augment NK activity, whereas ribonuclease treatment had no effect. Sharma et al. (125) showed that NK activity could be augmented if human peripheral blood lymphocytes were cocultured with *Toxoplasma* antigen. Associated with the elevation in NK activity was a concomitant increase in interferon in the cell culture supernates. In addition, the NK cell augmenting effect of *Toxoplasma* antigen could be blocked by the presence of anti-*Toxoplasma* antibodies. More recently, Hauser and Tsai (229) provided further evidence that NK cells may be involved in resistance to *Toxoplasma*. In their studies, NK cells isolated from spleen cells from mice acutely infected with *T. gondii* had significantly greater cytotoxicity for extracellular RH tachyzoites than did control cells from uninfected mice. Hence, it has been shown that toxoplasmic infection in mice enhances natural killer cell activity and that those cells when potentiated are toxoplasmacidal.

3. Interferon Induction

It is well established that toxoplasma infection in mice induces production of interferon (124,162); however, the type of interferon produced has not been defined. The rapid rise in serum interferon parallels the rise in natural killer cell activity induced by toxoplasma infection. There are two mechanisms involved in *Toxoplasma*'s ability to induce interferon production: one that is not dependent on previous sensitization to *T. gondii* or *T. gondii* antigens (125), and one that is dependent on acquired immunity (223). Cocultivation of human mononuclear cells from patients without serological evidence of prior toxoplasma infection with *Toxoplasma* antigen resulted in significant production of interferon (125). Shirahata and Shimizu (223) cocultured murine splenocytes from mice acutely infected with *T. gondii* with *Toxoplasma* antigen and demonstrated that immune interferon was induced in splenocytes of mice as early as 4 days after infection. Because increased levels of interferon have been demonstrated in the serum of mice as early as 24 hr postinfection (124,162), there is probably a component to its induction that does not require an acquired immune response. The production of interferon early in infection is probably the manner in which natural killer and monocyte-macrophage function is potentiated, and this may occur prior to the development of acquired immunity.

Besides having the ability to augment the function of effector cells, interferon has also been found to have a direct effect on *Toxoplasma* multiplication within nonphagocytic cells. Both chicken and mouse beta-interferon suppressed the growth of *Toxoplasma* in homologous host cells (230). Human gamma- or beta-interferon had no effect on the proliferation of *Toxoplasma* within human fibroblasts (231). Shirahata and Shimizu (223) showed that a lymphokine with the physiochemical characteristics of gamma-interferon blocked the intracellular growth of *T. gondii* in L cells. Subsequently, it was shown that fibroblasts cocultured with recombinant purified gamma-interferon either prior to infection or after infection with *T. gondii* inhibited the intracellular multiplication of the organism (225,226). This effect of gamma-interferon has been shown to be due to the induction of an indoleamine 2,3-dioxgenase, which results in an increase in tryptophan degradation within the host cell (226,231a).

B. Humoral Immunity

Natural toxoplasma infection in humans results in an early rise in *Toxoplasma*-specific IgM antibody, which may persist for up to a year after infection (232), and a rise in IgG antibody, which is believed to persist for the life of the host. Perorally acquired *T. gondii* in mice is associated with the development of secondary IgA specific for *T. gondii* (232a). However, the actual role of humoral immunity in resistance to toxoplasma infection has been a subject of controversey. Passive transfer of serum containing high titers of anti-*Toxoplasma* antibodies to chronically infected mice has been reported to actively exacerbate the infection, as measured by increased parasitemia (233) and increased cyst rupture in the brains of these mice (234). In this respect, Kasper (117) also observed that passive transfer of a monoclonal antibody to the 30,000-dalton antigen exacerbated subsequent toxoplasma infection. Other investigators reported that passive transfer of immune serum had little or no effect on the course of infection (235). In contrast, Krahenbuhl et al. (195) demonstrated that passive transfer of mouse serum containing high titers of anti-*Toxoplasma* antibody conveyed considerable protection to mice infected with a relatively avirulent strain of *Toxoplasma*. Furthermore, in recent studies by Johnson et al. (120), passively transferred monoclonal antibodies specific to the 14,000- and 35,000-D membrane antigens conferred protection to mice infected with a moderately virulent strain of *T. gondii*. Subsequently, Sharma et al. (115) were able to confer protection against a moderately virulent strain of *T. gondii* by passive transfer of a monoclonal antibody specific to a cytoplasmic antigen. It is intriguing to speculate on the mechanisms involved in the variability in host protection with various monoclonal antibodies. The fact that some passively transferred antibodies protect mice from acute infection whereas others exacerbate infection may be analogous to a situation that other investigators described with different preparations of polyclonal antisera. Perhaps if the humoral response is predominantly directed against certain antigens, infection may be worsened rather than limited.

Further evidence that humoral immunity plays an important role in host resistance to infection was demonstrated by Frenkel and Taylor (236), who depleted neonatal mice of B cells by treatment with anti-u antiserum. All of the B-cell-depleted mice eventually died as a result of their infection, whereas 85% (10/12) of the untreated controls survived. Passively transferred hyperimmune serum protected 25% of B-cell-depleted mice. In addition, *Toxoplasma* could not be isolated from brains of the passively immunized surviving mice, suggesting that antibody may be important in controlling chronic toxoplasmosis but seems to have little influence on early resistance to infection.

Treatment of tachyzoites with antibody facilitates killing of the organisms by two mechanisms. Tachyzoites opsonized with polyclonal (237,238) or mono-clonal (118,119) anti-*Toxoplasma* antibody facilitate phagocystosis and killing of the organism by nonactivated macrophages. The majority of opsonized organisms are killed by nonactivated macrophages, and the multiplication of the survivors is significantly inhibited. Anti-*Toxoplasma* antibody in the presence of accessory factor results in increased permeability of the parasite membrane (239) and death of the organism. Early reports indicated that actuation of the alternative pathway of complement was involved in antibody-dependent killing of *T. gondii*. However, Suzuki et al. (240) reported a requirement for C4 and C2 components of complement, suggesting that the classical pathway was involved in the killing of *Toxoplasma*. Schreiber and Feldman (241) demonstrated in a definitive manner by using sera genetically deficient in the various individual complement components and highly purified human complement factors that an intact classical pathway of complement activation is necessary for antibody-dependent killing of *Toxoplasma*.

VIII. GENETIC VARIABILITY IN HOST RESISTANCE

The availability of syngeneic strains of mice has allowed the study of genetic aspects of susceptibility and resistance to toxoplasma infection (242,243). Williams et al. (244) showed that at least two genes, one linked to the H-2 and one linked to the H-13 locus, determined resistance as measured by mortality to toxoplasma infection. They reported that the B6 mice are more susceptible to low-dose infection with *T. gondii* than are BALB/C mice. Subsequently, Jones and Erb (245) evaluated the genetic susceptibility to toxoplasma infection by determining the effect of infection in various congeneic strains of mice and the number of brain cysts formed. By using 14 different strains they found that the strains that were resistant to the development of cysts had in common the d or s haplotype in the right-hand region of the H-2 complexes. BALB/C mice were found to have significantly fewer brain cysts than C57BL/6 mice. The authors hypothesized that this H-2 complex-linked resistance may be due to influences on the primary immune response, which affects the number of *Toxoplasma* organisms available to enter brain tissue and thereby form cysts. Suzuki and Kobayashi (160) and Brinkmann et al. (245a) demonstrated that the macrophage and B-cell immunosuppression associated with toxoplasma infection is controlled by both H-2-linked and nonlinked genes.

IX. HOST FACTORS ASSOCIATED WITH DISSEMINATED TOXOPLASMOSIS

There are a variety of neoplastic and nonneoplastic conditions associated with disseminated toxoplasmosis (10-13). Both the underlying diseases and the immunosuppression associated with these conditions are probably responsible for the severity of the infection. The lymphocyte-monocyte macrophage axis plays a dominant role in protection against intracellular pathogens. This aspect of the immune axis is depressed by corticosteroids and cytotoxic and antithymocyte drugs (246-248), and therefore these agents probably do play a role in the host's inability to control infection or allow the reactivation of latent infection with *T. gondii*. In addition, malignancies of the reticuloendothelial and hematological systems further compromise patients' cellular immunity and therefore are strongly associated with *T. gondii* infection. Not surprisingly, persons with Hodgkin's disease, who comprise 40% of all cases of severe toxoplasmosis in non-AIDS patients, have various abnormalities in their cell-mediated immune system.

Patients with the acquired immune deficiency syndrome (AIDS) have a striking propensity for the development of disseminated toxoplasmosis, in particular toxoplasmic encephalitis, and therefore the immunological abnormalities associated with AIDS will be discussed in more detail. Finally, a group of patients in whom *Toxoplasma* has caused tremendous concern comprises fetuses and neonates; however, this subject has already been comprehensively reviewed (24) and will not be discussed here.

A. Pharmacological Agents

Active *T. gondii* infection has rarely been clinically suspected or diagnosed prior to the patient receiving immunosuppressive therapy (13). Most cases of disseminated toxoplasmosis in the non-AIDS immunocompromised host had been receiving corticosteroids. Corticosteroids profoundly decrease the number of peripheral lymphocytes and in particular the helper T-cell subpopulation (249). The egress of monocytes (250) and polymorphonuclear leukocytes (251) from the circulation is depressed with chronic corticosteroid administration. In addition, the presence of corticosteroids abrogates the ability of lymphokines to activate normal murine peritoneal macrophages (252,253). However corticosteroids have no effect on the ability of the macrophages, once activated, to inhibit the replication of *T. gondii*. Cytotoxic agents, including cyclophosphamide, also suppress cell-mediated immune function. Cyclophosphosphamide, is a cycle-specific agent that is especially toxic to proliferating cells. It inhibits T-cell lymphocyte proliferation, thereby decreasing the number of committed lymphocytes to a specific antigen as well as decreasing the number of cells available for sensitization. It also has a depressive effect on the numbers of monocytes and polymorphonuclear leukocytes. In most cases of Hodgkin's disease, both cytotoxic drugs and corticosteroids have been administered together and in proximity to the development of toxoplasmic encephalitis. Both corticosteroids and cyclophosphamide have been shown to have an adverse effect on resistance to *T. gondii* infection (see Section X).

The use of cyclosporin in place of other immunosuppressive agents in transplant recipients has been associated with a reduction in the incidence of infectious complications in these patients. In heart transplant recipients, the use of cyclosporin has significantly reduced the incidence of rises in *Toxoplasma* antibody titers in comparison with other immunosuppressive regimens (29). This may be due to the intrinsic anti-*Toxoplasma* activity of cyclosporin (257,258) in addition to its immunosuppressive action.

B. Hodgkin's Disease

Hodgkin's disease has been associated with numerous defects in cell-mediated immunity. In patients with Hodgkin's disease there is lymphocyte depletion of lymphoid tissue as well as peripheral lymphopenia (259). In addition to this quantitative disorder, qualitative abnormalities in T-cell dysfunction have been demonstrated both in vivo and in vitro. These abnormalities in cell-mediated immunity may persist for as long as 10 years after cessation of antineoplastic therapy. Depression in various parameters of cell-mediated immunity has been associated with the neoplasm prior to the initiation of antineoplastic therapy and is further aggravated by radiation and chemotherapy.

In vivo abnormalities indicative of impaired cell-mediated immunity include prolonged skin homograft survival (260,261) and diminished delayed skin hypersensitivity reactions (262-266). Whereas abnormalities in delayed hypersensitivity responses to "recall" antigens are seen in only a minority of patients and are related to the extent of the neoplasm (264), the majority of patients are unable to develop delayed hypersensitivity to neoantigens (266). Various in vitro parameters of T-lymphocyte function have also been shown to be depressed in patients with Hodgkin's disease, including lymphocyte proliferation in response to mitogens (267-272), soluble antigens (273,274), and both allogenic (272) and autologous (273) mixed leukocyte reactions. Depression in lymphocyte function has been attributed to serum factors (273) and to plastic adherent mononuclear cells (273,274) and T cells (275). Monocytes from patients with Hodgkin's disease have been shown to suppress lymphocyte function through the production of prostaglandin E2 (276). Gaines et al. (273) demonstrated that lymphocytes from three individuals with untreated Hodgkin's disease who had previous serological evidence of *Toxoplasma* infection had a depressed proliferative response to *Toxoplasma* antigen. Subsequently, McLeod and Estes (277) found that the lymphoproliferative response to *Toxoplasma* antigen was depressed in six of eight patients with treated Hodgkin's disease and chronic latent *T. gondii* infection.

There is evidence that mononuclear effector cell function is abnormal in patients with Hodgkin's disease. It has been shown that skin test reactivity in anergic patients with Hodgkin's disease cannot be rendered positive to tuberculin by passive transfer of lymphoid cells or transfer factor from normal tuberculin-positive donors. This suggests that these patients were unable to mount the inflammatory response necessary to express a delayed hypersensitivity reaction. Ward and Berenberg (278) demonstrated that in the sera of patients with Hodgkin's disease there was an excessive amount of potent chemotactic factor inactivator, which inactivates leukotactic mediators that are complement-derived. This factor inactivated chemotactic factors for both neutrophils and monocytes. Steigbigel et al. (279) found no abnormality in the ability of polymorphonuclear leukocytes, monocytes, or monocyte-derived macrophages from untreated patients with Hodgkin's disease to kill various pathogens including *Listeria monocytogenes* and *Salmonella typhimurium*. McLeod and Estes (280) found no significant differences in monocyte toxoplasmacidal activity between patients with Hodgkin's disease and control subjects. Furthermore, when monocytes were cocultured with chemotherapeutic agents commonly used in the treatment of Hodgkin's disease, there was no alteration in the ability of these phagocytes to eliminate intracellular *T. gondii*. In contrast to monocyte function, both natural killer activity and antibody-dependent cell-mediated cytotoxicity of splenocytes and peripheral blood lymphocytes from patients with Hodgkin's disease have also been found to have depressed activity (281).

C. Acquired Immune Deficiency Syndrome

Numerous abnormalities of the immune system characterize patients with AIDS. Severe lymphoid and peripheral lymphocytopenia has been one of the hallmarks of this syndrome. Lymphocyte depletion of the T4 (helper/inducer) subset of T cells is most pronounced (282), resulting in a lowered ratio of T4 to T8 (suppressor/cytotoxic) T cells.

In addition to severe lymphopenia, numerous qualitative abnormalities in

T-lymphocyte function have been reported. As the syndrome progresses, delayed hypersensitivity to various antigens has been absent. Lymphocyte proliferation of whole mononuclear cells in response to T-cell mitogens and soluble antigens including *Toxoplasma* lysate antigen, and in the autologous and allogenic mixed leukocyte reaction has been depressed, as has been their ability to produce inter-leukin 2, macrophage activating factor, and gamma-interferon (282–285). Mononuclear cells from patients with AIDS cocultured with mitogens or specific antigens, including *Toxoplasma* antigen, were not able to produce the lympho-kine necessary to activate monocyte-derived macrophages to inhibit the intra-cellular multiplication of *T. gondii* or *Chlamydia psittaci*. In contrast, staphylo-coccal enterotoxin was able to induce mononuclear cells from AIDS patients to produce gamma-interferon, whereas production of gamma-interferon by these cells in response to mitogens and microbial antigens (including *Toxoplasma* anti-gen) was virtually absent.

Separation of T lymphocytes into their subpopulations (T4 and T8) is neces-sary in order to differentiate whether the abnormalities demonstrated above are due to quantitative depletion of subpopulations of T cells or to a qualitative disorder of the various subpopulations of T cells in responding to various stimuli. Furthermore, separating T cells into their subpopulations and then coculturing these subpopulations in fixed proportions would help to define whether a suppressor T-cell mechanism is involved in the depressed immune response. When T4 and T8 positive lymphocytes are separated and quantitatively adjusted, lymphocyte proliferation of both subpopulations to mitogens is intact, as is their ability to produce interleukin 2 and express the interleukin 2 receptor, however, the response to soluble antigens such as tetanus toxoid is severely diminished (286). Thus, the T-lymphocyte populations responsible for recognition of soluble antigens have been either destroyed or severely functionally impaired. Positively selected T4 lymphocytes from AIDS patients have also been found to respond normally in the allogenic mixed lymphocyte reaction. Further cell-mixing studies are needed to determine the actual relationship of the T4 to T8 cells in the depression of various parameters in cell-mediated immunity.

Patients with AIDS also have marked B-lymphocyte dysfunction. Abnormal-ities in B-lymphocyte function became obvious in the first cases of toxoplasmic encephalitis described in AIDS patients in whom there was no significant rise in anti-*Toxoplasma* antibody titers in response to severe infection. In studies by Lane et al. (287), it was determined that AIDS patients had a polyclonal activa-tion of B lymphocytes with a higher number of spontaneous plaque-forming cells in their peripheral blood than did homosexual or heterosexual controls. However, the B lymphocytes of AIDS patients did not respond to the T-cell-dependent B-cell mitogen, pokeweed mitogen, or to the T-cell-independent mitogen *Staphylococcus aureus* Cowan strain. Furthermore, T4 lymphocytes from AIDS patients were unable to provide help in the pokeweek-mitogen-induced B-cell differentiation assay. These experiments point to a combined defect in both the T4 helper/inducer subpopulation and the B cell itself.

Effector cell dysfunction has also been reported in AIDS patients. Monocytes from AIDS patients are able to effectively kill *T. gondii*, and killing by monocyte-derived macrophages from AIDS patients can be enhanced with gamma-interferon (283). Thus, the severe immune abnormalities in patients with AIDS have complicated both the serological diagnosis of toxoplasma infection and the ability to control the infection with chemotherapeutic agents.

X. PATHOGENESIS OF TOXOPLASMOSIS

Our knowledge of the pathogenesis of toxoplasma infection in the immuno-compromised host is largely dependent on studies in animal models of infection. There have been few prospective studies of groups of immunocompromised patients at high risk for the development of toxoplasmosis. Knowledge of the pathogenesis in humans must be gleaned from a myriad of case reports and short series of cases. The pathogenesis of the disease in any patient is dependent on several host factors, including whether the infection has been recently acquired or is a result of the reactivation of a latent infection; the nature and severity of the patient's immunocompromising illness and whether it is ultimately reversible; and the cellular and humoral immune status of the patient in regard to *T. gondii*. Although the tachyzoite is not thought to have any proclivity to infect a particular organ, the brain, heart, and skeletal muscle of latently infected animals have greater numbers of cysts than other organs. Remington (288) noted that the number of cysts in the brains of chronically infected rats and mice was greater than in organs such as liver, spleen, and kidney.

A. Animal Models

Because toxoplasma infection in the nonimmunocompromised adult is usually asymptomatic, our knowledge of the pathogenesis of the early infection comes from experimental infection in animals. After infection via the oral route by ingestion of tissue cysts or oocysts, the organism is released within the gastro-intestinal tract and invades the intestinal epithelium (17). *Toxoplasma* multiplies intracellularly, causes cellular disruption, and then invades adjacent cells. The tachyzoites are disseminated throughout the body from the initial site of infection through the lymphatics and the vascular system. Tachyzoites are able to invade all cell types, and therefore organisms have been demonstrated in all tissue types. In humans, parasitemia has been demonstrated for up to a year after acute toxoplasma infection (67), and tissue cysts have been found in multiple organs (17). McLeod et al. (155) studied the histopathological response of mice orally infected with *Toxoplasma* tissue cysts. They noted the presence of tachyzoites in mesenteric lymph nodes as early as 2 days after peroral infection. Eight days after infection, foci of inflammatory cells were found in the lungs, brain, and heart of infected mice. Tachyzoites were most prominent in the brain, where they were found in association with foci of necrosis and inflammation. Clusters of epitheloid histocytes found in the spleens were reminiscent of the epitheloid histocytes present in the lymph nodes during lymphadenopathic toxoplasmosis in humans (155). Small foci of small and large lymphocytes were found within the hepatic lobules in association with degenerating and necrotic hepatic cells. The observation of McLeod et al. of larger numbers of tachyzoites in the brain of mice acutely infected compared with other organs is reminiscent of the earlier study of Frenkel (289). He observed that *Toxoplasma* tachyzoites were cleared less efficiently from brains of mice than from extraneural sites. He postulated that the blood-brain barrier allowed the organisms to proliferate in the environment free of antibody, at a time when they were being destroyed in extraneural sites. With the development of cell-mediated and humoral immunity, tachyzoites are destroyed and are not demonstrable in tissues of the host. The tissue cyst becomes the only demonstrable form of the organism.

There is evidence to suggest that in the chronically infected animal, active recurrent infection is responsible for the lifelong persistence of antibodies and cell-mediated immunity to *Toxoplasma*. Recurrent episodes of parasitemia have been documented by recovery of *Toxoplasma* organisms from blood of immunocompetent mice (68), guinea pigs (290), rabbits (291), and humans (67) for as long as 8 months after the infection. Lainson (72) and Van der Waaj (292) sequentially studied the development of tissue cysts in the brains of mice infected with *Toxoplasma* and found that daughter cysts develop in close proximity to larger cysts. No inflammatory reaction accompanied this process. Wanko et al. (73) noted that in mice infected over a 60-day period two distinct subpopulations of cysts developed that could be differentiated on the basis of size. Conley and Jenkins (293) also noted populations of large and small cysts in mice infected with *T. gondii*. However, the smaller cysts were accompanied by a focus of inflammatory cells. These studies suggest recurrent rupturing of cysts, with the release of organisms and the formation of new cysts. This sequence may cause persistent antigenic stimulation, which may account for the persistence of high titers of antibody and cell-mediated immunity as well as organism-associated immunosuppression. This organism-induced immunosuppression may be further accentuated when there is underlying immunosuppression, which aggravates the rate of cyst rupture.

The inflammatory process found in acutely infected animals is not necessarily associated with the presence of antigens or organisms. McLeod et al. (155) found that many of the inflammatory lesions in lymphoid tissues and livers of acutely infected mice had no associated antigen or organisms. In contrast, Conley and

Jenkins (293) studied the anatomical relationship of *Toxoplasma* organisms or antigens to the inflammatory response in brains of infected mice. Using an immunohistochemical stain, they found that initially tachyzoites were seen in proximity to small vessels and that this was followed several days later by a perivascular infiltrate of mononuclear cells. The mononuclear cells formed microglial nodules in proximity to tachyzoites or toxoplasmal antigens. Cysts were found in the periphery of the microglial nodules and were remote from any inflammatory response. Frenkel and Escajadillo (293a) also demonstrated that the formation of the microglial nodule is anatomically associated with the presence of tissue cysts, bradyzoites, or lysed organisms.

The effect of immunosuppression on the pathogenesis of severe disseminated toxoplasmosis has been studied by numerous investigators. However, Frenkel et al. (294,295) first provided convincing experimental evidence that perturbation of the cell-mediated immune system by immunosuppression resulted in the recrudescence of infection. This recrudescent infection is similar to that seen in humans. In these studies, chronically infected hamsters treated with cortisone and total body irradiation developed encephalitis, pneumonitis, and retinochoroiditis. Histologically, the encephalitis was a focal necrotizing process consistent with the rupturing of single or groups of tissue cysts in close proximity to one another. This caused the release of tachyzoites, which resulted in the infection of surrounding neurons and astrocytes and an inflammatory infiltrate. The centers of the inflammatory foci were composed of necrotic tissue, and toward the periphery there were large numbers of tachyzoites. Vollmer et al. (295a) showed that depletion of CD4 positive T cells in mice chronically infected with *T. gondii* results in severe central nervous system damage due to toxoplasma infection with only minor systemic findings.

Acute infection in mice immunocompromised by treatment with cortisone (296), antilymphocyte serum (297), antithymocyte serum (298,299), monoclonal antibodies directed against the CD4 T cells (295a), or 6-mercaptopurine (296) results in decreased resistance to infection and severe disseminated infection, including diffuse meningoencephalitis. Animals that had received cortisone or antilymphocyte serum developed prolonged parasitemia. Histopathologically, mice had evidence of widespread disseminated infection, which included diffuse infection of the brain and meninges.

B. Human Studies

In humans, the pathogenesis of the infection in the immunocompromised host can be inferred from a variety of case reports or small series of cases and from the experimental finding described above. In the first review of toxoplasmosis in the immunocompromised host, Ruskin and Remington (10) called attention to 81 cases of toxoplasmosis in the compromised host. Neurological manifestations of infection dominated the clinical picture in more than half the patients. Although *Toxoplasma* was reported in association with a variety of underlying conditions, cancer of the reticuloendothelial system accounted for more than 50% of the conditions associated with disseminated toxoplasmosis. The most common malignancy associated with toxoplasmic encephalitis is Hodgkin's disease. The combination of the immunological abnormalities associated with Hodgkin's disease and the chemotherapy which consists of corticosteroids and cytotoxic agents, seems to greatly enhance the possibility of the development of severe toxoplasma infection. Indeed, only a small minority of patients with Hodgkin's disease (13) or other reticuloendothelial malignancies develop toxoplasmosis prior to receiving chemotherapy or remote from from their last chemotherapy. Both the corticosteroids and cytotoxic chemotherapy as well as the underlying Hodgkin's disease impact greatly on the cellular immune function and therefore may diminish the host's ability to respond adequately to acute infection or allow the recrudescence of a latent infection.

It is difficult to discern in Hodgkin's disease or other immunocompromising illnesses which mode of pathogenesis, new acute infection or recrudescence, is more prominent. Certain patients with severe disseminated toxoplasmosis have no detectable anti-*Toxoplasma* antibody at the time of diagnosis of toxoplasmic encephalitis, suggesting the acute onset of infection (11,300–302). In addition, the relationship of the onset of severe toxoplasma infection to the duration of the underlying malignancy varied from 2 months to 8 years, and in some instances occurred when the patient was not receiving chemotherapy and was in remission (12,303). In one patient with acute myelocytic leukemia, the patient seroconverted and developed severe toxoplasmic encephalitis while in remission. The acute acquisition of toxoplasma infection was also dramatically shown in four patients with acute leukemia who received granulocyte transfusions from two patients with chronic myelogenous leukemia. All four patients developed serological and clinical evidence of acute toxoplasma infection (26).

The most convincing evidence regarding recrudescence of infection as the pathogenic mechanism involved in toxoplasmosis are the recent studies of disseminated toxoplasmosis in AIDS patients (60) and bone marrow recipients (44, 304,305). In six patients with bone marrow transplantation and disseminated toxoplasmosis, *Toxoplasma* antibody was present prior to transplantation (44, 304,305), suggesting that reactivation of a latent infection is the likely source of active disease. Similarly, in a series of 27 patients with central nervous system toxoplasmosis and AIDS, serological tests for *Toxoplasma* antibody were available in 15 patients between 1 and 6 months prior to the onset of cerebral disease. All 15 patients had *Toxoplasma* antibody prior to the onset of toxoplasmic encephalitis (60). These data suggest that in this group of patients, toxoplasmic encephalitis resulted from recrudescence of a latent infection.

Frenkel et al. (295) suggested that the lesions of recrudescence are limited for the most part to the brain. In the immunocompromised patient, after a cyst rupture, the organism multiplies and gives rise to a focal lesion without the impeding force of an intact immune system. This evolves into a focal necrotizing encephalitis. In contrast, the immune system outside the central nervous system is still effective in controlling the infection. This hypothesis may explain why in 50% of the immunocompromised patients with disseminated toxoplasmosis central nervous system disease is the most prominent manifestation of infection (10).

In contrast to these studies, in cardiac transplant recipients there is strong epidemiological evidence that the donor heart is the principal source of infection (28-30,306). Cardiac transplant recipients who were seronegative for *Toxoplasma* antibodies before cardiac transplantation and received a heart from a seropositive donor developed severe life-threatening infection. Clinically significant disease did not develop in those patients who were seropositive prior to transplantation (29). In addition, of four renal transplant recipients who developed toxoplasmic encephalitis and in whom *Toxoplasma* serology was available prior to transplantation, none had *Toxoplasma* antibody prior to transplantation (45,75,307). In these cases, as in the series described by Siegel et al. (26) of transfusion-associated toxoplasmosis, the infection was widespread, with multiple organs involved.

XI. PATHOLOGY

The histopathological changes associated with toxoplasma infection in the immunocompromised host are variable, depending on whether the infection is acutely acquired or a recrudescence of a latent infection, as well as on the type and severity of the underlying immunocompromising conditions. Knowledge of the protean histopathological presentations of *Toxoplasma* is important because of its ability to mimic other disease processes.

A. Lymph Nodes

In general, lymphadenopathy is not a prominent manifestation of toxoplasmosis in the immunocompromised host. However, toxoplasmic lymphadenopathy may resemble a lymphoreticular disorder. Two patients who were treated with chemotherapy and/or radiotherapy for lymphosarcoma died of disseminated toxoplasmosis (308,309). At autopsy, and in retrospect, the diagnosis of lymphosarcoma was incorrect. Similarly, another patient was incorrectly treated for a malignant reticuloendotheliosis and died of severe disseminated toxoplasmosis (38). In contrast, Miettinen and Franssila (310) pointed out that while the histological differential diagnosis between toxoplasmosis and malignant lymphoma is usually not difficult, atypical lymphoid hyperplasia with epitheloid cell proliferation in patients with Hodgkin's disease, mainly lymphocyte predominance nodular type, are the most frequent differential diagnositic problems with lymph node toxoplasmosis. Dorfman and Remington (311) found an excellent correlation of serological evidence of acute toxoplasma infection with the histopathological changes of the lymph node that occur as a result of toxoplasmosis. Pathological criteria included follicular hyperplasia associated with the presence of irregular clusters of epitheloid histocytes, usually located in the cortical and paracortical zones or within the germinal center and characteristically encroaching upon and blurring the margins of the germinal centers. In addition, subcapsular and trabecular sinuses were distended by "monocytoid" cells. These "monocytoid" cells have been identified as IgG-bearing B lymphocytes. The ability of *Toxoplasma* to induce striking changes in mononuclear cell morphology is not confined to the lymph node. The *Toxoplasma*-associated inflammatory response to intracerebral infection may be so atypical as to cause difficulty in differentiating reactive changes from malignant lymphoma (see the following section).

B. Brain

The histopathological changes in humans with toxoplasmic encephalitis are variable. The changes can vary from a well-localized indolent granulomatous process (37,312,313) to a widely diffuse necrotizing encephalitis (11,37,47,75). The degree of localization and degeneration of the infectious process is dependent on the severity of the underlying immunodeficiency. In patients who are severely immunocompromised and left untreated, the ability to contain the infection and develop an organized encapsulated abscess is diminished. The lesions can be unifocal or multifocal and may vary in size from microscopic (53) to involving almost an entire cerebral hemisphere (11,37,47,314). Both the white matter and gray matter as well as every part of the central nervous system may be involved. There is a propensity for the lesions of toxoplasmic encephalitis to localize in the basal ganglia, the corticomedullary interface, the thalamus, and the white matter (315,316). The pituitary gland may also be involved either as a focal area of infection or as part of an extensive encephalitic process (11, 317). The leptomeninges are usually not involved except as part of a localized reaction of an underlying cortical process.

Necrotizing lesions are not dependent on the host's inflammatory response. Severe necrotizing processes may occur with minimal or no inflammation, suggesting that unimpeded proliferation or *Toxoplasma* causes lysis and destruction of infected cells. In addition to the ability of the organism to infect any cell in the central nervous system (including neurons, glial cells, vascular endothelial cells, pericytes, and astrocytes), nonspecific changes such as vacuolization within neurons and Purkinje cells and loss of Nissl substance may occur (307,318–321).

Infection with *Toxoplasma* causes vascular proliferation and endothelial hyperplasia associated with a perivascular inflammatory infiltrate (Fig. 3) (313, 321-323). There may be a profound response of microglial cells in various stages of activation, which form nodules (12,38,295,300,307,318). These microglial nodules may not be associated with any other evidence of acute inflammation; however, in the same patients, in areas of the brain remote from these nodules, there may be a large area of necrosis. Areas of severe necrosis do not invariably occur, and the only histopathological manifestation of toxoplasmic encephalitis may be a severe gliotic reaction (319) or the presence of microglial nodules scattered through the brain, cerebellum, and spinal cord (53). By using routine histopathological stains, it is occasionally possible to demonstrate *Toxoplasma* tachyzoites adjacent to the microglial nodule (53). However, Conley et al. (323) have shown that tachyzoites or *Toxoplasma* antigen were invariably associated with microglial nodules but were not found in the surrounding parenchyma. Histopathologically, the microglial nodule associated with toxoplasmic encephalitis cannot be differentiated from the microglial nodule seen in viral encephalitis, and in certain situations the only way to differentiate a viral encephalitis from a toxoplasmic encephalitis is by immunohistochemical staining (323).

The response to *Toxoplasma* infection is most often a granulomatous reaction with an admixture of lymphocytes, plasma cells, macrophages, and occasional neutrophils (11,60,324). Perivascular round cell infiltrates are prominent and are found in and around the granulomatous lesions but may also be found in areas without associated focal lesions. The perivascular infiltrate, both round cells and polymorphonuclear leukocytes, can encroach on the vessels, causing a vasculitis with frank necrosis of the arterial walls and intraluminal thrombosis (60,73, 313). This may result in infarction and hemorrhage. The area of necrosis can become extensive and is dependent on the severity of the underlying immunosuppression as well as on whether or not anti-*Toxoplasma* chemotherapy has been administered. At the periphery of the areas of necrosis, free tachyzoites, pseudocysts, and cysts are identifiable (Fig. 7). It may be necessary to use immunospecific stains to identify the tachyzoite, especially in areas free of necrosis or significant inflammation. This histological pattern has been seen in both AIDS patients and non-AIDS patients with toxoplasmic encephalitis.

In histopathologically characterizing the focal toxoplasmic encephalitis in AIDS patients, Post et al. (315) noted the lesions to have three distinct zones. The central zone was described as an amorphous, avascular, necrotic area containing four identifiable organisms. When vessels were seen, they were necrotic and occluded by fibrinous thrombi. The intermediate zone was engorged with blood vessels, exhibited spotty necrosis, and contained numerous free extracellular and intracellular tachyzoites but rarely cysts. There was perivascular cuffing by round cells and endothelial cell swelling and proliferation. In the outer zone, necrosis was rare, vascular lesions were minimal, and the prominent form of the

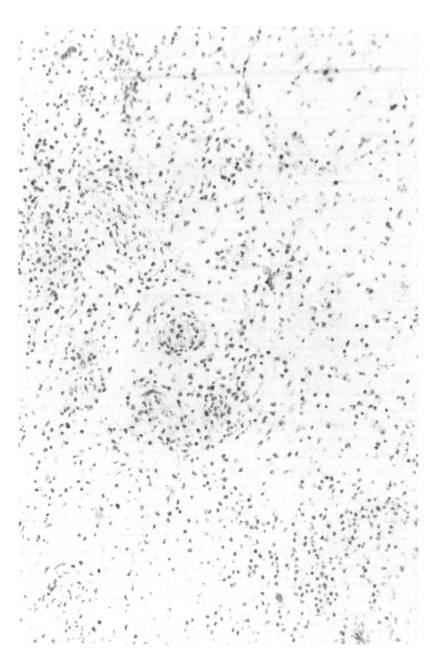

Figure 3 Cellular infiltrate in biopsy specimen of the brain of a patient with AIDS and toxoplasmic encephalitis. Notice the perivascular infiltrate. (Courtesy: F. Fromowitz.)

organism was the cysts. Luft et al. (324) noted a similar histological pattern in brain specimens from patients with toxoplasmic encephalitis that had AIDS or were otherwise immunocompromised. In a study utilizing the peroxidase–antiperoxidase immunohistochemical method, tachyzoites and *Toxoplasma* antigens have been easily recognized, even though cerebral examination of the biopsy sections stained with standard histological stains were inadequate for diagnosis (324). The value of the immunoperoxidase technique becomes clearly evident upon examination of the center of the necrotic focus, which contains coagulated debris. In these instances the immunoperoxidase stain identified what appears to be remnants of the organism.

Navia et al. (60) further defined the histopathological abnormalities seen with *Toxoplasma* by correlating the pathology with the chronicity of infection and length of chemotherapy. In patients who had undergone surgical biopsy or autopsy 14 days before the diagnosis of encephalitis, the lesion was characterized as poorly demarcated areas of necrosis containing a variable number of petechiae and surrounded by acute and chronic inflammatory cells, reactive astrocytes, and macrophages. There was prominent vascular proliferation and endothelial hyperplasia and frank vasculitis. Grossly, the abscess was characterized by areas of softening and discoloration with edema. Routine hematoxylin and eosin sections revealed many *T. gondii* tachyzoites located at the periphery of the abscess. In patients treated for 2 weeks or longer, the lesions consisted of large, well-demarcated areas of central coagulation necrosis surrounded by a thin rim of tightly packed lipid-laden macrophages. Cysts and tachyzoites were identified adjacent to the organizing abscess in only three of seven (42%) patients studied. Chronic abscesses were seen in patients treated for 4 weeks to 11 months. Chronic abscesses were noted that were small (less than 0.5 cm in diameter) cystic spaces that contained small numbers of lipid-laden and hemosiderin-containing macrophages with surrounding gliosis. Rare *Toxoplasma* cysts were noted in adjacent brain tissue. Most of these patients (five of six) had both organizing and chronic abscesses.

Occasionally, the cellular response to *Toxoplasma* has been so intense and atypical that it resembled an intracerebral lymphoma. In these instances the cellular response is described as composed of pelomorphic lymphocytes, plasma cells, reticulohistocytes, and giant cells (Figs. 3 & 4) (39,316,325). This has been found to occur in patients who had undergone renal transplantation (39) and in those with AIDS (315,325a). Recently, Fromowitz et al. (325) attempted to define parameters to differentiate primary cerebral lymphoma from the reactive pleomorphic round cell infiltrate in toxoplasma infection. In this report, the authors noted that the histopathology of a specimen from a patient with toxoplasmic encephalitis showed that in most areas the infiltrate was clearly reactive but not consistently vasocentric. The lymphocytes showed variable but distinct cytological atypia. The cells were larger than usual; many had irregular or

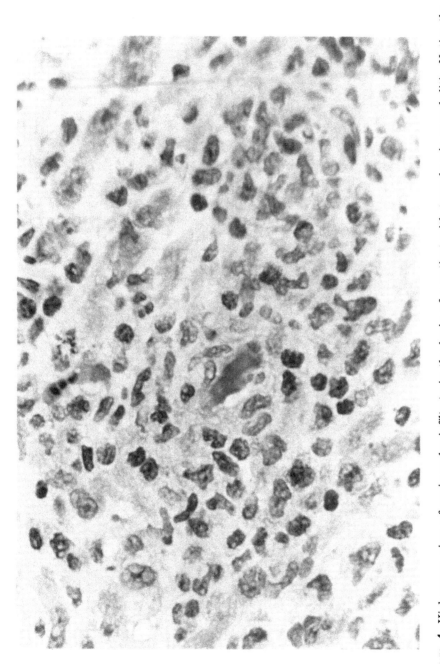

Figure 4 High-power view of perivascular infiltrate in the brain of a patient with toxoplasmic encephalitis. Notice the atypical nature of the cells. (Courtesy: F. Fromowitz.)

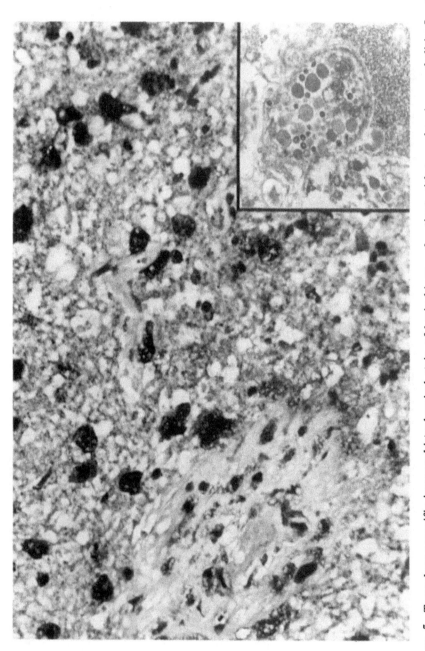

Figure 5 *Toxoplasma*-specific immunohistochemical stain of brain biopsy of patient with toxoplasmic encephalitis. *Inset:* Electron micrograph of *T. gondii* seen in this brain biopsy. (Courtesy: F. Fromowitz.)

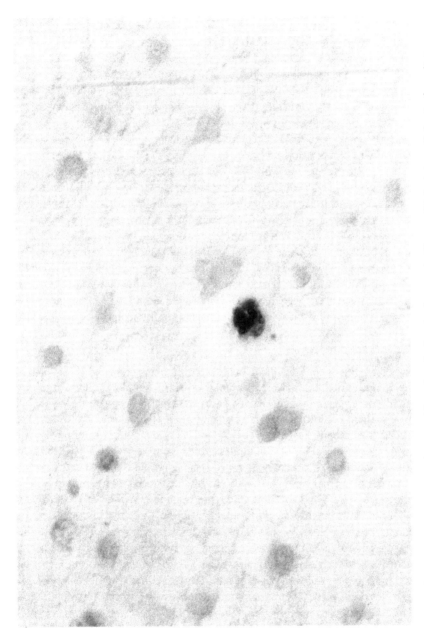

Figure 6 *Toxoplasma*-specific immunohistochemical stain demonstrating multiple intracellular tachyzoites.

cerebriform nuclei, and a few had small nucleoli. Histocytes and endothelial cells were large with nuclear lobulation or multinucleation with prominent nucleoli simulating Reed-Sternberg cells. Immunospecific staining of the cell surface markers revealed the cellular infiltrate to be composed of T lymphocytes, B lymphocytes, and histocytes. Reticulin, which is usually associated with lymphoma, was focally abundant. These findings were compared to the histopathology of a B-cell lymphoma from an AIDS patient. At the periphery of the lesion, where the cell density was diminished, there was involvement of Virchow-Robin space, making the infiltrate appear perivascular and reactive. However, the overall cellular composition revealed a dense round cell infiltrate that extended diffusely as closely packed cells. The lymphoma cells were large with round, oval, or indented nuclei containing either a prominent single central nucleus or a few smaller nucleoli located on the nuclear membrane. Reticulin was sparse. Reed-Sternberg cells were present. Immunohistochemical staining revealed a monoclonal B-cell lineage. The authors felt that the only way to differentiate the highly atypical areas of reactive T-cell changes in response to *Toxoplasma* from the changes seen with a B-cell lymphoma was by careful immunohistochemical staining. In addition, it was felt that this was particularly important when small amounts of tissue were available such as in needle biopsy, which may not necessarily give the morphological information necessary for an appropriate diagnosis.

C. Retinochoroiditis

Retinochoroiditis is an infrequent manifestation of disseminated toxoplasmosis in the compromised host. Gross examination of the retina is similar to that seen on fundoscopic examination. In the histopathological examination of an eye from a patient with toxoplasmic choroiditis, Nicholson and Wolchek (326) described the salient features. The patient developed retinochoroiditis after receiving corticosteroids for 18 months for a vague systemic illness. Grossly, multiple focal areas of cheesy, white, perivascular retinal necrosis occurred along the course of the arteries and veins in all quadrants. Scattered intraretinal hemorrhages were apparent, and the vitreous humor was clear. Microscopic examination confirmed the gross examination of severe necrotic disease in proximity to the retinal veins and arteries. Retinal necrosis involving nerve fiber and ganglion cell layers occurred adjacent to both arteries and veins. At the margin of each perivascular retinal necrosis, *Toxoplasma* cysts were identified. In addition, at the interface between the normal and necrotic inner retina, free tachyzoites were seen. There was not inflammatory infiltrate surrounding the areas of perivascular necrosis. The outer retinal layer was well preserved in general; however, in the areas where there was full thickness necrosis of the sensory retina, plasma cells and lymphocytes infiltrated the choroid. Cysts were also identified in pigment epithelial cells as well as in histologically normal portions of the retina. Rarely, clusters of free organisms were present in areas where there was no evidence of tissue necrosis. The optic nerve was atrophic, and both cysts and tachyzoites were present in the prelaminar, laminar, and anterior retrolaminar portion of the nerve.

D. Myocarditis

Toxoplasmic myocarditis has been reported to occur in numerous immunocompromised patients; however the histopathological description is scant. In the case described by Wertlake and Winter (327), toxoplasmic myocarditis occurred in a patient with acute lymphoblastic leukemia who had no evidence of encephalitis. Histopathologically, the heart was found to contain numerous tissue cysts and free organisms. Many of the cysts were surrounded by a prominent inflammatory reaction consisting predominantly of lymphocytes and plasmacytes. There were similar areas of inflammation in the area of the right bundle branch of the conducting system and the pericardium, although no cysts were seen at these sites.

In heart transplant recipients who develop myocarditis, the pathological changes due to *Toxoplasma* are more difficult to discern from rejection of the allograft (30,328). In addition, because the transplanted heart is the source of infection, a myocarditis may be the initial manifestation of acute infection. In a report by Luft et al. (328), two cases of toxoplasmic myocarditis were described that were diagnosed by endomyocardial biopsy. Microscopic examination of the myocardium revealed areas of focal necrosis, edema, and an inflammatory cell infiltrate containing plasma cells, macrophages, lymphocytes, and eosinophils. The presence of eosinophils, in particular, may be an indicator of toxoplasma infection, in contrast to rejection. *Toxoplasma* organisms are usually within the myocytes but may also be seen extracellularly. The intact pseudocyst was found to elicit little inflammatory reaction, but once the tachyzoites were released, a corresponding inflammatory reaction was seen.

E. Other Organs

Toxoplasma has been demonstrated in numerous other organs including the testes, skeletal muscle, bone marrow, gastrointestinal tract, liver, pancreas, lymph nodes, thyroid, skin, and lung (10-13). However, the pathological discussion of involvement at these organs is not extensive and therefore will be only briefly reviewed.

Toxoplasmic pneumonitis is associated with the development of hyaline membranes, thickened alveolar septae containing a sparse round cell infiltrate, and large prominent alveolar lining cells (321,329-331). Alveolar capillaries may become markedly congested, and hemosiderin-laden macrophages may be found within the alveoli. Parasites can be found within the alveolar lining cells and

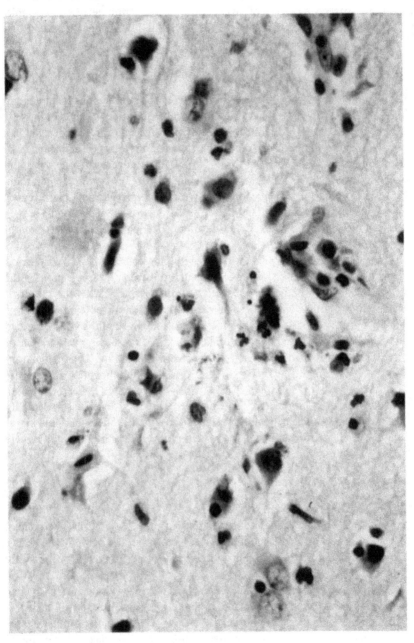

Figure 7 Low-power view of *Toxoplasma*-specific immunohistochemical stain demonstrating free tachyzoites and intracellular tachyzoites forming a pseudocyst.

within intraalveolar macrophages (321) and may cause multiple foci of necrosis with destruction of the normal pulmonary architecture (321,332).

Rash has been associated with acute toxoplasmosis, but in most instances the diagnosis of these exanthems being due to *T. gondii* has relied on serological diagnosis of infection. In instances where the organism has been identified, it has been found most frequently in the dermis with a strong inflammatory reaction (333–336). However, organisms have been identified in both the dermis and epidermis (333–336). The extent of the inflammatory infiltrate is variable and probably depends on the underlying immunosuppression of the host. Necrosis, vasculitis, perivasculitis, periadnexal inflammation, and granulomas have all been associated with toxoplasma infection of the skin (333–336).

Toxoplasmic myositis has been reported to occur in both immunocompromised and nonimmunocompromised hosts (337,338). Histopathologically, interstitial and perivascular infiltration of mononuclear cells may be noted, especially in areas of necrotic muscle fibers. *Toxoplasma gondii* cysts and pseudocysts may be seen within muscle fibers either at the edge of areas of necrosis or in skeletal muscle fibers without associated inflammation (337,338).

XII. CLINICAL MANIFESTATIONS

A. Immunocompetent Host

Acute toxoplasma infection in the immunocompetent host is totally asymptomatic in 80–90% of patients (338,339). The spectrum of clinical manifestations of acquired toxoplasmosis range from asymptomatic lymphadenopathy to acute fulminant disease, at time resulting in death. Asymptomatic lymphadenopathy is the most common sign of infection and may be localized or generalized. The nodes are discrete, nontender or of variable tenderness, and nonsuppurative. Cervical lymphadenopathy is most common, although any group of nodes may be involved (340). Mesenteric or retroperitoneal lymph nodes may be involved and associated with fever and intraabdominal pain (339,340). The lymphadenopathy may occasionally be associated with a mononucleus-like syndrome with symptoms including fever, malaise, night sweats, myalgia, sore throat, maculopapular rash, and hepatosplenomegaly. Peripheral blood smear may reveal an atypical lymphocystosis. Although the lymphadenopathy syndrome is usually self-limited with symptoms resolving within a month and lymphadenopathy resolving within several months, symptoms may persist or recur for up to a year (341).

The majority of cases of toxoplasmic retinochoroiditis are the result of congenital infection, but acquired retinochoroiditis is being reported with increased frequency (B. Luft, manuscript in preparation). This usually produces symptoms of blurred vision, pain, photophobia, scotoma, and epiphora. With

Table 2 Clinical Features of Toxoplasmosis in the Normal and Immunocompromised Host

---

Normal host
Common
  Asymptomatic (90%)
  Isolated lymphadenopathy (10%)
Uncommon
  Choriorotinitis
Rare
  Encephalitis
  Myocarditis
  Pneumonitis
  Hepatitis
Immunocompromised host
Common
  Toxoplasmic encephalitis
  Myocarditis
  Pneumonitis

---

acute acquired toxoplasmic retinochoroditis, the lesions are unilateral and may resemble the posterior uveitis of tuberculosis, leprosy, histoplasmosis, or syphilis.

Acquired toxoplasmosis may rarely be associated with multiple organ involvement (339). The most prominent is central nervous system disease with or without concomitant involvement of the lung, heart, liver, and muscle. This occurs as a result of diffuse and uncontrolled dissemination of the organism throughout the body (13). As a result, patients may present with nonspecific neurological symptoms such as confusion, seizures, disorientation, and lethargy. Patients may also complain of symptoms and signs of fever, arthralgia, myalgia, and maculopapular rash. Muscle biopsy may reveal evidence of myositis (337,338). Cardiac involvement may be associated with congestive heart failure and electrocardiographic abnormalities due to arrhythmias (327). *Toxoplasma* has also been implicated as a cause of diffuse interstitial pneumonitis in the healthy adult (341a,341b,341c,342).

Toxoplasma infection localized to the brain has also been described (13). These patients tend to have focal symptoms such as headache, blurred vision, weakness. Acute toxoplasmic chorioretinitis may precede the neurological sequelae of acute toxoplasma infection. *Toxoplasma* has also been implicated in the etiology of hepatitis (343), polymyositis (337), and myocarditis (344); however, in most of these instances the diagnosis was not definitively substantiated.

B. Immunocompromised Host

1. Central Nervous System Toxoplasmosis

Signs and symptoms of encephalitis are the predominant manifestation of toxoplasma infection in the immunocompromised host (10,13). The clinical manifestations of toxoplasmic encephalitis are divided between two patterns of presentation. The initial neurological symptoms in one group include focal abnormalities such as focal seizures, hemiparesis, hemiplegia, hemisensory loss, cerebellar tremor, homonymous hemianopsia, cranial nerve palsies, diplopia, blindness, personality changes, and severe headache not responsive to analgesics. The clinical pattern in the other group is characterized by general symptoms and signs of central nervous system dysfunction including weakness, myoclonus, confusion, lethargy, disorientation, headache, and coma. Signs of meningeal inflammation are variable. As the disease progresses, patients may develop signs of focal neurological disease. The development of focal neurological defects may be due to the multifocal nature of this necrotizing infection as well as the association of edema and vasculitis with infarction and hemorrhage with active infection (see Section XI.B). The manifestations of toxoplasmic encephalitis vary between an insidious and subacute process and one that evolves over weeks to an acute confusional state or focal neurological deficit accompanied by headache. In Hodgkin's disease patients who remained untreated, the course of the infection from initial manifestation of encephalitis to death varies from 13 days to 3½ months (13).

The clinical presentation of toxoplasmic encephalitis in patients with Hodgkin's disease is evenly divided between the focal and the nonfocal patterns of presentation. In contrast, patients who develop toxoplasmic encephalitis following organ or bone marrow transplantation usually have nonfocal central nervous system abnormalities. In general, localizing neurological signs tend to occur late in the course of the infection or not at all (13). The course of encephalitis in transplant patients is variable and ranges from an indolent, progressive process over several months (13,29,39,313,314) to fulminant disease (13,40, 307, 345) that results in death within several weeks. Fever often but not invariably occurs with the encephalitis.

AIDS patients with toxoplasmic encephalitis have presented most often with symptoms and signs of a diffuse encephalopathy. However, upon careful neurological examination, focal neurological abnormalities are found in the majority of patients. Toxoplasmic encephalitis may be the initial manifestation of their immunodeficiency or can occur later following another opportunistic infection. Many patients may initially complain of anorexia, weight loss, and malaise, which reflects their underlying immunodeficiency (14). In 9 of 27 patients with AIDS and toxoplasmic encephalitis described by Navia et al. (60), global cognitive impairment associated with impaired recent memory, attention deficit, and slowness of verbal and motor responses was found prior to the onset of toxoplasmosis. These abnormalities were reminiscent of the AIDS-related dementia syndrome believed to be caused by HIV infection of the central nervous system. Furthermore, after successful treatment for toxoplasmosis, patients may continue to deteriorate neurologically in a manner that resembles the AIDS-related subacute encephalitis (60). In these cases there has been a failure to identify *Toxoplasma* after repeat brain biopsy (60,316). This pattern of neurological dysfunction, cognitive impairment with preserved consciousness, which is associated with the AIDS-associated dementia has been found to occur in 66% of patients with AIDS and toxoplasmic encephalitis.

Toxoplasma can infect any cell in the brain, but specific focal neurological symptoms vary, depending on the areas of the brain affected. However, there is a tendency for *Toxoplasma* to cause disease in the brain stem, basal ganglia, and the pituitary. With brain-stem involvement, neurological symptoms such as ataxia, limb dysmetria, and cranial nerve palsies are not uncommon. Choreiform movements and choreoathetosis have been found in patients with basal ganglia infection. Acquired hydrocephelus may also develop (316a). Blindness may occur as a result of chorioretinitis or involvement of the visual cortex of the brain. Lesions of the pituitary and hypothalmus have been mentioned in cases of central nervous system toxoplasmosis (11), but no evidence of functional pituitary insufficiency has been demonstrated. Recently, Milligan et al. (317) described a patient with panhypopituitarism due to toxoplasma infection of the pituitary.

Although *Toxoplasma* is capable of infecting all tissues and therefore all organs, the most prominent clinical manifestations of toxoplasma infection is encephalitis; however, other organs including the heart, lungs, muscle, eye, and skin may be simultaneously involved. The manifestations of other organ involvement will be discussed below. In addition, concomitant infection with other pathogens including *Pseudomonas, Candida, Cryptococcus, Aspergillus, Mycobacterium tuberculosis, Herpes zoster, Herpes simplex,* and cytomegalovirus has been reported in non-AIDS immunocompromised hosts. In patients with AIDS, concomitant systemic and/or cerebral infection with *Pneumocystis carinii,* cytomegalovirus, *Mycobacterium tuberculosis, Mycobacterium avium-intracellulare, Candida,* and *Cryptosporidium* has been reported. Therefore, it may be difficult to discern in patients with toxoplasmic encephalitis whether systemic symptoms of other organ involvement are due to *Toxoplasma* or to a concomitant infection with another pathogen.

2. Retinochoroiditis

Retinochoroiditis is an unusual manifestation of toxoplasma infection in the immunocompromised host. However, it is important to be cognizant of it since it may be a harbinger of more extensive disease. Ophthalmoscopic examination reveals mild vitreous haze overlying a yellowish-white raised intraretinal lesion with irregular border. In addition, there may be perivascular retinal inflammation associated with an anterior uveitis. There are usually retinal scars consistent with recurrent infection. Either one eye or both eyes may be involved. Blurred vision, scotoma, and photophobia may be prominent symptoms. Impairment of vision may occur as a result of macular involvement, infection of the optic nerve, retinal vein occlusion, or vitreitis (300,346-351).

Toxoplasmic retinochoroiditis has been reported to occur in patients receiving corticosteroids (326) with Hodgkin's disease (300,348), lymphoma (349), angioimmunoblastic lymphadenopathy (347), AIDS (346,350,351), and cardiac and renal transplantation (29,345). Retinochoroiditis may be the initial manifestation of systemic toxoplasma infection or may occur together with encephalitis. AIDS patients may develop toxoplasmic retinochoroiditis either without evidence of encephalitis or 4 months before the onset of neurological symptoms (351). Renal and cardiac transplant recipients had chorioretinitis of unknown etiology 2 and 5 months after transplantation, respectively, prior to the development of toxoplasmic encephalitis (345).

3. Systemic Toxoplasmosis

The systemic manifestations of toxoplasma infection are difficult to discern because the criteria for diagnosis are frequently based on a rise in antibody titer without any histopathological or microbiological confirmation of active infection. As will be discussed in Section XIII.A, the use of serological change as the sole criterion for diagnosis may be misleading in that immunocompromised patients may have serological changes without any manifestations of active infection. Recently, Hakes and Armstrong (352) analyzed 25 patients with neoplastic disease and *T. gondii* infection. In over 48% of these patients, fever was the sole manifestation of infection, and the diagnosis was made on the basis of serological criteria. In this situation, it is impossible to discern whether the fever was due to active *Toxoplasma*, other infectious etiologies, or the patients' underlying disease. This is underscored by the fact that in the series of patients described by Hakes and Armstrong (352), 7 of 17 patients improved spontaneously, and 9 improved while receiving sulfadiazine and pyrimethimine therapy (the remaining patient did not improve with therapy but survived). It is clear that stringent serological and microbiological criteria should be adopted for the diagnosis of *Toxoplasma* in immunocompromised hosts and that such criteria will vary from one patient population to another.

Myocarditis, pneumonitis, and hepatitis due to *Toxoplasma* have been frequently noted upon histopathological examination of autopsy material. However, clinical manifestations of severe organ involvement have been infrequently mentioned in case reports and series of cases. It is important to be aware of infection in these organs, since it may occur independently of central nervous system involvement. Abnormal liver function tests have been noted in patients with acute infection, and disease may progress to frank hepatitis with death due to hepatic failure (10-12). Interstitial pneumonia associated with fever and shortness of breath may occur in as many as 32% of immunocompromised patients with toxoplasmosis (330). Chest X-ray abnormalities may simulate interstitial pulmonary edema, although there may also be a combination of interstitial and intraalveolar infiltrates with air-space consolidation. *Toxoplasma* has also been noted to have a multinodular appearance on chest X-ray. Frequently, enlarged hilar nodes are also present (329-331,333). Pulmonary infection with *T. gondii* may occur concomitantly with that of other pathogens (352b,352a). Bronchoalveolar lavage has been found to be useful in the diagnosis of pulmonary toxoplasmosis (352c).

Toxoplasmic myocarditis has two manners of presentation in the immunocompromised host. In the heart transplant recipient, the cardiac allograft is the source of infection. Toxoplasmic myocarditis may initially manifest itself as cardiac rejection uncontrolled or actually worsened with increasing immunosuppression. Associated with this is progressive congestive heart failure. Since the heart is the initial source of infection, there may be no other manifestations of systemic infection; however, if the infection is untreated, these manifestations will occur (328). In other immunocompromised hosts, toxoplasmic myocarditis may manifest itself as intractable congestive heart failure and/or cardiac arrythmias. The electrocardiogram may show low voltage and ST-T wave changes. Arrhythmias including sinus bradycardia, atrial fibrillation, and heart blocks may be present (327).

Cutaneous manifestations of toxoplasmosis have been reported to occur. The lesions may be nodular, purpuric, papulopustular, lichenoid, vegetating, and erythema multiforme-like lesions (333-336,352d).

XIII. DIAGNOSIS

A. Serology

The diagnosis of acute acquired toxoplasmosis in the noncompromised host can be established by the demonstration of seroconversion from a negative to positive titer or a fourfold rise in antibody titer (24,353). The dye test and the conventional indirect fluorescent antibody titer rise within the first 2 weeks after infection and continue to rise to usually $\geqslant 1:1024$. The presence of high titers by the Sabin-Feldman dye test (DT) antibody or conventional indirect fluorescent antibody (IFA) technique ($>1:1024$) is suggestive of acute infection; however, a

Table 3   Serological Evidence of Acute Infection

Normal host

Demonstration of anti-*Toxoplasma* IgM antibody measured by IgM-IFA or IgM ELISA

Fourfold rise in anti-*Toxoplasma* IgG antibody titer as measured by the Sabin-Feldman dye test or the IgC-IFA

Immunocompromised host

Seroconversion in anti-*Toxoplasma* antibody

Demonstration of local anti-*Toxoplasma* antibody production

Presence of anti-*Toxoplasma* antibody in a patient with focal or multifocal encephalitis (usually requires biopsy for definitive diagnosis)

---

high titer antibody may persist for years after acute infection (353). Therefore, in patients who have stable high titer antibody, the presence of high IgM antibody titer by the IgM-IFA (titer $> 1:80$) or the double sandwich IgM enzyme linked immunosorbent assay (ELISA) (354) may be useful. However, IgM antibody when measured by the IgM ELISA (354) may remain elevated for up to a year after acute infection (177,354a). Furthermore, because high titer, high affinity anti-*Toxoplasma* IgG antibody may competitively inhibit the binding of IgM antibody in the IgM-IFA test, a negative IgM IFA where *Toxoplasma* infection is highly suspected should be confirmed with the highly sensitive double sandwich IgM ELISA (354).

Complement fixation test titers rise after dye test and IFA antibody (355). This assay may be useful to demonstrate rising titers when the dye test and IFA titers are elevated and stable. Other tests that have proved useful for assaying for the presence of antibody are the agglutination test (356) and the conventional IgG ELISA.

In the immunocompromised host, interpretation of the serological data is dependent on an understanding of the degree of underlying immunosuppression, the serological status of the patient prior to the development of symptoms indicative of acute *Toxoplasma* infection, and knowledge of the pathogenesis of *Toxoplasma* infection in the risk group to which the patient belongs.

Luft et al. (29) performed a prospective study on heart transplant recipients to determine the usefulness of antibody serology in predicting the development of significant disease due to *Toxoplasma*. In this study, 50% of patients with serological evidence of toxoplasma infection prior to cardiac transplantation developed significant rises in IgG antibody titers after transplantation, and in 50% of those patients there was a significant elevation in IgM antibody titers.

None of these patients developed significant illness due to *Toxoplasma*. In contrast, patients who were seronegative for *Toxoplasma* antibody prior to transplantation and received a heart from a seropositive donor seroconverted and developed severe symptomatic disease. The manifestations of the infection could be delayed for as long as 9 months after transplantation. Nagington and Martin (36) at Papworth Hospital in England described four seronegative heart transplant recipients who received hearts from seropositive donors. Three developed significant morbidity due to *Toxoplasma*; however, only two of the three seroconverted. The third patient did not develop significant antibody titers to *T. gondii* but died with disseminated toxoplasmosis. These authors estimated that one of six transplant recipients will be seronegative for *T. gondii* and receive a heart from a seropositive donor in England. At Stanford University Hospital it is estimated that 1 in 14 will fall into this category (9d). Similarly, four renal transplant recipients who developed significant infection due to *T. gondii* were seronegative prior to transplantation, suggesting that the toxoplasma infection was acquired posttransplantation (13). Therefore, in the heart transplant recipients it is important to know the serological status of both the recipient and the donor prior to transplantation. Because the likelihood of disease due to *T. gondii* is high in a seronegative recipient who receives a heart from a seropositive donor, the patient should be followed prospectively for seroconversion or for the development of symptoms or signs that may be attributable to disseminated *T. gondii* infection. In addition, the cardiac pathologist should be alerted to examine endomyocardial biopsies with particular care for evidence of active toxoplasmic myocarditis (328).

It is apparent that serological tests may reveal changes in antibody titers without necessarily being indicative of active infection. Therefore, serological rises in antibody titers alone in immunocompromised patients cannot be used as a sole diagnostic criterion of active infection due to *T. gondii*, especially if the clinical manifestations of infection are nonspecific. Recently, Peacock et al. (357) described a patient with chronic myelogenous leukemia and fever who was documented to have a striking and significant rise in antibody titers to *Toxoplasma* without specific evidence of infection. At autopsy, careful and systematic histopathological examination of all the major organs revealed no evidence of toxoplasma infection except a *Toxoplasma* tissue cyst. Similarly, Vogel and Lunde (358) demonstrated high titers of *Toxoplasma* antibody in patients with underlying malignancy, especially in patients with chronic myelogenous leukemia, without evidence of active infection. Kusne et al. (358c) noted similar rises in antibody titers in a patient without clinical evidence of toxoplasmosis post liver transplantation and were also able to fortuitously isolate the organism from the blood of the patient. Therefore, clinicians should be careful in making a diagnosis of toxoplasmosis in patients with underlying immunocompromising conditions with nonspecific signs such as persistent fever and malaise. In these situations, confirmation of active *Toxoplasma* should be sought by detection of parasitemia by inoculation of peripheral blood buffy coats into fibroblast tissue culture (359) or mice.

In contrast to rises in antibody titers in some immunocompromised patients without any definite signs or symptoms of active toxoplasmic infection, other immunocompromised patients with fulminant toxoplasmosis may have low or negative dye test or IFA titers (<1:1024) and show no rise in antibody titer with serial specimens (11–13,301,302,352).

Luft and Remington (13) reviewed the serological data of 10 patients with various immunocompromising illnesses and toxoplasmic encephalitis who had serological tests performed at the Palo Alto Medical Foundation. In these 10 patients—Hodgkin's disease (one patient), lymphoma (one patient), primary amyloidosis (one patient), hairy cell leukemia (one patient), and bone marrow (one patient), renal (one patient), or cardiac (four patients) transplants—dye test antibody titers varied between 1:16 and 1:16,000, and IgM antibody could be detected in 8 out of 10 patients. Similarly, Lunde et al. (360) found that patients with leukemia and active *T. gondii* infection all had IgM and/or precipitating antibody to *T. gondii*.

In bone marrow transplant recipients and patients with AIDS, the serological diagnosis of toxoplasmosis is even more formidable. All bone marrow transplant patients with toxoplasmosis who had serological studies prior to transplantation had antibody to *Toxoplasma* at that time (304,305). However, antibody titers did not rise with the development of clinical disease due to *T. gondii*. In two bone marrow transplant recipients who developed toxoplasmic encephalitis, there was a drop in antibody titer from 1:1024 and 1:16 prior to transplantation to 1:64 and no detectable antibody, respectively, with the development of encephalitis (304,339). Similarly, all AIDS patients with toxoplasmic encephalitis who had serological studies performed on serum samples prior to the development of encephalitis had antibody to *Toxoplasma* at that time (60). In addition, rises in antibody titer could be demonstrated in only a minority of cases of AIDS patients with toxoplasmic encephalitis (60,324). Luft et al. (324) studied the antibody response of 38 patients with AIDS and toxoplasmic encephalitis and found dye test titers to range between negative and 1:8192. Approximately one-fifth had antibody titers of 1:1024 or greater. A significant rise in antibody titer was demonstrated in only 2 of 16 patients; however, serum samples and changes in antibody titers may have occurred earlier in the course of the disease. Wong et al. (52) demonstrated a rise in antibody titer in a patient with AIDS and toxoplasmic encephalitis when antibody titer at the onset of symptoms was compared with the antibody titer obtained 2 months prior to the onset of symptoms. Navia et al. (60) showed a significant rise in antibody titers in 5 of 15 (33%) AIDS patients with toxoplasmic encephalitis when antibody titers prior to onset of cerebral disease were compared with titers at the onset of symptomatic toxoplasmosis. Twenty-eight percent had titers of 1:1024 or greater, and 12% had titers of 1:16 or below. The agglutination test seems to be a more sensitive indicator of active disease, especially when used in conjunction with the dye test (290). However, as demonstrated by Luft et al. (290), 44% of patients with AIDS and toxoplasmic encephalitis will have low (<1:512) antibody titers no matter what serological test is performed.

It is clear that the interpretation of serological tests for toxoplasmosis is not uniform but is dependent on the clinical situation and the clinician's interpretation of the pathogenesis of infection in the particular patient. The interpretation of serological tests in the heart transplant patient is far different from that in the bone marrow transplant patient. Furthermore, serological tests must be correlated with other diagnostic techniques including radiographic and other laboratory abnormalities as well as the clinical situation. Serological tests stimulate the clinician to consider the diagnosis and then act to confirm the diagnosis. In the seronegative heart transplant recipient who has received a heart from a seropositive donor, *Toxoplasma* should be strongly considered as a possible etiological agent for an atypical allograft rejection or encephalitis even if seroconversion has not occurred in the recipient. *Toxoplasma* should be considered a possible etiological agent of myocarditis, pneumonitis, myositis, and encephalitis in all bone marrow transplant recipient and AIDS patients who had evidence of latent infection prior to the onset of symptoms. In other immunocompromised hosts, paticularly those with malignancies of the reticuloendothelial system, toxoplasma infection should be suspected if IgM antibody is present if there is a DT or IFA titer of $\geqslant 1:1024$ and the clinical and radiographic picture is consistent with toxoplasmosis. However, a significant number of cases of toxoplasmosis will not meet these serological criteria, and in such patients histopathological confirmation of the diagnosis is necessary. The need for histopathological confirmation becomes obvious when one considers that between 10 and 60% of the population has detectable antibody to *T. gondii*.

B. Detection of Antibody, Antigen, and the Organism in Body Fluids

The detection of *Toxoplasma* antigen in the serum of acutely infected patients may provide a rapid means of diagnosing infection. It may be particularly important in immunocompromised patients in whom active disease is not always associated with rises in antibody titers. By using an enzyme-linked immunoassay, circulating *Toxoplasma* antigens in cases of acute acquired toxoplasmosis, antigen has been detected in the serum and/or urine samples in various animal models of infection as early as 2 days after infection (140,361,362). Mice acutely infected with either a virulent or avirulent strain of *T. gondii* have detectable levels of nucleoside triphosphate hydrolase as a circulating antigen (362a). *Toxoplasma* antigen has also been demonstrated in ocular fluid of rabbits experimentally infected with *Toxoplasma* (141). Antigen can be detected in the sera of acutely infected humans (139,142). In one study, *Toxoplasma* antigen was detected in 15 of 23 sera tested from 22 patients with acute toxoplasmosis (139). In addition, *Toxoplasma* antigen has been recently detected in serum immune complexes of patients acutely infected with *T. gondii* (145). The ELISA method was also found to be useful in the detection of antigen in tissues of animals acutely infected with *T. gondii*. Shepp et al. (305) recently described isolation of *Toxoplasma* from the blood of three bone marrow transplant patients, two of whom ultimately were documented to have invasive disease due to *T. gondii*. In this study they isolated the organism in a tissue culture routinely used to isolate cytomegalovirus.

Determination of *Toxoplasma* antibodies in the cerebrospinal fluid may be useful in the diagnosis of toxoplasmic encephalitis. However, the presence of *Toxoplasma* antibody in and of itself is not diagnostic of toxoplasmic encephalitis. For example, in a study by Amato Neto et al. (363) of 20 neurologically normal patients with toxoplasmic lymphadenopathy, all had positive dye test titers in their cerebrospinal fluid. Therefore, it is important to establish whether or not the antibody present in the cerebrospinal fluid is produced locally. Methods for determination of local antibody production in the cerebrospinal or aqueous humor can be evaluated by the following formula:

$$C = \frac{\text{antibody titer body fluid}}{\text{antibody titer serum}} \times \frac{\text{concentration of globulin serum}}{\text{concentration of globulin body fluid}}$$

In the nonimmunocompromised host, if C is greater than 8, local antibody production has occurred (364–366). Recently, Potasman et al. (367) demonstrated that in 7 of 10 patients with toxoplasmic encephalitis and AIDS there was evidence of local production of anti-*Toxoplasma* antibody. However, in this study, evidence of local product *Toxoplasma*-specific immunoglobulin was determined if C was greater than 1. Perhaps in immunocompromised hosts less stringent criteria are necessary because of abnormalities in immunoglobulin production. Navia et al. (60) and Wong et al. (52) noted that three AIDS patients in whom serial cerebrospinal fluid and serum titers were available demonstrated a greater than fourfold rise in CSF antibody titers in the presence of unchanged serum titers. However, one must be cautious in the interpretation of these results, because a small amount of nonspecific leakage of immunoglobulin from the blood into the cerebrospinal fluid will have relatively greater effect on the cerebrospinal fluid antibody titer with no effect on the serum titer.

C. Radiology and Nuclear Medicine

The radiological manifestations of disseminated toxoplasmosis are confined to radiological abnormalities of the lung (329–331,333) and central nervous system (13). The lungs are not frequently involved with toxoplasmosis; however, when they are involved, the early stages of the disease resemble those of interstitial pulmonary edema. In some cases, the infiltrates may have a focal distribution with consolidation or the chest radiograph may show a diffuse bilateral nodular process. Hilar adenopathy frequently occurs.

Prior to the advent of computerized axial tomography and nuclear magnetic resonance imaging, radiological and nuclear medicine diagnostic procedures were relatively insensitive in detecting central nervous system toxoplasmosis in the immunocompromised host. Brain scans or angiography demonstrated abnormalities in only 55% of patients (13).

Computerized axial tomography (CAT) has been found to be extremely useful in the diagnosis of toxoplasmic encephalitis. It has successfully demonstrated abnormalities due to *Toxoplasma* in patients with no underlying immunosuppression; with lymphoma or leukemia; and with bone marrow, heart, and renal transplants; as well as in patients with AIDS (13). Characteristics of the abnormalities seen on CAT scan are varied and depend on the ability of the host to immunologically respond to the infection as well as on the pathogenesis (acute acquired infection or recrudescence of a latent infection) of the infectious process itself. The CAT scan has shown the lesions of toxoplasmic encephalitis to be rounded, single, or multiple, and isodense or hypodense. Post (315) described the CAT scan abnormalities in 31 patients with toxoplasmic encephalitis and AIDS studied at the University of Miami School of Medicine. In over 80% of these patients, the lesions were multiple (between 2 and 11 lesions), with deep and superficial contrast-enhancing lesions located in both cerebral hemispheres. The corticomedullary junction and the basal ganglia were the most common sites of involvement, although any part of the central nervous system may be involved. The lesions were frequently associated with edema and mass effect. Contrast enhancement, either ring or nodular enhancement, was demonstrated in over 90% of patients (Fig. 8). The lesions varied in size, and some had multiple central areas of lucency within the central area of the lesion. In contrast to these findings, others have occasionally reported the CAT scan to be normal at a time when there were clinical signs of encephalitis. In these instances, however, it is not clear whether the CAT scan was performed in the manner described by Post (315). Both Whelan (316) and Post (315) suggested that a delayed double dose CT study may be a more sensitive means of diagnosing toxoplasmic encephalitis in AIDS patients. This method takes maximum advantage of any damage to the blood-brain barrier and optimizes the diffusion of contrast into the lesion. Post et al. (368) prospectively compared results of CAT scans performed immediately after infusion of contrast material with those of CAT scans performed 1 hr after infusion. In 41 instances, 25 patients had both immediate and delayed studies performed. The delayed CAT scan was superior in 75% of the cases and showed a greater number of enhancing lesions and/or a larger size to the lesions. In several cases, the immediate CAT scan was negative or showed only edema whereas the delayed study demonstrated enhancing lesions. Therefore, the delayed double dose CAT scan, if not contraindicated, would be the preferable procedure to detect early disease.

The CAT scan may underestimate or not detect the extent of a histopatho-

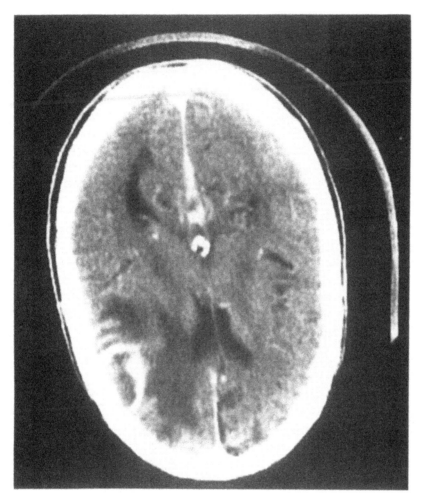

Figure 8 CAT scan of patient with toxoplasmic encephalitis. Large ring enhancing lesions and edema are characteristic of toxoplasmic encephalitis.

logical process with minimal inflammatory response. This may be particularly true if the infection is acquired acutely and disseminated throughout the brain. This is in contrast to the CAT scan appearance when the host is capable of developing enough of a response to limit the infection, and therefore this local process may present in a ring and/or nodular contrast-enhancing configuration. The CAT scan may reveal an abnormality without any evidence of cerebral dysfunction. Recently, magnetic resonance imaging (MRI) has been found to be useful in the diagnosis of toxoplasmic encephalitis (369). It has detected lesions in patients with active toxoplasmic encephalitis whose CAT scans were without abnormality (Fig. 9). Therefore, it is recommended that an MRI be performed on patients with neurological symptoms and antibody to *Toxoplasma* whose CAT scan shown no abnormality.

The CAT scan is useful for the assessment of therapy, especially in those patients started on empirical treatment for toxoplasmic encephalitis. Patients with encephalitis should respond both clinically and radiographically within 2 weeks of institution of therapy (368). However, the use of corticosteroids can reduce the degree of contrast enhancement and edema as well as having a therapeutic effect on lymphomatous process, thus making interpretation of response to therapy difficult. In addition, there are no pathognomonic features that would radiologically differentiate toxoplasmic encephalitis from other inflammatory and noninflammatory diseases including infections caused by *Candida, Aspergillus,* and mcobacteria as well as primary intracerebral lymphoma, Kaposi's sarcoma, or metastatic tumor.

D. Biopsy

Toxoplasma gondii has been identified in biopsy specimens of the bone marrow (370), myocardium (268), skeletal muscle (337, 338), lung (329–331,333), and brain (14,323,324). Although disseminated toxoplasma infeection occurs with increased frequency in non-AIDS immunocompromised hosts, especially those with malignancy of the reticuloendothelial system, it accounts for a very small minority of all causes of infection in these patient populations. Therefore, diagnosis of *Toxoplasma* on biopsy specimen requires a high index of suspicion. In two situations, generalizations can be made regarding the indications for biopsy and the interpretation of biopsy results.

1. Endomyocardial Biopsies

Endomyocardial biopsies have been shown to be especially useful in the diagnosis of toxoplasmic myocarditis in heart transplant recipients. In allograft recipients who were seronegative prior to transplantation and received a heart from a seropositive donor, all endomyocardial biopsies taken to evaluate rejection should also be examined for evidence of toxoplasmic myocarditis by both hematoxylin and eosin stain and immunospecific stains for *Toxoplasma. Toxoplasma* should be suspected in recalcitrant rejection episodes and histopathological specimens that contain eosinophils within the inflammatory infiltrate. Clearly parasitized myofibers may not be in proximity to an inflammatory infiltrate, and inflammation may only occur upon rupturing of the infected myofiber (328).

2. Brain Biopsy

Brain biopsy is essential for the diagnosis of toxoplasmic encephalitis in the non-AIDS immunocompromised host for several reasons. Although toxoplasmic encephalitis occurs with greater frequency in patients with various underlying immunocompromising conditions, it is the etiological agent of central nervous system infection in only a small minority of non-AIDS immunocompromised patients. Toxoplasmic encephalitis comprised 5% of intracerebral infections in patients with malignancy seen at the Memorial Sloan-Kettering Cancer Center between 1955 and 1972 (31) and approximately 2% of central nervous system infections in immunocompromised patients from 1969 to 1979 at Massachusetts General Hosptial (32). As mentioned, serological test results are not reliable indicators of active clinical toxoplasma infection because titers rise with certain forms of immunosuppression without active disease and do not rise in others in which there is fulminant disease. Furthermore, radiological changes that occur with *T. gondii* infection are not pathognomonic but may occur with various infectious and noninfectious intracerebral processes that occur more commonly than *Toxoplasma* in the non-AIDS immunocompromised host. Therefore, it is strongly suggested that accessible intracerebral lesions in a non-AIDS immuno-compromised host be biopsied.

The decision to biopsy intracerebral lesions in AIDS patients has been a source of controversy (371,372). Proponents of early biopsy of intracerebral lesions in AIDS patients point out that the etiologies of intracerebral disease in AIDS patients are numerous and include encephalitis due to *Toxoplasma, Aspergillus, Candida*, and mycobacteria as well as neoplastic processes such as primary intracerebral lymphoma and Kaposi's sarcoma. In addition, therapy for *Toxoplasma* is prolonged, lasting 6 months or longer, and is fraught with numerous side effects, including leukopenia and skin rash. If therapy is discontinued, there is a high rate of recurrence. In addition, if corticosteroids are given concomitantly with anti-*Toxopolasma* therapy, it is not possible to differentiate the therapeutic effect of the anti-*Toxoplasma* chemotherapy from the corticosteroid-induced decrease in edema and contrast enhancement on CAT scan. Also, corticosteroids may have an antineoplastic effect in patients with intracerebral lymphoma. In contrast, others feel that brain biopsy in AIDS patients who have anti-*Toxoplasma* antibody and characteristic contrast-enhancing lesions on CAT scan is not necessary until a therapeutic trial of anti-*Toxoplasma* chemotherapy has been undertaken. These investigators would biopsy patients

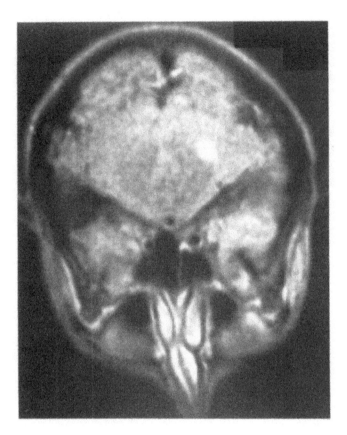

Figure 9 MRI of brain of patient with toxoplasmic encephalitis who had no abnormalities noticed on CT scan. Note a lesion in each hemisphere.

only if a therapeutic response is not established within 10-14 days of therapy. Their feeling, although not yet substantiated in the literature, is that the correlation of an intracerebral focal abnormality with toxoplasma infection is very high if the patient has anti-*Toxoplasma* antibody. Furthermore, some centers have reported a high morbidity and mortality associated with brain biopsy. Unfortunately, the value of brain biopsy in AIDS patients is purely conjectural at this time because a systematic study of patients in a center where immunohistological procedures on biopsy specimens are readily performed has not been done.

Biopsy has proved diagnostic by histopathological examination in only 50% of reported cases of toxoplasmic encephalitis, but the organism could be isolated in other cases by inoculation of the specimen into mice (13,372a). The CAT scan and MRI are useful for the localization of accessible lesions. Post (315)

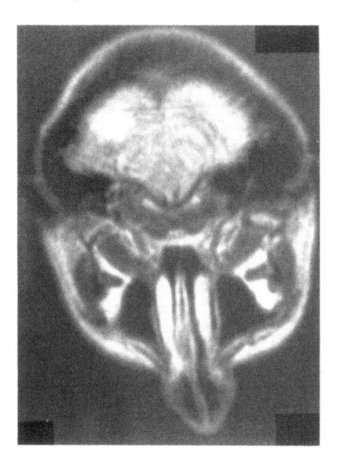

found that coronal views are more likely to demonstrate the extent of the lesion to be biopsied; however, the MRI may prove even more sensitive (369). Both intraoperative sonography and needle biopsy with a stereotactic device have proved useful for the diagnosis of deep lesions.

It is clear that *T. gondii* may be present as an encephalitic process without being evident by histopathological stain. This is poignantly demonstrated in the cases in which histopathological stains did not demonstrate *T. gondii* but the organism was isolated by mouse inoculation (372a). Immunohistological stains may provide a more sensitive technique for demonstrating *Toxoplasma*, particularly the tachyzoites or *Toxoplasma* antigens (323). This is particularly important because the histological changes associated with *Toxoplasma* may closely resemble those of a viral encephalitis, and tachyzoites may be difficult to distinguish from necrotic debris. Furthermore, pseudocysts and cysts that are easily identifiable by histopathological stains may not be present during active infec—tion or may be present only at the periphery of the lesion or within normal brain. This problem becomes more acute when sterotactic biopsies are performed because of the small sample that is obtained from a very localized area. Because organisms identifiable by histopathological stains may be present only in the periphery of the severely necrotizing process, identifiable pathogens may be missed. Therefore, in patients with encephalitis of unknown etiology, immunohistological studies for *T. gondii* should be performed if histology, as determined by conventional stains, is negative. Furthermore, in these situations, response to therapy may be the only way to make a presumptive diagnosis of toxoplasmic encephalitis short of a wider excisional biopsy.

Significant difficulty may arise in differentiating a primary cerebral lymphoma from the reactive round cell infiltrate in toxoplasma infection. Kersting and Newman (39) described a renal transplant recipient in whom a neoplasm resembling a lymphoma was found containing *T. gondii*. They felt that this process was not a lymphoma but represented an atypical response to *T. gondii*. Subsequently, two patients with AIDS whose biopsies of intracerebral lymphoma and received radiotherapy died. At autopsy, diffuse toxoplasmic encephalitis was present; no evidence of lymphoma was found (316). In a report from the University of California at San Francisco Medical Center, two patients with AIDS were reported to have both toxoplasmic encephalitis and primary central nervous system lymphoma in the same needle biopsy (57). Recently, Fromowitz et al. (325) described the similarities in the morphological appearance of the reactive lymphocytes and monocytes occasionally seen in response to *T. gondii* infection to those of intracerebral lymphoma. In one case of toxoplasmic encephalitis, the distribution and composition of cells were clearly reactive, but in some areas the infiltrate was highly atypical and not vasocentric. Lymphocytes showed cytological atypia larger than usual and containing irregular cerebriforn nuclei. Histocytes and endothelial cells were large, and some showed nuclear lobulation of multinucleation with prominent nuclei resembling Reed-Sternberg cells. In contrast to the monoclonal B cells seen in primary B-cell lymphoma of the central nervous system, atypical cells were found that consisted of predominant T-cell, macrophage, and polyclonal B-cell populations. Immunohistological stains may be invaluable in distinguishing a primary intracerebral lymphoma from a cellular reaction to *T. gondii*. Therefore, it is recommended that if the needle biopsy does not definitively diagnose *T. gondii* infection or lymphoma, further tissue should be obtained for more extensive immunohistological studies with pathogen- and cell-specific antibodies. The effort and expense of these procedures is justified, since response to appropriate therapy may be expected to prolong the useful life of these patients.

XIV. TREATMENT

Treatment for toxoplasma infection is reserved for patients who develop acute acquired infection during pregnancy and for immunocompromised patients with evidence of active disease due to *Toxoplasma*. It is relatively rare that a normal host requires therapy for toxoplasmosis. In almost all instances the infection is self-limited in the nonimmunocompromised host. One possible exception is infection acquired during laboratory accident, which may be more virulent and therefore require therapy promptly. Therapy for toxoplasmosis should be instituted in those immunocompromised patients in whom there is histopathological evidence of active infection. Empirical therapy should be instituted in seropositive immunocompromised patients who are primarily predisposed to developing toxoplasmic encephalitis and have a characteristic lesion on cerebral axial tomography that is inaccessible to biopsy or when there is a contraindication to biopsy. Immunocompromised patients with serological evidence of recently acquired infection may develop a clinical syndrome consistent with diffuse systemic and cerebral involvement and should be started on anti-*Toxoplasma* therapy whether or not there is evidence of abnormalities on CAT scan.

Heart transplant recipients who are seronegative for *Toxoplasma* antibodies and receive an allograft from a seropositive donor may initially present with toxoplasmic myocarditis. In these instances, toxoplasmic myocarditis may be mistaken for rejection of the allograft. Therefore, heart transplant recipients who seroconvert after transplantation should be treated early with anti-*Toxoplasma* therapy. AIDS patients also have a striking propensity toward developing toxoplasmic encephalitis, and therefore special recommendations may be made for the initiation of empirical therapy. Patients with AIDS and central nervous system signs or symptoms should be studied with both CAT scan and serological tests for *Toxoplasma*. If the CAT scan reveals a focal abnormality and serological tests are positive, empirical therapy for *T. gondii* should be instituted pending a brain biopsy if the lesion is accessible. If the CAT scan is normal, magnetic resonance imaging (MRI) should be performed to determine a focal abnormality. In patients who are started on empirical therapy, a therapeutic response within 10 days should be sought as confirmation of the diagnosis. However, if the patient has been placed on corticosteroids, clinical improvement or resolution of radiographic abnormalities does not provide evidence that the changes are due to specific anti-*Toxoplasma* therapy. Corticosteroids can give dramatic transient improvement in disease caused by other infectious and noninfectious processes including lymphoma. In the case of lymphoma, reduction in peritumoral edema may be dramatic, and the steroids may have a direct cytotoxic effect on the tumor cells as well. Therefore, when corticosteroids are used concomitantly with anti-*Toxoplasma* chemotherapy, serial CAT scans after the discontinuation of corticosteroids should be obtained to determine that the radiographic abnormality does not exacerbate.

The exact duration of chemotherapy necessary to place the infection in remission has not been established in controlled, prospective studies and is probably dependent on the level of immunosuppression caused by the underlying illness. Treatment is usually continued for 4-6 weeks after resolution of all signs and symptoms. Because chemotherapy against *Toxoplasma* is active only against multiplying *Toxoplasma* tachyzoites and not against the tissue cysts, it is suggested that chemotherapy be continued until an adequate cell-mediated immune response against *Toxoplasma* has been restored. This is necessary to prevent the high risk of recrudescence of serious toxoplasmosis in patients who continue to be severely immunocompromised (e.g., AIDS patients) (60,372a).

A. Specific Therapy

1. Pyrimethamine Plus Sulfonamide

Pyrimethamine, a 2,4-diaminopyrimidine, is one of the cornerstones in the current therapy of significant toxoplasma infection. Pyrimethamine inhibits the activity of the enzyme dihydrofolate reductase, thereby interrupting the synthesis of tetrahydrofolate, which is necessary for normal nucleic acid synthesis. It has a higher affinity to the dihydrofolate reductase of the parasite than to the mammalian cell, making it an effective chemotherapeutic agent. However, its activity is limited to the replicating tachyzoites; there has been no activity demonstrated against the tissue cyst or the nonreplicating tachyzoite form of the organism. In tissue culture, pyrimethamine at a concentration of 0.5 μg/ml inhibited the multiplication of RH *Toxoplasma* and caused striking morphological alterations. When added in combination with an ineffective level of sulfadiazine (15 μg/ml), a level of 0.1 μg/ml was highly active against *Toxoplasma* (373-375). However, in these studies, levels of paraaminobenzoic acid and folate were above physiological levels, and therefore it is possible that lower levels of both pyrimethamine and sulfonamide may be effective.

The effectiveness of pyrimethamine as a sole agent in the treatment of toxoplasmosis is limited by the potential bone marrow toxicity of the drug and the low therapeutic levels achieved in the serum and cerebrospinal fluid of patients. After oral administration of 50 mg of pyrimethamine, a plasma level of approximately 0.3 μg/ml is achieved (376). The cerebrospinal fluid concentration is approximately 10-25% of that achieved in the serum according to a study of the pharmacokinetics of pyrimethamine in patients with meningeal leukemia. In rats and dogs the brain tissue level is approximately 2.6 times the serum level. Thus, the achieved levels of pyrimethamine in the serum and cerebrospinal fluid of patients may not be much more (and may be even less) than the minimal concentration found to be effective when used alone in a tissue culture system, which emphasizes the relative necessity of using pyrimethamine in conjunction with sulfadiazine or trisulfapyrimidines. Furthermore, in patients with AZOS the measured serum levels are not predictable on the basis of oral dosage (376a).

Sulfonamides inhibit dihydrofolic acid synthetase and thereby interfere with the use of paraaminobenzoic acid by the parasite. When used in conjunction with pyrimethamine, sulfonamides cause a "sequential blockade" of folic acid metabolism and act synergistically against *Toxoplasma*.

Among the sulfonamides, sulfadiazine, sulfamethazine, and sulfamerazine have been found to be equally effective in their activity against *Toxoplasma*. Sulfathiazole, sulfapyridine, sulfadimetine, and sulfisoxazole are less active and are therefore not recommended (377). After a 4-g oral dose of sulfadiazine, the peak serum drug is between 40 and 60 μg/ml, and about 90-95% of the drug is in active form (378). Sulfadiazine readily penetrates into normal cerebrospinal fluid and may attain a concentration of about one-half that of the serum (379). From these data it is evident that pyrimethamine and sulfadiazine or trisulfapyrimidine are most effective when used together. Sulfadiazine is well absorbed from the gastrointestinal tract and achieves peak serum levels within 3-6 hr after ingestion. The serum half-life of the drug is about 2-3 hr. The usual dose of sulfadiazine or triple sulfonamides is 6-8 g/day given in four equally divided doses for an adult, or 100 mg/kg body weight per day for a child given in four to six equal doses. However, the minimum amount of sulfonamide necessary to achieve its maximal synergistic effect in the clinical situation has not been established. Therapy with pyrimethamine, which has a half-life of 4 days, should be initiated with a loading dose of 200 mg/day, followed by 50-75 mg/day. After several weeks of therapy with good clinical response, the dose of medication may be tapered to 25-50 mg/day while monitoring for any evidence of recrudescence of active infection. In situations where there has not been a satisfactory response or where pyrimethamine is to be used alone because of an adverse reaction to sulfonamide, a dose of 100 mg/day should be considered with careful monitoring of hematological toxicity.

Pyrimethamine is a folic acid antagonist and when used in anti-*Toxoplasma* doses may cause significant bone marrow suppression. Folinic acid (leucovorin) is transported across human cell membranes but not across *Toxoplasma* cell membranes and therefore may be a useful adjunct to prevent the bone marrow toxicity of pyrimethamine but maintain its therapeutic efficacy. In contrast, folic acid seems to have an adverse effect on the action of pyrimethamine and sulfadiazine (380). Folinic acid at a dose of 5-10 mg/day should be given orally or parenterally along with pyrimethamine. Other less serious side effects with pyrimethamine include gastrointestinal distress, headaches, and a bad taste in the mouth.

The clinical response of immunocompromised patients with toxoplasmosis to treatment with pyrimethamine and sulfonamides has been dependent on whether the diagnosis is made and therapy is initiated in a prompt manner. In a literature review of toxoplasmosis in the compromised host, Ruskin and Remington noted that only 20 of 81 immunocompromised patients with toxoplasmosis were treated and of these, 80% responded to therapy. Luft and Remington (13) reviewed 11 cases from the literature of toxoplasmic encephalitis in the non-AIDS immunocompromised host who received therapy with pyrimethamine and sulfadiazine and found that seven responded to therapy. In the cases in which there was a poor response to therapy, there were extenuating circumstances, including discontinuation of therapy because of leukopenia and delay in diagnosis of infection. In contrast, in a recent review of the experience at Memorial Sloan-Kettering Cancer Center with toxoplasmic encephalitis in AIDS patients, 12 of 14 patients who responded to therapy and survived for more than 2 months had their sulfonamide discontinued during the course of therapy. Four of these patients experienced relapse while being treated with pyrimethamine alone (three patients) or with pyrimethamine in conjunction with clindamycin (one patient) (352). In the instances when sulfonamides cannot be continued, consideration should be given to the use of pyrimethamine alone (75 mg/day) in combination with clindamycin (see below).

2. Trimethoprim Plus Sulfamethoxazole

Trimethoprim, a 2,4-diaminopyrimidine, plus sulfamethoxazole has been found to have synergistic activity against *Toxoplasma*. The ability of trimethoprim to inhibit catalytic activity of the dihydrofolate reductase enzyme of *Toxoplasma* and its ability to inhibit the replication of *Toxoplasma* in vitro are markedly less than those of comparable amounts of pyrimethamine (381). Therefore, therapy with trimethoprim plus sulfamethoxazole cannot be considered optimal combination therapy for the treatment of toxoplasmosis, and the efficacy of this regimen may be due to the activity of sulfamethoxazole alone. This combination should not be used for life-threatening toxoplasma infection in the compromised host.

3. Clindamycin

The toxoplasmacidal activity of clindamycin has been demonstrated in mice infected with either a virulent or avirulent strain of *Toxoplasma* (382). Recently, clincamycin has been shown to be effective in a murine model of toxoplasmic encephalitis (383). There have been several reports of patients with AIDS and toxoplasmic encephalitis for whom treatment with pyrimethamine and clindamycin yielded apparent improvement. It is unclear what role clindamycin played in the observed improvement, since pyrimethamine is active when used alone. Prospective controlled studies are needed to assess clindamycin's role in the treatment of this disease.

4. Spiramycin

Spiramycin, a macrolide antibiotic, used commonly in Europe for the prevention of transplacental transmission of toxoplasmosis (383a), has not been fully evaluated for a role in treatment or prophylaxis in immunocompromised patients. However, one small study of four patients (three AIDS, one bone marrow transplant) revealed that spiramycin was not efficacious for prophylaxis or treatment of these patients (383b).

B. Experimental Agents

1. Trimetrexate

Trimetrexate, a dihydrofolate reductase inhibitor, is a new highly lipid soluble antineoplastic agent. Kovacs et al. (384,384a) have demonstrated that trimetrexate potently inhibited the catalytic activity of *Toxoplasmic* dihydrofolate reductase, had a higher affinity for *Toxoplasma* dihydrofolate reductase than did pyrimethamine or trimethoprim, and inhibited the replication of *Toxoplasma* at lower concentration of drug than trimethoprim or pyrimethamine. Further controlled studies are necessary to determine whether this highly active dihydrofolate reductase inhibitor in conjunction with folinic acid is a more effective and less toxic drug than pyrimethamine.

2. Arprinocid

Arprinocid, 6-amino-9-(2-chloro-fluorebenzyl)purine is an anticoccidial effective in chickens infected with various species of coccidia including *Eimeria tenella* (385), a coccidian closely related to *Toxoplasma*. The drug is a specific inhibitor of hypoxanthine transmembrane transport and inhibits the incorporation of hypoxanthine into nucleic acids of *E. tenella*, embryonic chick kidney epithelial cells, and HeLa cells. This mode of action may be particularly important vis-à-vis *Toxoplasma* in view of the data of Perotto et al. (76) suggesting that *Toxoplasma* is unable to produce purines de novo and that it utilizes hypoxanthine transport as a source of purines (386). Arprinocid also inhibits the dihydrofolate reductase of *E. tenella*. In addition, the major metabolite arprinocid 1-N oxide has potent anticoccidian activity (387). Recently, Luft (83) demonstrated that arprinocid is a highly potent toxoplasmacidal agent in the treatment of mice infected with either the virulent RH or less virulent C56 strain of *Toxoplasma*. Arprinocid protected mice against infection with 10^6 times the lethal dose of *Toxoplasma* and was able to eradicate the infection from cell tissue. In addition, arprinocid completely protected (0% mortality) mice that were infected with the C56 strain of *Toxoplasma* and severely immunocompromised with either cyclophosphamide or corticosteroids, whereas 100% of similarly infected cyclophosphamide- and corticosteroid-treated control mice died. The therapeutic efficacy of this drug was maintained when as little as 0.1 mg of arprinocid was given to mice daily. On a weight-to-weight basis, arprinocid was found to be 10–100 times more active than pyrimethamine in vivo. Further studies are necessary to determine the relative safety of arprinocid in humans.

3. Roxithromycin

Roxithromycin, a macrolide antibiotic, is a long-acting oral antibiotic that is active against *Toxoplasma* in animal models of infection (388,388a). Mice infected with either the less virulent C56 or the RH strain of *Toxoplasma* had significantly lower mortality ($p < 0.001$) than untreated controls. Similarly, roxithromycin has been able to significantly protect mice infected with C56 *Toxoplasma* and immunocompromised with either cyclophosphamide or corticosteroids. Interestingly, roxithromycin has been shown to be able to completely eradicate infection from mice infected with the RH strain but is unable to do so in mice infected with the less virulent C56 strain of *Toxoplasma*. Roxithromycin has also been found to act synergistically with gamma-interferon in a murine model of toxoplasmic encephalitis (388b). Because of its apparent safety in phase I studies, roxithromycin may become a useful agent in the treatment of toxoplasmosis.

C. Immunotherapy

1. Interferon

The control of severe toxoplasma infection is ultimately dependent on the development of an adequate cell-mediated immune response to the pathogen. With the development of recombinant genetic engineering techniques to manufacture lymphokines that enhances cell-mediated immune function, immunotherapy alone or in conjunction with specific chemotherapy may be useful in reversing this relapsing illness in the severely immunocompromised host. Gamma-interferon has been shown to augment natural killer cell activity and to activate macrophages (see Section VI). Both of these effector cells have been implicated as having a prominent role in host resistance to toxoplasma infection. In studies of the effect of interferon administration on host resistance to acute toxoplasma infection, McCabe et al. (389) demonstrated that interferon fully protected or significantly prolonged the life of mice infected with *T. gondii*. These interferon-treated mice also had enhanced antibody synthesis and earlier activation of macrophages. Further studies are needed to determine whether interferon is a useful adjunct in combination with chemotherapeutic agents in the treatment of significant toxoplasma infection.

2. Interleukin 2

Recombinant interleukin 2 facilitates the development of cytotoxic T cells (390) and natural killer cell activity (391) as well as antigen-induced T-cell proliferation (392). Chan and Luft (388) showed that splenocytes from animals acutely infected with *T. gondii* had a diminished capacity to produce interleukin 2.

Sharma et al. (393) has recently demonstrated that administration of interleukin 2 (IL2) significantly protected mice against mortality due to a lethal infection with *T. gondii*. Administration of IL2 enhanced survival and reduced the number of cysts formed in the brain of infected animals. There was no difference in antibody synthesis specific to *T. gondii* or reversal in the suppression of lymphocyte transformation associated with acute infection. However, natural killer cell activity was potentiated in mice that received interleukin 2. Administration of interleukin 2 may prove useful as adjunctive therapy or as a method to specifically restore a particular defect in selected immunocompromised hosts.

XV. PREVENTION

Immunocompromised patients should be serologically tested for evidence of previous toxoplasma infection and should be advised by their physician of the appropriate method to prevent infection with *Toxoplasma*, especially if there is no serological evidence of previous infection. Specifically, because the infection is usually transmitted by ingestion of meat that contains the cyst form of the organism or foods contaminated with oocysts, attempts should be made to eradicate the infectious organism from food. The tissue cyst can be rendered noninfectious by cooking meat thoroughly until well done or by freezing meat at -20°C for 24 hr prior to use. After handling raw meat, hands should be washed with soap and water. Eggs should not be eaten raw. Unpasteurized goat's milk and cheese should be avoided. The patient should avoid contact with cat feces or foods potentially contaminated with oocysts. Fruits and vegetables should be washed, because flies, cockroaches, and other copraphagious insects serve as transport hosts for *T. gondii* oocysts, and their access to food should be prevented. The patient should be educated that the oocysts may remain in the environment in an infectious state for a prolonged period of time (24).

ACKNOWLEDGMENT

The author gratefully acknowledges Jack S. Remington for teaching him the nuances involved in the biology and clinical manifestations of this disease which are hopefully reflected in this chapter.

REFERENCES

1. Nicolle, C., and Manceaux, L. Sur un protozoaire nouveau de Gondi:, *Toxoplasma. Arch. Inst. Pasteur (Tunis)* 2:97 (1909).
2. Splendore, A. Un nuovo protozoa parassita dei conigli. Incontrato nelle lesioni anatomchie d'una malattia che ricorda in molti punti il kala-azar dell'uomo. *Rev. Soc. Sci, (Sao Paulo)* 3:109 (1908).

3. Janku, J. Pathogenesa a pathologicka anatomie tak nazvaneho vrozeneho kolobomu zlute sdvrny v oku normalne velikem a mikropthalmickem s nalezem parazitu v sitnici. *Cesk. Parasitol. 6*:9 (1929).

4. Frenkel, J. K. Pursuing *Toxoplasma. J. Infect. Dis. 122*:553 (1970).

5. Wolf, A., and Cowen, D. Grandulomatous encephalomyleitis due to encephalitozoan (encephalitozoic encephalomyelitis). A new protozoan disease of man. *Bull. Neurol. Inst. NY 6*:306 (1937).

6. Sabin, A., and Olitski, P. *Toxoplasma* and obligate intracellular parasitism. *Science 85*:336 (1937).

7. Paige, B. H., Cowen, D., and Wolff, A. Toxoplasmic encephalitis. V. Further observations of infantile toxoplasmoses: intra-uterine inception of the disease: visceral manifestation. *Am. J. Dis. Child. 63*:474 (1942).

8. Sabin, A. B., and Feldman, H. A. Dyes as microchemical indicators of a new immunity phenomenon affecting a protozoan parasite (*Toxoplasma*). *Science 108*:660 (1948).

9. Wilson, C. B., and Remington, J. S. What can be done to prevent congenital toxoplasmosis? *Am. J. Obstet. Gynecol. 138*:357 (1980).

10. Ruskin, J., and Remington, J. S. Toxoplasmosis in the compromised host. *Am. Intern. Med. 84*:193 (1976).

11. Townsend, J., Wolinsky, J. S., Baringer, J. R., and Johnson, P. C. Acquired toxoplasmosis. *Arch. Neurol. 32*:335 (1975).

12. Vietzke, W. M., Gelderman, A. H., Grimley, P. M., and Valsamin, M. P. Toxoplasmosis complicating malignancy. *Cancer 21*:816 (1968).

13. Luft, B. J., and Remington, J. S. Toxoplasmosis of the central nervous system. In *Current Clinical Topics in Infectious Diseases* (J. S. Remington and M. N. Swartz, eds.). McGraw-Hill, New York, 1985, p. 315.

14. Luft, B. J., Conley, F. K., Remington, J. S., et al. Outbreak of CNS toxoplasmosis in Western Europe and North America. *Lancet 1*:78 (1983).

15. Luft, B. J., and Remington, J. S. Acute toxoplasma infection among family members of patients with acute lymphadenopathic toxoplasmosis. *Arch. Intern. Med. 144*:53 (1984).

16. Wallace, G. D. The role of the cat in the natural history of *Toxoplasma gondii. Am. J. Trop. Med. Hyg. 22*:313 (1973).

17. Frenkel, J. K. Toxoplasmosis: paraiste life cycle, pathology and immunology. In *The Coccidia* (D. M. Hammond, ed.). University Park Press, Baltimore, 1973, p. 343.

18. Teutsch, S. M., Juranek, D. D., Sulzer, A., et al. Epidemic toxoplasmos associated with infected cats. *New Engl. J. Med. 300*:695 (1979).

19. Benson, M. W., Takafuji, E. T., Lemon, S. M., et al. Oocyst transmitted toxoplasmosis associated with the ingestion of contaminated water. *New Engl. J. Med. 307*:666 (1982).

20. Wallace, G. D. Serologic and epidemiologic observations on toxoplasmosis on three Pacific atolls. *Am. J. Epidemiol. 90*:103 (1969).

21. Weinman, D., and Chandler, A. H. Toxoplasmosis in men and swine: an investigation of the possible relationship. *JAMA 161*:229 (1956).

22. Desmonts, G., Couvreur, J., Alison, F., Baudelot, J., Gerbeaux, J., and Lelong, M. Etude epidemiologique sur la toxoplasmose: de l'influence de la cuisson des viandes de boucherie sur la frequence de l'infection humaine. *Rev. Fr. Etud. Clin. Biol. 10*:952 (1965).

23. Kean, B. H., Kimball, A. C., and Christenson, W. N. An epidemic of acute toxoplasmosis. *JAMA 208*:1002 (1969).

24. Remington, J. S., and Desmonts, G. Toxoplasmosis. In *Infectious Diseases of the Fetus and Newborn Infant* (J. S. Remington and J. O. Klein, eds.). W. B. Saunders, Philadelphia, 1983, p. 143.

25. Sacks, J. J., Roberto, R. R., and Brooks, W. F. Toxoplasmosis infection associated with goat's milk. *JAMA 248*:1728 (1982).

26. Siegel, S. E., Lunde, M. N., Gelderman, A. H., et al. Transmission of toxoplasmosis by leukocyte transfusion. *Blood 37*:388 (1971).

27. Neu, H. C. Toxoplasmosis transmitted at autopsy. *JAMA 202*:284 (1967).

28. Ryning, F. W., McLeod, R., Maddox, J. C., et al. Probable transmission of *Toxoplasma gondii* by organ transplantation. *Ann. Intern. Med. 90*:47 (1979).

29. Luft, B. J. Primary and reactivated *Toxoplasma* infection in patients with cardiac transplants: clinical spectrum and problems in diagnosis in a defined population. *Ann. Intern. Med. 99*:27 (1983).

30. Rose, A. C., Vys, C. J., Novitsky, D., Cooper, D. K. C., and Barnard, C. N. Toxoplasmosis of donor and recipient hearts after heterotopic cardiac transplantation. *Arch. Pathol. Lab. Med. 107*:368 (1983).

31. Chernik, N. L., et al. Central nervous system infectious in patients with cancer. *Medicine 52*:563 (1973).

32. Hooper, D. C., et al. Central nervous system infection in the chronically immunosuppressed. *Medicine 61*:166 (1982).

33. McLeod, R., et al. Toxoplasmosis presenting as a brain abscess. *Am. J. Med. 67*:711 (1979).

34. Britt, R. H., et al. Intracranial infection in cardiac transplant recipients. *Ann. Neurol. 9*:107 (1981).

35. Stinson, E. B., et al. Infectious complications following cardiac transplantation in men. *Ann. Intern. Med. 74*:22 (1971).

36. Nagington, J., and Martin, A. L. Toxoplasmosis and heart transplantation. *Lancet, 2679* (1983).

37. Tavolato, B., et al. Toxoplasma encephalitis in the adult. *Acta Neurol. (Napoli) 33*:321 (1978).

38. Budzilovich, G. N. Acquired toxoplasmosis. *Am. J. Clin. Pathol. 25*:66 (1971).

39. Kersting, G., and Newman, J. "Malignant lymphoma" of the brain following renal transplantation. *Acta Neuropathol. VI (Suppl)*:131 (1975).

40. Rhodes, R. H., et al. Disseminated toxoplasmosis with brain involvement in renal allograft recipient. *Bull. Los Angeles Neurol. Soc. 42*:16 (1977).

41. Ghatak, N. R., et al. Toxoplasmosis of the CNS in the adult. *Arch. Pathol. 89*:337 (1970).

42. Flament-Durand, J., et al. Toxoplasmic encephalitis and amyositis during

treatment with immunosuppressive drugs. *Acta Clin. Belg.* 22:44 (1967).

43. Reynolds, E. S., et al Generalized toxoplasmosis following renal transplantation. *Arch. Intern. Med.* 118:401 (1966).

44. Lowenberg, B., et al. Fatal cerebral toxoplasmosis in a bone marrow transplant recipient with leukemia. *Transplantation* 35:30 (1983).

45. Guibeau, J. C., et al. Aspects tomodensitometriques d'un de toxoplasmose intracranienne chez un immunon deprime. *J. Radiol. (Paris)* 64:347 (1983).

46. Emerson, R. G., et al. Toxoplasmosis: a treatable neurologic disease in the immunologically compromised patient. *Pediatrics* 67:653 (1981).

47. Fisher, M. A., Levy, J., Helfrich, M., Luft, B. J., August, C. S., and Starr, S. E. Detection of *Toxoplasma gondii* in the spinal fluid of a bone marrow transplant recipient. (submitted for publication)

48. Anthony, C. W. Disseminated toxoplasmosis in a liver transplant patient. *J. Am. Med. Wom. Assoc.* 27:601 (1977).

49. Tilney, N. L., Kohler, T. R., and Strom, T. B. Cerebromeningitis in immunosuppressed recipients of renal allografts. *Ann. Surg.* 195:104 (1982).

50. Shroter, G. P. J., Hoelscher, M., Putnam, C. W., Porter, K. A., Hansbrough, J. F., and Starzl, T. E. Infections complicating orthotopic liver transplantation. A study emphasizing graft-related septicemia. *Arch. Surg.* 111:1337 (1976).

51. Winston, D. J., Gale, R. P., Meyer, D. V., and Young, L. S. Infectious complication of human bone marrow transplantation. *Medicine (Baltimore)* 58:1 (1979).

52. Wong, B., Gold, J. W. M., Brown, D. E., et al. Central nervous system toxoplasmosis in homosexual men and parenteral drug abusers. *Ann. Intern. Med.* 100:36 (1984).

53. Hooper, A. D. Acquired toxoplasmosis: report of a case with autopsy findings. *AMA Arch. Pathol.* 64:1 (1957).

54. Vieira, J., et al. Acquired immune deficiency in Haitians: opportunistic infections in previously health Haitian immigrants. *New Engl. J. Med.* 308:125 (1983).

55. Moskowitz, L. B., et al. Unusual causes of death in Haitians residing in Miami. High prevalence of opportunistic infections. *JAMA* 250:1187 (1983).

56. Clumeck, N., et al. Acquired immunodeficiency syndrome in African patients. *New Engl. J. Med.* 310:492 (1984).

57. Levy, R. M., Bredesen, D. E., and Rosenblum, M. L. Neurological manifestations of the acquired immunodeficiency syndrome (AIDS). Experience of UCSF and review of the literature. *J. Neurosurg.* 62:475 (1985).

58. Snider, W. D., et al. Neurological complications of acquired immunodeficiency syndrome. Analysis of 50 patients. *Ann. Neurol.* 14:403 (1983).

59. Chan, J. C., et al. Toxoplasma encephalitis in recent Haitian entrants. *South. Med. J.* 76:211 (1983).

60. Navia, B. A., Petito, C. K., Gold, J. W., Cho, E., Jordan, B. D., and Price, R. W. Cerebral toxoplasmosis complicating the acquired immune deficiency

syndrome: clinical and neuropathalogical findings in 27 patients. *Ann. Neurol. 19*:224 (1986).

61. Dubey, J. P., Miller, N. L., and Frenkel, J. K. The *Toxoplasma gondii* oocyst from cat feces. *J. Exp. Med. 133*:636 (1970).

62. Stagno, S., Dykes, A. C., Ames, C. S., Head, R. A., Juranek, D. P., and Walls, K. An outbreak of toxoplasmosis linked to cats. *Pediatrics 65*:706 (1980).

63. Kasper, L. H., and Ware, P. L. Recognition and characterization of stage specific oocyst/sporozoite antigens of *Toxoplasma gondii* by human antisera. *J. Clin. Invest. 75*:1570 (1985).

64. Rawal, B. D. Toxoplasmosis: a dye test survey on sera from vegetarians and meat eaters in Bombay. *Trans. R. Soc. Trop. Med. Hyg. 53*:61 (1959).

65. Jacobs, L., Remington, J. S., and Melton, N. L. The resistance of the encysted form of *Toxoplasma gondii*. *J. Parasitol. 46*:11 (1960).

66. Talice, R. V., Gurri, J., Royal, J., et al. Investigationes sobre la toxoplasmosis en el uruguey; sobrevida da *Toxoplasma gondii* en sengre human *in vitro. An. Fac. Med. Montevideo 42*:143 (1957).

67. Miller, M. J., Aronson, W. J., and Remington, J. S. Late parasitemia in asymptomatic acquired toxoplasmosis. *Ann. Intern. Med. 71*:139 (1969).

68. Remington, J. S., Melton, M. L., and Jacobs, L. Induced and spontaneous recurrent parasitemia in chronic infections with avirulent strains of *Toxoplasma gondii*. *J. Simmunol. 87*:578 (1961).

69. Krahenbuhl, J. L., Blazovek, A. A., and Lysenko, M. G. In vivo and in vitro studies of delayed hypersensitivity to *Toxoplasma gondii* in guinea pigs. *Infect. Immun. 3*:260 (1971).

70. Jones, T. C., Bierz, K. A., and Erb, P. *In vitro* cultivation of *Toxoplasma gondii* cysts in astrocytes in the presence of gamma interferon. *Infect. Immun. 51*:147 (1986).

71. Frenkel, J. K., and Friedlander, S. *Toxoplasmosis.* Public Health Service publication No. 141. U.S. Gov. Printing Office, Washington, D.C., 1951.

72. Lainson, R. Observations on the development and nature of pseudocysts and cysts of *Toxoplasma gondii*. *Trans. R. Soc. Trop. Med. Hyg. 12*:221 (1958).

73. Wanko, T., Jacobs, L., and Gavin, M. A. Electron microscopy study of toxoplasma cysts in mouse btain. *J. Protozool. 9*:235 (1962).

74. Carver, B. K., and Golman, M. Staining *Toxoplasma gondii* with fluorescence-labeled antibody. III. The reaction in frozen and paraffin sections. *Am. J. Clin. Pathol. 32*:159 (1959).

75. Meija, G., et al. Transmission of toxoplasmosis by renal transplant. *Am. J. Kidney Dis. 2*:615 (1983).

76. Perotto, J., Keister, D. B., and Gelderman, A. H. Incorporation of precursors into *Toxoplasma* DNA. *J. Protozool. 18*:470 (1971).

77. Scholtyseck, E., Mehlhorn, H., and Friedloft, K. The fine structure of the conoid of sporozoa and related organisms. *Z. Parasitenk. 34*:68 (1970).

78. Jones, T. C. Multiplication of toxoplasmosis in enucleate fibroblasts. *Proc. Soc. Exp. Biol. Med. 142*:1268 (1973).

79. Sethi, K. K., Pelster, B., Piekarski, G., and Brandish, H. Multiplication of *Toxoplasma gondii* in enucleated L cells. *Nature New Biol. 242*:255 (1973).

80. Schwartzman, J. D., and Pfefferkorn, E. R. Pyrimidine synthesis by intracellular *Toxoplasma gondii. J. Parasitol. 67*:150 (1981).

81. Asai, T., O'Sullivan, W. J., Kobayashi, M., et al. Enzymes of the de novo pyrimidine biosynthetic pathway in *Toxoplasma gondii. Mol. Biochem. Parasitol. 7*:89 (1983).

82. Pfefferkorn, E. R., and Pfefferkorn, L. C. *Toxoplasma gondii*: specific labeling of nucleic acids of intracellular parasites in Lesch-Nyhan cells. *Exp. Parasitol. 41*:95 (1977).

83. Luft, B. J. Potent *in vivo* activity of arprinocid, a purine analog, against murine toxoplasmosis. *J. Infect. Dis. 154*:692 (1986).

84. Pfefferkorn, E. R.,and Pfefferkorn, L. C. *Toxoplasma gondii*: growth in the absence of host cell protein synthesis. *Exp. Parasitol. 52*:129 (1981).

85. Takeuchi, T., Fujiwara, T., and Akao, S. Na^+, K^+-dependent ATPase activity and effect of K^+ on in vitro protein synthesis and NAD pyrophosphorylase in *Toxoplasma gondii. J. Parasitol. 66*:591 (1980).

86. Miayagami, T., Takei, Y., Matsumoto, Y., et al. An *in vitro* study on the toxoplasmacidal activity of lonomycin in host cells. *J. Antibiot. 24*:218 (1981).

87. Frenkel, J. K., and Smith, D. D. Inhibitory effects of mesensin on shedding of *Toxoplasma* oocysts by cats. *J. Parasitol. 68*:851 (1982).

88. Melton, M. C., and Sheffield, H. G. Activity of the anticoccidial compound, lasalocid against *Toxoplasma gondii* in cultured cells. *J. Parasitol. 61*:713 (1975).

89. Prince, J. B., Koven-Quinn, M. A., Remington, J. S., and Sharma, S. D. Cell free synthesis of *Toxoplasma gondii* antigens. *Mol. Biochem. Parasitol. 17*: 163 (1985).

90. Bloomfield, M. M., and Remington, J. S. Comparison of three strains of *Toxoplasma gondii* by polyacrylamide-gel electrophoresis. *Trop. Geogr. Med. 22*:367 (1970).

91. Handman, E., Goding, J. W., and Remington, J. S. Detection and characterization of membrane antigens of *Toxoplasma gondii. J. Immunol. 124*: 2578 (1980).

92. Towbin, H., Staehlin, T., and Gordon, J. Electrophoretic transfer of proteins from polyacrylamide gels to nitrocellulose sheets: procedure and some application. *Proc. Natl. Acad. Sci. USA 76*:4350 (1979).

93. Johnson, A. M., McDonald, P. J., and Neoh, S. H. Molecular weight analysis of the major polypeptides and glycopeptides of *Toxoplasma gondii. Biochem. Biophys. Res. Commun. 100*:934 (1981).

94. Ogata, K., Kaschara, T., Shiori-Nakano, K., et al. Immunoenzymatic detection of three kinds of 43,000 molecular weight antigens by monoclonal antibodies in the insoluble freaction of *Toxoplasma gondii. Infect. Immun. 43*:1047 (1984).

95. Kasper, L. H., Crabb, J. H., and Pfefferkorn, E. R. Purification of a major protein of *Toxoplasma gondii* by immunoabsorption with a monoclonal antibody. *J. Immunol. 130*:2407 (1983).

96. Rodriguez, C., Afchain, D., Capron, A., Dissous, C., and Santoro, F. Major surface protein of *Toxoplasma gondii* (p 30) contains an immunodominant region with repetitive epitopes. *Eur. J. Immunol. 15*:747 (1985).

97. Lindenschmidt, E. G. Demonstration of immunoglobulin M class antibodies to *Toxoplasma gondii* antigenic component p 35000 by enzyme-linked antigen immunosorbent assay. *J. Clin. Microbiol. 24*:1045 (1986).

98. Potasman, I., Araujo, E., and Remington, J. S. Toxoplasma antigens recognized by naturally occurring human antibodies. *J. Clin. Microbiol. 24*:1050 (1986).

98a. Santoro, F., Afchain, D., Pierce, R., Cesbron, J. Y., Ovalque, G., and Capran, A. Serodiagnosis of toxoplasma infection using a purified parastie protein (p 30). *Clin. Exp. Immunol. 62*:262 (1985).

99. Brzosko, W. J., Dymowska, Z., and Urbanek-Szufnara, K. Electron microscopic immunomorphology of *Toxoplasma gondii. Exp. Med. Microbiol. 22*:252 (1970).

100. Johnson, A. M., Haynes, W. D., Leppard, P. J., et al. Ultrastructural and biochemical studies on the immunohistochemistry of *Toxoplasma gondii* antigens using monoclonal antibodies. *Histochemistry 77*:209 (1983).

101. Handman, E., and Remington, J. S. Serological and immunochemical characterization of monoclonal antibodies to *Toxoplasma gondii. Immunology 40*:579 (1980).

102. Johnson, A. M., McNamara, P. J., Neoh, S. H., et al. Hybridous secreting monoclonal antibody to *Toxoplasma gondii. Aust. J. Exp. Biol. Med. Sci. 59*:303 (1981).

103. Pande, P. G., Shukla, R. R., and Sekarich, P. C. A heteroglycan from *Toxoplasma gondii. Nature 180*:644 (1961).

104. Mauras, G., Dodeur, M., Laget, P., et al. Partial resolution of the sugar content of *Toxoplasma gondii* membrane. *Biochem. Biophys. Res. Commun. 97*:906 (1980).

105. Sethi, K. K., Rahman, A., Pelster, B., and Brandis, H. Search for the presence of lectin binding sites on *Toxoplasma gondii. J. Parasitol. 63*: 1076 (1977).

106. Mineo, J. R., Camargo, M. E., and Ferreira, A. W. Enzyme linked immunosorbent assay for antibodies to *Toxoplasma gondii* polysaccharides in human toxoplasmosis. *Infect. Immun. 27*:283 (1980).

107. Camargo, M. E., Ferreira, A. W., Mineo, J. R., Takiguti, C. K., and Nakahara, O. S. Immunoglobulin G and immunoglobulin M enzyme linked immunosorbent assays and defined toxoplasmosis serological patterns. *Infect. Immun. 21*:55 (1978).

108. Naot, Y., Guptill, D. R., Mullenax, J., and Remington, J. S. Characterization of *Toxoplasma gondii* antigens that react with human immunoglobulin M and immunoglobulin G antibodies. *Infect. Immun. 41*:331 (1983).

109. Partanen, P., Turnen, H. J., Paasivuo, R., et al. Identification of antigenic components of *Toxoplasma gondii* by an immunoblotting technique. *FEBS Lett. 158*:252 (1983).

110. Ehrlich, H. A., Rodgers, G., Vaillancort, P., et al. Identification of antigen

specific immunoglobulin M antibody associated with acute *Toxoplasma* infection. *Infect. Immun. 41*:683 (1983).

111. Sharma, S. D., Mullenax, J., Araujo, F. G., et al. Western blot analysis of the antigens of *Toxoplasma gondii* recognized by human IgM and IgG antibodies. *J. Immunol. 131*:977 (1983).

112. Partanen, P., et al. Immunoblot analysis of *Toxoplasma gondii* antigens by human immunoglobulins G, M and A antibodies at different stages of infection. *J. Clin. Microbiol. 20*:133–135 (1984).

113. Lunde, M. N., and Jacobs, L. Antigenic differences between endozoites and cystozoites of *Toxoplasma gondii. J. Parasitol. 69*:806 (1983).

114. Kasper, L. H., Bradley, M. S., and Pfefferkorn, E. R. Identification of stage specific sporozoite antigens of *Toxoplasma gondii* by monoclonal antibodies. *J. Immunol. 132*:443 (1984).

115. Sharma, S. D., Araujo, F. G., and Remington, J. S. Toxoplasma antigen isolated by affinity chromatography with monoclonal antibody protects mice against lethal infection with *Toxoplasma gondii. J. Immunol. 133*: 2818 (1984).

116. Araujo, F., and Remington, J. S. Partially purified antigen preparations of *Toxoplasma gondii* protect against lethal infection in mice. *Infect. Immun. 45*:122 (1984).

117. Kasper, L. H. An expected response to vaccination with a purified major membrane tachyzoite antigen (p 30) of *Toxoplasma gondii. J. Immunol. 134*:3426 (1985).

118. Hauser, W. E., Jr., and Remington, J. S. Effect of monoclonal antibodies on phagocytosis and killing of *Toxoplasma gondii* by normal macrophages. *Infect. Immun. 32*:637 (1981).

119. Sethi, K. K., Endo, T., and Brandis, H. *Toxoplasma gondii* trophozoites precoated with specific monoclonal antibodies cannot survive within normal murine macrophages. *Immunol. Lett. 2*:343 (1981).

120. Johnson, A. M., McDonald P. J., and Neoh, S. H. Monoclonal antibodies to *Toxoplasma* cell membrane surface antigens protect mice from toxoplasmosis. *J. Protozool. 30*:351 (1983).

121. Cutchins, E. C., and Warren, J. Immunity patterns in the guinea pig following *Toxoplasma* infection and vaccination with killed *Toxoplasma. Am. J. Trop. Med. Hyg. 5*:197 (1956).

122. Krahenbuhl, J. L., Ruskin, J., and Remington, J. S. The use of killed vaccines in immunization against an intracellular parasite: *Toxoplasma gondii. J. Immunol. 108*:425 (1972).

123. Araujo, F. G., and Remington, J. S. Protection against *Toxoplasma gondii* in mice immunized with *Toxoplasma* cell fractions, RNA and synthetic polyribonucleotides. *Immunology 27*:711 (1974).

124. Hauser, W. E., Jr., Sharma, S. D., and Remington, J. S. Augmentation of NK cell activity by soluble and particulate fractions of *Toxoplasma gondii. J. Immunol. 131*:458 (1983).

125. Sharma, S. D., Verhoef, J., and Remington, J. S. Enhancement of human natural killer cell activity by subcellular components of *Toxoplasma gondii. Cell. Immunol. 86*:317 (1984).

126. Werk, R. How does *Toxoplasma gondii* enter host cells? *Rev. Int. Dis. 7*: 449 (1985).

127. Jones, T. C., Yeh, S., and Hirsch, J. G. The interaction between *Toxoplasma gondii* and mammalian cells. I. Mechanism of entry and intracellular fate of parasite. *J. Exp. Med. 136*:1157 (1972).

128. Ryning, F. W., and Remington, J. S. Effect of cytochalasin D on *Toxoplasma gondii* cell entry. *Infect. Immun. 20*:739 (1978).

129. Silva, S. R. L., Meirelles, S. S. L., and de Souza, W. Mechanism of entry of *Toxoplasma gondii* into vertebrate cells. *J. Submicrosc. Cytol. 14*:471 (1982).

130. Schwartzman, J. D., and Pfefferkorn, E. R. Immunfluorescent localization of myosin at the anterior pole of the coccidian, *Toxoplasma gondii*. *J. Protozool. 30*:657 (1983).

131. Nichols, B. A., and O'Connor, R. Penetration of mouse peritoneal macrophages by the protozoan *Toxoplasma gondii*. New evidence for active invasion and phagocytosis. *Lab. Invest. 44*:324 (1981).

132. Wilson, C. B., Tsai, V., and Remington, J. S. Failure to trigger the oxidative burst by normal macrophages. Possible mechanism for survival of intracellular pathogens. *J. Exp. Med. 151*:328 (1980).

133. Murray, H. W., and Cohn, Z. A. Macrophage oxygen-dependent antimicrobial activity. III. Enhanced oxidative metabolism as an expression of macrophage activation. *J. Exp. Med. 152*:1596 (1980).

134. Murray, H. W., Nathan, C. F., and Cohn, Z. A. Macrophage oxygen-dependent antimicrobial activity. IV. Role of endogenous scavengers. *J. Exp. Med. 152*:1610 (1980).

135. Jones, T. C., and Hirsch, J. G. The interaction between *Toxoplasma gondii* and mammalian cells II. The absence of lysosomal fusion with phagocytic vacuols containing living parasites. *J. Exp. Med. 136*:1173 (1972).

135a. Jones, T. C., Yel, S., and Hirsch, J. G. The interaction between *Toxoplasma gondii* and mammalian cells I. Mechanism of entry and intracellular fate of the parasite. *J. Exp. Med. 136*:1157–1172 (1972).

135b. Sibley, L. D., Werdner, E., and Krahenbuhl, J. L. Phagosome acidification blocked by intracellular *Toxoplasma gondii*. *Nature (Lond.) 315*:416–419 (1985).

135c. Sibley, L. D., Krahenbuhl, J. L., Adams, G. M. W., and Weidner, E. *Toxoplasma* modifies macrophage phagosomes by secretion of a vesicular network rich in surface proteins. *J. Cell. Biol. 103*:867–874 (1986).

136. Dzbenski, T. H., and Zielinska, E. Antibody induced formation of caps in *Toxoplasma gondii*. *Experimentia 32*:454 (1976).

137. Dubrametz, J. F., Rodriguez, C., and Ferreira, E. *Toxoplasma gondii* Redistribution of monoclonal antibodies during host cell invastion. *Exp. Parasitol. 59*:24 (1985).

138. Dubrametz, J. F., Dissous, C., and Ferreira, E. *Toxoplasma gondii*: liberation d'une proteine 25 kD associee a l'invasion de la cellule-hote. *J. Protozool. 29*:303 (1982).

139. Araujo, F. G., and Remington, J. S. Antigenemia in recent acquired acute toxoplasmosis. *J. Infect. Dis. 141*:144 (1980).

140. Hughes, H. P. A., and Van Knappen, F. Characterization of a secretory antigen from *Toxoplasma gondii* and its role in circulating antigen production. *Int. J. Parasitol. 12*:433 (1982).
141. Rollins, D. F., Talbara, K. F., O'Connor, R., Araujo, F. G., and Remington, J. S. Detection of toxoplasmal antigen and antibody in ocular fluids in experimental ocular toxoplasmosis. *Arch. Ophthalmol. 101*:455 (1983).
142. Araujo, F. G., Handman, E., and Remington, J. S. Use of monoclonal antibodies to detect antigens of *Toxoplasma gondii* in serum and other body fluids. *Infect. Immun. 30*:12 (1980).
143. Siegel, J. P., and Remington, J. S. Circulating immune complexes in toxoplasmosis: detection and clinical correlates. *Clin. Exp. Immunol. 52*:157 (1983).
144. Raisman, R. E., and Neva, F. A. Detection of circulating antigen in acute experimental infections with *Toxoplasma gondii. J. Infect. Dis. 132*:44 (1975).
145. van Knappen, F., et al. Demonstration of *Toxoplasma* antigen containing complexes in active toxoplasmosis. *J. Clin. Microbiol. 22*:645 (1985).
146. Strickland, G. T., Ahmed, A., and Sell, K. W. Blastogenic response of *Toxoplasma*-infected mouse spleen cells to T- and B-cell mitogens. *Clin. Exp. Immunol. 22*:167 (1975).
147. Huldt, G. Studies on experimental toxoplasmosis. *Ann. NY Acad. Sci. 177*:146 (1971).
148. Huldt, G., Gard, S., and Olovson, S. G. Effect of *Toxoplasma gondii* on the thymus. *Nature 244*:301 (1973).
149. Hibbs, J. B., Jr., Lambert, L. H., Jr., and Remington, J. S. Activated macrophage mediated nonspecific tumor resistance associated with immunosuppression. *J. Reticuloendothial Soc. 13*:368 (1973).
150. Buxton, D., Reid, H. W., and Pow, I. Immunosuppression in toxoplasmosis: studies in mice with a clostridial vaccine and louping-ill virus vaccine. *J. Comp. Pathol. 89*:375 (1979).
151. Buxton, D., Reid, H. W., Finlayson, J., Pow, I., and Anderson, I. Immunosuppression in toxoplasmosis: studies in sheep with vaccines for chlamydial abortion and louping-ill virus. *Vet. Rec. 109*:559 (1981).
152. Hibbs, J. B., Jr., Remington, J. S., and Stewart, C. C. Modulation of immunity and host resistance by microorganisms. *Pharmacol. Ther. 8*:37 (1980).
153. Chan, J., Siegel, J. P., and Luft, B. J. Demonstration of T-cell dysfunction during acute *Toxoplasma* infection. *Cell. Immunol. 98*:422 (1986).
154. McLeod, R., Van Le, L., and Remington, J. S. *Toxoplasma gondii* lymphocyte function during acute infection in mice. *Exp. Parasitol. 54*:55 (1982).
155. McLeod, R., Estes, R. G., Mack, D. G., and Cohen, H. Immune response of mice to ingested *Toxoplasma gondii*: a model of *Toxoplasma* infection acquired by ingestion. *J. Infect. Dis. 149*:234 (1984).
156. Suzuki, Y. N., Watanabe, N., and Kobayashi, A. Nonspecific suppression of primary antibody responses and presence of plastic-adherent suppressor cells in *Toxoplasma gondii*–infected mice. *Infect. Immun. 34*:30 (1981).

157. Suzuki, Y., Watanabe, N., and Kobayashi, A. Nonspecific suppression of initiation of memory cells in *Toxoplasma gondii*-infected mice. *Infect. Immun. 34*:36 (1981).
158. Suzuki, Y., and Kobayashi, A. Suppression of unprimed T and B cells in antibody responses by irradiation resistant and plastic adherent suppressor cells in *Toxoplasma gondii*-infected mice. *Infect. Immun. 40*:1 (1983).
159. Suzuki, Y., and Kobayashi, A. Macrophage-mediated suppression of immune responses in *Toxoplasma* infected mice I. Inhibition of proliferation of lymphocytes in primary antibody responses. *Cell. Immunol. 85*: 417 (1984).
160. Suzuki, Y., and Kobayashi, A. Macrophage-mediated suppression of immune responses in *Toxoplasma*-infected mice. II. Both H-2 linked and nonlinked control of induction of suppressor macrophages. *Cell. Immunol. 91*:375 (1984).
161. Luft, B. J., Chan, J., and Yazdani-Buicky, M. Isolation of suppressor T-cells during acute murine toxoplasmosis. (submitted for publication)
161a. Jones, T. C., Alkan, S., and Erb, P. Spleen and lymph node cell populations, *in vitro* cell proliferation and interferon and α production during the primary immune response to *Toxoplasma gondii. Parasite Immunol. 8*: 619–629 (1986).
162. Hauser, W. E., Jr., Sharma, S. D., and Remington, J. S. Natural killer cells induced by acute and chronic *Toxoplasma* infection. *Cell. Immunol. 69*: 1330 (1982).
163. Kamiyama, T., and Hagiwara, T. Augmented followed by suppressed levels of natural cell-mediated cytotoxicity in mice infected with *Toxoplasma gondii. Infect. Immun. 36*:628 (1982).
164. Kamiyama, T., and Tatsumi, M. Effect of *Toxoplasma* infection on the sensitivity of mouse thymocytes to natural killer cells. *Infect. Immun. 42*: 789 (1983).
165. Beverley, J. K. A., and Henry, L. Histopathological changes caused by congenital toxoplasmosis in mice. *Lyon Med. 225*:883 (1971).
166. Frenkel, J. K. Pathogenesis, diagnosis, and treatment of human toxoplasmosis. *JAMA 140*:369 (1949).
167. Jacobs, L., Naquin, H., Hoover, R., and Woods, A. C. A comparison of toxoplasmic skin tests, the Sabin-Feldman dye tests, and the complement fixation tests for toxoplasmosis in various forms of ureitis. *Bull. Johns Hopkins Hosp. 99*:1 (1956).
168. Remington, J. S., Barnett, C. G., Meikel, M., and Lunde, M. Toxoplasmis and infectious mononucleosis. *Arch. Intern. Med. 110*:744 (1962).
169. Anderson, S. E., Jr., Krahenbuhl, J. L., and Remington, J. S. Longitudinal studies of lymphocyte response to toxoplasma antigen in humans infected with *T. gondii. J. Clin. Lab. Immun. 2*:293 (1979).
170. Johnson, W. D., Jr. Chronological development of cellular immunity in human toxoplasmosis. *Infect. Immun. 33*:948 (1981).
171. Luft, B. J., Kansas, G., Engleman, E. G., and Remington, J. S. Functional and quantitative alterations in T-lymphocyte subpopulations in acute toxoplasmosis. *J. Infect. Dis. 150*:761 (1984).

171a. Luft, B. J., Pedrotti, P. W., and Remington, J. S. In vitro generation of adherent mononuclear suppressor cells to *Toxoplasma* antigen. *Immunology 63*:643 (1988).

172. Luft, B. J., Pedrotti, P., Engleman, E., and Remington, J. S. Identification of functionally active suppressor (Leu-7) T-cells during acute infection with *Toxoplasma gondii J. Infect. Dis. 155*:1033, (1987).

173. Yano, A., Norose, K., Yamashita, K., Aozai, F., Sugane, K., Segawa, K., and Hayashi, S. Immune response to *Toxoplasma gondii*–an analysis of suppressor T-cells in a patient with symptomatic acute toxoplasmosis. *J. Parasitol. 73*:954–961 (1987).

174. Dewaele, M., Thielmans, C., and Van Camp. B. Immunoregulatory T-cells in mononucleosis and toxoplasmosis. (letter) *New Engl. J. Med. 305*: 228 (1981).

174a. Dewaele, M., Naessens, A., Foulon, W., and Van Camp, B. Activated T-cells with suppressor/cytotoxic phenotype in acute *Toxoplasma gondii* infection. *Clin. Exp. Immunol. 62*:256 (1985).

175. Sklenar, I., Jones, T. C., Alkan, S., and Erb, P. Association of symptomatic human infection with *Toxoplasma gondii* with imbalance of monocytes and antigen-specific T-cell subsets. *J. Infect. Dis. 153*:315 (1986).

176. Kaufman, H. E., Melton, M. L., Remington, J. S., and Jacobs, L. Strain differences of *Toxoplasma gondii*. *J. Parasitol. 45*:189 (1959).

177. Kaufman, H. E., Remington, J. S., and Jacobs, L. Toxoplasmosis: the nature of virulence. *Am. J. Ophthalmol. 46*:255 (1958).

178. Jacobs, L., and Melton, M. Modifications in virulence of a strain of *Toxoplasma gondii* by passage in various hosts. *Am. J. Trop. Med. Hyg. 3*:447 (1954).

179. Melton, M. L., and Jacobs, L. Repeated enhancement in virulence of a strain of *Toxoplasma* by passage in mice. *J. Parasitol. 41 (suppl)*:21 (1955).

180. Matsubayoshi, H., and Akao, S. Morphological studies on the development of the *Toxoplasma* cyst. *Am. J. Trop. Med. Hyg. 12*:321 (1963).

181. Lycke, E., and Norrby, R. Demonstration of a factor of *Toxoplasma gondii* enhancing the penetration of *Toxoplasma* parasites into cultured host cell penetration of *Toxoplasma gondii*. *J. Bacteriol. 93*:53 (1967).

182. Norrby, R., and Lycke, E. Factors enhancing the host-cell penetration of *Toxoplasma gondii*. *J. Bacteriol. 93*:53 (1967).

183. Norrby, R. Host cell penetration of *Toxoplasma gondii*. *Infect. Immun. 2*: 250 (1970).

184. Lycke, E., Norrby, R., and Remington, J. S. Penetration-enhancing factor extracted from *Toxoplasma gondii* which increases its virulence for mice. *J. Bacteriol. 96*:785 (1968).

185. Lycke, E., Carlberg, K., and Norrby, R. Interactions between *Toxoplasma gondii* and its host cells: function of the penetration enhancing factor of *Toxoplasma*. *Infect. Immun. 11*853 (1975).

186. Schwartaman, J. D. Inhibition of penetration enhancing factor of *Toxoplasma gondii* by monoclonal antibodies specific for rhoptries. *Infect. Immun. 51*:760 (1986).

187. Ruskin, J., and Remington, J. S. Immunity and intracellular infection: resistance to bacteria in mice infected with a protozoa. *Science 160*:72 (1968).
188. Gentry, L. O., and Remington, J. S. Resistance against *Cryptococcus* conferred by intracellular bacteria and protozoa. *J. Infect. Dis. 123*:22 (1971).
189. Hibbs, J. B., Lambert, L. H., and Remington, J. S. Resistance to murine tumors conferred by chronic infection with intracellular protozoa, *Toxoplasma gondii* and *Besnoitia jellisoni*. *J. Infect. Dis. 124*:587 (1971).
190. Hibbs, J. B., Lambert, L. H., and Remington, J. S. Possible role of macrophage mediated nonspecific cytotoxicity in tumor resistance. *Nature (New Biol.) 235*:48 (1972).
191. Hibbs, J. B., Lambert, L. H., and Remington, J. S. Control of carcinogenesis: possible role for the activated macrophage. *Science 177*:998 (1972).
192. Frenkel, J. K. Adoptive immunity to intracellular infection. *J. Immunol. 98*:1309 (1967).
193. Shirahatz, T., Shimizu, and Suzuki, N. Effects of immune lymphcyte products and serum antibody on the multiplication of *Toxoplasma* in murine peritoneal macrophages. *Z. Parasitenkd. 49*:11 (1976).
194. Jones, T. C. Macrophages and intracellular parasitism. *J. Reticuloendothel. Soc. 15*:439 (1974).
195. Krahenbuhl, J. L., Ruskin, J., and Remington, J. S. The use of killed vaccines in immunization against an intracellular parasite: *Toxoplasma gondii*. *J. Immunol. 198*:425 (1972).
196. Hatizi, A., and Modabber, F. Z. Effect of cyclophosphamide on *Toxoplasma gondii* infection: reversal of the effect by passive immunization. *Clin. Exp. Immunol. 33*:389 (1978).
197. Lindberg, R. E., and Frenkel, J. K. Toxoplasmosis in nude mice. *J. Parasitol. 63*:219 (1977).
198. Frenkel, J. K., and Taylor, D. W. Toxoplasmosis in immunoglobulin M-suppressed mice. *Infect. Immun. 38*:360 (1982).
199. Pavia, C. S. Protection against experimental toxoplasmosis by adoptive immunotherapy. *J. Immunol. 137*:2985–2990 (1986).
199a. Suzuki, Y., and Remington J. S. Dual regulation of resistance against *Toxoplasma gondii* infection by Lyt2[+] and Lyt1[+], L374[+] cells in mice. *J. Immunol. 140*:3943 (1988).
200. Chinchilla, M., and Frenkel, J. K. Mediation of immunity to intracellular infection (*Toxoplasma* and *Besnoitia*) within somatic cells. *Infect. Immun. 19*:999–1012 (1978).
201. Chinchilla, M., and Frenkel, J. K. Specific mediation of cellular immunity to *Toxoplasma gondii* in somatic cells of mice. *Infect. Immun. 46*:862–866 (1984).
202. Reyes, L., and Frenkel, J. K. Specific and nonspecific mediation of protective immunity to *Toxoplasma gondii*. *Infect. Immun. 55*:856–863 (1987).
202a. McCabe, R. E., Luft, B. J., and Remington, J. S. Effect of murine interferon gamma on murine toxoplasmosis. *J. Infect, Dis. 150*:961 (1984).

202b. Suzuki, Y., Orellona, M. A., Schreiber, R. D., and Remington, J. S. Interferon γ: the major mediator of resistance against *Toxoplasma gondii*. *Science 240*:516 (1988).

203. Remington, J. S. Krahenbuhl, J. L., and Mendenahll, J. W. A role for activated macrophages in resistance to infection with *Toxoplasma*. *Infect. Immun. 6*:829 (1972).

203a. Khan, I. A., Smith, K. A., and Kasper, L. H. Induction of antigen specific cytotoxic T-cell splenocytes by a major membrane protein (p30) of *T. gondii. Clin. Res. 36*:456A (1988).

204. Williams, D. M., Sawyer, S., and Remington, J. S. Role of activated macrophages in resistance of mice to infection with *Trypanosoma cruzi. J. Infect. Dis. 134*:610 (1976).

205. Krahenbuhl, J. L., and Remington, J. S. The role of activated macrophages in specific and nonspecific cytostasis of tumor cells. *J. Immunol. 113*:507 (1974).

206. Krahenbuhl, J. L., and Remington, J. S. *In vitro* induction of nonspecific resistance in macrophages by specifically sensitized lymphocytes. *Infect. Immun. 4*:327 (1971).

207. Sethi, K. K., Pelster, B., Suzuki, N., Pierkerski, G., and Brandis, H. Immunity to *Toxoplasma gondii* induced *in vitro* in nonimmune mouse macrophages with specifically immune lymphocytes. *J. Immunol. 115*: 1151 (1975).

208. Anderson, S. E., Jr., and Remington, J. S. Effect of normal and activated human macrophages on *Toxoplasma gondii. J. Exp. Med. 139*:1154 (1974).

209. Anderson, S. E., Jr., Bautista, S., and Remington, J. S. Induction of resistance to *Toxoplasma gondii* in human macrophages by soluble lymphocyte products. *J. Immunol. 117*:381 (1976).

210. Nathan, C. F., Murray, H. W., Wiebe, M. E., and Rubin, B. Y. Identification of interferon as the lymphokine that activated human macrophage oxidative metabolism and antimicrobial activity. *J. Exp. Med. 158*:670 (1983).

211. Murray, H. W., Spitelny, G. L., and Nathan, C. F. Activation of mouse peritoneal macrophages in vitro and in vivo in interferon γ. *J. Immunol. 134*:1619 (1985).

211a. Sethi, K. K., Omato, Y., and Frandis, H. Contributions of immune infection (IFNα) in lymphokine reduced anti-Toxoplasma activity: studies with recombinant murine interferon-α. *Immunobiology 170*:270–283 (1985).

212. McLeod, R., Bensch, K. G., Smith, S. M., and Remington, J. S. Effects of human peripheral blood monocytes, monocyte-derived macrophages and spleen mononuclear phagocytes on *Toxoplasma gondii. Cell. Immunol. 54*: 330 (1980).

213. Wilson, C. B., and Remington, J. S. Activity of human blood leukocytes against *Toxoplasma gondii. J. Infect. Dis. 140*:890 (1979).

214. Murray, H. W., and Cohn, Z. A. Macrophage oxygen-dependent antimicrobial activity I. Susceptibility of *Toxoplasma gondii* to oxygen intermediates. *J. Exp. Med. 150*:938 (1979).

215. Locksley, R. M., Wilson, C. B., and Klebanott, S. J. Role of endogenous and acquired peroxidase in the toxoplasmacidal activity of human and murine mononuclear phagocytes. *J. Clin. Invest.* 69:1099 (1982).

216. Murray, H. W., Jungbanich, C. W., Nathan, C. F., and Cohn, Z. A. Macrophage oxygen-dependent antimicrobial activity. II: The role of oxygen intermediates. *J. Exp. Med. 150*:950 (1979).

217. Wilson, C. B., and Haas, J. E. Cellular defenses against *Toxoplasma gondii* in newborns. *J. Clin. Invest. 73*:1606 (1984).

217a. Catterall, J. R., Sharma, S. D., and Remington, J. S. Oxygen independent killing by alveolar macrophages. *J. Exp. Med. 163*:1113–1131 (1986).

217b. McCabe, R. E., and Remington, J. S. Mechanisms of killing *Toxoplasma gondii* by rat peritoneal macrophages. *Infect. Immun.* 52:151–155 (1986).

218. Nakagawara, A., Nathan, C. F., and Cohn, Z. A. Hydrogen peroxide metabolism in human monocytes during differentiation *in vitro*. *J. Clin. Invest. 68*:1243 (1981).

219. Locksley, R. M., and Klebanoff, S. J. Oxygen-dependent microbicidal systems of phagocytes and host defense against intracellular protozoa. *J. Cell Biochem. 22*:173 (1983).

219a. Locksley, R. M., Nelson, C. S., Fankhauser, J. E., and Klebanoff, S. J. Loss of granule myeloperoxidase during *in vitro* culture of lumen monocytes correlates with decay in antiprotozoa activity. *Am. J. Trop. Med. Hyg. 36*:541–548 (1987).

220. McLeod, R., and Remington, J. S. Inhibition or killing of an intracellular pathogen by activated macrophages is abrogated by TLCK or aminophylline. *Immunology 39*:599 (1980).

221. Murray, H. W., Rubin, B. Y., Carriero, S. M., Harris, A. M., and Jaffee, E. R. Human mononuclear phagocyte anti protozool mechanisms: oxygendependent vs independent activity against intracellular *Toxoplasma gondii J. Immunol. 134*:1982 (1985).

222. Matsumoto, Y., Nagasawa, H., Sabruai, H., Sasaki, S., and Suzuki, N. Mouse spleen cell derived *Toxoplasma* growth inhibitory factor. Its effect on *Toxoplasma* multiplication in the mouse kidney cell. *Zentralbl. Bakteriol. Parasitenkd. Infektionskr. Hyg Abt 1 Orgin Reike A 250*:383 (1981).

223. Shirahata, T., and Shimizu, K. Production and properties of immune interferon from spleen cell cultures of toxoplasma infected mice. *Microbiol. Immunol. 24*:1109 (1980).

224. Shirahata, T., and Shimizu, K. Growth inhibition of *Toxoplasma gondii* in cell cultures treated with murine type II interferon. *Jap. J. Vet. Sci. 44*: 865 (1982).

225. Pfefferkorn, E. R., and Guyre, P. M. Inhibition of growth of *Toxoplasma gondii* in cultured fibroblasts by human recombinant gamma interferon. *Infect. Immun. 44*:211 (1984).

226. Pfefferkorn, E. R. Interferon γ blocks the growth of *Toxoplasma gondii* in human fibroblasts by inducing the host cells to degrade tryptophan. *Proc. Natl. Acad. Sci. USA 81*:908 (1984).

227. Hatcher, F. M., and Kuhn, R. E. Destruction of *Trypanosoma cruzi* by natural killer cells. *Science 218*:295 (1982).

228. Murphy, J. W., and McDaniel, D. O. In vitro effects of natural killer (NK) cells on *Cryptococcus neoformans*. In *NK Cells and Other Natural Effector Cells* (R. B. Herberman, ed.). Academic Press, New York, 1982, p. 1105.

229. Hauser, W. E., Jr., and Tsai, V. Acute *Toxoplasma* infection of mice induces spleen NK cells that are cytotoxic for *T. gondii* in vitro. *J. Immunol. 136*:313 (1986).

230. Remington, J. S., and Merigan, T. C. Interferon: protection of cells infected with an intracellular protozoan (*Toxoplasma gondii*). *Science 161*:804 (1968).

231. Shmunis, G., Weisserbacker, M., Chowchuvech, E., Sawicki, L., Galin, M. A., and Baron, S. Growth of *Toxoplasma gondii* in various tissue cultures treated with In. Cn or interferon. *Proc. Soc. Exp. Biol. Med. 143*: 1153 (1973).

231a. Pfefferkorn, E. R., Eckel, M., and Rebhun, S. Interferon a suppresses the growth of *Toxoplasma gondii* in human fibroblasts through starvation for tryptophan. *Mol. Biochem. Parasitol. 20*:215–224 (1986).

232. Naot, Y., Guptill, D. R., and Remington, J. S. Duration of IgM antibodies to *Toxoplasma gondii* after acute acquired toxoplasmosis. *J. Infect. Dis. 145*:770 (1982).

232a. McLeod, R., and Mack, D. G. Secretory IgA specific for *Toxoplasma gondii*. *J. Immunol. 136*:2640–2643 (1986).

233. Eichenwald, H. F. Experimental toxoplasmosis II. Effect of sulfadiazine and antiserum on congenital toxoplasmosis in mice. *Proc. Soc. Exp. Biol. Med. 71*:45 (1949).

234. Werner, H., Masihi, K. N., and Meingassner, J. G. Investigation on immune serum therapy on cysts of *Toxoplasma gondii* in latent infected mice. *Zentrobl. Bakteriol. 242*:405 (1978).

235. Foster, B. G., and McCulloch, W. F. Studies of active and passive immunity in animals inoculated with *Toxoplasma gondii*. *Can. J. Microbiol. 14*:103 (1968).

236. Frenkel, J. K., and Taylor, D. W. Toxoplasmosis in immunoglobulin M-suppressed mice. *Infect. Immun. 38*:360 (1982).

237. Anderson, S. E., Jr., Bautista, S. C., and Remington, J. S. Specific antibody-dependent killing of *Toxoplasma gondii* by normal macrophages. *Clin. Exp. Immunol. 26*:375 (1976).

238. Jones, T. C., Len, L., and Hirsch, J. G. Assessment in vitro of immunity against *Toxoplasma gondii*. *J. Exp. Med. 141*:466 (1975).

239. Feldman, H. A. The relationship of *Toxoplasma* antibody activator to the serum-properdin system. *Ann. NY Acad. Sci. 66*:263 (1956).

240. Suzuki, M., Tsunematsu, Y., and Torisu, M. Studies on the accessory factor for *Toxoplasma* dye test. Essential role of complement. *J. Parasitol. 57*: 294 (1971).

241. Schreiber, R. D., and Feldman, H. A. Identification of the activator system for antibody to *Toxoplasma* as the classical complement pathway. *J. Infect. Dis. 141*:366 (1980).

242. Araujo, F. G., Williams, D. M., Grumet, F. C., and Remington, J. S. Strain dependent differences in murine susceptibility to *Toxoplasma. Infect. Immun. 13*:1528 (1976).

243. Kamei, K., Sato, K., and Tsunematsu, Y. A strain of mouse highly susceptible to *Toxoplasma. J. Parasitol. 62*:714 (1976).

244. William, D. M., Grumet, F. C., and Remington, J. S. Genetic control of murine resistance to *Toxoplasma gondii. Infect. Immun. 19*:416 (1978).

245. Jones, T. C., and Erb, P. H-2 complex-linked resistance in murine toxoplasmosis. *J. Infect. Dis. 151*:739 (1985).

245a. Brinkman, V., Sharma, S. D., and Remington, J. S. Different regulation of the L3T4-T cell subset by B Cells in different mouse strains bearing the H-2^K haplotype. *J. Immunol. 137*:2991–2997 (1986).

246. Balow, J. E. Cyclophosphamide suppression of established CMI. *J. Clin. Invest. 56*:65 (1970).

247. Butler, W. T., and Rossen, R. D. Effects of corticosteroids on immunity in man. *J. Clin. Invest. 52*:2629 (1973).

248. Thomas, F., Wolf, J., Thomas, J., et al. Specific immunosuppression in cardiac allographing using antithymocyte globulin and soluble transplantation antigen. *Ann. Thorac. Surg. 18*:241 (1979).

249. Fauci, A. S., and Dale, D. C. The effect of *in vivo* hydrocortisone on subpopulations of human lymphocytes. *J. Clin. Invest. 53*:240 (1974).

250. Haynes, B. F., and Fauci, A. S. The differential effect of *in vivo* hydrocortisone on the kinetics of subpopulations of human peripheral blood thymus-derived lymphocytes. *J. Clin. Invest. 61*:703 (1978).

251. Fauci, A. S., Dole, D. C., and Balow, J. E. Glucocorticosteroids therapy: mechanisms of action and clinical considerations. *Ann. Intern. Med. 84*: 304 (1976).

252. Masur, H., Murray, H. W., and Jones, T. C. Effect of hydrocortisone on macrophage response to lymphokine. *Infect. Immun. 35*:709 (1982).

253. Fauci, A. S., Wolff, S. M., and Johnson, J. S. Effect of cyclophosphamide upon the immune response in Wegener's granulomatosis. *New Engl. J. Med. 285*:1493 (1971).

254. Preiksaitis, J. K., Rosno, S., Grumet, C., and Merigan, T. C. Infections due to herpesviruses in cardiac transplant recipients: role of donor heart and immunosuppressive therapy. *J. Infect. Dis. 147*:974 (1983).

255. Dummer, J. S., Herdy, A., Poorsetter, A., and Ho, M. Early infections in kidney, heart, and liver transplant recipients on cyclosporine. *Transplantation 36*:259 (1983).

256. Najarian, J. S., Ferguson, R. M., Sutherland, D. E. R., Rynasiewicz, J. J., and Simmons, R. L. A prospective trial of the efficacy of cyclosporine in renal transplantation at the University of Minnesota. *Transplant Proc. 15*: 438 (1983).

257. McCabe, R. E., Luft, B. J., and Remington, J. S. The effects of cyclosporine A on *Toxoplasma gondii in vivo* and *in vitro. Transplantation 41*: 611 (1986).

258. Mack, D. G., and McLeod, R. New micromethod to study the effect of antimicrobial agents on *Toxoplasma gondii* comparison of sulfadoxine and

sulfadiazine individually and in combination with pyrimethanine and study of clindamycin, metronidazole, and cyclosporine. A. *Antimicrob. Ag. Chemother. 26*:31 (1984).

259. Zacharski, L. R., and Linman, J. W. Lymphocytopenia: its causes and significance. *Mayo Clin. Proc. 46*:168 (1971).

260. Green, I., and Carson, P. F. A study of skin homografting in patients with lymphoma. *Blood 14*:235 (1959).

261. Miller, D. G., Lizardo, J. G., and Snyderman, R. K. Hemalogous and heterologous skin transplantation in patients with lymphomatous disease. *J. Natl. Cancer Inst. 26*:569 (1969).

262. Sokol, J. E., and Primikiro, M. The delayed skin test response in Hodgkin's disease and lymphosarcoma. *Cancer 14*:597 (1969).

263. Eltringham, J. S., and Kaplan, H. S. Impaired delayed hypersensitivity response in 154 patients with untreated Hodgkin's disease. *Natl. Cancer Inst. Monogr. 36*:127 (1973).

264. Aisenberg, A. C. Studies on delayed hypersensitivity in Hodgkin's disease. *J. Clin. Invest. 41*:1964 (1962).

265. King, G. W., Yanes, B., Hurtubise, P. E., et al. Immune function of successfully treated lymphoma patients. *J. Clin. Invest. 57*:1451 (1976).

266. Engleman, E. G., Benike, C. J., Hoppe, R. T., and Kaplan, H. S. Autologous mixed lymphocyte reaction in patients with Hodgkin's disease: evidence for a T-cell defect. *J. Clin. Invest. 66*:149 (1980).

267. Brown, R. S., Haynes, B. A., Foley, H. T., Godwin, H. A., Berard, C. W., and Carbone, P. P. Hodgkin's disease. Immunologic clinical and histologic features in 50 untreated patients. *Ann. Intern. Med. 67*:291 (1967).

268. Bobrove, A. M., Fuks, Z., Strober, S., and Kaplan, H. S. Quantitation of T- and B-lymphocytes and cellular immune function in Hodgkin's disease. *Cancer 36*:169 (1975).

269. Hersh, E. M., and Oppneheim, J. J. Impaired *in vitro* function in untreated Hodgkin's disease. *New Engl. J. Med. 290*:181 (1974).

270. Levy, R., and Kaplan, H. S. Impaired lymphocyte function in untreated Hodgkin's disease. *New Engl. J. Med. 290*:181 (1974).

271. Faughet, G. B. Quantitation of immunocompetence in Hodgkin's disease. *J. Clin.Invest. 56*:951 (1975).

272. Goodwin, J. S., Messner, R. P., Barkhurst, A. D., Peake, G. T., Saiki, J., and Williams, R. C., Jr. Prostaglandin-producing suppressor cells in Hodgkin's disease. *New Engl. J. Med. 297*:963 (1977).

273. Gaines, J. D., Gilmer, A., and Remington, J. S. Deficiency of antigen recognition in Hodgkin's disease. *Natl. Cancer Inst. Monogr. 36*:117 (1973).

274. De Gost, G. C., Halie, M. R., and Nieureg, H. O. Immunological responsiveness against two primary antigens in untreated patients with Hodgkin's disease. *Eur. J. Cancer 11*:213 (1975).

275. Hillinger, S. M.,and Herzig, G. P. Impaired cell mediated immunity in

Hodgkin's disease mediated by suppressor lymphocyte and monocytes. *J. Clin. Invest. 61*:1620 (1978).

276. Twomey, J. J., Laughter, A. H., Farrow, S., and Douglass, C. C. Hodgkin's disease: an immunodepleting and immunosuppressive disorder. *J. Clin. Invest. 56*:467 (1975).

277. McLeod, R., and Estes, R. Role of lymphocyte blastogenesis to *Toxoplasma gondii* antigens in containment of chronic, latent *T. gondii* infection in humans. *Clin. Exp. Immunol. 62*:24 (1985).

278. Ward, P. A., and Berenberg, J. L. Defective regulation of inflammatory mediators in Hodgkin's disease. *New Engl. J. Med. 290*:76 (1980).

279. Steigbigel, R. T., Lambert, L. H., Jr., and Remington, J. S. Polymorphonuclear leukocyte, monocyte, and macrophage bactericidal function in patients with Hodgkin's disease. *J. Lab. Clin. Med. 88*:54 (1976).

280. McLeod, R., and Estes, R. Microbicidal activity of peripheral blood monocytes from patients with Hodgkin's disease for *Toxoplasma gondii. J. Infect. Dis. 146*:565 (1982).

281. Gupta, S., and Fernandes, G. Natural killing in patients with Hodgkin's disease. In *NK Cells and Other Natural Effector Cells* (R. B. Herberman, ed.). Academic Press, New York, 1982, p. 1201.

282. Fauci, A. S., Macher, A. M., Longo, D. L., et al. Acquired immunodeficiency syndrome: epidemiologic, clinical immunologic, and therapeutic considerations. *Ann. Intern.Med. 100*:92 (1983).

283. Murray, H. W., Rubin, B. Y., Masur, H., et al. Impaired production of lymphokines and immune gamma-interferon in the acquired immunodeficiency syndrome. *New Engl. J. Med. 310*:883 (1984).

284. Gupta, S., and Safai, B. Deficient autologues mixed lymphocyte reaction in Kaposi's sarcoma associated with deficiency of Leu 3-positive responder cells. *J. Clin. Invest. 71*:296 (1983).

285. Prince, H. E., Kermani-Arab, V., and Fahey, J. L. Depressed interleukin-2 receptor expression in acquired immune deficiency and lymphadenopathy syndrome. *J. Immunol. 133*:1313 (1986).

286. Lane, H. C., Depper, J. M., Greene, W. C., Whalen, G., Waldmann, T. A., and Fauci, A. S. Qualitative analysis of immune function in patients with the acquired immunodeficiency syndrome. Evidence for a selective defect in soluble antigen recognition. *New Engl. J. Med. 313*:79 (1985).

287. Lane, H. C., Masur, H., Edgar, L. C., et al. Abnormalities of B lymphocyte activation and immunoregulation in patients with the acquired immunodeficiency syndrome. *New Engl. J. Med. 309*:453 (1983).

288. Remington, J. S., et al. Studies on chronic toxoplasmosis: the relation of infective dose to residual infection and to the possiibility of congenital transmission. *Am. J. Ophthalmol. 46*:261 (1958).

289. Frenkel, J. K. Pathogenesis of toxoplasmosis with a consideration of cyst rupture in *Besnoitia* infection. *Surv. Ophthalmol. 6*:799 (1961).

290. Huldt, G. Experimental toxoplasmosis. Parasitemia in guinea pigs. *Acta Pathol. Microbiol. Scand. 58*:457 (1963).

291. Ito, S., Tsunoda, K., Suzuki, K., and Tsutsumi, Y. Demonstration by microscopy of parasitemia in animals experimentally infected with *Toxoplasma gondii. Natl. Inst. Anim. Health Q (Tokyo) 6*:8 (1966).

292. Van der Waaj, D. Formation, growth and multiplication of *Toxoplasma gondii* cysts in mouse brains. *Trop. Geogr. Med. 11*:345 (1959).

293. Conley, F. K., and Jenkins, K. A. Immunohistological study of the anatomic relationship of *Toxoplasma* antigens to the inflammatory response of mice chronically infected with *Toxoplasma gondii. Infect. Immun. 31*: 1184 (1981).

293a. Frenkel, J. K., and Escajadillo, A. Cyst rupture as a pathogenic mechanism of toxoplasmic encephalitis. *Am. J. Trop. Med. Hyg. 36*:517–522 (1987).

294. Frenkel, J. K. Effects of cortisone total body irradiation and mitogen mustered on chronic, latent toxoplasmosis. *Am. J. Pathol. 33*:618 (1957).

295. Frenkel, J. K., Nelson, B. M., and Arias-Stelle, J. Immunosuppression and toxoplasmic encephalitis: clinical and experimental aspects. *Hum. Pathol. 6*:97 (1975).

295a. Vollmer, T. L., Waldo, M. K., Steinman, L., and Conley, F. K. Depletion of T-4[+] lymphocytes with monoclonal antibody reactivated toxoplasmosis in the central nervous system: a model of superinfection in AIDS. *J. Immunol. 138*:3737–3741 (19xx).

296. Stahl, W. Modification of subclinical toxoplasmosis in mice by cortisone, t-mercaptopurine and splenectomy. *Am. J. Trop. Med. Hyg. 15*:869 (1966).

297. Nakayama, I., and Aoki, I. The influence of antilymphocyte serum on the resistance of mice to *Toxoplasma gondii. Jap. J. Parasitol. 19*:537 (1970).

298. Strannegard, O., and Lycke, E. Effect of antithymocyte serum on experimental toxoplasmosis in mice. *Infect. Immun. 5*:769 (1972).

299. Stahl, W. Effect of heterologous antithymocyte serum on *Toxoplasma gondii* infection in mice. I. Potentiation of primary nonlethal infection. *Jap. J. Parasitol. 27*:231 (1978).

300. Toussaint, D., and Vanderhaeghen, J. J. Ocular toxoplasmosis, trigeminal herpes zoster and pulmonary tuberculosis in a patient with Hodgkin's disease. *Ophthalmologica 171*:237 (1975).

301. Slavick, H. E., and Lipman, I. J. Brainstem toxoplasmosis complicating Hodgkin's disease. *Arch. Neurol. 34*:636 (1977).

302. Mazer, S., et al. Unusual computed tomographic presentation of cerebral toxo plasmosis. *AJNR 4*:458 (1983).

303. Green, J. A. Favorable outcome of CNS toxoplasmosis occurring in a patient with untreated Hodgkin's disease. *Cancer 45*:808 (1980).

304. Lowenberg, B., et al. Fatal cerebral toxoplasmosis in a bone marrow transplant recipient with leukemia. *Transplantation 35*:30 (1983).

305. Shepp, D. H., Hackman, R. C., Conley, F. K., Anderson, J. B., and Meyers, J. D. *Toxoplasma gondii* reactivation identified by a detection of parasitemia in tissue culture. *Ann. Intern. Med. 103*:218 (1985).

306. Nagington, J., and Martin, A. L. Toxoplasmosis and heart transplantation. *Lancet 2*:679 (1983).
307. Cohen, S. N. Toxoplasmosis in patient receiving immunosuppressive therapy. *JAMA 211*:657 (1970).
308. O'Reilly, M. J. J. Acquired toxoplasmosis: an acute fatal case in a young girl. *Med. J. Aust. 2*:968 (1954).
309. Barlotta, F. M. Toxoplasmosis, lymphoma or both? *Ann. Intern. Med. 70*: 517 (1969).
310. Miettinen, M., and Franssila, K. Malignant lymphoma simulating lymph node toxoplasmosis. *Histopathology 6*:129 (1982).
311. Dorfman, R. F., and Remington, J. S. Value of lymph node biopsy in the diagnosis of acute acquired toxoplasmosis. *New Engl. J. Med. 289*:878 (1973).
312. Koeze, T. H., and Klinger, G. H. Acquired toxoplasmosis. *Arch. Neurol. 11*:191 (1964).
313. Ghatak, N. R., and Sawyer, D. R. A morphologic study of opportunistic cerebral toxoplasmosis. *Acta Neuropathol. 42*:217 (1978).
314. Rabinowicz, T. A case of acquired toxoplasmosis in the adult. In *Toxoplasmosis* (D. Hertscl ed.). Hans Huber, Bern, 1971.
315. Post, M. J., et al. Toxoplasma encephalitis in Haitian adults with acquired immunodeficiency syndrome. *Am. J. Roentgenol. 140*:861 (1983).
316. Whelan, M. A., et al. Acquired immunodeficiency syndrome: cerebral computed tomographic manifestations. *Radiology 149*:477 (1983).
316a. Nolla-Sallas, J., Ricart, C., D'Ohlaberringue, L., Gali, F., and Lamorca, J. Hydrocepholis: an unusual CT presentation of cerebral toxoplasmosis in a patient with acquired immunodeficiency syndrome. *Eur. Neurol. 27*: 130 (1987).
317. Milligan, S. A., Katz, M. S., Craven, P. C., Strandberg, D. A., Russell, I. J., and Becker, R. A. Toxoplasmosis presenting as parhypopituitarism in a patient with the acquired immunodeficiency syndrome. *Am. J. Med. 77*: 760 (1984).
318. Nery-Guimares, F. Toxoplasmose humane meningoencefalomielite toxoplasmica. *Mem. Inst. Oswaldo Cruz 38*:257 (1943).
319. Alenghat, J. P., et al. Computed tomography in opportunistic cerebral toxoplasmosis: report of two cases. *Comput. Tomog. 5*:231 (1981).
320. Ghatak, N. R., and Zimmerman, H. M. Fine structure of *Toxoplasma* in the brain. *Arch. Pathol. 95*:276 (1983).
321. Gleason, T. H., and Hamlin, W. B. Disseminated toxoplasmosis in the compromised host. *Arch. Intern. Med. 134*:1059 (1974).
322. Togretti, F. Neurological toxoplasmosis presenting as a brain tumor. *J. Neurosurg. 56*:716 (1982).
323. Conely, F. K., et al. *Toxoplasma gondii* in infection of the central nervous system. *Hum. Pathol. 12*:690 (1981).
324. Luft, B. J., et al. Toxoplasmic encephalitis in patients with the acquired immunodeficiency syndrome (AIDS) and other immunocompromising diseases. *JAMA 252*:913 (1984).

325. Fromowitz, F., Rush, T. J., Peress, N., and Luft, B. J. Toxoplasmic encephalitis resembling intracerebral lymphoma. (submitted for publication).

325a. Luft, B. J., Fromowitz, F., Peress, N., Eilbott, D., Burger, H., and Weiser, B. Immunohistochemical and *in situ* hybridization analysis of cellular infiltrate occurring in toxoplasmic encephalitis and AIDS. IV. International Conference on AIDS, 1988, p. 395.

326. Nicholson, D. H., and Wolchek, E. B. Ocular toxoplasmosis in an adult receiving long-term corticosteroid therapy. *Arch. Ophthalmol. 94*:248 1976).

327. Wertlake, P. T., and Winter, T. S. Fatal toxoplasma myocarditis in an adult patient with acute lymphocyte leukemia. *New Engl. J. Med. 237*:438–440 (1965).

328. Luft, B. J., Billingham, M., and Remington, J. S. Endomyocardial biopsy in the diagnosis of toxoplasmic myocarditis. *Transplant Proc. 18*:1871 (1986).

329. Couvreur, J. Lepoumon et al toxoplasmose. *Rev. Fr. Mal. Resp. 3*:525 (1975).

330. Catterall, J. R., Hofflin, J. S., and Remington, J. S. Pulmonary toxoplasmosis. *Am. Rev. Resp. Dis. 133*:794–705 (1986).

331. Tourani, J. M., Israe-Biet, D., Veret, A., and Andriew, J. M. Unusual pulmonary infection in a puzzling presentation of AIDS. *Lancet 1*:989 (1985).

332. Prosmane, O., Chalquoi, J., Sylvestre, J., and Lefebvre, R. Small nodular pattern in the lungs due to opportunistic toxoplasmosis. *J. Assoc. Can. Radiol. 35*:186 (1984).

333. Leyva, W. H., and Santa Cruz, D. J. Cutaneous toxoplasmosis. *J. Am. Acad. Dermatol. 14*:600 (1986).

334. Justus, J. Cutaneous manifestations of toxoplasmosis. *Curr. Probl. Dermatol. 4*:24 (1972).

335. Binazei, M., and Papini, M. Cutaneous toxoplasmosis. *Int. J. Dermatol. 19*: 332–335 (1980).

336. Topi, G., Gandolfo, L. D., Giacalone, B., et al. Acquired cutaneous toxoplasmosis. *Dermatologica 167*:24 (1983).

337. Greenlee, J. E., Johnson, W. D., Campa, J. F., Adelman, L. S., and Sande, M. A. Adult toxoplasmosis presenting as polymyositis and cerebellar atoxic. *Ann. Intern. Med. 82*:367 (1975).

338. Remington, J. S. Toxoplasmosis in the adult. *Bull. NY Acad. Med. 50*: 211 (1974).

339. Faruqi, A. M. A., Frank, M., Rosvali, et al. Acute acquired toxoplasmosis. *South. Med. J. 69*:1234 (1976).

340. Kean, B. H. Clinical toxoplasmosis: 50 years. *Trans. R. Soc. Trop. Med. Hyg. 66*:549 (1972).

341. McCabe, R. E., Brooks, R. G., Dorfman, R. F., and Remington, J. S. Clinical spectrum in 107 cases of toxoplasmic lymphadenopathy. *Rev. Infect. Dis. 9*:754–774 (1987).

341a. LeTan Vinh, Barbet, J. P., Mace, B., Rousset, S., and Huault, B. La pneumonie toxoplasmique avec generalisation. *Sem. Hop. Paris 56*:744–750 (1980).

341b. Ludlam, G. B., and Beattie, C. D. Pulmonary toxoplasmosis? *Lancet 2*: 1136–1138 (1963).

341c. Michel, O., and Sergysels, R. Acute pulmonary toxoplasmosis with alveolitis of T suppressor lymphocyte type. *Thorax 41*:972–973 (1986).

342. Ludlum, G. B., and Beattie, C. P. Pulmonary toxoplasmosis. *Lancet 2*: 1136 (1963).

343. Vischer, T. L., Bernheim, C., and Engelbrecht, E. Two cases of hepatitis due to *Toxoplasma gondii. Lancet 2*:917 (1967).

344. Theologides, A., and Kennedy, B. J. Toxoplasmic myocarditis and pericarditis. *Am. J. Med. 47*:169 (1969).

345. Best, T., and Finlayson, M. Two forms of encephalitis in opportunistic toxoplasmosis. *Arch. Pathol. Lab. Med. 103*:693 (1979).

346. Friedman, A. H. The retinal lesions of the acquired immunodeficiency syndrome. *Trans. Am. Ophthalmol. Soc. 82*:447 (1984).

347. Launais, B., Laurent, G., Berchkroun, S., Moulin, J. J., Pris, J., Bec, P., and Monnier, J. Manifestations meningo-encephaliques et chorioretiniennes de la toxoplasmose chez un malade immunodeprime. *Sem Hop. Paris 1*: 40 (1983).

348. Hoerni, B., Vallat, M., Durand, M., and Pesme, D. Ocular toxoplasmosis and Hodgkin's disease: report of two cases. *Arch. Ophthalmol. 96*:62 (1978).

349. Yeo, J. H., Jacobiec, F. A., Iwamato, T., et al. Opportunistic toxoplasmic retinochoroiditis following chemotherapy for systemic lymphoma. A light and electron microscopic study. *Arch. Ophthalmol. 90*:885 (1983).

350. Perke, D. W. Diffuse toxoplasmic retinochoroiditis in a patient with AIDS. *104*:571 (1986).

351. Weiss, A., Margo, C. E., Ledford, D. K., Lockey, R. F., and Brinser, J. H. Toxoplasmic retinochoroiditis as an initial manifestation of the acquired immunodeficiency syndrome. *Am. J. Ophthalmol. 101*:248 (1986).

352. Hakes, T. B., and Armstrong, D. Toxoplasmosis: problems in diagnosis and treatment. *Cancer 52*:1535 (1983).

352a. Theologides, A., and Lee, J. C. Concomitant opportunistic infection with *Toxoplasma*, pneumocystis and cytomegalvirus. *Mim. Med. 53*:615–619 (1970).

352b. Luna, M. A., and Lectiger, B. Disseminated toxoplasmosis and cytomegalovirus infection complicating Hodgkin's disease. *Am. J. Clin. Pathol. 55*:499–505 (1971).

352c. Maguire, G. P., Tatz, J., Giose, R., and Ahmed, T. Diagnosis of pulmonary toxoplasmosis by bronchoalveolar lavage. *NY state J. Med. 78*:204–250 (1986).

352d. Pinkerton, H., and Weinman, D. Toxoplasma infection in man. *Arch. Pathol. 30*:374 (1940).

353. Krahenbuhl, J. L., and Remington, J. S. Immunology of toxoplasma and toxoplasmosis. In *Immunology of Parasitic Infections* (S. Cohen and K. S. Warren, eds.). Blackwell Scientific, Oxford, England, 1982, p. 356.

354. Naot, Y., and Remington, J. S. An enzyme-linked immunosorbent assay for detection of IgM antibodies to *Toxoplasma gondii*. Use for diagnosis of acute acquired toxoplasmosis. *J. Infect. Dis. 142*:757 (1980).

354a. Brooks, R. G., McCabe, R. E., and Remington, J. S. Role of serology in the diagnosis of toxoplasmic lymphadenopathy. *Rev. Infect. Dis. 9*:775–782 (1987).

355. Welch, P. C. Serologic diagnosis of acute lymphadenopathic toxoplasmosis. *J. Infect. Dis. 142*:256 (1980).

356. Desmonts, G., and Remington, J. S. Direct agglutination test for diagnosis of *Toxoplasma* infection: method for increasing sensitivity and specificity. *J. Clin. Microbiol. 11*:562 (1980).

357. Peacock, J. E., Folds, J., Orringer, E., Luft, B. J., and Cohen, M. S. *Toxoplasma gondii* and the compromised host: antibody response in the absence of clinical manifestations of disease. *Arch. Intern. Med. 143*: 1235 (1983).

358. Vogel, C. L., and Lunde, M. N. Toxoplasma serology in patients with malignant diseases of the reticuloendothelial system. *Cancer 25*:537 (1969).

358a. Kusne, S., Dummer, J. S., Ho, M., Whiteside, T., Robin, B. S., Mekowe, L., Esquivel, C. O., and Starzl, T. E. Self limited *Toxoplasma* parasitemia after liver transplantation. *Transplantation 44*:457 (1987).

359. Hofflin, J. M., and Remington, J. S. Tissue culture isolation of *Toxoplasma* from blood of a patient with AIDS. *Arch. Intern. Med. 145*:925 (1985).

360. Lunde, M. N., Gelderman, H. H., Hayes, S. L., and Vogel, C. L. Serological diagnosis of active toxoplasmosis complicating malignant disease. *Cancer 25*:37 (1970).

361. Turenen, H. J. Detection of soluble antigens of *Toxoplasma gondii* by a four-layer modification of an enzyme immunoassay. *J. Clin. Microbiol. 17*: 768 (1983).

362. Raizman, R. E., and Neva, F. A. Detection of circulating antigen in acute experimental infections with *Toxoplasma antigen*. *J. Infect. Dis. 132*:44 (1975).

362a. Asai, T., Kim, T., Kobayashi, M., and Kojima, S. Detection of nucleoside triphosphate hydrolase as a circulating antigen in sera of mice infected with *Toxoplasma gondii*. *Infect. Immun. 55*:1332–1335 (1987).

363. Amato Neto, V., et al. The Sabin Feldman test in the spinal fluid of patients with acquired toxoplasmosis. *Rev. Inst. Med. Trop. Sao Paulo 18*: 80 (1976).

364. Silverstein, A. M. Doyne Memorial Lecture 1974: Immunogenic uveitis. *Trans. Ophthalmol. Soc. UK 94*:496–516 (1974).

365. Witmer, R. Clinical implications of aqueous humor studies in uveitis. *Trans. Ophthalmol. Soc. UK 94*:496–516 (1974).

366. Desmonts, G. Definitive serological diagnosis of ocular toxoplasmosis. *Arch. Ophthalmol. 76*:839 (1966).

367. Potasman, I., Resnick, L., Luft, B. J., and Remington, J. S. Intrathecal production of antibodies against *T. gondii* in patients with toxoplasmic encephalitis and AIDS. (submitted for publication).

368. Post, M. J., Kursonoglu, S. J., Hensley, G. T., Chan, J. C., Moskowitz, L. B., and Hoffman, T. A. Cranial CT in acquired immunodeficiency syndrome: spectrum of diseases and optimal contrast enhancement technique. *Am. J. Roentgenol. 145*:929 (1985).

369. Post, M. J. D., Sheldan, J. J., Hensley, G. T., Soila, K., Tobias, J. A., Chan, J. C., Quencer, R. M., and Moskowitz, L. B. Central nervous system disease in acquired immunodeficiency syndrome: prospective correlation using CT, MR imaging and pathologic studies. *Radiology 158*:141 (1986).

370. Finch, E. S. Intercurrent infection with *Toxoplasma*: organisms found in the bone marrow of a patient with advanced reticulosarcoma. *Med. J. Aust. 2*:965 (1954).

371. Pitchenick, A. E., Fischl, M. A., and Walls, K. W. Evaluation of cerebral mass lesions in acquired immunodeficiency disease. *New Engl. J. Med. 308*:1099 (1983).

372. Levy, R. M., Pons, V. G., and Rosenblum, M. L. Intracerebral mass lesions in the acquired immunodeficiency syndrome (AIDS). *New Engl. J. Med. 309*:1454 (1983).

372a. Wanke, C., Tuazon, C. V., Kovacs, A., Dina, T., Davis, D. D., Barton, N., Katz, D., Lunde, M., Levy, C., Conley, F. K., Lane, H. C., Fauci, A. S., and Magur, H. *Toxoplasma* encephalitis in patients with acquired immune deficiency syndrome: diagnosis and response to therapy. *Am. J. Trop. Med. Hyg. 36*:509 (1987).

373. Eyles, D. E., and Coleman, N. Synergistic effect of sulfadiazine and daraprim against experimental toxoplasmosis in the mouse. *Antibiot. Chemother. 3*:483 (1953).

374. Eyles, D. E., and Coleman, N. An evaluation of the curative effects of pyrimethamine and sulfadiazine, alone and in combination, on experimental mouse toxoplasmosis. *Antibiot. Chemother. 5*:529 (1955).

375. Sheffield, H. G., and Melton, M. L. Effect of pyrimethamine and sulfadiazine on the fine structure and multiplication of *Toxoplasma gondii* in cell cultures. *J. Parasitol. 61*:704 (1975).

376. Stickney, D. R., Simmons, W. S., DeAngelis, R. L., Rundles, R. W., and Nichol, S. A. Pharmacokinetics of pyrimethamine (PRM) and 2,4-diamine-5(3'4'-dichlorophenyl)-6-methylpyrimidine (DMP) relevant to meningeal leukemia. *Proc. Am. Assoc. Cancer Res. 14*:52 (1973).

376a. Weiss, L. M., Harris, C., Berger, M., Tanowitz, B., and Wittner, M. Pyrimethamine concentrations in serum and cerebrospinal fluid during treatment of acute *Toxoplasma* encephalitis in patients with AIDS. *J. Infect. Dis. 155*:480 (1988).

377. Eyles, D. E., and Coleman, N. The relative activity of the common

sulfonamides against experimental toxoplasmosis in the mouse. *Am. J. Trop. Med. Hyg.* 2:54 (1953).

378. Bullows, J. G. M., and Ratish, H. D. A therapeutic and pharmacological study of sulfadiazine, monomethylsulfadiazine and dimethylsulfadiazine in lobar pneumonia. *J. Clin. Invest.* 23:676 (1944).

379. Today's Drugs, sulphonamides, *Brit. Med. J.* 2:674 (1968).

380. Frenkel, J. K., and Hitchings, G. H. Relative reversal by vitamin (p-amino-benzoic, folic, and folinic acids) of the effects of sulfadiazine and pyrimethamine on *Toxoplasma*, mouse and man. *Antibiot. Chemother.* 7: 630 (1957).

381. Grossman, P. L., and Remington, J. S. The effect of trimethoprim and sulfamethoxozole on *Toxoplasma gondii in vitro* and *in vivo*. *Am. J. Trop. Med. Hyg.* 28:445 (1979).

382. Araujo, F. G., and Remington, J. S. Effect of clindamycin on acute and chronic toxoplasmosis in mice. *Antimicrob. Agents Chemother.* 5:647 (1974).

383. Hofflin, J. M., and Remington, J. S. Clindamycin and murine intracerebral toxoplasmosis. (abstr. 1115) In Program and Abstracts of the 25th Interscience Conference on Antimicrobial Agents and Chemotherapy, American Society for Microbiology, Washington, D.C., 1985.

383a. Desmonts, G., and Douvreur, J. Congenital toxoplasmosis: a prospective study of the offspring of 542 women who acquired toxoplasmosis during pregnancy. Pathophysiology of congenital disease. In *Perinatal Medicine, Sixth European Congress* (O. Thalhammer, K. Baumgarten, and A. Pollak, eds.). George Thieme, Stuttgart, 1979, pp. 51–60.

383b. Leport, C., Vilde, J. L., Kattamal, C., Regnier, B., and Matherson, S. Failure of spiramycin to prevent neurotoxoplasmosis in immunosuppressed patients. *JAMA* 255:2290 (1986).

384. Kovacs, J. A., Allegra, C. J., Chabner, B. A., Drake, J. C., Swan, J. C., Parillo, J. E., and Masur, H. Potent *in vitro* and *in vivo* anti-*Toxoplasma* activity of the new lipid soluble antifolate trimetrexate. *Clin. Res.* 34: 522A (1986).

384a. Allegra, C. J., Kovacs, J. A., Drake, J. C., Swan, J. C., Chabner, B. A., and Masur, H. Potent *in vitro* and *in vivo* antitoxoplasma activity in the lipid soluble antifolate trimetrexate. *J. Clin. Invest.* 79:478–482 (1987).

385. Ruff, M. D., Anderson, W. I., and Reid, W. M. Effect of the anticoccidial arprinocid on production, sporulation and infectivity of *Eimeria* oocysts. *J. Parasitol.* 64:306 (1978).

386. Wang, C. C., Tolman, R. L., Simashkevich, P. M., and Stotish, R. L. Arprinocid, an inhibitor of hypoxanthine-guanine transport. *Biochem. Pharmacol.* 28:2249 (1979).

387. Wang, C. C., Simashkevich, P. M., and Fan, S. S. The mechanism of anticoccidial action of aprinocid-1-N-oxide. *J. Parasitol.* 67:137 (1981).

388. Chan, J., and Luft, B. J. Rothromycin (RU28965): an effective drug in the treatment of murine toxoplasmosis. *Antimicrob. Ag. Chemother.* (in press).

388a. Luft, B. J. *In vivo* and *in vitro* activity of roxithromycin against *Toxoplasma gondii* in mice. *Eur. J. Clin. Microbiol. 6*:479 (1987).

388b.Hofflin, J. M., and Remington, J. S. *In vivo* synergism of roxithromycin (RU965) and interferon against *Toxoplasma gondii. Antimicrob. Ag. Chemother. 31*:346 (1987).

389. McCabe, R. E., Luft, B. J., and Remington, J. S. Effect of murine interferon gamma on toxoplasmosis. *J. Infect. Dis. 150*:961 (1984).

390. Wagner, H., Hardt, C., Heeg, K., and Rolinghoff, M. T-cell derived helper factor allows *in vivo* induction of cytotoxic T-cells in nu/nv mice. *Nature 284*:278 (1980).

391. Hefneider, S. H., Conlon, J., Henney, C. S., and Gillis, S. In vivo interleukin 2 administration augments the generation of alloreactive T-lymphocytes and resident natural killer cells. *J. Immunol. 130*:122 (1983).

392. Hoffenbach, A., Lagrange, P. H., and Bach, M. A. Deficit of interleukin 2 production associated with impaired T-cell proliferative responses in *Myobacterium lepromurium* infection. *Infect. Immun. 39*:109 (1983).

393. Sharma, S. D., Hofflin, S. D., and Remington, J. S. *In vivo* recombinant interleukin 2 administration enhances survival against a lethal challenge with *Toxoplasma gondii. J. Immunol. 135*:4160 (1985).

5

Cryptosporidium spp.

WILLIAM L. CURRENT
Lilly Research Laboratories, A Division of Eli Lilly and Company, Indianapolis, Indiana

I. INTRODUCTION

Protozoans of the genus *Cryptosporidium* are small (2-6 μm, depending on stage in life cycle) coccidian parasites that infect the mucosal epithelium of a variety of animals, including humans (1-3). Until recently, infections with *Cryptosporidium* spp. were considered rare in animals, and in humans they were thought to be the result of an opportunistic pathogen of immunodeficient persons outside its normal host range (4-8). Our concept of this coccidian has changed within the past few years to that of a significant and widespread cause of gastrointestinal illness in several animal species, especially calves, lambs, and humans (1-3).

In immunocompetent human beings, at least one species (*C. parvum*) of this protozoan genus may produce mild to severe diarrhea lasting from several days to more than a month (9,10). In immunodeficient persons, especially those with the acquired immune deficiency syndrome (AIDS), cryptosporidiosis usually presents a prolonged, life-threatening choleralike illness (9,11). Diarrhea in many of these patients often becomes irreversible, and the fluid loss is excessive; 3-6 liters/day is common, and as much as 17 liters of watery feces per day has been reported (12). Recent reports of respiratory (13) and biliary (14) cryptosporidiosis demonstrate that this intracellular protozoan is not confined to the gastrointestinal tract of immunodeficient persons. To date, no effective therapy has been found (12); thus, the finding of cryptosporidiosis in the immunodeficient host often carries an ominous prognosis.

The recent recognition of *Cryptosporidium* spp. as a widespread pathogen of humans and animals has spawned over 200 articles between 1983 and 1987. No attempt has been made in this chapter to discuss all of the data contained in these publications; however, it does address much of our present understanding of the biology of *Cryptosporidium* spp. and the diseases it produces in the immunocompetent and immunodeficient host.

II. THE ORGANISM

A. Taxonomy and History

The taxonomic classification (15) of the small intracellular protozoans assigned to the genus *Cryptosporidium* is presented in Table 1. Other true coccidia (Eimeriorina) known to infect humans include *Toxoplasma gondii, Isospora belli,* and *Sarcocystis* spp. Clarke, in 1895, may have been the first to observe a species to *Cryptosporidium* (16). It is possible that the minute organisms he called "swarm spores" lying free upon the gastric epithelium of mice were the motile merozoites of *C. muris,* the type species named by Tyzzer 12 years later (17). Three years after creating the genus, Tyzzer described the life cycle of *C. muris* (18) infecting the gastric glands of mice, and in 1913 he described a second species, *C. parvum,* whose developmental stages were confined to the small intestine of the same host (19). During the ensuing 70 years, an additional 18 species of *Cryptosporidium* were named on the basis of oocyst morphology

Table 1   Classification of *Cryptosporidium* spp. (15)

Classification	Name	Biological characteristics
Phylum	Apicomplexa	Apical complex with polar rings, rhoptries, micronemes, conoid, and subpellicular microtubules
Class	Sporozoasida	Locomotion of invasive organisms by body flexion, gliding, or undulation
Subclass	Coccidiasina	Life cycle with merogony, gametogony, and sporogony
Order	Eucoccidiorida	Merogony present; in vertebrates
Suborder	Eimeriorina	Male and female gametes develop independently
Family	Cryptosporidiidae	Homoxenous (one host life cycle), with development just under surface membrane of host cell; oocyst without sporocysts and with four sporozoites; microgametes without flagella

(oocysts containing no sporocysts and four free sporozoites) and on the assumption that they were as host-specific as the closely (taxonomically) related coccidia assigned to the genus *Eimeria* [see Refs. 3 and 15 for the list of names].

Only a few of the 20 named species of *Cryptosporidium* are now considered to be valid. Five species of *Cryptosporidium—C. ameviae, C. crotali, C. ctenosauris, C. lamporpeltis,* and *C. vulpis*—are no longer considered valid because they were described from oocysts found in the feces of their hosts, and these environmentally resistant life-cycle forms are now recognized as the sporocyst stage of parasites belonging to the genus *Sarcocystis*. Successful cross-transmission of infections by oral inoculation of oocysts obtained from calves, cats, lambs, and humans to one or more different hosts have resulted in *C. angi, C. bovis, C. cuniculus,* and *C. felis* being considered invalid species (these are probably *C. parvum*, see below). The lack of host specificity exhibited by isolates from mammals prompted several investigators to consider *Cryptosporidium* as a single-species genus (1,20). A more realistic approach was presented by Levine (15), who consolidated the 20 named organisms into four species—one each for those infecting fish (*C. nasorum*), reptiles (*C. crotali*), birds (*C. meleagradis*), and mammals (*C. muris*). Although additional documentation is needed to determine the number of species infecting fish, reptiles, birds, and mammals, information now available in the published literature indicates that this consolidation is not correct for a number of reasons. As mentioned earlier, *C. crotali* (21) is considered to be a species of *Sarcocystis* (22,23). There are at least two valid species, *C. baileyi* (24) and *C. meleagradis* (25), infecting birds. Also, Cryptosporidium species producing oocysts indistinguishable from *C. muris* and *C. parvum*, both originally described by Tyzzer (18,19), are known to infect calves (*C. muris* in the stomach; *C. parvum* in the small intestine). On the basis of oocyst morphology, it is *C. parvum*, not *C. muris*, that is associated with all of the previously well-documented cases of cryptosporidiosis in mammals (26). Thus, at the present time, the species with oocysts measuring 4–5 μm that produces clinical illness in humans and other mammals should be referred to as *C. parvum*, or as *Cryptosporidium* sp. if there is not enough morphological, life-cycle, and/or host-specificity data to relate it to Tyzzer's description (19). I have adopted this conservative approach, realizing that careful studies of the proposed differences in host specificity, sites of infection, and pathogenicity among mammalian isolates (1–3) may result in the validation of additional species. Along with this conservative approach, the designation of a particular parasite obtained from a mammalian host as an isolate rather than a strain is preferable.

B. Life Cycle

Three years after his 1907 report (17) of the type species, *C. muris*, in the gastric glands of laboratory mice, Tyzzer presented much of its life cycle in amazing detail (18). The most notable features of this classic investigation, as well as his subsequent report (19) of *C. parvum* infecting the small intestine of laboratory mice, included descriptions of a single generation of schizogony, micro- and macrogametogony, fertilization, oocyst wall formation, sporogony, excystation, and experimental transmission by oocysts. Approximately 60 years later, Tyzzer's statement (18), "It is remarkable that an organism so minute should show so great structural variation and present modes of propagation analogous to those found in organisms very much larger," was confirmed by an ultrastructural study of *C. wrairi* in the guinea pig (27). Because Vetterling et al. (23,27) did not find oocysts in the feces of infected guinea pigs. they suggested that the oocysts described by Tyzzer were second-generation meronts containing four merozoites. This discrepancy was resolved in part when Pholenz et al. (28), studying naturally infected calves, and Iseki (29), investigating naturally infected cats, found sporulated oocysts within enterocytes and free in the feces. More recently, Angus et al. (30) reported that their isolate of *Cryptosporidium* sp. produced oocysts in experimentally infected guinea pigs. They proposed that the extended, incomplete, endogenous development of *C. wrairi* reported by Vetterling et al. (23) may have been the behavior of the organism in a species that is perhaps not the natural host. Although the existence of oocysts was no longer questioned by these authors, they could not agree on the number of generations of meronts.

The studies discussed above, along with more recent investigations of the development of calf and human isolates of *C. parvum* in mice (31), chicken embryos (32), and cell culture (33), and of *Cryptosporidium baileyi* in chickens (24) have revealed that, like those of the other true coccidia (Eimeriorina), the life cycle of *Cryptosporidium* spp. can be divided into six major developmental events: excystation (release of infective sporozoites from oocysts), merogony (asexual replication), gametogony (gamete formation), fertilization, oocyst wall formation, and sporogony (sporozoite formation). Since the life cycles of *C. parvum* and *C. baileyi* differ primarily in the number of types of meronts, the remaining life-cycle discussion will concentrate on the former species infecting humans and other mammals. The life cycle of *C. parvum* is illustrated in Figure 1*A*. Comparative morphological details of sporozoites, sporocysts, and oocysts of coccidia assigned to the families Eimeriidae, Sarcocystidae, and Cryptosporiidae are illustrated in Figure 1*B*. Photomicrographs and transmission electron micrographs of developmental stages of this parasite in the mucosal epithelium of the ileum of experimentally infected mice are shown in Figures 2–26 and 28–48. Additional details of the life cycle of *C. parvum* are presented below, with an emphasis on those events that have been confused or misinterpreted in the literature.

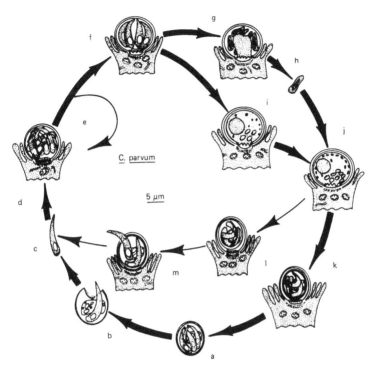

Figure 1*A*   Life cycle of human and calf isolates of *Cryptosporidium parvum* in experimentally infected mice. (a) Sporulated oocyst in feces. (b) Excystation within intestine. (c) Free sporozoite in intestine before penetration of the microvillous region of an ileal enterocyte. (d) Type I meront (six or eight merozoites). (e) Recycling of type I merozoite to form more type I meronts. (f) Type II meront (four merozoites). (g) Microgamont, with approximately 16 microgametes. (h) Microgamete fertilizes macrogamete (i) to form zygote (j). Approximately 80% of the zygotes form thick-walled oocysts (k) that sporulate within the host cell. Almost all thick-walled oocysts pass unaltered in the feces; they are the resistant forms that transmit the infection to another host. About 20% of the zygotes do not form an oocyst wall; their sporozoites are surrounded only by a unit membrane (l). Sporozoites within autoinfective, thin-walled oocysts (l) are released into the intestinal lumen (m) and reinitiate the endo-genous cycle (at c).

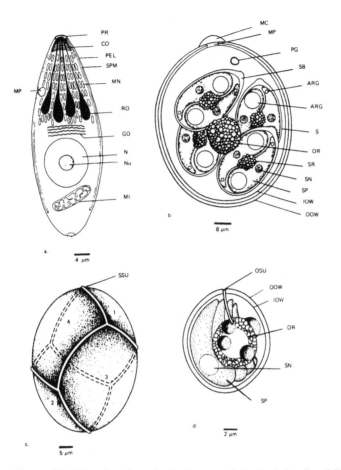

Figure 1B Line drawings depicting morphological details of life-cycle stages of coccidian parasites assigned to the families Eimeriidae, Sarcocystidae, and Cryptosporiidae. (a) Coccidian sporozoite showing organelles that are typical of invasive forms of organisms assigned to the phylum Apicomplexa. The apical complex is made up of the polar ring (PR), conoid (CO), micronemes (MN), and rhoptries (RO). (Redrawn from Ref. 168.) (b) Oocyst of an *Eimeria* sp. (family Eimeriidae). The oocyst wall is composed of inner (IOW) and outer (OOW) layers and contains a micropyle (MP) through which bile salts and proteolytic enzymes enter. Oocysts of *Eimeria* spp. contain four sporocysts (S), each with two sporozoites (SP), whereas oocysts of *Isopera* spp. and *Sarcocystis* spp. contain two sporocysts, each with four sporozoites. (Redrawn from Ref. 169.) (c) Sporocyst of *Sarcocystis* sp. The sporocyst wall is composed of four plates (1–4) joined by sporocyst wall plate sutures (SSU). (Redrawn from Ref. 170.) (d) Oocyst of *Cryptosporidium parvum* showing the inner (IOW) and outer (OOW) oocyst walls surrounding four free sporozoites (SP) and a granular oocyst

1. Excystation

Excystation, the release of infective sporozoites from environmentally resistant oocysts, is a key event in the life cycle of every true coccidian. This infection-initiating event usually occurs in the lumen of the gastrointestinal tract following ingestion of oocysts by a suitable host. In most coccidian species examined to date, excystation may also be triggered in vitro by exposing oocysts to conditions that simulate the gastrointestinal environment of the host (i.e., reducing conditions, CO_2, host body temperature, bile salts, and trypsin). Much of our understanding of this process is based on in vitro excystation studies of coccidian species belonging to the families Eimeriidae (34,35) and Sarcocystidae (36–38) whose oocysts possess sporocysts, each containing infective sporozoites (Fig. 1*B*). Such investigations have suggested that there may be two major steps in excystation. The first step is alteration of oocyst wall permeability, allowing influx of proteolytic enzymes and bile salts. This can be triggered by exposure to host body temperature and CO_2 and is often accomplished by a peeling away or dissolving of the micropyle, a thinning of the oocyst wall at one pole. This step can also be accomplished by removing the oocyst wall with a tissue grinder, releasing sporocysts. The second step is the release of sporozoites from sporocysts by the action of pancreatic enzymes and/or bile salts. Sporozoites of eimeriid coccidia (e.g., *Eimeria* spp. and some *Isospora* spp.) escape through an opening in one pole of the sporocysts that is formed by degradation of a plug, the Stieda body (Fig. 1*B*). It is believed that trypsin degrades the Stieda body and that bile salts stimulate sporozoite motility. Species of coccidia assigned to the family Sarcocystidae have sporocysts whose walls are composed of four plates joined by sutures. Trypsin and/or bile salts cause dissolution of the sutures, allowing sporozoites to escape between the collapsed plates.

The name *Cryptosporidium* was chosen by Tyzzer (18) because the oocysts of *C. muris* contained no sporocysts surrounding the sporozoites; that is, the sporozoites were naked or free within the oocyst wall. Oocysts of *C. parvum* release their sporozoites within the small intestine of experimentally inoculated mice (2,31) and in vitro when incubated in solutions containing a bile salt and

---

residuum (OR). A single suture (OSU) spanning approximately one-third the circumfrence of the oocyst occurs in the oocyst wall near the anterior of the sporozoites. (Redrawn from Ref. 26.) Abbreviations: ARG, anterior refractile granule; CO, conoid; GO, Golgi apparatus; IOW, inner oocyst wall; MC, micropyle cap; MI, mitochondrion; MN, microneme; MP, micropyle; N, nucleus; NU, nucleolus; OOW, outer oocyst wall; OR, oocyst residuum; OSU, oocyst wall suture; PEL, pellicle; PG, polar granule; PR, polar ring; PRG, posterior refractile globule; RO, rhoptry; S, sporocyst; SB, Stieda body; SN, sporozoite nucleus; SP, sporozoite; SR, sporozoite residuum; SSU, sporocyst wall suture.

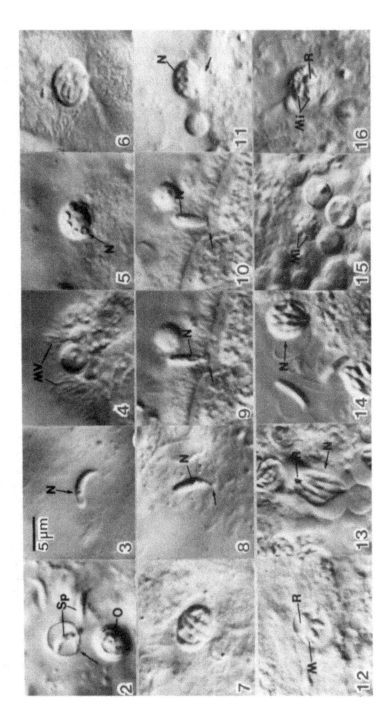

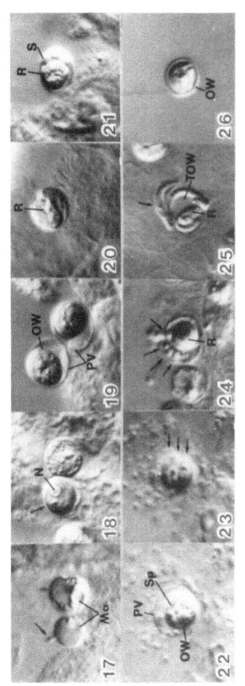

Figure 2-26   [Legend on p. 290.]

Figures 2-26 Nomarski interference contrast photomicrographs of developmental stages of *C. parvum* in mucosal scrapings of the small intestines of experimentally infected suckling mice. 2. Sporozoites (Sp) free and excysting from opening (arrow) in oocyst wall and an intact oocyst (O), 8 hr postinoculation. 3. Free sporozoite showing posterior location of the nucleus (N). 4. Uninucelate meront surrounded by hypertrophied microvilli (MV). 5. Immature type I meront with six nuclei (N) in focus. 6. Mature type I meront with eight merozoites. 7. Mature type I meront with six merozoites. All merozoites are in focus; the meront was flattened with coverslip pressure. 8. Merozoite attached to host cell. Arrow points to site of host-parasite attachment. Note position of the nucleus (N). 9. Merozoite penetrating into microvillous border of an enterocyte. The nucleus (N) of the merozoite is located near the middle of the cell. The anterior of the parasite has formed an invagination of the microvillous border of the host cell (arrow). 10. Merozoite in Figure 9, photographed several minutes later, showing a later phase of penetration into the microvillous border. The parasite nucleus (N) has migrated posteriorly, and there is a prominent band of material (arrow) in the host cell cytoplasm just beneath the parasite. 11. Immature type II meront with four nuclei (N) near the periphery. Arrow points to the attachment of the meront to the base of the PV. 12. Type II meront with four merozoites (M) budding from the residuum (R). 13. Mature type II meront with four merozoites and the small residuum (R). 14. Mature type II meronts showing arrangement of merozoites like segments of an orange. Nuclei (N) of the merozoites are aligned in the center of the meront. 15. Microgamont with microgametes (Mi) beginning to bud from the surface. 16. Microgamont with microgametes (Mi) free in the PV and a large residuum (R) attached to the base of the PV. 17. Two macrogametes (Ma), each with an attached microgamete. Arrow points to microgamete in focus. 18. Macrogamete containing a large eccentric nucleus (N) and a microgamete (arrow). 19. Two unsporulated oocysts with thick walls (OW). Oocysts are within prominent parasitophorous vacuoles (PV). 20. Early stage of sporogony showing separation of a granular oocyst residuum (R) from the sporont. 21. Oocyst with an oocyst residuum (R) and four sporoblasts (S). 22. Sporulated oocyst within a parasitophorous vacuole (PV). Note the thick oocyst wall (OW) and four sporozoites, one of which is seen in a longitudinal optical section (SP). 23. Different optical section of oocyst in Figure 21 showing the other three sporozoites (arrows). 24. One of only a few thick-walled oocysts observed releasing sporozoites (arrows). Note the large oocyst residuum (R) and the posterior of an escaping sporozoite within the oocyst. 25. One of many oocysts with a thin oocyst wall (membrane) (TOW), which readily ruptured, releasing sporozoites. Note the characteristic posterior position of the sporozoite nucleus (arrow) and the oocyst residuum (R). 26. Thick-walled oocyst free in intestinal lumen. Note the prominent thick oocyst wall (OW). [Adapted from Current and Reese (31).]

Table 2 Effects of Preincubation in Reducing Atmosphere and of Sodium Taurocholate (Bile Salt) and Trypsin on Excystation of Oocysts of a Human Isolate (Ref. 9, case 14) of *Cryptosporidium parvum*[a]

Treatment group	Preincubation[b]	Incubation[c]			Percent excystation[d]
	Cys-HC1 + CO_2	PBS only	Trypsin	Bile salt	
A	+	0	+	+	73
B	0	0	+	+	64
C	0	0	+	0	34
D	0	0	0	+	29
E	0	+	0	0	2.5

[a]Oocysts had been stored in 2.5% $K_2 Cr_2 O_7$ at 4°C for 3 months prior to excystation studies.

[b]Preincubation of oocysts was in 0.02 M cystein-HC1 in normal saline in an atmosphere of 50% CO_2 for 16 hr at 37°C.

[c]Incubation was in 0.75% (w/v) sodium taurocholate (bile salt) and/or 0.25% (w/v) trypsin in phosphate-buffered saline (PBS, pH 7.4) or in PBS only at 37°C for 90 min in an atmosphere of air.

[d]Percent excystation was determined microscopically and is expressed as the number of empty oocysts (excysted) observed in two separate counts of 100 total (excysted plus intact) oocysts.

trypsin (39). Data presented in Table 2 suggest that, at mammalian body temperature, sodium taurocholate plus trypsin are the major factors stimulating excystation of *C. parvum* sporozoites in vitro. These data also demonstrate that, unlike oocysts of many *Eimeria* and *Isospora* spp., preincubation of *C. parvum* oocysts in a reducing solution and 50% CO_2 to alter oocyst wall permeability is not necessary for excystation to occur. Similar findings have been reported by others (39). Fayer and Leek (40) reported that excystation of sporozoites of *C. parvum* readily occurs by incubating oocysts in water at $37°C$ and that exposure to reducing conditions followed by bile salts and pancreatic enzymes was not necessary. If this were true, warm water (~$37°C$) could be used as an effective disinfectant. It is possible that these authors may not have been measuring excystation, but rather the structural and functional integrity of the oocyst wall suture (see below). Storage of partially cleaned oocysts in water usually results in the growth of bacteria and fungi, which release, among other things, a variety of proteolytic enzymes. With time, these microbial enzymes may degrade the oocyst wall suture so that it no longer prevents rapid influx of water when these forms are placed in a warm, hypoosmotic environment. This may explain the authors' (40) observations of a higher percentage of excysted (= osmotically ruptured) oocysts incubated in water compared to those incubated in saline. Data presented in Table 3 demonstrate that only a small percentage of oocysts will rupture when placed in warm water and that sporozoites released from oocysts incubated in water do not remain viable (Table 2); they quickly become short and swollen and begin to rupture. These data also suggest that 2.5% potassium dichromate is better than water as a long-term storage medium for oocysts. The use of antibiotics in water may also increase the survival time of oocysts.

The oocyst walls of *C. parvum* from calves and humans (31), *C. muris* from calves (26) and mice (18), and *C. baileyi* from chickens (24) have a single suture at one pole that spans one-third to one-half the circumfrence of the oocysts (Fig. 1B). During excystation, the suture dissolves partially, and the adjacent margins of the oocyst wall separate and form a cleftlike opening through which the sporozoites escape (Figs. 2 and 27). Similar observations have been reported in a scanning electron microscopic study of sporozoites excysting from oocysts of a calf isolate of *C. parvum* (41).

Based on the chemical and physical stimuli promoting excystation of *Cryptosporidium* oocysts and on the presence of a suture in the oocyst wall, one may conclude that these resistant forms are similar to sporocysts of sarcocystid coccidia. These observations prompted Reduker et al. (41) to postulate that *Cryptosporidium*, like *Sarcocystis*, may be passed from the host as sporocysts. Others (42,43) have proposed that these resistant forms should be called sporocysts because they contain naked sporozoites when passed from the host. Our

Table 3 In Vitro Excystation of a Human Isolate (Ref. 9, case 14) of *Cryptosporidium parvum* at Different Times after Storage at 4°C in 2.5% (w/v) $K_2Cr_2O_7$, Tap Water with Antibiotics, or Tap Water

Storage medium	Time of storage (days)	Preincubation (H_2O, 4 hr, 37°C)		Incubation (EF, 1 hr, 37°C)[a]	
		% Excystation[b]	Sporozoites per 100 oocysts[c]	% Excystation[b]	Sporozoites per 100 oocysts[d]
H_2O	1	2.0	0.5	86.8	117.5
	14	4.5	3.8	91.3	144.8
	28	3.8	2.5	82.3	178.3
	56	5.5	7.0	86.5	179.3
	100	14.8	6.3	79.8	86.3
	140	9.5	12.8	79.5	21.3
H_2O + antibiotics[e]	1	2.3	1.0	82.5	122.3
	14	4.0	2.8	92.0	173.3
	28	1.3	0.5	92.5	183.3
	56	7.5	12.8	82.3	133.3
	100	5.0	8.5	85.8	88.0
	140	9.5	4.8	78.0	51.5

Table 3 In Vitro Excystation of a Human Isolate (Ref. 9, case 14) of *Cryptosporidium parvum* at Different Times after Storage at $4°C$ in 2.5% (w/v) $K_2Cr_2O_7$, Tap Water with Antibiotics, or Tap Water (Continued)

Storage medium	Time of storage (days)	Preincubation (H_2O, 4 hr, $37°C$)		Incubation (EF, 1 hr, $37°C$)[a]	
		% Excystation[b]	Sporozoites per 100 oocysts[c]	% Excystation[b]	Sporozoites per 100 oocysts[d]
2.5% $K_2Cr_2O_7$	1	1.3	1.5	92.5	136.0
	14	0.8	0.5	90.3	182.5
	28	2.50	0.5	94.8	196.3
	56	6.3	5.5	93.0	185.8
	100	10.8	6.0	87.3	101.8
	140	13.0	5.8	94.0	81.0

[a]Incubation was in excystation fluid (EF) composed of 0.75% (w/v) sodium taurocholate plus 0.25% (w/v) trypsin in Hank's balanced salt solution. Incubation for 1 hr at $37°C$ occurred following the 4-hr preincubation in water at $37°C$.

[b]Percent excystation is expressed as the mean percentage of excysted (empty) oocysts observed microscopically in four samples of 100 total (excysted plus intact) oocysts obtained from each sample at each time.

[c]Sporozoites per 100 oocysts is the mean number of sporozoites counted while observing 100 total oocysts in four separate samples. Sporozoites released during preincubation were short, swollen, and nonmotile and appeared dead.

[d]Sporozoites per 100 oocysts are mean values determined as described in footnote c. Most sporozoites released during incubation in EF were long, slender, and motile.

[e]Antibiotics added to water were penicillin (500 IU/ml), streptomycin (500 μg/ml), and amphotericin B (125 μg/ml).

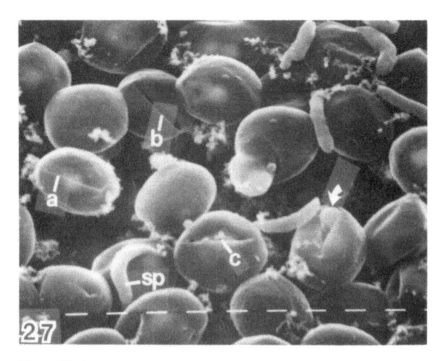

Figure 27 Scanning electron micrograph of oocysts of a human isolate of *C. parvum* (Ref. 7, case 14). Oocysts were cleaned and concentrated from the feces of an experimentally infected calf, preincubated in H_2O at $37°C$ for 2 hr, and then incubated in 0.25% trypsin plus 0.75% sodium taurocholate (w/v) in PBS (pH 7.4) for 40 min at $37°C$. Parasites were then deposited on Nucleopore filters, fixed with 3% (w/v) glutaraldehyde in phosphate buffer (pH 7.4), and processed for scanning electron microscopy. The oocyst wall suture begins to dissolve, forming an indention (a). Further dissolution results in the formation of a cleft (b), which widens (c). Sporozoites (sp) escape through the widened cleft (arrow). Lines at the bottom of the micrograph each represent 1.0 µm.

studies of oocyst wall development (31) (reviewed below) and sporulation within host cells (26,32,33) demonstrate that it is not technically correct to refer to these forms as sporocysts. If these resistant forms were true sporocysts, the bilayered oocyst wall would disappear soon after it is formed and a similar-appearing sporocyst wall would then have to be constructed. Since these events do not occur during oocyst wall formation and sporogony of *C. parvum* (31), the resistant forms of *Cryptosporidium* spp. passed from the host should be referred to as oocysts (thick-walled oocysts).

2. Merogony

Merogony is the asexual replicative phase culminating in the formation and release of invasive merozoites that begins soon after sporozoites (Figs. 3 and 27) of *Cryptosporidium* spp. take up residence in the microvillous region of host epithelial cells. Sporozoite and merozoite invasion of host cells are similar (Figs. 8–10 and 31). After becoming surrounded by a host-cell-derived parasitophorous vacuole membrane, these invasive forms round up into uninucleate meronts (Figs. 4 and 32). Uninucleate meronts and subsequent developmental stages assume an intracellular, extracytoplasmic position within the host cell: intracellular, because each parasite is surrounded by a host-cell-derived parasitophorous vacuole membrane; extracytoplasmic, because all developmental stages are confined to the microvillous region of the host cell (Figs. 28–48). A network of microfilaments, similar to those comprising the terminal web of the host cell, forms beneath the parasite and may play a role in preventing its relocation into the perinuclear region, the area occupied by intracellular forms of most other coccidian species.

Following nuclear divisions, meront nuclei migrate to the periphery and merozoites begin to form by a budding process (ectomerogony) (Figs. 4, 11, 12, and 34–36). Fully formed merozoites have an apical complex (Fig. 1*B*) composed of micronemes, rhoptries, a conoid, and preconoidal rings (Figs. 37 and 38). Such organelles are found commonly in invasive forms of other coccidian species. Merozoites and sporozoites of *C. parvum* lack subpellicular microtubules and conodial rings, the proposed microtubule organizing center for these subpellicular supportive elements that are so prominent in invasive forms of other coccidia. Type I merozoites of *C. parvum* may recycle or they may form type II meronts whose merozoites do not recycle but develop directly into gamonts (sexual stages) (29–31).

3. Gametogony and Fertilization

The majority of type II merozoites of *C. parvum* that enter host cells develop into macrogametes, whereas the remainder form microgamonts (Fig. 39) which produce microgametes, the male counterpart of the sexual cycle. Each microgamont produces approximately 16 bullet-shaped, nonflagellated microgametes (Figs. 15,16, and 40) which attach to (Fig. 17) and penetrate (Fig. 18) macrogametes. Although observation of fusion of macro- and micronuclei has not been reported for any species of *Cryptosporidium*, it is assumed that fertilization occurs prior to formation of the oocyst wall. Macrogametes are characterized by the presence of polysaccharide storage granules (amylopectin) in the basilar region of the cell (Fig. 41) and two types of wall forming bodies near the periphery (Fig. 42).

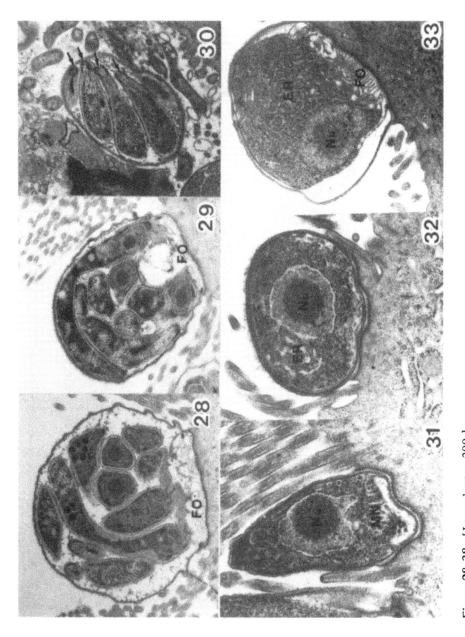

Figure 28–38 [Legend on p. 299.]

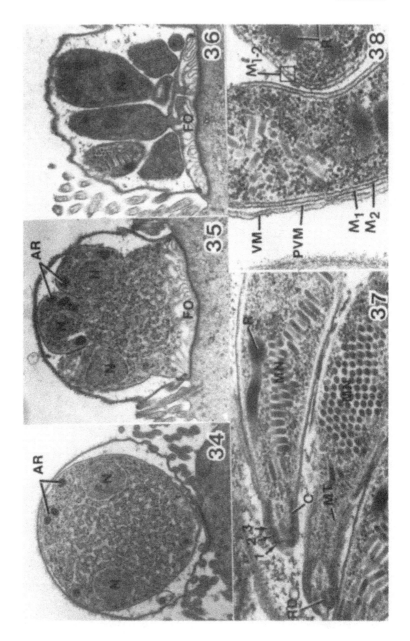

Figures 28–38 Transmission electron micrographs (TEM) of meronts in the microvillous region (Figs. 28–30 ×11,000) and TEM showing major features of merogony and merozoite fine structure (Figs. 31–38). **28.** Type I meront with eight merozoites, two of which are in the final stages of budding from the residuum. The basilar portion of the residuum is modified into a feeder organelle (FO). **29.** Type I meront with six merozoites and a feeder organell (FO) within the parasitophorous vacuole. **30.** Section through anterior of the four merozoites (arrows) of a type II meront. **31.** Merozoite in final stages of penetrating into microvillous region. Note the nucleus with a large nucleolus (NU) and the vacuolated cytoplasm previously occupied by micronemes (MN). ×22,250. **32.** Early uninucleate meront with dilated endoplasmic reticulum (ER) and a nucleus with a large nucleolus (NU). ×17,350. **33.** Late-stage uninucleate meront with extensive ER and an eccentric nucleus with a nucleolus (NU) that is less prominent than that of the previous stage. The plasma membrane of the parasite has folded extensively to form the feeder organelle (FO) at the base of the PV. ×15,200. **34.** Meront with two nuclei (N) without nucleoli and with anlagen of the rhoptries or micronemes (AR) near the periphery. ×12,000. **35.** Type II meront showing three of four merozoites budding from the surface opposite the feeder organelle (FO). Within each budding merozoite is a nucleus (N) and an anlagen of rhoptries or micronemes (AR). ×12,500. **36.** Nearly mature type II meront with three merozoites free in the PV and one in the final stages of budding from the feeder organelle (FO). Merozoite nuclei have prominent nucleoli (Nu). ×15,200. **37.** Higher resolution of anterior portion of type II merozoites shown in Figure 30. The apical complex is composed of three preconoidal rings (arrows 1, 2, 3), a conoid (C), two rhopties (R), and numerous micronemes (MN). Note the microtubule (MT) accompanying what appears to be a duct from a rhoptry (RD) leading to a nipple like projection at the anteriormost end. ×34,260. **38.** Section through the posterior of several merozoites showing the arrangement of membranes. VM, outer villous membrane; PVM, parasitophorous vacuole membrane; M_1, outer plasma membrane of merozoite; M_2, inner plasma membrane present only in the posterior half of the merozoite (note its absence in Fig. 37). Rhopties (R) and micronemes can also be seen. ×45,250. [Adapted from Current and Reese (31).]

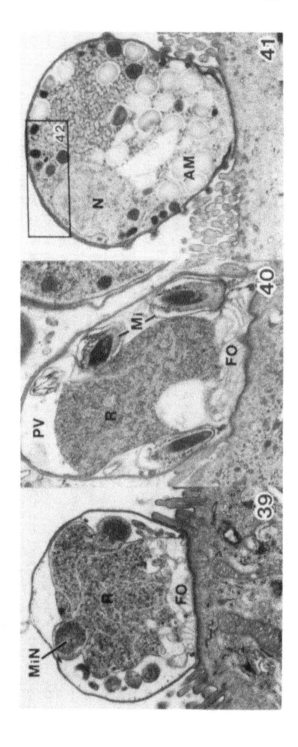

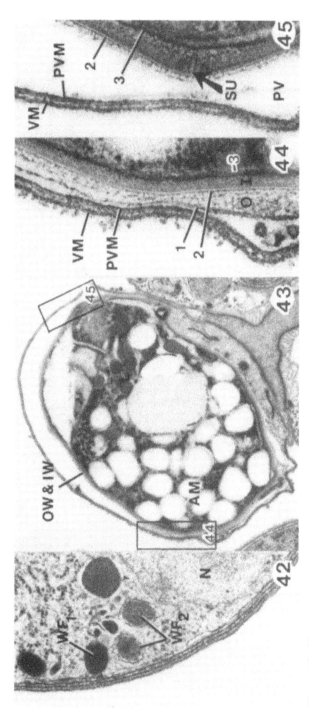

Figure 39–48 [Legend on p. 303.]

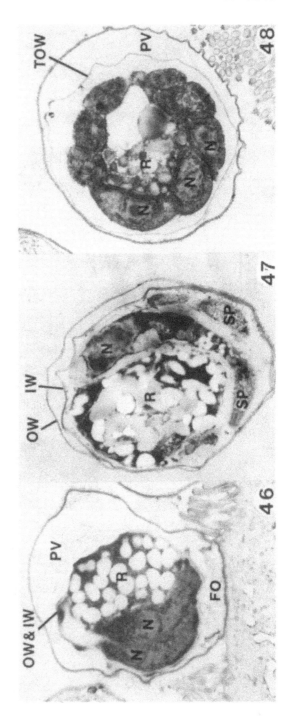

Figures 39–48 Transmission electron micrographs of sexual stages of *C. parvum* in enterocytes. **39.** Immature microgamont with compact nuclei (MiN) near the periphery of what will be the large residuum (R) whose basilar region has formed the feeder organelle (FO). ×16,000. **40.** Nearly mature microgamont with microgametes (Mi) free in the parasitophorous vacuole (PV) and budding from the residuum (R). The parasite membrane nearest the host cell has folded extensively to form the feeder organelle (FO). ×18,800. **41.** Macrogamete with an eccentric nucleus (N) and an accumulation of amylopectin-like bodies (AM) near the feeder organelle. ×16,700. **42.** Enlargement of the boxed portion of the macrogamete in Figure 41 showing two types of wall-forming bodies (WF$_1$, WF$_2$). Membranes surrounding the macrogamete include, from outside to inside, the villous membrane, the parasitophorous vacuole membrane, the outer plasmalemma of the parasite (1), and a short segment of membrane 2 forming just beneath membrane 1. ×43,000. **43.** Unsporulated, thick-walled oocyst within a PV. Amylopectin-like granules (AM) are numerous, and some smaller lipid-like bodies are present. The arrangement of membranes associated with the outer (OW) and inner (IW) oocyst walls in the boxed areas are shown in Figures 44 and 45. ×17,500. **44.** The oocyst is contained in two host cell membranes, the villous membrane (VM) and the parasitophorous vacuole membrane (PVM). The outer wall (O) of the oocyst is limited by parasite membranes 1 and 2, whereas the inner wall (I) is limited by membranes 2 and 3. ×85,000. **45.** Portion of oocyst with membrane 1 and a portion of the outer oocyst wall missing. The suture (SU) in the inner oocyst wall represents the site of oocyst wall collapse during excystation (see Fig. 2). VM, villous membrane; PVM, parasitophorous vacuole membrane; 2 and 3, membranes 2 and 3 of oocyst wall; PVM, parasitophorous vacuole membrane. ×85,000. **46.** Sporulated, thick-walled oocyst within a parasitophorous vacuole (PV). Two of the four sporozoites with posteriorly located nuclei (N) and a residuum (R) with amylopectin-like granules are enclosed within the outer and inner oocyst walls (OW&IW). The feeder organelle (FO) is still firmly attached to the base of the PV. ×12,000. **47.** Thick-walled oocyst shed in feces. The outer (OW) and inner (IW) oocyst walls surround the sporozoites (SP) and residuum (R), both of which contain amylopectin-like granules. Note the posterior position of the sporozoite nucleus (N). ×15,000. **48.** Thin-walled autoinfective oocyst within a parasitophorous vacuole (PV). The thin oocyst wall (TOW) consists of a single unit membrane surrounding the four sporozoites (three of their nuclei [N] are labeled) and the residuum (R) containing many amylopectin-like granules. ×15,000. [Adapted from Current and Reese (31).]

4. Oocyst Wall Formation and Sporogony

Macrogametes become oocysts when one or more layers of the oocyst wall are formed (Figs. 43–45). The oocyst wall is composed of two layers and three unit membranes. Apparently, type I wall-forming bodies fuse with membrane 2 and release their contents between membranes 1 and 2 to form the outer layer of oocyst wall. Similarly, it is believed that type II wall-forming bodies fuse with membrane 3 and release their contents between membranes 2 and 3 to form the inner layer of the oocyst wall. During excystation, a suture in the inner oocyst wall (Fig. 45) dissolves, and the oocyst wall collapses inwardly to form an opening through which the sporozoites exit (Fig. 27).

The process of oocyst wall formation occurs in approximately 80% of the oocysts of C. parvum and results in the production of thick-walled oocysts (31, 32). Thick-walled oocysts sporulate within the host cell (Fig. 46), and virtually all of them pass unaltered through the gut of the host (Fig. 47). These thick-walled forms, the oocysts that are detected in the feces of infected animals, are highly resistant and maintain their infectivity for mice and cell cultures for up to 16 months if stored at 4°C in a 2.5% aqueous solution of potassium dichromate (2,31). Thick-walled oocysts are the environmentally resistant forms that transmit the infection from one susceptible host to another.

In addition to the thick-walled form, transmission electron microscopy has revealed the presence of a thin-walled oocyst (Fig. 48) in enterocytes of mice experimentally infected with C. parvum (2,31). In contrast to the resistant forms, which have two distinct layers in the oocyst wall, the four sporozoites and residuum of the thin-walled oocysts are surrounded by only a single unit membrane. Soon after the thin-walled oocysts are released from the host cell, this unit membrane ruptures, and the freed sporozoites penetrate into adjacent epithelial cells and reinitiate the endogenous cycle (2,31). Autoinfective, thin-walled oocysts are not passed in the feces. Similar autoinfective, thin-walled oocysts of C. parvum are also produced in experimentally infected chicken embryos (32).

Cryptosporidium parvum can also complete its developmental cycle in extraintestinal sites. Respiratory and biliary infections of C. parvum have been reported in AIDS patients (13,14). Introduction of oocysts of a calf isolate of C. parvum into the trachea and eyes of suckling pigs resulted in infections of the tracheal and conjunctival epithelium, respectively (44). Introduction of oocysts of C. baileyi isolated from the gastrointestinal tract of chickens into the eyes and nares of 1-day-old and 1-month-old chickens results in infections of the respiratory conjunctival epithelia (44a). Thick-walled oocysts are also produced in each of these extraintestinal sites, suggesting a developmental cycle similar to that observed in the gastrointestinal tract.

The presence of autoinfective oocysts (~20% of the oocysts found in host cells), along with type I meronts that recycle, are life-cycle features of C. parvum that make it unique among the coccidia infecting warm-blooded vertebrates. It is believed that these two features explain why a small number of oocysts can produce severe infections in susceptible hosts and why immunodeficient persons may develop persistent, life-threatening infections in the absence of repeated oral exposure to thick-walled oocysts. The lack of host and organ specificity and the zoonotic potential of *C. parvum* are features that also make the epidemiology of this protozoan intriguing.

C. Epidemiology

Since *Cryptosporidium* was recognized only recently as a human pathogen, our knowledge of its epidemiology is somewhat limited and is confined to information relative to its mode of transmission, potential sources of infection, and prevalence in humans and domesticated animals. Studies of experimental infections in farm and laboratory animals have clearly shown that cryptosporidiosis in mammals is transmitted by oocysts (thick-walled) of *C. parvum* (26) that are fully sporulated and infective at the time they are passed in the feces (2,9,31). Oocysts of *C. parvum*, like those of other coccidian species, are resistant to most disinfectants used in hospitals and laboratories (1). Infectivity of *Cryptosporidium* sp. oocysts was reported to be destroyed by ammonia, formal saline (45), freeze-drying, and exposure (30 min) to temperatures below freezing ($-20°C$) and above $65°C$ [1]. Full-strength commercial bleach is used as a disinfectant in our laboratory. Exposure of oocysts to full-strength bleach (5.25% sodium hypochlorite) for 10 min or longer at room temperature destroys their infectivity for suckling mice (unpublished data). However, if one uses bleach as a disinfectant, the final concentration should be above 70%. Since incubation of oocysts in solutions of 20% commercial bleach (1.05% sodium hypochlorite) for 12 min in an ice bath did not prevent subsequent release of viable sporozoites under conditions of in vitro excystation (39), routine chlorination of drinking water should have no effect on the infectivity of *Cryptosporidium* sp. oocysts. Although heat (hot water $>80°C$ or autoclaving) and full-strength bleach may destroy infectivity of *Cryptosporidium* sp. oocysts, a disinfectant for medical instruments that cannot tolerate such harsh treatments is needed.

Recent studies have clearly shown that calves are a source of human infection (9,46,47), and it has been suggested that companion animals such as rodents, puppies, and kittens are also reservoir hosts (9,10). This, coupled with a large list (Table 4) of animals reported to be infected with what is believed to be a parasite that readily crosses species barriers, led to the view that zoonotic transmission accounts for most human infection. This view is probably correct for persons living and working in environments where they are exposed to fecal contamination from potential reservoir hosts. However, zoonotic transmission

Table 4   Some Animals Reported to Be Infected with *Cryptosporidium* spp.

Animal species	Ref.
Fishes	
Naso tang (*Naso lituratus*)	147
Carp (*Cyprinus carpio*)	148
Reptiles	
Red-bellied black snake (*Pseudechis porphyriacus*)	149
Corn snake (*Elaphae guttata*)	150
Timber rattlesnake (*Crotalus horridus*)	150
Trans-pacos ratsnake (*Elephae subocularis*)	150
Madagascar boa (*Sansinia madagascarensis*)	150
Birds	
Chicken (*Gallus gallus*)	107–110
Turkey (*Meleagris gallopavo*)	111,112,151,152
Peafowl (*Pavo cristatus*)	113
Bobwhite quail (*Colinus virginianus*)	114,115
Black-throated finch (*Poephila cincta*)	153
Domestic goose (*Anser anser*)	154
Red-lored parrot (*Amazona autumnalis*)	155
Mammals	
Humans (*Homo sapiens*)	1–14,46–72
Macaques (*Macaca fascincularis*)	156
(*Macaca radiata*)	156
(*Macaca mulatta*)	156
Goat (*Capra hircus*)	9
Calf (*Bos taurus*)	89–91
Lamb (*Ovis aries*)	96–100
Swine (*Sus scrofa*)	102–104
Horse (*Equis caballus*)	105,106
Roe deer (*Capreolus capreolus*)	157
Red deer (*Cervus elaphus*)	152,158
White tail deer (*Odocolleus virginianus*)	159
Fox squirrel (*Sciurus niger*)	160
Gray squirrel (*Sciurus carolinensis*)	159

Table 4 Some Animals Reported to Be Infected with *Cryptosporidium* spp. (Continued)

Animal species	Ref.
Flying squirrel (*Glaucomys volans*)	159
13-Lined ground squirrel (*Spermophilus tridecemlineatus*)	159
Pocket gopher (*Geomys bursarius*)	159
Chipmunk (*Tamias striatus*)	159
Woodchuck (*Marmota monax*)	159
Beaver (*Castor canadensis*)	159
Muskrat (*Ondatra zibethicus*)	159
Nutrina (*Myocastor coypus*)	159
Cottontail rabbit (*Sylvilagus floridanus*)	159
Domestic rabbit (*Oryctolagus cuniculus*)	161
Exotic undulates (~14 species)	116
Domestic dog (*Canis familiaris*)	9,162
Coyote (*Canis latrans*)	159
Red fox (*Vulpes vulpes*)	159
Grey fox (*Orocyon cinereoargenteus*)	159
Domestic cat (*Felis catus*)	9,27,163
Striped skunk (*Mephitis mephitis*)	159
Raccoon (*Procyon lotor*)	164
Black bear (*Ursus americanus*)	159

does not explain the large number of infections among urban dwellers whose exposure to animal feces is minimal.

Evidence has been accumulating rapidly that person-to-person transmission of cryptosporidiosis is common. An accidental infection of a researcher demonstrated that a human isolate of *C. parvum* could be transmitted from one person to another (48). Outbreaks of cryptosporidiosis have been reported among children in day care centers (49,50), several hospital-acquired infections have been investigated (10,51), at least one large waterborne outbreak has been documented (52), and this protozoan appears to be a cause of traveler's diarrhea (53,54).

Soon after the waterborne outbreak noted above (52) was investigated, a preliminary study in conjunction with F. W. Schaefer of the Environmental

Protection Agency demonstrated that oocysts of *C. parvum* can be recovered from water samples by high-volume orlon filters [55] used to trap cysts of *Giardia lamblia* (unpublished data). Similar water-filtration methods, coupled with an immunofluorescent detection technique, resulted in the recovery and identification of *Cryptosporidium* sp. oocysts from the secondary effluent of a sewage treatment plant in Tucson, Arizona (56). *Cryptosporidium* sp. oocysts have also been identified by an immunofluorescence detection procedure in materials filtered from several rivers in western Washington (57).

The epidemiological features of cryptosporidiosis emphasized above—transmission by an environmentally resistant cyst (oocyst), the identification of numerous potential reservoir hosts for zoonotic transmission, the demonstration of person-to-person transmission, and documentation of waterborne transmission—are very similar to those of human giardiasis that came to light during the past decade. The importance of *G. lamblia* as a widespread cause of diarrheal illness in humans has been recognized for several years, and *Cryptosporidium* is now ascending a similar recognition curve. A review (2) of the data presented in 15 of the first large-scale surveys to determine the prevalence of *Cryptosporidium* oocysts in stool specimens obtained from selected populations in areas of Australia (58), Costa Rica (59,60), the United Kingdom (61), the United States (62,63), Brazil (64), Peru (65), South Africa (66), Bangladesh (67), Spain (68), Denmark (69), Central Africa (70), Liberia (71), and Haiti (72) suggested that this protozoan is an important, widespread cause of diarrheal illness in humans. In the majority of the studies, *Cryptosporidium* sp. was the most common parasite found, and in several this protozoan was considered to be the most significant of all known enteropathogens causing diarrheal illness. Other findings common to these 15 surveys were that children had a significantly higher prevalence of cryptosporidiosis than did adults and that infections were often seasonal, with a higher prevalence during the warmer, wetter, months. From the viewpoint of infection control, another interesting finding was that small numbers of oocysts may be present in the feces for up to 2 weeks following resolution of diarrhea.

A more complete picture of the overall geographical distribution and prevalence of human cryptosporidiosis was revealed in a recent review (3) of 36 large-scale surveys, including the 15 mentioned above, that employed standard diagnostic techniques to demonstrate the presence of *Cryptosporidium* sp. oocysts in stool specimens. Most of the stool specimens examined in the 36 surveys (see Ref. 3 for references) were from selected populations, such as children or adults who seek medical attention for diarrhea or other gastrointestinal symptoms; the remainder were specimens routinely submitted to a particular diagnostic laboratory. These surveys suggest that *Cryptosporidium* sp. is associated with diarrheal illness in all areas of the world and that it is more prevalent in less developed regions. For example, prevalence rates reported in surveys from

Europe (1-2%) and North America (0.6-4.3%) were lower than those reported in surveys from Asia, Australia, Africa, and Central and South America (3-20%). Data from all 36 surveys confirm that in many areas *Cryptosporidium* sp. is among the top three or four enteric pathogens identified and that there appears to be a higher prevalence of infection during the warmer, more humid months.

In light of the information just reviewed, physicians, veterinarians, and others involved in educating the public of risk factors associated with the transmission of infectious diseases should broaden their educational role to include crypto-sporidiosis. This role should be approached aggressively because of the apparently high prevalence of the disease, because of the large number of potential reservoir hosts, and because persons with compromised immune systems may develop life-threatening cryptosporidiosis (see below). It is important that physicians recognize when the disease is present in their patients, and it is equally important that veterinarians recognize when the infectious agent is present in farm and companion animals so that persons at high risk of developing serious illness can be warned. The typical symptoms in humans and clinical signs in animals are reviewed in Section IV.A and techniques to diagnosie crypto-sporidiosis in Section IV.B.

D. Growth and Metabolism

All species of *Cryptosporidium* that have been studied are obligate intracellular parasites that complete their life cycle within the microvillous region of the mucosal epithelium of several organs, especially those of the gastrointestinal tract. Because *C. parvum* exhibited little host specificity for mammals, and because other species of coccidia have been grown in chicken embryos, we attempted its cultivation in ovo. After techniques were developed to purify oocysts from feces, sterilize the purified preparation, and obtain viable sporozoites, the attempted chicken embryo cultivation of *C. parvum* was successful (32). Both human and calf isolates of *C. parvum* completed their entire life cycle, from sporozoite to sporulated oocyst, in the endoderm cells of the chorio-allantoic membrane (CAM) of chicken embryos incubated at 35–41°C. The morphology, time of appearance, and sequence of development of *C. parvum* in cells of the CAM on days 1-8 after sporozoite inoculation were similar to those reported in ileum enterocytes of mice inoculated orally with oocysts of the same species (Figs. 2-48) (30). Subsequent to this report we found that the source of chicken embryos is very important. Virtually all embryos (both White Leghorn and broilers) obtained from one source supported development of large numbers of parasites, whereas only a small percentage (10-20%) of embryos from two other sources would support parasite growth. The reason(s) for this difference in suitability of embryos from different sources has not been resolved.

With access to the proper source of chicken embryos, the in ovo cultivation system can be manipulated for use in screening candidate therapeutic agents. It has been disappointing, however, that this method of cultivation has not resulted in a system for obtaining large numbers of purified parasites, free from the bacteria and other intestinal contaminants associated with *C. parvum* grown in laboratory animals. Most oocysts of *C. parvum* were retained in cells of the CAM and were not released into the allantoic fluid. Numerous attempts to recover purified oocysts from infected CAM tissues have been somewhat disappointing.

More recently, we have been able to cultivate and transfer from embryo to embryo a *C. baileyi* originally isolated from chickens (unpublished data). The life cycle, including morphology, timing, and sequence of developmental stages, of the *C. baileyi* grown in chicken embryos is similar to that occurring in the gut of experimentally infected chickens (24). Unlike *C. parvum*, whose oocysts remain in endoderm cells of the CAM, many oocyts of the species isolated from chickens are released in the allantoic fluid. Large numbers of infective oocysts can be collected and purified from the allantoic fluid, allowing continuous propagation in embryos.

Complete development, from sporozoite to infective oocyst, in cell culture has also been reported for a human isolate of *C. parvum* (33). This parasite completed its life cycle in several cell types (human fetal lung, porcine kidney, and primary chicken kidney); however, the number of oocysts produced in cell culture was considerably less than in experimentally infected mice or chicken embryos. Development of *C. parvum* in human fetal lungs (HFL) cells was similar to that observed in mice during the first 3 days following inoculation of oocysts. However, on days 4–8 after inoculation, the number of parasites in HFL cells decreased whereas the number increased in enterocytes of infected mouse ileum. This difference was attributed to the presence of thin-walled oocysts in mice (31) and the absence of these autoinfective forms in cell culture (33). To date, I am not aware of anyone who has been able to manipulate infected cell cultures so that *C. parvum* would produce autoinfective oocysts. Without such an autoinfective cycle, it is very difficult to recover enough oocysts for passage of *C. parvum* from cell culture to cell culture.

Although very little is known about the metabolism of *Cryptosporidium* spp., the unique ultrastructural features of the parasite may provide some direction for studies of this topic. The intracellular-extracytoplasmic location of the parasite, its so-called feeder organelle, and its lack of structurally identifiable mitochondria are interesting features that merit investigation.

As discussed earlier (Section II.B), *Cryptosporidium* spp. reside within a parasitophorous vacuole that is confined to the microvillous region of enterocytes. Parasites grown in chicken embryos and in cultured cells also assume a similar intracellular, extracytoplasmic position. Thus, regardless of host-cell type, developmental stages of *Cryptosporidium* spp. are confined to a parasitophorous vacuole that bulges outward beneath the host-cell surface and that is apparently prevented from migrating into the perinuclear region by a dense network of filaments that form beneath its base in the host-cell cytoplasm. The portion of the parasite separated from the host-cell cytoplasm by the microfilamentous sheet undergoes extensive membrane folding to form what has been called the feeder organelle. To date, I am not aware of any physiological evidence of nutrient transport into the parasite through this unique species-to-species interface.

Not only is there an absence of knowledge concerning the site(s) of nutrient transport and the identity of nutrients incorporated by *Cryptosporidium* sp., but there is also a void in our understanding of the metabolic pathways that provide the energy required by this rapidly dividing parasite. The apparent absence of structurally identifiable mitochondria in all developmental stages and the presence of large amounts of stored polysaccharide (amylopectin granules) in sporozoites suggest that a glycolytic pathway supplies most of the energy for these invasive forms. The resistance of intracellular forms of *Cryptosporidium* spp. to a vast number of drugs, many of which are metabolic poisons, may be due to the compound not gaining access to the parasite or to the presence of unique metabolic pathways. Exploitation of the chicken embryo and cell culture models may provide some important information concerning the metabolism of this protozoan parasite.

E. Immunology and Virulence

Relatively little is known about the immunology and virulence of *Cryptosporidium* spp. The void in our understanding of such things as the major antigenic components of the *C. parvum* and how the organism responds to host defense mechanisms is probably due to the difficulty of obtaining large numbers of purified parasites and the absence of a good laboratory animal model. The lack of understanding of factors that may increase or decrease the virulence of *Cryptosporidium* sp. can be attributed to the taxonomic confusion clouding the genus and to the paucity of research addressing the topic.

During 1985 and 1986 we succeeded in purifying large numbers of oocysts of *C. parvum* (human isolate) from calf feces and *C. baileyi* from chicken embryos (Fig. 49). These oocysts were used to immunize rabbits, and oocyst/sporozoite polypeptides separated by SDS-polyacrylamide gel electrophoresis (SDS-PAGE) were probed with the immune rabbit serum in an attempt to construct an antigenic library. Preliminary results of western blot analysis (Fig. 50) demonstrate that more than 40 oocyst/sporozoite antigens of both species of *Cryptosporidium* can be resolved by SDS–PAGE. These Western blots also demonstrate distinct banding patterns for the two species and a high degree of antigenic cross-reactivity. The importance of the various oocyst/sporozoite antigens and their role in stimulating host immunity merits further investigation,

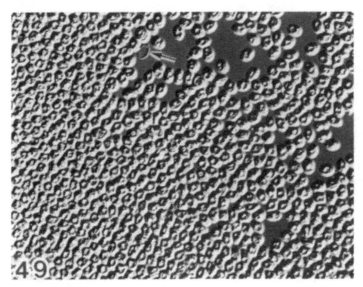

Figure 49 Nomarski interference micrograph of a wet mount of purified *Cryptosporidium baileyi* oocysts prior to freeze–thaw cycles (see legend for Fig. 50). These oocytes (measuring 6.2 X 4.6 μm) were obtained from chicken embryos inoculated previously with sporozoites of an isolate obtained from chickens (24). Arrow points to an empty oocyst.

as does the development of techniques for the recovery of large numbers of other developmental stages of the parasite.

Evading or suppressing host defense mechanisms has been shown to be of major importance to the survival of many parasite species. The way in which *Cryptosporidium* evades host defense mechanisms is unknown. In immunocompetent humans (2), suckling calves (9), and suckling mice (9), a primary gastrointestinal infection apparently stimulates an immune response of sufficient magnitude to clear the parasites and to render the host resistant for several months to oral challenge with infective oocysts. This suggests that *C. parvum* has not evolved elaborate mechanisms to evade or suppress the host immune response. Development of an immunocompetent adult rodent model for cryptosporidiosis is needed to pursue these and other important host–parasite interactions.

Differences in the virulence of various mammalian isolates of *C. parvum* and in their infectivity for laboratory and/or farm animals have been reported (see Ref. 2 for examples). It is possible that such differences in virulence may be responsible, at least in part, for differences in the severity of human cryptosporidiosis. Carefully controlled studies that eliminate differences in host factors

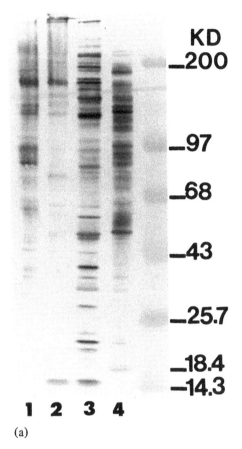

KD
_200

_97

_68

_43

_25.7

_18.4
_14.3

1 2 3 4

(a)

Figure 50 Western blot (enzyme immunotransfer blot) of oocyst/sporozoite antigens of two species of *Cryptosporidium*. Oocysts of *C. parvum* were purified from the feces of experimentally infected calves. Oocysts of *Cryptosporidium baileyi* were purified from the allantoic fluid of infected chicken embryos (Fig. 49). Oocysts were placed in 10 mM TRIS buffer (pH 8.0) with 2 mM phenyl methyl sulfonyl fluoride and ruptured by three freeze–thaw cycles (liquid nitrogen, $+40°C$). Following centrifugation ($15,000 \times g$, 30 min), the protein concentration of the supernate (soluble antigen) was determined (165). The soluble antigen and the pellet (membrane-enriched antigen) were placed in sample buffer containing SDS and 2-mercaptoethanol and boiled for 5 min. Lanes of 5–15% gradient, SDS-polyacrylamide slab gel were loaded with 20 μl of soluble (lanes 3 and 4) or membrane-enriched (lanes 1 and 2) oocyst/sporozoite antigen (~500 μg protein/ml), electrophoresed, and transblotted onto nitro-cellulose. The nitrocellulose sheets were probed with a 1:100 dilution of antisera from rabbits immunized with freeze–thaw-disrupted oocysts of *C. parvum*. The horseradish peroxidase-conjugated, affinity purified, goat anti-rabbit IgG (KPL

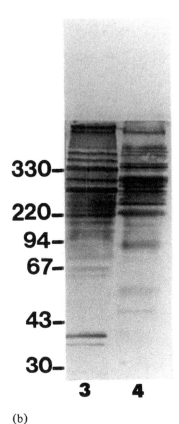

(b)

Figure 50 (Continued)

Laboratories) was diluted 1:1000. Further details of the procedures used are outlined elsewhere (166,167). (*a*) Lanes: 1, membrane-enriched antigens of *C. baileyi*; 2, membrane-enriched antigens of *C. parvum*; 3, soluble antigens of *C. parvum*; 4, soluble antigens of *C. baileyi*. (*b*) SDS was included in the transfer buffer to facilitate transfer to the high molecular weight antigens seen here. Lane 3, soluble antigens of *C. parvum*. Lane 4, soluble antigens of *C. baileyi*.

such as immune status, genetic background, nutritional status, and general health are needed to define the virulence factors associated with *Cryptosporidium* spp.

III. THE HOST

A. Host Defense Mechanisms

The extent of our knowledge of host defense mechanisms as it applies to cryptosporidiosis can be discussed from the standpoint of age resistance of the host or the development of acquired immunity. It is not easy, however, to separate these two factors, and future studies are likely to show that they often operate in conjunction to protect the host from clinical illness.

It has been our experience that virtually all suckling rodents—mice, rats, cotton rats, guinea pigs, and hamsters—develop heavy intestinal infections following oral inoculation of oocysts of calf and human isolates of *C. parvum* (2,9, 31). However, adults of these species cannot be infected, or they develop very mild infections with only a few parasites scattered through the mucosa of the ileum (46). Our attempts to develop an adult immunosuppressed mouse *C. parvum* model using cyclophosphamide therapy were disappointing. Immunosuppressive therapy did not increase the percentage of adult mice that developed infections nor did it result in heavier infections following challenge with *C. parvum*. Several of the immunosuppressed mice did, however, shed a small number of oocysts for several days beyond the normal patent period (unpublished data). Similar results—heavy infections in all neonates and very light infections in about half of the adults—were obtained following oral inoculation of oocysts of *Cryptosporidium* sp. into athymic nude mice and their immunocompetent, heterozygous littermates (73). The reasons for the apparently decreased susceptibility of older rodents is unknown, and its occurrence in other animals has not been sufficiently investigated. The absence of cryptosporidiosis in adult cattle has been attributed to age resistance; however, it may also be due to acquired immunity, since most calves are exposed to *Cryptosporidium* during the first month of life. Age resistance does not appear to be a significant factor in human cryptosporidiosis because infections occur in both children and adults.

In humans, the major factor controlling the susceptibility to and severity of cryptosporidiosis appears to be the immune status of the host. Immunocompetent persons usually have short-term (less than 2 weeks) gastrointestinal illness following oral exposure to oocysts, whereas individuals with immunodeficiencies may develop a prolonged, life-threatening gastrointestinal, respiratory, or hepatic infection (2). Such prolonged, life-threatening infections have been reported in patients undergoing immunosuppressive chemotherapy and in persons with congenital (e.g., hypogammaglobulinemia) and acquired (AIDS) immune deficiencies (see Section IV.A for additional details and references). Since at least one of the persons with hypogammaglobulinemia and prolonged crypto-sporidiosis was reported to have normal T-cell function (9), and since some AIDS patients with prolonged infections had high antibody titers to *Crypto-sporidium* (74), one may argue that both humoral and cell-mediated immunity are involved in the clearance of a gastrointestinal infection.

Our previous studies have demonstrated that most immunocompetent persons have serum antibodies specific to *Cryptosporidium* sp. that are detectable by an indirect immunofluorescent antibody assay for several months following recovery from gastrointestinal cryptosporidiosis (74). One of these individuals had an indirect immunofluorescent titer greater than 1:80 approximately 2 years after recovery. Serum obtained from this individual 2-3 months following recovery recognized more than 20 sporozoite/oocyst antigens of *C. parvum* separated by SDS-PAGE electrophoresis (unpublished data). Since *C. parvum* is apparently confined to the microvillous region of the intestinal mucosa of immunocompetent persons, it is difficult to support the concept that serum antibodies may play a major role in acquired immunity, especially since such a role has not been well established by extensive laboratory investigations of the development of immunity to other species of coccidia (75). It is more probable that local antibodies (intestinal IgA) coupled with cell-mediated immune mechanisms are required for the clearance of parasites from the gut. The importance of T cells for recovery from gastrointestinal cryptosporidiosis was suggested recently by a study monitoring the course of experimentally induced *C. parvum* infections in suckling athymic nude mice and their heterozygous, immunocompetent littermates. The immunocompetent white mice did not develop diarrhea and stopped shedding oocysts 21-30 days after inoculation, whereas the T-cell-deficient nude littermates developed diarrhea and shed oocysts in their feces until they died or until the experiment was terminated on day 56. It is doubtful that the immune mechanisms responsible for recovery from a primary infection and for resistance to subsequent oocyst challenge will be resolved until an immunocompetent adult rodent *Cryptosporidium* sp. model is developed.

B. Pathogenesis and Pathology

Most of our limited knowledge of the pathology and pathogenesis of human cryptosporidiosis has been derived from histological studies of intestinal tissues obtained from immunodeficient persons with the disease. In such patients, developmental stages of the protozoan have been found in the pharynx, esophagus, stomach, duodenum, jejunum, ileum, appendix, colon, and rectum (4-7,11, 12,124). Postmortem examination of three patients revealed that the jejunum was the most heavily infected region of the gut in all cases (7,8,78).

Histological lesions reported in heavily infected regions of the small intestine obtained from humans included villous atrophy, an increase in crypt length, and

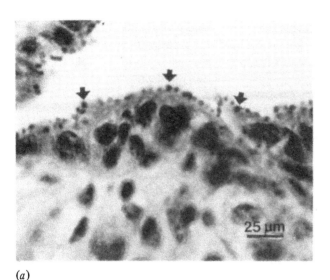

(*a*)

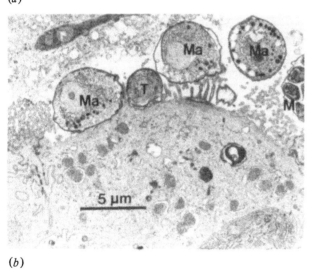

(*b*)

Figure 51 (*a*) Histological section (stained with H&E) of the ileum of a calf infected with *C. parvum*. Note the numerous endogenous stages of the parasite (arrows) in the microvillous region of cuboidal enterocytes covering a blunt villus. (*b*) Transmission electron micrograph showing endogenous stages of *C. parvum* in ileal enterocytes of an experimentally infected mouse. Ma, macrogametes; M, mature meront; T, uninucleate meront (trophozoite).

mild to moderate mononuclear cell infiltration of the lamina propria (4–8) (see Fig. 51). Similar microscopic lesions have been reported in the small intestine of experimentally infected mice (73), pigs (76), and lambs (77) and in the small (79) and large (80) intestines of germ-free calves monoinfected with *C. parvum*. Heine et al. (79) proposed that malabsorption due to villous atrophy of the small intestine was the basis for cryptosporidia-induced diarrhea in these germ-free calves. In a subsequent study, Pholenz et al. (80) reported that gnotobiotic calves monoinfected with *C. parvum* also had extensive colonization of the spiral colon by the parasite and that infected regions had marked erosion of epithelium. Thus, it appears that malabsorption and impaired digestion in the small intestine coupled with malabsorption in the large intestine are the major factors responsible for diarrhea in calves with cryptosporidiosis. Malabsorption has also been reported in immunsuppressed humans with cryptosporidiosis (8,11). However, the secretory (often described as choleralike) diarrhea common to many immunodeficient persons with cryptosporidiosis would suggest hypersecretion into the gut. Slow marker intestinal profusion tests of a patient with AIDS and a *Cryptosporidium* infection of the entire small bowel suggested profuse fluid secretion into the duodenum and proximal jejunum and normal reabsorption of water and sodium in the ileum and colon (81). At present, the pathophysiological mechanism(s) of *Cryptosporidium*-induced diarrhea are poorly defined. Definitive, systematic studies of the mechanisms by which *Cryptosporidium* sp. and its metabolites or toxins may alter normal intestinal function of a susceptible animal model are needed.

IV. THE DISEASE

A. Clinical Features

Gastrointestinal illness has been attributed to *Cryptosporidium* infections in a variety of animals, particularly calves and humans. Clinical features of cryptosporidiosis occurring in these two mammalian species as well as a variety of other animals are discussed below.

1. Calves

The role of *Cryptosporidium* sp. (*C. parvum*) as a cause of gastrointestinal illness in calves was first presented in the literature by Panciera et al. in 1971 (82). From 1976 to 1979, papers published by researchers in Iowa (28), Canada (83), and South Dakota (84) presented data supporting the view that *C. parvum* is a cause of neonatal bovine diarrhea. All of these studies relied on the recognition of endogenous stages of the parasite in the microvillous border of tissues obtained during necropsy. With the development of techniques to demonstrate oocysts in the feces (see Section IV.B), numerous papers have appeared within the past 10 years demonstrating that *Cryptosporidium* infections are prevalent and widespread in young calves [for representative papers, see Refs. 82-92].

Most cases of cryptosporidiosis in calves are reported as a diarrheal illness resulting in low to moderate mortality and moderate to high morbidity in animals 5-15 days of age. *Cryptosporidium* frequently occurs along with other enteropathogens of the neonatal calf diarrhea complex, such as rotavirus, coronavirus, enterotoxogenic *E. coli*, and *Salmonella* spp. In such multiple infections, the enteropathogens may act in combination to increase morbidity and mortality. High mortality also may occur when calves with cryptosporidiosis are exposed to extremely cold temperatures (84,93). Postmortem examination of these animals reveals that death is usually due to starvation (84,93). Apparently, malabsorption due to cryptosporidiosis prevents calves fed diets that are formulated for warm weather from meeting the additional energy demand when environmental temperatures are unusually low. Thus, when cryptosporidiosis is associated with high calf mortality, concurrent infections with other enteropathogens, cold weather, and perhaps poor management practices should be considered.

Difficulty in separating or identifying the roles of the different components of the neonatal calf diarrhea complex, along with the finding of asymptomatic *Cryptosporidium* sp. infections has led some to question the role of this coccidian as a primary pathogen (94). The controversy as to whether *Cryptosporidim* sp. is a true enteropathogen in the absence of other agents of enteric disease in calves has, to my satisfaction, been resolved. The typical clinical signs of diarrhea and malabsorption, and the characteristic lesions of villous blunting, atrophy, and fusion noted in naturally and experimentally infected animals also occur in gnotobiotic calves monoinfected with *C. parvum* (79). Heine et al. (79) suggested that malabsorption caused by villous atrophy resulting from accelerated loss of epithelium was the basis for *Cryptosporidium*-induced diarrhea in these calves. Similar findings also have been published for gnotobiotic pigs (95) and gnotobiotic lambs (96) that were reported to be moninfected with *C. parvum*. Thus, it appears that most of the *C. parvum* isolates studied to date are primary pathogens that cause diarrhea in calves. As with any primary enteropathogen, one should expect to find some animals infected with *C. parvum* that have no clinical signs of illness. The finding of large numbers of infected calves without diarrhea in a herd would suggest that different isolates of *C. parvum* may vary markedly in their virulence. Such differences in virulence have been suggested by others (1,94).

2. Sheep, Goats, Pigs, and Horses

Several other mammals commonly raised on farms have been reported to be susceptible to *Cryptosporidium* sp. (*C. parvum*) infection. Diarrhea associated with high morbidity and mortality has been attributed to natural (97,98) and experimentally induced (96,99–101) *Cryptosporidium* sp. infections in suckling lambs. As with calves, *Cryptosporidium* sp. appears to be an important cause of neonatal diarrhea in lambs. Young goats may also develop severe diarrhea following oral inoculation with *Cryptosporidium* sp. oocysts (9).

Natural (102,103) and experimentally induced (104) cryptosporidiosis in young pigs have also been associated with diarrheal illness. However, cryptosporidiosis appears to occur less frequently and to be a less severe disease in young pigs than in calves, lambs, and goats.

Cryptosporidiosis has been associated with diarrheal illness and mortality in immunodeficient foals (105) and nonfatal diarrhea in immunocompetent foals (106). The role of *Cryptosporidium* sp. as a cause of neonatal equine diarrhea merits further investigation.

3. Poultry

Cryptosporidium spp. have been reported to be recovered from the gastrointestinal and respiratory tracts of poultry. Intestinal (bursa of Fabricius and cloaca) cryptosporidiosis appears to be common among broiler chickens and has not been associated with overt clinical diseases (107–109). When the organism colonizes the epithelium of the upper respiratory tract of broilers, however, it can cause significant respiratory disease (110). Respiratory cryptosporidiosis, responsible for high morbidity and mortality, has also been reported for turkeys (111,112) and peacock chicks (113).

During the past several years I have been made aware of several outbreaks of respiratory cryptosporidiosis in broiler houses, particularly in the southeastern United States, most of which have resulted in increased morbidity and mortality. Several producers have suggested that respiratory cryptosporidiosis may also contribute to airsacculitis condemnation of broilers during processing. Although it is not known why sudden outbreaks of respiratory cryptosporidiosis occur, recent studies (44a) have shown that the same species of parasite commonly found in the bursa of Fabricius of broilers (*C. baileyi*) can produce respiratory disease in chickens and turkeys. Approximately a week after intratracheal inoculation of *C. baileyi* oocysts isolated from the bursa of Fabricius of commercial broilers, young turkeys and chickens may develop respiratory disease associated with extensive colonization of the mucosal epithelium by the parasite (unpublished data).

In addition to turkeys and chickens, the quail is another commercially reared species that is susceptible to clinical cryptosporidiosis. High mortality of young, commercially raised quail has been attributed to cryptosporidiosis of the small intestine (114) and the upper respiratory tract (115).

4. Companion and Wild Animals

Numerous other species of animals have been reported to be infected with *Cryptosporidium* spp. Of particular interest to physicians, veterinarians, and others interested in the epidemiology of cryptosporidiosis are clinical (usually diarrhea) and nonclinical infections reported in companion animals such as rodents, puppies, and kittens and in the wild mammals such as raccoons, foxes, coyotes, beavers, muskrats, and squirrels (Table 3). Cryptosporidiosis has also been reported as an important cause of neonatal diarrhea in exotic undulates raised in captivity (116).

5. Humans

The most common clinical feature of cryptosporidiosis in immunocompetent and immunodeficient persons is diarrhea, and it is this symptom that most often leads to diagnosis. Characteristically, the diarrhea is profuse and watery, it may contain mucus but rarely blood and leukocytes, and it is often associated with weight loss. A recent summary (3) of the clinical features of cryptosporidiosis recorded in case reports of persons with gastrointestinal cryptosporidiosis revealed that 63 of 67 patients with AIDS or AIDS-related complex (ARC), 16 of 17 persons with other immunodeficiencies, and 31 of 35 immunocompetent individuals had diarrhea. Other less common clinical features included abdominal pain, nausea and vomiting, and low-grade fever (<39°C). Occasionally, nonspecific symptoms such as myalgia, weakness, malaise, headache, and anorexia are reported (1-3). Severity of these symptoms may wax and wane in individual patients and often parallel the intensity of oocyst shedding (1-3). The duration of symptoms and outcome typically vary according to the immune status of the host. AIDS patients usually experience a prolonged, life-threatening illness, whereas most immunocompetent individuals experience a short-term illness with complete, spontaneous recovery. However, the clinical presentation of gastrointestinal cryptosporidiosis does not always fit within these two divergent categories. Persons with the clinical and laboratory features of AIDS have been known to clear *Cryptosporidium* sp. infections after several months of diarrhea, and persons reported to be immunocompetent have had prolonged infections lasting more than a month (10). Mild and even asymptomatic infections may occur in immunocompetent persons (9) as well as in patients with AIDS (117).

Immunocompetent Persons. Most of the 18 cases of cryptosporidiosis in immunocompetent humans reported prior to 1983 (46,47,128-132) and the numerous cases reported since then (48-54,58-72) describe a self-limited choleralike illness or a short-term, flulike, gastrointestinal illness. The most commonly reported symptoms in immunocompetent individuals with cryptosporidiosis are profuse, watery diarrhea (choleralike) and abdominal cramping, nausea, vomiting, low-grade fever, anorexia, and headache (flulike). Of the symptoms reported for 586 patients in 36 large-scale surveys (see Ref. 3 for references),diarrhea was the most commonly reported clinical feature (92%), followed by nausea and vomiting (51%), abdominal pain (45%), and low-grade fever (36%).

In most well-nourished persons, diarrheal illness due to *Cryptosporidium* sp. infection lasts from 3-12 days. Occasionally, these patients may require fluid replacement therapy, and occasionally the diarrheal illness may last for more than 2 weeks. In poorly nourished persons, especially children less than 2 years old, oral and parenteral rehydration therapy are often required because of extensive fluid loss. Although it is not common, young malnourished children with cryptosporidiosis may have diarrhea lasting for more than 3 weeks. Diarrheal illness is a major cause of morbidity and mortality, especially in young children living in developing countries. Estimates of Walsh and Warren suggest that in Asia, Africa, and Latin America there are as many as 5 billion episodes of diarrhea and 5-10 million diarrhea-associated deaths annually (133). Although recent surveys demonstrate that cryptosporidiosis is a major cause of diarrheal illness worldwide (2,3,58-72), it is not clear to what extent this protozoal disease contributes to morbidity and mortality. Additional, detailed studies employing the proper diagnostic tools should define more celarly the impact of cryptosporidiosis on human health in developing and developed countries.

Immunodeficient Persons. In the most severely immunodeficient hosts, such as patients with AIDS, diarrheal illness due to *Cryptosporidium* infection of the gastrointestinal tract becomes progressively worse and may be a major factor leading to death (9,11,13,14,120-122). It is believed that infection usually begins with the organism colonizing the ileal mucosa and develops into a life-threatening condition when a large portion of the gastrointestinal epithelium supports a virtual monolayer of parasites (2). Of the gastrointestinal pathogens identified in persons with AIDS, *Cryptosporidium* in the most ominous in its effects on morbidity and its contributions to mortality (123). Fluid loss by patients with AIDS and gastrointestinal cryptosporidiosis is often extensive; as noted above, 3-6 liters of diarrheic stool per day is common, and as much as 17 liters of watery feces per day has been reported (12).

Prolonged, life-threatening infections have also been documented in individuals on immunosuppressive chemotherapy (4,7,118,119) and persons with congenital immunodeficiencies such as hypogammaglobulinemia (5,8,9). However, in instances where the cause of immunosuppression is removed, patients may resolve their infections. For example, one child on immunosuppressive chemotherapy for lymphoblastic leukemia experienced two episodes of severe diarrhea due to cryptosporidiosis; both resolved spontaneously following withdrawal of immunosuppressive therapy (118). It also appears that persons at either end of the age spectrum or with nutritional deficiencies may respond like patients with immunodeficiencies (67,70).

In the immunodeficient person, *Cryptosporidium* infection is not always confined to the gastrointestinal tract. Acute and gangrenous cholecystitis in AIDS patients has been attributed to *Cryptosporidium* infections of the biliary tree and gall bladder epithelium (14,124,125). Respiratory tract infections with

Cryptosporidium sp. have been associated with chronic coughing, dyspnea, bronchiolitis, and pneumonitis in persons with AIDS (13,126) and in an infant with severe combined immune deficiency (127). Diarrhea and respiratory infection attributed to *Cryptosporidium* infection have also been associated with the acute phase of measles, a cause of transient immunosuppression (123a,123b). The importance of *Cryptosporidium* sp. as a cause of pulmonary and hepatic disease in immunodeficient and perhaps in immunocompetent persons merits further investiation.

B. Diagnosis

Prior to 1980, diagnosis of human cryptosporidiosis required identification of the small spherical endogenous stages of *Cryptosporidium* sp. in the microvillous region of the intestinal mucosa obtained by biopsy and subsequent processing for examination by light or electron microscopy (Fig. 51). Such invasive, time-consuming procedures are no longer required, since a variety of techniques have been developed for identifying *Cryptosporidium* sp. oocysts in fecal specimens (9,85,137-140). Intestinal biopsy may still be useful to determine the region of the gut infected with *Cryptosporidium* sp. and to ascertain histopathological changes that may occur in the affected region.

1. Specimen Collection and Treatment

Biopsy specimens should be fixed appropriately and submitted for histological or cytological processing and examination. Fecal specimens can be submitted as fresh material, in 10% formalin, or in sodium acetate–acetic acid–formalin (SAF) preservatives. Most of the recommended stains for demonstrating *Cryptosporidium* oocysts cannot be performed from stool preserved in polyvinyl alcohol (PVA) fixative. Because many clinical laboratories are now using a single collection vial (PVA) from which routine examinations for parasites can be performed, a vial of 10% formalin may have to be included in the system to accommodate requests for *Cryptosporidium*.

The number of oocysts can vary from specimen to specimen; thus, multiple stool samples should be submitted, particularly in the case of mild infections. In formed stools, the number of oocysts present is usually small, and they are often difficult to find.

Because respiratory cryptosporidiosis has been reported in immunodeficient patients (13,126,127), sputum samples from such patients with undiagnosed respiratory illness should be placed in 10% formalin and examined for *Cryptosporidium* oocysts using one of the techniques described below.

2. Identification of Oocysts

Oocysts seen in direct smears or concentration procedures are generally round and measure from 4 to 6 μm. Unless the numbers are many and the viewer is experienced in identifying *Cryptosporidium* oocysts, it is easy to confuse these resistant forms of the parasite with yeast cells. Depending on the type and quality of the optics used, internal details such as the four sporozoites and the granular oocyst residuum (Figs. 16, 46–48, and 52) may or may not be visible.

Fecal specimens obtained from most hosts (animals and humans) with the watery diarrhea typical of gastrointestinal cryptosporidiosis should contain large numbers of oocysts, and the use of most published concentration (9,85) or staining (134-139) techniques developed for identification of *Cryptosporidium* oocysts should result in a positive diagnosis. However, some fecal samples contain only a few oocysts, making it difficult for the medical microbiologist or the veterinary diagnostician to decide if one or two *Cryptosporidium*-like bodies seen in a stained fecal smear warrant a positive diagnosis. This is especially true for poorly prepared, acid-fast-stained smears because of the small spherical objects other than *Cryptosporidium* oocysts in some stool samples that may appear to be acid-fast. Increased sensitivity can be achieved by using one of several oocyst concentration techniques such as Sheather's sugar flotation (85). Material concentrated from stool samples can be examined prior to (9) or after (134) staining.

The routine stains (trichrome, iron hematoxylin) used for stool diagnosis of other parasites are not acceptable for the identification of *Cryptosporidium* oocysts. Several widely used techniques for demonstrating *Cryptosporidium* sp. oocysts in fecal specimens from animals and humans are modified acid-fast staining (134-136), negative staining (137,138), and Sheather's sugar flotation (9,85). Acid-fast staining procedures are effective because they stain the oocyst wall red and contaminating yeast cells take on the background stain. The negative staining procedure employs a stain, such as Kinyouin's modified carbol fuchsin or safranin, that stains everything (including yeast) except the oocysts. The oocysts are bright and refractile, because they contain water and are covered with immersion oil (Fig. 52). *Cryptosporidium* oocysts concentrated by Sheather's sugar solution are bright and refractile when viewed with phastcontrast microscopy; yeasts are not refractile (Fig. 52). Although the last two procedures are used routinely in our research laboratory, acid-fast staining is usually the method of choice for the clinical laboratory. All three procedures are relatively simple, rapid, and inexpensive and will allow one to distinguish *Cryptosporidium* oocysts from the yeasts commonly found in stool specimens. As noted previously, considerable experience is required with the concentration and staining procedures to obtain an accurate diagnosis. For this reason, the use of polyclonal or monoclonal antibodies that are specific for *Cryptosporidium* oocysts should be helpful in providing a more sensitive method of detecting organisms by less experienced technicians. Fluorescent detection of *Cryptosporidium* oocysts in human fecal specimens by the use of monoclonal antibodies has been reported recently (140).

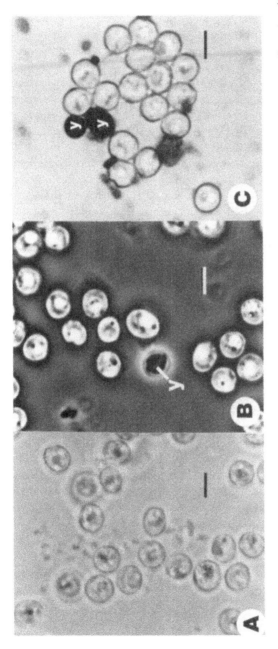

Figure 52 Oocysts of *C. parvum* from fecal specimens. (A) Bright-field photomicrograph of Sheather's sugar flotation (85). (B) Phase-contrast photomicrograph of Sheather's sugar flotation (9). Oocysts are bright and refractile, and contain one to six prominent dark granules. Yeasts (y) are not refractile. (C) Kinyoun's carbol fuchsin negative stain (137,138) of oocysts in fecal smear. Oocysts are bright and refractile, whereas yeasts (y) are darkly stained. Bars represent 5 μm.

Any laboratory faced with the task of diagnosing cryptosporidiosis should have one or more persons who become familiar with two techniques, one technique to be used as the primary diagnostic procedures and the other as a back-up procedure for specimens that give confusing results with the first method. Good quality, *Cryptosporidium*-positive fecal specimens should be available while laboratory personnel are becoming familiar with the techniques of choice and as a reference source while the diagnostic procedures are performed. Many laboratories may obtain good reference specimens through routine submissions. If stool samples containing *Cryptosporidium* sp. oocysts are stored cold (4°C) in either 2.5% potassium dichromate or 10% formalin, they should remain useful for at least 12 months (2).

Now that several rapid, inexpensive, and reliable techniques for identifying *Cryptosporidium* oocysts in fecal specimens are available, cryptosporidiosis should be considered in the routine diagnosis of diarrheal illness in humans. If supervisors of clinical laboratories choose not to consider cryptosporidiosis in the routine diagnosis of diarrheal illness, they should at least consider it for all specimens of watery diarrhea, even if the specific evaluation is not requested by a physician. Veterinarians and veterinary diagnosticians may consider incorporating these diagnostic procedures into health-monitoring programs for pets, especially if the pet owners are immunocompromised. Physicians may consider the use of these diagnostic procedures prior to placing patients on immunosuppressive chemotherapy. Delaying immunosuppressive chemotherapy until after a mild or subclinical *Cryptosporidium* sp. infection is resolved may avoid a life-threatening diarrheal illness.

3. Serodiagnosis

Antibodies specific to *Cryptosporidium* have been detected by an indirect immunofluorescent antibody (IFA) procedure in the sera of persons who recovered from confirmed infections (74), and the IFA procedure has been used for the presumptive diagnosis of cryptosporidiosis in two clusterings of cases (10,52). Specific anti-*Cryptosporidium* IgG and or IgM were also detected by an enzyme-linked immunosorbent assay in 95% of patients with cryptosporidiosis at the time of medical presentation and in 100% within 2 weeks of presentation (140a). Several serological surveys have reported that more than 50% of persons with no known infection may have *Cryptosporidium*-specific IgG, suggesting that infection at some time during life is common (140a,140b). The use of these serodiagnostic techniques has thus far been limited to only a few laboratories, and additional evaluation is needed to ascertain if they will be of any use for clinical diagnosis.

C. Treatment

Treatment of cryptosporidiosis in a previously healthy, immunocompetent person is usually not necessary, since the duration of diarrhea almost always is less than 20 days and since clinical symptoms and oocyst shedding resolve spontaneously. On the other hand, cryptosporidiosis can be prolonged and life-threatening in immunodeficient patients, and an effective therapy is needed. To date, treatment of cryptosporidiosis in immunodeficient persons has been frustrating and unsuccessful in most cases; there have been no controlled studies and all therapeutic information is based on isolated reports. The list of unsuccessful attempts to treat cryptosporidiosis in immunodeficient persons is growing rapidly. Many of these attempts have been reviewed in recent papers (3,11,141,142) and are listed in Table 5. Some therapies reported to be of value in the treatment of cryptosporidiosis in immunodeficient persons are discussed below.

1. Antimicrobial/Antiparasite Agents

Of the numerous antimicrobial and antiparasitic drugs administered to immunodeficient persons with intestinal cryptosporidiosis, spiramycin is the only one reported to have some efficacy; spiramycin, a macrolide antibiotic, administered orally at 3 g/day was reported to control diarrhea in nine patients with AIDS and cryptosporidiosis (143). However, some of these AIDS patients continued to shed *Cryptosporidium* sp. oocysts in their feces. Other physicians have reported to me that spiramycin therapy is of little value in the treatment of cryptosporidiosis in persons with AIDS. These conflicting reports may be explained, in part, by a report that spiramycin therapy may control diarrhea in some patients treated for cryptosporidiosis early in the progression of AIDS but does not appear to have any effect on the course of clinical cryptosporidiosis in patients who have progressed into the later stages of AIDS (144). Carefully controlled studies are needed to determine if spiramycin therapy is effective in the treatment of cryptosporidiosis in immunodeficient persons.

2. Immunomodulation

The major factor determining the severity and duration of a *Cryptosporidium* infection appears to be the immune status of the host. Discontinuing immunosuppressive chemotherapy, allowing restoration of the immune function, has resulted in clearance of cryptosporidiosis from the intestinal tract of several patients (4,118,119). These findings suggest that immunomodulation or passive transfer of antibodies or lymphocytes may be of value in the treatment of cryptosporidiosis in immunodeficient patients.

I know of at least one patient who has been given serum from three persons with high antibody titers to *C. parvum*. In addition, lymphocytes were obtained from immune donors, irradiated, and given to the patient, who had hypogammaglobulinemia and cryptosporidiosis. Passive transfer of immune serum and lymphocytes had no effect on the course of cryptosporidiosis in this immunodeficient patient.

Mata et al. (60) reported a lower incidence of cryptosporidiosis in breast-fed

Table 5 Antimicrobial/Antiparasitic Agents and Preventive Modalities Used for *Cryptosporidium* Infections[a]

Amphotericin B (h)	Glucose + amino acids (h)
Ampicillin (h,a)	Gluten-free diet (h)
Amprolium (h,a)	Halofuginone (a)
Arpinocin (a)	Indometacin (h)
Bismuth salicylate (h)	Interferon (h)
Bleomycin (a)	Interleukin 2 (h)
Bovine transfer factor (h)	Iodoquinol (h)
Cabenicillin (h)	Ipronidazole (a)
Cefamandole (h)	Ivermectin (a)
Chloramphenicol (a)	Ketoconazole (h)
Chloroquine (h)	Lactose-free diet (h)
Cholestyramine (h)	Lasalocid (a)
Cimetadine (h)	Levamisol (h)
Clindamycin (h)	Lincomycin (a)
Clondine (h)	Loperamide (h)
Clopidol (a)	Mepacrine (h)
Cloxacillin (h)	Methylbenzoquate (a)
Colistin (h)	Metronidazole (h,a)
Cotrimoxazole (h)	Monensin (a)
Decoquinate (a)	Naproxyn (h)
Difluoromethyl-ornithine (h,a)	Neomycin (a)
Diloxanide furoate (h)	Nicarbazin (a)
Dimetridazole (a)	Nystatin (a)
Dinitolmide (a)	Paragonic (h)
Diphenoxylate HCl (h)	Paramomycin (h)
Doxycycline (h)	Penicillin (h)
Emtryl (a)	Pentamidine (h)
Enterolyte N (a)	Phenamidine (a)
Erythromycin (a)	Piperazine (a)
Ethopabate (a)	Primaquine (h)
Furaltadone (a)	Pyrimethamine (h)
Furazolidone (h,a)	Quinacrine (h,a)
Gamma globulin (h)	Quinine (h)
Gentamicin (h,a)	Robenidine (a)

Table 5 Antimicrobial/Antiparasitic Agents and Preventive Modalities Used for
Cryptosporidium Infections (Continued)

Salinomycin (h,a)	Thiabendazole (h)
Septrin (h)	Trimethoprim (h,a)
Spectinomycin (a)	Trimethoprimsulfamethoxazole (h,a)
Spiramycin (h)	Tincture of opium (h)
Streptomycin (h)	Trinamide (a)
Sulfonamides (h,a)	Vancomycin (h)
Tetracycline (h)	Zoaquin (a)

h denotes use reported in humans; a denotes use reported in animals other than humans.
Source: Adapted in part from Ref. 3.

infants compared to babies fed artificial diets and suggested that lactogenic
immunity may be of some value in preventing cryptosporidiosis in neonates.
Lactogenic immunity doses not appear to play a role in altering the course of
cryptosporidiosis in suckling calves or mice. In our research facility, calves are
routinely infected by mixing oocysts of *C. parvum* with the first liter of colostrum fed. These calves then receive an additional 1-2 liters of colostrum during
the next 36 hr. High antibody titers (primarily IgG) were found by indirect
immunofluorescence (10,74,122) in three of four of the colustrum samples
examined. The presence or absence of colostrum antibodies against *Cryptosporidium* sp. had no apparent effect on the course of cryptosporidiosis in these
calves (unpublished data). Similarly, female mice that recovered from neonatal
cryptosporidiosis and that were challenged orally with *C. parvum* oocysts during
gestation did not confer protective lactogenic immunity to their offspring that
were challenged with *C. parvum* oocysts (145). Bovine colostrum containing
antibodies (IgG) to *Cryptosporidium* sp. administered orally for several days was
of no value in the treatment of cryptosporidiosis in one patient with AIDS
(145a). Additional studies are needed to determine the role of lactogenic immunity in preventing cryptosporidiosis in neonates.

Transfer factor prepared from lymphoid cells obtained from calves immune
to *C. parvum* was recently reported to be effective in the treatment of cryptosporidiosis in several AIDS patients (146). Oral administration of the bovine
transfer factor resulted in resolution of diarrhea in six of seven patients with
cryptosporidiosis and AIDS. Four of these patients also stopped shedding
Cryptosporidium sp. oocysts in their feces. One patient showed no symptomatic
or parasitological improvement during or following bovine transfer factor
therapy. More extensive studies are needed to confirm the results obtained in

this small number of AIDS patients and to determine if transfer factor therapy is of any value in the treatment of cryptosporidiosis in persons with AIDS and other types of immunodeficiencies.

3. Supportive Therapy

Oral or parenteral rehydration therapy is often required by both immuno-deficient and immunocompetent persons with severe cryptosporidial diarrhea, especially young children. Parenteral nutrition may help sustain the nutritional status of some immunodeficient patients with persistent cryptosporidiosis; however, this procedure has not been successful in sustaining many persons with AIDS and cryptosporidiosis. Until an effective drug is found to treat crypto-sporidiosis, supportive care with oral or intravenous hydration therapy is the only therapeutic intervention available to most clinicians.

4. Prevention

It is well established that cryptosporidiosis is transmitted by environmentally resistant oocysts via the fecal-oral route common to other enteric pathogens (1-3). In addition to direct transmission from human to human or from animal to human (see Table 3 for possible reservoir hosts), infection is also acquired through ingestion of contaminated food or water containing viable oocysts (1-3). Measures to prevent infection include good personal hygiene, proper disposal of fecal material, proper treatment of drinking water, and avoidance of contact with infected hosts. These measures have been effective against other feces-borne enteropathogens and should be successful in eliminating transmission of *Cryptosporidium* infections.

REFERENCES

1. Tzipori, S. Cryptosporidiosis in animals and humans. *Microbiol. Rev. 47*: 48–96 (1983).
2. Current, W. L. *Cryptosporidium* and cryptosporidiosis. In *Acquired Immune Deficiency Syndrome* (M. S. Gottlib, and J. E. Groopman, eds.). UCLA Symposia on Molecular and Cellular Biology, New Series, *16*:355–373 (1984).
3. Fayer, R., and Unger, B. L. P. *Cryptosporidium* spp. and cryptosporidiosis. *Microbiol. Rev. 50*:458–483 (1986).
4. Meisel, J. L., Perera, D. R., Meligro, C., and Rubin, C. E. Overwhelming watery diarrhea associated with *Cryptosporidium* in an immunosuppressed patient. *Gastroenterology 70*:1156–1160 (1976).
5. Lasser, K. H., Lewin, K. J., and Ryning, F. W. Cryptosporidial enteritis in a patient with congenital hypogammaglobulinemia. *Human Pathol. 10*:234–240 (1979).
6. Stemmerman, G. N., Hayaski, T., Glober, G. A., Oishi, N., and Frankel, R. I. Cryptosporidiosis: report of a fatal case complicated by disseminated toxoplasmosis. *Am. J. Med. 69*:637–642 (1980).

7. Weisburger, W. R., Hutcheon, D. F., Yardley, J. H., Roche, J. C., Hillis, W. D., and Charache, P. Cryptosporidiosis in an immunosuppressed renal-transplant recipient with IgA deficiency. *Am. J. Clin. Pathol.* 72:473–478 (1979).

8. Sloper, K. S., Dourmashkin, R. R., Bird, R. B., Slavin, G., and Webster, A. B. D. Chronic malabsorption due to cryptosporidiosis in a child with immunoglobulin deficiency. *Gut.* 23:80–82 (1982).

9. Current, W. L., Reese, N. C., Ernst, J. V., Bailey, W. S., Heyman, M. B., and Weinstein, M. D. Human cryptosporidiosis in immunocompetent and immunodeficient persons: studies of an outbreak and experimental transmission. *New Engl. J. Med.* 308:1252–1257 (1983).

10. Koch, K. L., Phillips, D. J., Aber, R. C., and Current, W. L. Cryptosporidiosis in hospital personnel: evidence for person-to-person transmission. *Ann. Intern. Med.* 102:593–596 (1985).

11. Navin, T. R., and Juranek, D. D. Cryptosporidiosis: clinical, epidemiologic, and parasitologic review. *Rev. Infect. Dis.* 6:313–327 (1984).

12. Centers for Disease Control. Cryptosporidiosis: assessment of chemotherapy of males with acquired immune deficiency syndrome (AIDS). *Morb. Mortal. Wkly. Rep.* 31:589–592 (1982).

13. Forgacs, P., Tarshis, A., Ma, P., Federman, M., Mele, L., Silverman, M. L., and Shea, J. A. Intestinal and bronchial cryptosporidiosis in an immunodeficient homosexual man. *Ann. Intern. Med.* 99:793–794 (1983).

14. Guarda, L. A., Stein, S. A., Cleary, K. A., and Ordonez, N. G. Human cryptosporidiosis in the acquired immune deficiency syndrome. *Arch. Pathol. Lab. Med.* 107:562–566 (1983).

15. Levine, N. D. Taxonomy and review of the coccidian genus *Cryptosporidium* (Protozoa: Aplicomplexa). *J. Protozool.* 31:94–98 (1984).

16. Clarke, J. J. A study of coccidia met with in mice. *J. Microsc. Sci.* 37:277–302 (1895).

17. Tyzzer, E. E. A sporozoan found in the peptic glands of the common mouse. *Proc. Soc. Exp. Biol. Med.* 5:12–13 (1907).

18. Tyzzer, E. E. An extracellular coccidium *Cryptosporidium muris* (gen. et sp. nov.) of the gastric glands of the common mouse. *J. Med. Res.* 23:487–509 (1910).

19. Tyzzer, E. E. *Cryptosporidium parvum* (sp. nov.), a coccidian found in the small intestine of the common mouse. *Arch. Protistenkd.* 26:394–418 (1912).

20. Tzipori, S., Angus, K. W., Campbell, I., and Gray, E. W. *Cryptosporidium*: evidence for a single-species genus. *Infect. Immun.* 30:884–886 (1980).

21. Triffit, M. J. Observations on two new species of coccidia parasitic in snakes. *Protozoology* 1:19–26 (1925).

22. Hoare, C. A. Studies on some new ophidian and avian coccidia from Uganda, with a revision of the classification of the *Eimeriidae. Parasitology* 25:359–388 (1933).

23. Vetterling, J. M., Jarvis, H. R., Merrill, T. G., and Sprinz, H. *Cryptosporidium wrairi* sp. n. from the guinea pig *Cavia porcellus*, with an emendation of the genus. *J. Protozool. 18*:243–247 (1971).

24. Current, W. L., Upton, S. J., and Haynes, T. B. The life cycle of *Cryptosporidium baileyi* n. sp. (Apicomplexa, Cryptosporidiae) infecting chickens. *J. Parasitol. 33*:289–196 (1986).

25. Slavin, D. *Cryptosporidium meleagridis* (sp. nev). *J. Comp. Pathol. 62*: 262–266 (1955).

26. Upton, S. J., and Current, W. L. The species of *Cryptosporidium* (Apicomplexa: Cryptosporiidae) infecting mammals. *J. Parasitol. 71*:625–629 (1985).

27. Vetterling, J. M., Takeuchi, A., and Madden, P. A. Ultrastructure of *Cryptosporidium wrairi* from the guinea pig. *J. Protozool. 18*:248–260 (1971).

28. Pholenz, J., Bemrick, W. J., Moon, H. W., and Cheville, N. F. Bovine cryptosporidiosis: a transmission and scanning electron microcopic study of some stages in the life cycle of the host-parasite relationship. *Vet. Pathol. 15*:417–427 (1978).

29. Iseki, M. *Cryptosporidium felis* sp. n. (Protozoa: Eimeriorina) from the domestic cat. *Jap. J. Parasitol. 28*:285–307 (1979).

30. Angus, K. W., Hutchison, G., and Munro, H. M. C. Infectivity of a strain of *Cryptosporidium* found in the guinea pig (*Cavia porcellus*) for guinea pigs, mice and lambs. *J. Comp. Pathol. 95*:151–165 (1985).

31. Current, W. L., and Reese, N. C. A comparison of endogenous development of three isolates of *Cryptosporidium* in suckling mice. *J. Protozool. 33*:98–108 (1986).

32. Current, W. L., and Long, P. L. Development of human and calf *Cryptosporidium* in chicken embryos. *J. Infect. Dis. 148*:1108–1113 (1983).

33. Current, W. L., and Haynes, T. B. Complete development of *Cryptosporidium* in cell culture. *Science 224*:603–605 (1984).

34. Doran, D. J., and Farr, M. M. Excystation of the poultry coccidium *Eimeria acervulina*. *J. Protozool. 9*:154–161 (1962).

35. Nyberg, P. A., Bauer, D. H., and Knapp, S. E. Carbon dioxide as the initial stimulus of excystation of *Eimeria tenella* oocysts. *J. Protozool. 15*:144–148 (1968).

36. Fayer, R., and Leek, R. G. Excystation of *Sarcocystis fusiforms* sporocysts from dogs. *Proc. Helminthol. Soc. Wash. 40*:294–296 (1973).

37. Christie, E., Pappas, P. W., and Dubey, J. P. Ultrastructure of excystment of *Toxoplasma gondii* oocysts. *J. Protozool. 25*:438–443 (1978).

38. Box, E. P., Marchiondo, A. A., Duszynski, D. W., and Davis, C. P. Ultrastructure of *Sarcocystis* sporocysts from passerine birds and opossums: comments on the classification of the genus *Isospora*. *J. Parasitol. 66*:68–74 (1980).

39. Reduker, D. W., and Speer, C. A. Factors influencing excystation in *Cryptosporidium* oocysts from cattle. *J. Parasitol. 71*:112–115 (1985).

40. Fayer, R., and Leek, R. G. The effects of reducing conditions, medium, pH,

temperature, and time on in vitro excystation of *Cryptosporidium*. *J. Protozool. 31*:567–569 (1984).

41. Reduker, D. W., Speer, C. A., and Blixt, J. A. Ultrastructure of *Cryptosporidium* oocysts and excysting sporozoites as revealed by high resolution scanning electron microscopy. *J. Protozool. 32*:708–711 (1985).

42. Brandler, U. Licht- und elektronenmikroskopische Untersuchungen der Entwicklung von *Cryptosporidium* sp. in Darm experimentell infizierter Mäuse. *Vet. Med. Diss.*, München, 1982, 54 pp.

43. Goebel, E., and Brandler, U. Ultrastructure of microgametogenesis, microgametes, and gametogony of *Cryptosporidium* sp. in the small intestine of mice. *Protistologica 18*:331–334 (1982).

44. Heine, J., Moon, H. W., Woodmansee, D. B., and Pholenz, J. F. L. Experimental tracheal and conjunctive infections with *Cryptosporidium* sp. in pigs. *Vet. Parasitol. 17*:17–25 (1984).

44a. Blagburn, B. L., Lindsay, D. S., Giambrone, J. J., Sunderman, C. A., and Hoerr, F. J. Experimental cryptosporidiosis in broiler chickens. *Poultry Sci. 66*:442–449 (1987).

45. Campbell, I., Tzipori, S., Hutchison, G., and Angus, K. W. The effect of disinfectants on survival of *Cryptosporidium* oocysts. *Vet Rec. 111*:414–415 (1982).

46. Reese, N. C., Current, W. L., Ernst, J. V., and Bailey, W. S. Cryptosporidiosis of man and calf: a case report and results of experimental infections in mice and rats. *Am. J. Trop. Med. Hyg. 31*:226–229 (1982).

47. Anderson, B. C., Donndelinger, T., Wilkins, R. M., and Smith, J. Cryptosporidiosis in a veterinary student. *J. Am. Vet. Med. Assoc. 180*:408–409 (1982).

48. Blagburn, B. L., and Current, W. L. Accidental infection of a researcher with human *Cryptosporidium*. *J. Infect. Dis. 148*:772–773 (1983).

49. Alpert, G., Bell, L. M., Kirkpatrick, C. E., Budnick, L. D., Campos, J. M., Friedman, H. M., and Poltkin, S. A. Cryptosporidiosis in a day care center. *New Engl. J. Med. 311*:860–861 (1984).

50. Centers for Disease Control. Cryptosporidiosis among children attending day care centers—Georgia, Pennsylvania, Michigan, California, New Mexico. *Morb. Mortal. Wkly. Rep. 33*:599–601 (1984).

51. Baxby, D., Hart, C. A., and Taylor, C. Human cryptosporidiosis: a possible case of hospital cross infection. *Br. Med. J. 287*:1760–1761 (1983).

52. D'Antonio, R. G., Winn, R. E., Taylor, J. P., Gustafson, T. L., Current, W. L., Rhodes, M. M., Gary, G. W., and Zajac, R. A. A waterborne outbreak of cryptosporidiosis in normal hosts. *Ann. Intern. Med. 103*:886–888 (1986).

53. Soave, R., and Ma, P. Cryptosporidiosis traveler's diarrhea in 2 families. *Arch. Intern. Med. 145*:70–72 (1985).

54. Jokipii, L., Pohjola, S., and Jokipii, A. M. M. *Cryptosporidium*: a frequent finding in patients with gastrointestinal symptoms. *Lancet 1*:358–361 (1983).

55. Jakubowski, W., and Erikson, T. H. Methods for detection of *Giardia* cysts in water supplies. In *Waterborne Transmission of Giardiasis*, U.S.-EPA, EPA-60019-79-001 (W. Jakubowski and J. C. Hoff, eds.). National Technical Information Service, Springfield, Va., 1979.

56. Sterling, C. R., and Arrowood, M. J. Detection of *Cryptosporidium* sp. infections using a direct immunofluorescent assay. *Pediatr. Infect. Dis. 5*: 5139–5142 (1986).

57. Ongerth, J. E., and Stibbs, H. H. Detection of *Cryptosporidium* in water by using polyproylene cartridge filters. *Appl. Environ. Microbiol. 53*:672–676 (1987). 60th Ann. Meeting, Am. Soc. Parasitol., Athens, Ga., Aug. 4–8, 1985, Abstr. No. 100.

58. Tzipori, S., Smith, M., Birch, C., Barnes, G., and Bishop, R. Cryptosporidiosis in hospital patients with gastroenteritis. *Am. J. Trop. Med. Hyg. 32*: 931–934 (1983).

59. Mata, L., Bolaños, H., Pizarro, D., and Vives, M. Cryptosporidiosis in children from some highland Costa Rican rural and urban areas. *Am. J. Trop. Med. Hyg. 33*:24–29 (1984).

60. Mata, L., Bolaños, H., Pizarro, D., and Vives, M. Cryptosporidiosis en niños de Costa Rica: estudio transversal y longitudinal. *Rev. Biol. Trop. 32*:129–135 (1984).

61. Hart, C. A., Baxby, D., and Blundell, N. Gastroenteritis due to *Cryptosporidium*: a prospective survey in a children's hospital. *J. Infect. 9*:264–270 (1984).

62. Holley, P., Westphal, M., and Dover, C. Cryptosporidiosis—a common cause of parasitic diarrhea in children. *Pediatr. Res. 19*:296 (1985).

63. Richter, J. M., Wolfsen, J. S., Waldron, M. A., and McCarthy, D. M. Cryptosporidiosis in immunocompetent patients. *Gastroenterology 88*:1555 (1985).

64. Weikel, C. S., Johnson, L. I., DeSousa, M. A., and Cuerrant, R. L. Cryptosporidiosis in northeastern Brazil: association with sporadic diarrhea. *J. Infect. Dis. 151*:963–965 (1985).

65. Seegar, J. K., Gilman, R. H., Galarza, T., Black, R. E., Brown, K. H., Demarini, J. C., and Rojas, V. *Cryptosporidium*—an important agent of infantile diarrhea in Peru. 33rd Ann. Meeting. Am. Soc. Trop. Med. Hyg., Boston, 1984, Abstr. No. 369.

66. Smith, G. *Cryptosporidium* in association with diarrheal disease in South Africa. *S. Afr. Med. J. 67*:442 (1985).

67. Shahid, N. S., Rahaman, A. S. M.H., Anderson, B. C., Mata, L. J., and Sanyal, S. C. Cryptosporidiosis in Bangladesh. *Br. Med. J. 290*:114–115 (1985).

68. Portus, M., Serra, T., Botet, J., and Gallego, J. Cryptosporidiosis humana en España. *Med. Clin. 84*:462 (1985).

69. Holten-Andersen, W., Gerstoft, J., Henriksen, S. A., and Pedersen, N. S. Prevalence of *Cryptosporidium* among patients with acute enteric infections. *J. Infect. 9*:277–282 (1984).

70. Bogaerts, J., Lepage, P., Rouvony, D., and Vandepitte, J. *Cryptosporidium* spp., a frequent cause of diarrhea in central Africa. *J. Clin. Microbiol. 20*: 874–876 (1984).
71. Hojlyny, N., Molbak, K., Jepsen, S., and Hansson, A. P. Cryptosporidiosis In Liberian children. *Lancet 1*:734 (1984).
72. Pape, J. W., Levine, E., Marshall, F., Bealieu, M. E., and Johnson, W. D. Cryptosporidiosis in Haitian children. *Clin. Res. 33*:414 (1985).
73. Heine, J., Moon, H. W., and Woodmansee, D. B. Persistent *Cryptosporidium* infection in congenitally athymic (nude) mice. *Infect. Immun. 43*:856–859 (1984).
74. Campbell, P. N., and Current, W. L. Demonstration of serum antibodies to *Cryptosporidium* sp. in normal and immunodeficient humans with confirmed infections. *J. Clin. Microbiol. 18*:165–169 (1983).
75. Rose, M. E. Host immune responses. In *The Biology of the Coccidia* (P. L. Long, ed.). University Park Press, Baltimore, 1982, pp. 329–371.
76. Moon, H. W., and Bemrick, W. J. Fecal transmission of calf cryptosporidia between calves and pigs. *Vet. Pathol. 18*:248–255 (1981).
77. Angus, K. W., Tzipori, S., and Gray, E. W. Intestinal lesions in specific pathogen-free lambs associated with a *Cryptosporidium* from calves with diarrhea. *Vet. Pathol. 19*:587–592 (1982).
78. Boothe, C. C., Slavin, G., and Dourmashkin, R. R. Immunodeficiency and cryptosporidiosis. Demonstration at the Royal College of Physicians of London. *Br. Med. J. 281*:1123–1127 (1983).
79. Heine, J., Pholenz, J. F. L., Moon, H. W., and Woode, G. N. Enteric lesions and diarrhea in gnotobiotic calves monoinfected with *Cryptosporidium* species. *J. Infect. Dis. 150*:768–775 (1984).
80. Pholenz, J. F. L., Woode, G. N., and Woodmansee, D. Typhlitis and colitis in gnotobiotic calves experimentally infected with 10^8–10^9 chemically purified *Cryptosporidium* oocysts. Conf. of Research Workers in Animal Disease, Chicago, Nov. 12–13, 1984, Abstr. No. 273.
81. Andrean, T., Modigliani, R., Charpentier, Y., Calian, A., Brouet, J. C., Liance, M., Lachance, J. R., Messing, B., and Vernisse, B. Acquired immunodeficiency with intestinal cryptosporidiosis: possible transmission by Haitian whole blood. *Lancet*, May 28, 1187–1191 (1983).
82. Panciera, R. J., Thomassen, R. W., and Garner, F. M. Cryptosporidial infection in a calf. *Vet. Pathol. 8*:479–484 (1971).
83. Morin, M., Larivière, S., and Lallier, R. Pathological and microbiological observations made on spontaneous cases of acute neonatal calf diarrhea. *Can. J. Comp. Med. 40*:228–240 (1976).
84. Bergeland, M. E., Johnson, D. D., and Shave, H. Bovine cryptosporidiosis in the north central United States. *Am. Assoc. Vet. Labor. Diagnost., 22nd Ann. Proc.*, 1979, pp. 131–138.
85. Anderson, B. C. Patterns of shedding of cryptosporidial oocysts in Idaho calves. *J. Am. Vet. Med. Assoc. 178*:982–984 (1981).
86. Pearson, G. R., and Logan, E. F. Demonstration of cryptosporidia in the

small intestine of a calf by light, transmission electron and scanning electron microscopy. *Vet. Rec. 103*:212–213 (1978).

87. Morin, M., Larviere, S., Lallier, R., et al. Neonatal calf diarrhea: pathology and microbiology of spontaneous cases in dairy herds and incidence of the enteropathogens implicated as etiological agents. *Int. Symp. Neonatal Diarrhea, Vet. Infect. Dis. Org. 2*:347–368 (1978).

88. Tzipori, S., Campbell, I., Sherwood, D., et al. An outbreak of calf diarrhoea attributed to cryptosporidial infection. *Vet. Rec. 107*:579–580 (1980).

89. Tzipori, S., Smith, M., Halpin, C., Angus, K. W., Sherwood, D., and Campbell, I. Experimental cryptosporidiosis in calves: clinical manifestations and pathological findings. *Vet. Rec. 112*:116–120 (1983).

90. Pivont, P., Meuiner, J., Lefevre, F., Baudouin, P., Bughin, J., and Antoine, H. Frèquence des cryptosporidies dans les matières fecales des veaux d'un clientèle vètèrinaire. *Ann. Med. Vet. 128*:369–374 (1984).

91. Leek, R. G., and Fayer, R. Prevalence of *Cryptosporidium* infections, and their relation to diarrhea in calves on 12 dairy farms in Maryland. *Proc. Helminthol. Soc. Wash. 51*:360–361 (1984).

92. Pearson, G. R., and Logan, E. F. The pathology of neonatal enteritis in calves with observations in *E. coli*, rotavirus, and *Cryptosporidium. Ann. Rech. Vet. 14*:422–426 (1983).

93. Haynes, T. B., Lauerman, L. H., Klesius, P. H., Mitchell, F. M., Long, I. R., and Ellis, A. C. Cryptosporidiosis in newborn calves. *Am. Assoc. Vet. Parasitol., 29th Ann. Proc.*, 1984, Abstr. No. 66.

94. Fayer, R., Ernst, J. V., Miller, R. G., and Leek, R. G. Factors contributing to clinical illness in calves experimentally infected with a bovine isolate of *Cryptosporidium. Proc. Helminthol. Soc. Wash. 52*:64–70 (1985).

95. Tzipori, S., Smith, M., Makin, T., and Haplin, C. Enterocolitis in piglets caused by *Cryptosporidium* sp. purified from calf feces. *Vet. Parasitol. 11*: 121–126 (1982).

96. Snodgrass, D. R., Angus, K. W., and Gray, E. W. Experimental cryptosporidiosis in germ-free lambs. *J. Comp. Pathol. 94*:141–152 (1984).

97. Angus, K. W., Appleyard, W. T.,Menzies, J. D., Campbell, I., and Sherwood, D. An outbreak of diarrhea associated with cryptosporidiosis in naturally reared lambs. *Vet. Rec. 110*:129–130 (1982).

98. Tzipori, S., Angus, K. W., Campbell, I., and Clerihew, L. W. Diarrhea due to *Cryptosporidium* infection in artificially reared lambs. *J. Clin. Microbiol. 14*:100–105 (1981).

99. Tzipori, S., Sherwood, D., Angus, K. W., Campbell, I., and Gordon, M. Diarrhea in lambs: experimental infections with enterotoxigenic *Escherichia coli*, rotavirus, and *Cryptosporidium* sp. *Infect. Immun. 33*:401–406 (1981).

100. Tzipori, S., Angus, K. W., Campbell, I., and Gray, E. W. Experimental infection of lambs with *Cryptosporidium* isolated from a human patient with diarrhoea. *Gut 23*:71–74 (1982).

101. Tzipori, S., Angus, K. W., Gray, E. W., Campbell, I., and Allan, F. Diarrhea in lambs experimentally infected with *Cryptosporidium* isolated from calves. *Am. J. Vet. Res. 42*:1400-1404 (1981).
102. Kennedy, G. A., Kreitner, G. L., and Strafuss, A. C. Cryptosporidiosis in three pigs. *J. Am. Vet. Med. Assoc. 170*:348-350 (1977).
103. Links, I. J. Cryptosporidial infection of piglets. *Aust. Vet. J. 58*:60-62 (1982).
104. Moon, H. W., Schwartz, M. J., Welch, M. J., McCann, P. P., and Runnels, P. L. Experimental fecal transmission of human cryptosporidiosis to pigs, an attempted treatment with an ornithine decarboxylase inhibitor. *Vet. Pathol. 19*:700-707 (1982).
105. Gibson, J. A., Hill, M. W. M., and Huber, M. J. Cryptosporidiosis in Arabian foals with severe combined immunodeficiency. *Aust. Vet. J. 60*: 378-379 (1983).
106. Gajadhar, A. A., Caron, J. P., and Allen, J. R. Cryptosporidiosis in two foals. *Can Vet. J. 26*:132-134 (1985).
107. Fletcher, O. J., Munnell, J. F., and Page, R. K. Cryptosporidiosis of the bursa of Fabricius of chickens. *Avian Dis. 19*:630-639 (1975).
108. Randall, C. J. Cryptosporidiosis of the bursa of Fabricius and trachea in broilers. *Avian Pathol. 11*:95-102 (1982).
109. Itakura, C., Goryo, M., and Umemura, T. Cryptosporidial infection in chickens. *Avian Pathol. 13*:487-499 (1984).
110. Dhillon, A. S., Thacker, H. L., Dietzel, A. V., and Winterfield, R. W. Respiratory cryptosporidiosis in broiler chickens. *Avian Dis. 25*:747-751 (1981).
111. Hoerr, F. J., Ranck, F. M., and Hastings, T. F. Respiratory cryptosporidiosis in turkeys. *J. Am. Vet. Med. Assoc. 173*:1591-1593 (1978).
112. Glisson, J. R., Brown, T. P., Brugh, M., and Page, R. K. Sinusitis in turkeys associated with respiratory cryptosporidiosis. *Avian Dis. 28*:783-790 (1984).
113. Mason, R. W., and Hartley, W. J. Respiratory cryptosporidiosis in a peacock chick. *Avian Dis. 24*:771-776 (1980).
114. Hoerr, F. J., Current, W. L., and Haynes, T. B. Intestinal cryptosporidiosis in quail. 121st Ann. Meeting, Am. Vet. Med. Assoc., New Orleans, July 16-19, 1984).
115. Tham, V. L., Kniseberg, S., and Dixon, B. R. Cryptosporidiosis in quails. *Avian Pathol. 11*:619-626 (1982).
116. Heuschele, W. P., Janssen, D., Oosterhuis, J., Schofield, S., and Halligan, K. Etiology and prevention of neonatal diarrhea in hand-raised exotic ruminants. Conf. Research Workers in Animal Disease, Chicago, Nov. 11-13, 1984, Abstr. No. 271.
117. Zar, F., Geiseler, P. J., and Brown, V. A. Asymptomatic carriage of *Cryptosporidium* in the stool of a patient with acquired immune deficiency syndrome. *J. Infect. Dis. 151*:195 (1985).
118. Miller, R. A., Holmberg, R. E., and Clausen, C. R. Life-threatening diarrhea

caused by *Cryptosporidium* in a child undergoing therapy for acute lymphocytic leukemia. *J. Pediatr. 103*:256–259 (1983).

119. Lewis, I. J., Hart, C. A., and Baxby, D. Diarrhoea due to *Cryptosporidium* in acute lymphoblastic leukaemia. *Arch. Dis. Child. 60*:60–62 (1985).

120. Pitilka, S. D., Fainstein, V., Garza, D., Guarda, L., Boliver, R., Rios, A., Hopfer, R. L., and Mansell, P. A. Human cryptosporidiosis: spectrum of disease. Report of six cases and reviews of the literature. *Arch. Intern. Med. 143*:2269–2273 (1983).

121. Malebranche, R., Arnoux, E., Guérin, J. M., Piere, G. D., Laroche, A. C., Guichard, C. P., Elie, R., Morisset, P. H., Spira, T., Mandeville, R., Drotman, P., Seemayer, T., and Dupuy, J. P. Acquired immunodeficiency syndrome with severe gastrointestinal manifestations in Haiti. *Lancet* Oct. 15; 873–878 (1983).

122. Koch, K. L., Shankey, T. V., Weinstein, G. S., Dye, R. E., Abt, A. B., Current, W. L., and Eyster, M. E. Cryptosporidiosis in a patient with hemophilia, common variable hypogammaglobulinemia, and the acquired immunodeficiency syndrome. *Ann. Intern. Med. 99*:337–340 (1983).

123. Weinstein, W. M. The gastrointestinal tract as a target organ. In *The Acquired Immunodeficiency Syndrome* (M. S. Gottlieb, moderator). *Ann. Intern. Med. 99*:208–220 (1983).

123a. Mol. P., Mukashuma, S., Bogarts, J., Hemelhof, W., and Butzler, J. P. *Cryptosporidium* related to measles diarrhea in Rwanda. *Lancet 2*:42–43 (1984).

123b. Harari, M. D., West, B., and Dwyer, B. *Cryptosporidium* as a cause of laryngotracheitis in an infant. *Lancet 1*:1207 (1986).

124. Pitlik, S., Fainstein, V., Rios, A., Guarda, L., Mansell, P. W. A., and Hersh, E. M. Cryptosporidial cholecystitis. *New Engl. J. Med. 308*:976 (1983).

125. Blumberg, R. S., Kelsey, P., Perrone, T., Dickersin, R., Laquaglia, M., and Ferruci, J. Cytomegalovirus- and *Cryptosporidium*-associated acalculous gangrenous cholecystitis. *Am. J. Med. 76*:1118–1123 (1984).

126. Ma, P., Villanueva, T. G., Kaufman, D., and Gillooley, J. F. Respiratory cryptosporidiosis in the acquired immune deficiency syndrome. *JAMA 252*:1298–1301 (1984).

127. Kocoshis, S. A., Cibull, M. L., and Davis, T. E. Intestinal and pulmonary cryptosporidiosis in an infant with severe combined immune deficiency. *J. Pediatr. Gastroenterol. Nutr. 3*:149–157 (1984).

128. Nime, F. A., Burek, J. D., Page, D. L., Holscher, M. A., and Yardley, J. H. Acute enterocolitis in a human being infected with the protozoan *Cryptosporidium. Gastroenterology 70*:592–598 (1976).

129. Tzipori, S., Angus, K. W., Gray, E. W., and Campbell, I. Vomiting and diarrhea associated with cryptosporidial infection. *New Engl. J. Med. 303*: 818 (1980).

130. Fletcher, A., Sims, T. A., and Talbot, I. C. Cryptosporidial enteritis without general or selected immune deficiency. *Br. Med. J. 285*:22–23 (1982).

131. Babb, R. R., Differding, J. T., and Trollope, M. L. Cryptosporidia enteritis in a healthy professional athlete. *Am. J. Gastroenterol. 77*:833–834 (1982).
132. Centers for Disease Control. Human cryptosporidiosis—Alabama. *Morb. Mortal. Wkly, Rep. 31*:252–254 (1982).
133. Walsh, J. A., and Warren, K. S. Selective primary care. An interim strategy for disease control in developing countries. *New Engl. J. Med. 301*:967–974 (1979).
134. Garcia, L. S., Bruckner, D. A., Brewer, T. C., and Shimzu, R.Y. Techniques for the recovery and identification of *Cryptosporidium* oocysts from stool specimens. *J. Clin. Microbiol. 18*:185–190 (1983).
135. Ma, P., and Soave, R. Three step stool examination for cryptosporidiosis in ten homosexual men with protracted watery diarrhea. *J. Infect. Dis. 147*: 824–828 (1983).
136. Payne, P., Lancaster, L. A., Heinzman, M., and McCutchen, J. A. Identification of *Cryptosporidium* in patients with the acquired immunodeficiency syndrome. *New Engl. J. Med. 309*:614 (1983).
137. Heine, J. Eine einfache Nachweismethode fur Kryptosporidien in Kot, *Zbl. Vet. Med. B 29*:324–327 (1982).
138. Current, W. L. Human cryptosporidiosis. *New Engl. J. Med. 309*:1326–1327 (1983).
139. Baxby, D., Blundell, N., and Hart, C. A. The development and performance of a simple, sensitive method for detection of *Cryptosporidium* oocysts in faeces. *J. Hyg. (Camb.) 93*:317–324 (1984).
140. Garcia, L. S., Brewer, T. C., and Bruckner, D. A. Fluorescent detection of *Cryptosporidium* oocysts in human fecal specimens by using monoclonal antibodies. *J. Clin. Microbiol. 25*:119–121 (1987).
140a. Ungar, B. L. P., Soave, R., Fayer, R., and Nash, T. E. Enzyme immunoassay detection of immunoglobulin M and G antibodies to *Cryptosporidium* in immunocompetent and immunocompromised persons. *J. Infect. Dis. 153*:570–578 (1986).
140b. Tzipori, S., and Campbell, I. Prevalence of *Cryptosporidium* antibodies in 10 animal species. *J. Clin. Microbiol. 14*:455–456 (1981).
141. Soave, R. Therapy and prevention of coccidiosis. In *Microbiology 1984* (L. Leive and D. Schlessenger, eds.). Am. Soc. Microbiol., Washington, D.C., 1984, pp. 232–236.
142. Hart, A., and Baxby, D. Management of cryptosporidiosis. *J. Antimicrob. Chemother. 15*:3–4 (1985).
143. Portnoy, D., Whiteside, M. E., Buckley, E., and MacLeod, C. L. Treatment of intestinal cryptosporidiosis with spiramycin. *Ann. Intern. Med. 101*: 202–204 (1984).
144. Soave, R. Diagnosis, management, and prognosis of human cryptosporidiosis. 34th Ann. Meeting, Am. Soc. Trop. Med. Hyg., Miami, Fla., Nov. 3–7, 1985, Abstr. no. 135.
145. Moon, H. W. Intestinal cryptosporidiosis: pathogenesis and immunity.

10th International Symposium on Intestinal Microecology, Minneapolis, Minn., Oct. 2–3, 1985.

145a. Saxon, A., and Weinstein, W. Oral administration of bovine colostrum anti-cryptosporidia antibody fails to alter the course of human cryptosporidiosis. *J. Parasitol.* 73:413–415 (1987).

146. Louie, E., Borkowsky, W., Klesius, P. H., Haynes, T. B., Gordon, S., and Lawrence, H. S. Treatment of cryptosporidiosis with oral bovine transfer factor. ICAAC, Minneapolis, Minn., Sept. 29–Oct. 2, 1985, Abstr. No. 817.

147. Hoover, D. M., Hoerr, F. J., and Carlton, W. W. Enteric cryptosporidiosis in a naso tung, *Nasa lituratus* Bloch and Schneider. *J. Fish. Dis.* 4:425–428 (1981).

148. Pavlasek, I. *Cryptosporidium* sp. in *Cyrpinus carpio* Linne, 1758 in Czechoslavakia. *Folia Parasitol.* 30248 (1983).

149. McKenzie, R. A., Green, P. E., Hartley, W. J., and Pollitt, C. C. *Cryptosporidium* in a red-bellied black snake (*Pseudechis porphyriacus*). *Aust. Vet. J.* 54:365 (1978).

150. Brownstein, D. G., Strandberg, J. D., Montali, R. J., Bush, M., and Fortner, J. *Cryptosporidium* in snakes with hypertrophic gastritis. *Vet. Pathol.* 14:606–617 (1977).

151. Tarwid, J. N., Cawthorn, R. J., and Riddell, C. Cryptosporidiosis in the respiratory tract of turkeys in Saskatchewan. *Avian Dis.* 29:528–532 (1985).

152. Slavin, D. *Cryptosporidium meleagridis* (sp. nov.). *J. Comp. Pathol.* 65:262–266 (1955).

153. Gardiner, C. H., and Imes, G. D. *Cryptosporidium* sp. in the kidneys of a black-throated finch. *J. Am. Vet. Med. Assoc.* 185:1401–1402 (1984).

154. Proctor, S. J., and Kemp, R. L. *Cryptosporidium anserinum* sp. n. (Sporozoa) in a domestic goose *Anser anser* L., from Iowa. *J. Protozool.* 21.:664–666 (1974).

155. Doster, A. R., Mahaffey, E. A., and McClearen, J. R. Cryptosporidia in the cloacal corprodeum of red-lored parrots (*Amazona autumnalis*). *Avian Dis.* 23:654–661 (1979).

156. Wilson, D. W., Day, P. A., and Brummer, M. E. G. Diarrhea associated with *Cryptosporidium* spp. in juvenile macaques. *Vet. Pathol.* 21:447–450 (1984).

157. Korsholm, H., and Henriksen, S. A. Infection with *Cryptosporidium* in roe deer (*Caperolus caperolus*)—a preliminary report. *Nord. Vet. Med.* 36:266 (1984).

158. Tzipori, S., and Angus, K. W. Diarrhea in young red deer associated with infection with *Cryptosporidium*. *J. Infect. Dis.* 144:170–175 (1981).

159. Evans, R. H. Personal communication, Treehouse Wildlife Center, R.R. 1, Box 125E, Brighton, Ill. 62012, 1985.

160. Sandberg, J. P., Hill, D., and Ryan, M. J. Cryptosporidiosis in a gray squirrel. *J. Am. Vet. Med. Assoc.* 181:1420–1422 (1982).

161. Inman, L. R., and Takeuchi, A. Spontaneous cryptosporidiosis in an adult female rabbit. *Vet. Pathol. 16*:89–95 (1979).
162. Sisk, D. B., Gosser, H. S., and Styer, E. L. Intestinal cryptosporidiosis in two pups. *J. Am. Vet. Med. Assoc. 184*:835–836 (1984).
163. Poonacha, K. B., and Pippin, C. Intestinal cryptosporidiosis in a cat. *Vet. Pathol. 19*:708–710 (1982).
164. Carlson, B. L., and Nielsen, S. W. Cryptosporidiosis in a raccoon. *J. Am. Vet. Med. Assoc. 181*:1405–1406 (1982).
165. Bradford, M. M. A rapid and sensitive method for quantitation of microgram quantities of protein utilizing the principle of protein-dye binding. *Anal. Biochem. 72*:248–254 (1976).
166. Johnson, D. A., and Elder, J. H. Antibody directed to determinants of a Moloney virus derived MCF gp70 recognizes a thymic differentiation antigen. *J. Exp. Med. 159*:1751–1756 (1983).
167. Johnson, D. A., Gautsch, W. M., Sportsman, J. R., and Elder, J. H. Improved technique utilizing nonfat dry milk for analysis of proteins and nucleic acids transferred to nitrocellulose. *Gene Anal. Tech. 1*:3–4 (1984).
168. Levine, N. D. Introduction, taxonomy, and history. In *The Coccidia* (D. M. Hammond and P. L. Long, eds.). University Park Press, Baltimore, 1973.
169. Levine, N. D. Problems with the systematics of the "sporozoa." *J. Protozool. 8*:442–451 (1961).
170. Box, E. D., Marchiondo, A. A., Duszynski, D. W., and Davis, C. P. Ultrastructure of *Sarcocystis* sporocysts from passerine birds and opossums: comments on classification of the genus *Isospora. J. Parasitol. 66*:68–74 (1980).

6

Giardia lamblia

PHILLIP D. SMITH

Laboratory of Immunology, NIDR, National Institutes of Health, Bethesda, Maryland

I. INTRODUCTION

The protozoan parasite *Giardia lamblia* was first identified by the Dutch microscopist Anton van Leeuwenhoek in 1681. Reporting his findings in a letter to the Royal Society in London, van Leeuwenhoek drew attention to the possible association between intestinal disease and the organism he had identified (1). Despite the implication of this observation, *G. lamblia* was regarded as a nonpathogenic commensal for nearly 300 years. Even as recently as the 1950s, studies of the transmission of *G. lamblia* suggested that the parasite was nonpathogenic. However, during the last three decades an increased recognition that diarrheal diseases are a major cause of morbidity and mortality throughout the world, particularly in developing countries, has prompted new interest in the etiology and pathophysiology of diarrheal diseases. As a consequence of this interest, *G. lamblia* has become the subject of intense investigation. Facilitated by major advances in the clinical and basic sciences, this investigation has resulted in the recognition that *G. lamblia* is capable of causing gastrointestinal disease ranging from asymptomatic cyst passage to severe diarrhea with malabsorption. Recent investigation also has provided important insights into the biology of the parasite. In addition, complex issues regarding the immunology and pathophysiology of giardiasis are now being addressed. The importance of this renewed interest in *G. lamblia* is underscored by the fact that this parasite has become the most frequently identified intestinal parasite in the United States and many other regions of the world. Although many questions remain unanswered, remarkable advances in understanding *G. lamblia* and the disease it causes have occurred since van Leeuwenhoek's insightful report to the Royal Society.

II. THE ORGANISM

A. Life Cycle and Epidemiology

Giardia lamblia is a unicellular protozoan parasite that exists in two forms: the dormant cyst, which transmits disease to the host, and the motile flagellated trophozoite, which causes disease. There is no intermediate developmental stage outside the gastrointestinal tract of the host. Unlike other protozoan parasites such as *Toxoplasma gondii* (chapter 4), *Leishmania* spp., *Trypanosoma* spp., *Malaria* spp., or the coccidian protozoan *Cryptosporidium* (Chapter 5), *G. lamblia* is an extracellular protozoan. In this respect it resembles *Entamoeba histoloytica* (Chapter 7).

The clinically relevant phase of the parasite's life cycle appears to begin in the stomach (Fig. 1). Here normal physiological conditions including the acidity, oxidation-reduction potential, temperature, and presence of carbon dioxide are similar to the in vitro conditions that facilitate excystation (2,3). However, since trophozoites do not survive in an acidic environment, excystation likely is completed in the more alkaline proximal small intestine where colonization occurs. Here the trophozoite, which reproduces by binary fission, evades enzymatic degradation by unknown mechanisms and may survive for long periods of time. In view of the ability of bile and biliary lipids to promote trophozoite growth (4,5), apparently through enhanced membrane lipid (lecithin) uptake (6), the bile-rich proximal small intestine is a particularly suitable environment for colonization. In addition, luminal proteases in the proximal small intestine may participate in a novel host–parasite interaction by activating a lectin in *G. lamblia* most specific for mannose-6-phosphate, which then facilitates the binding of trophozoites to the glycosylated microvillous membrane of the intestinal surface (7). Between the proximal small intestine and colon trophozoites undergo encystation, a process augmented in vitro by primary bile salts (242), and the resulting cysts are eventually excreted. During periods of rapid intestinal transit, trophozoites also may be excreted, but they do not survive in the external environment.

The *Giardia* species that infect nonhuman mammals likely have a similar life cycle. In this regard, isolates of *G. lamblia* have been shown to infect a variety of hosts including mice (8,9), gerbils (10), rats (11,12), rabbits (13), and dogs (14,15), suggesting that the species that infects humans is not host-specific. The infections of these laboratory animals should provide convenient models for elucidating additional aspects of the parasite's life cycle. However, interpretation of host-specificity data is ultimately dependent on a sensitive system for taxonomic classification of *Giardia* species. Unfortunately, such a broadly acceptable system currently does not exist. In the past, minor morphological features including the position of cellular structures and the density of cellular material were used to

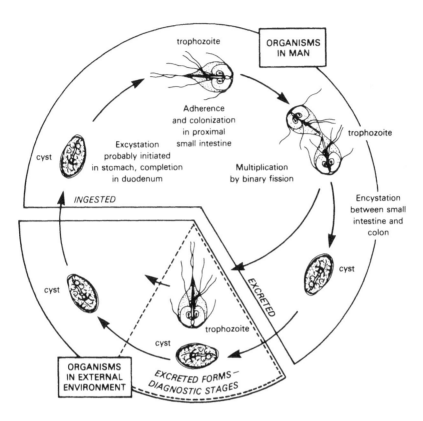

Figure 1 Life cycle of *G. lamblia*. (Adapted with permission from E. A. Meyer, *Microorganisms and Human Disease*, Appleton-Century-Crofts, New York, 1974.)

distinguish species of *Giardia* (16,17), but these differences more likely reflect variation in trophozoite maturity or fixation techniques. *Giardia* species also have been identified by combined analysis of trophozoite morphology and dimensions (morphometrics) (18,19). However, the reliability of these features for speciation of *Giardia* isolates has been questioned (20). The electrophoretic pattern of trophozoite enzymes also has been used to characterize different isolates of *Giardia* (21). More recent studies (22) have utilized restriction-endonuclease analysis of trophozoite DNA to distinguish different isolates of *Giardia* from humans and animals. Although some isolates from humans, a cat, and a beaver exhibit a common DNA banding pattern, the sensitivity of recombinant DNA analysis provides an important additional tool for identifying *Giardia* species. One feature common among various isolates of *G. lamblia* is the uniquely small set of ribosomal RNA components that have been shown by sequence analysis to be approximately 75% the size of bacterial and 65% the size of other protozoal rRNA species (23). Ultimately, a combination of these and perhaps more sensitive techniques should provide an accurate method for identifying different species and isolates of *Giardia*.

In contrast to the restricted geographical distribution of most other parasitic infections, infection of humans with *G. lamblia* occurs throughout the world. Moreover, it is estimated to infect between 2 and 25% of the world's population (24), making it one of the most common parasites of humans. Epidemiological studies have elucidated a number of factors that appear to contribute to this high prevalence. Fecal-oral transmission is one such factor. That this mode of transmission contributes to the prevalence of *G. lamblia* is supported by the high incidence of apparent person-to-person transmission among individuals more commonly exposed to fecal material such as infants in day care centers (25–27), close relatives of infants in day care centers (28), homosexuals (29–31), and patients in institutions for the mentally retarded (32,33). In addition, the inadequate personal hygiene that may accompany unsanitary living conditions would be expected to facilitate fecal-oral transmission of *Giardia*. This is reflected in the high prevalence rates in less developed regions of the world such as Bangladesh (34) and Tasmania (35). Although the fecal-oral route is the predominant mode of person-to-person transmission, food has been implicated as the vehicle of transmission in two epidemics of giardiasis attributed to infected food handlers (36,37).

Recently, *G. lamblia* was identified as the most common human intestinal parasite in the United States (38), particularly in mountainous regions such as Colorado (39), indicating that other factors contribute to its prevalence. A series of giardiasis epidemics in Oregon (40,41), the Rocky Mountain states (41–44), California (41), Pennsylvania (41), upstate New York (45), and Washington (46), have led to the elucidation of some of these factors. Epidemiological evaluation revealed that many of these outbreaks had the following features in common: (1) contaminated drinking water was implicated as the mode of transmission; (2) surface water originating from adjacent mountain streams (and not well water) supplied the water treatment facility; (3) chlorination was the principal, although ineffective, method of disinfection; (4) no filtration or defective filtration of the drinking water was in use at the time of the epidemic; and (5) beavers that were infected with *Giardia* were found in the watershed area of some epidemics. These findings suggest that beavers and possibly other animals serve as reservoir hosts for *Giardia* and contaminate streams that supply ineffective water treatment facilities. The apparent lack of strict host specificity of the parasite raises the possibility that the beavers were originally infected with *G. lamblia* from humans. Furthermore, the ability of cysts to survive at 0°C for long periods of time (2) suggests that the cysts would be capable of surviving in the cold water of mountainous environments inhabited by beavers and occasionally visited by humans. Some of these factors, in particular inadequate disinfection of drinking water, likely contribute to the acquisition of *G. lamblia* by tourists to other developed countries such as the Soviet Union (47,48). In summary, *G. lamblia* is acquired by several routes including fecal-oral transmission, contaminated water, and infrequently contaminated food. These modes of transmission apply to persons with adequate as well as inadequate personal hygiene living in temperate and tropical regions of the world.

B. Growth and Metabolism

Many of the recent studies on the biology of *G. lamblia* and the host response to the parasite were made possible by the painstaking work of investigators who developed the methods for cultivating the organism. The *Giardia* spp. first cultivated by Karapetyan in the early 1960s required the presence of yeast or fibroblasts (49,50). Subsequently, Meyer was able to isolate and axenically cultivate *Giardia* trophozoites from the rabbit, chinchilla, and cat (51) and then from a human (52). Visvesvara then adapted the organism to TP-S-1 medium (53), which had been developed for *Entamoeba histolytica* (54), and Keister further improved the cultivation technique by using TYI-S-33 medium supplemented with bile (55). Finally, Gillin defined the culture requirements for reducing agents, serum, temperature, ionic composition, and oxygen tension (56-58). Autoradiographic analysis of nuclear replication has revealed the generation time to be approximately 15 hr (59), but, depending on the isolate, it may be as short as 8 hr (60).

The ability to culture *G. lamblia* has made possible investigation into the metabolism of the organism. Previously, the low oxygen tension of its natural habitat and the absence of mitochondria (61) led to the presumption that *G. lamblia* was an aerotolerant anaerobe. However, recent studies indicate that the parasite actively respires in the presence of oxygen, transferring electrons from reduced substrates to molecular oxygen by an acid-extractable flavin, iron-sulfer protein system present in the particulate cell fraction (62,63). Metabolic inhibitor studies of respiration indicate the absence of a functional Krebs cycle and cytochrome-mediated oxidative phosphorylation (63). The significance of a respiratory system in an organism whose natural habitat is the relatively anaerobic environment of the small intestine is unclear. Carbohydrate metabolism also has been examined in *G. lamblia*, and endogenous as well as exogenous carbohydrates such as glucose are incompletely oxidized aerobically and anaerobically to ethanol, acetate, and CO_2; energy is generated by substrate-level phosphorylation (62-64). As for nucleotide requirements, *G. lamblia* appears to rely on the host for pyrimidines, since it is incapable of pryimidine biosynthesis (65).

C. Antigenic Components and Virulence

The ability to culture G. lamblia trophozoites also has facilitated investigation of the parasite's antigenic components. In the initial characterization of these components, we examined strains of G. lamblia from Afghanistan, Oregon, Ecuador, and Puerto Rico (66). Although polyacrylamide gel electrophoresis revealed gross similarity in the electrophoretic mobility of the protein bands (12,000–140,000 daltons) among the strains, crossed immunoelectrophoresis demonstrated several antigenic differences among the 37 anodic and one neutral antigen. In addition, employing trophozoites from each strain as antigen in enzyme-linked immunosorbent assays with 10 human antisera revealed significant qualitative and quantitative differences in the protein antigens among the strains. Recently, a polydisperse, high molecular weight, membrane-derived material, probably carbohydrate-free proteolipid residues that are released by trophozoites as excretory-secretory products, was identified as a potentially important antigenic component (67). In this regard, the Portland-1 isolate (Oregon) is the most antigenically diverse in comparison to the strains from Afghanistan, Ecuador, and Puerto Rico (66) and appears not to contain the major excretory-secretory product of the WB (Afghanistan) strain (67). Endonuclease restriction analysis of additional isolates has revealed significant differences in DNA banding patterns, indicating differences in nucleotide sequences among different isolates (22). These differences in DNA profiles appear to correlate, to some extent, with the variation in trophozoite surface antigens (68). More recent studies have identified a cysteine-rich 170-kD surface antigen which, in at least one Giardia isolate, undergoes antigenic variation in vitro (243), suggesting the intriguing possibility that antigenic variation in vivo may contribute to the variable clinical response among persons exposed to the same isolate.

In addition to the surface protein described above, a glycoprotein with a molecular weight of 82,000 possibly anchored in the plasma membrane and a 30–34,000-dalton antigen (85) were recently identified as a major surface antigen (69). Besides surface components and excretory-secretory products serving as potential antigens in host defense mechanisms, polypeptides in tubulin, the principal component of cytoskeletal microtubules, also have been identified as potential antigens in isolates of G. lamblia (70). Full characterization of the relevant membrane, cytoskeletal, and secretory antigens recognized by host defense mechanisms and the contribution of these components to the pathogenesis of giardiasis and the virulence of different isolates await future study.

III. THE HOST

A. Host Defense Mechanisms

Epidemiological, clinical, and experimental observations indicate that *G. lamblia* elicits a host immune response. The epidemiological observations of several outbreaks of giardiasis revealed that the incidence of infection and symptoms are lower among individuals repeatedly exposed to *G. lamblia* than among newly exposed individuals (39,43,71), indicating that prior exposure may provide partial resistance to infection. The clinical observations of an increased prevalence of *G. lamblia* in persons with certain immunoglobulin deficiencies (72–77) emphasize the potential importance of antibody in the host's response to the parasite. In addition, recent experimental studies in mice and humans confirm the presence of humoral and cellular immune responses to *Giardia*.

1. Antibody Responses

The presence of circulating antibodies to *G. lamblia* was first reported in 1976 by Ridley and Ridley (78). Using a crude preparation of cysts as antigen in an indirect immunofluorescence test, they detected antibodies to the cysts in patients with giardiasis and malabsorption. Subsequently, antibodies to cysts were detected by an immunodiffusion technique in patients who had been symptomatic for more than 2 years (79). We extended these preliminary findings with an indirect immunofluorescence (IIF) test (80) and an enzyme-linked immunosorbent assay (ELISA) (81) in controlled, blind protocols using cultured trophozoites as antigen and sera from well-characterized patients and control subjects. Circulating antibodies of the IgG isotype, which appeared to be direc- ted to the trophozoite surface and to have minimal cross-reactivity with other microorganisms, were detected in a high proportion of symptomatic patients. The presence of circulating IgG anti-*G. lamblia* antibodies in patients with symptomatic infection has been confirmed by others with both the IIF and ELISA assays (82,83). Also, the presence of anti-*Giardia* IgM antibodies in the serum of patients with symptomatic giardiasis indicates that *G. lamblia*, similar to other infectious agents, elicits an acute IgM response prior to the IgG response (84). In contrast, patients with AIDS do not exhibit an IgM response to *G. lamblia* during symptomatic infection (85), likely because of their impaired ability to mount de novo antibody responses (86). In addition to eliciting circu- lating antibodies, *G. lamblia* appears capable of eliciting secretory antiparasite antibodies (83). In this regard, the presence of IgA anti-*G. lamblia* antibodies in 79% of milk samples from Mexican women, in contrast to only 15% of samples from U.S. women, indicates that frequent exposure to the parasite probably contributes to the development of a secretory antibody response to *Giardia* (83).

Clinical and experimental evidence indicates that host antitrophozoite antibodies may contribute to protection against *G. lamblia*. The increased incidence of symptomatic infection in patients with various immunoglobulin deficiency diseases, in particular common variable hypogammaglobulinemia (72–76), supports this notion. Similarly, the apparent lower rate of infection in breast-fed, in contrast to formula-fed, infants in highly endemic regions (87) may be due in part to the presence of secretory IgA antiparasite antibodies in their mothers' milk (83), particularly when the mothers are infected with *Giardia* (244). The mechanism(s) by which antiparasite antibodies could participate in host defense against *G. lamblia* has been the subject of recent investigations. In vitro studies documenting the ability of immune serum, purified IgG from immune serum, and IgG specific antitrophozoite antibodies to augment macrophage and neutrophil adherence and/or phagocytosis of *Giardia* (88,89) suggest that one function of the antiparasite antibodies is opsonization of trophozoites, thereby facilitating effector cell–parasite interaction. In this regard, we have found that human granulocytes, which lack spontaneous cytotoxic activity toward *G. lamblia*, exhibit substantial cytotoxicity for the parasite in the presence of human IgG antitrophozoite antibodies (90). In addition, the ability of human sera, in particular sera containing anti-*G. lamblia* antibodies, to kill trophozoites by activation of complement via classical (91) and novel (245) pathway (91) suggests that a direct lethal effect of complement-fixing anti-*G. lamblia* antibodies also may be involved in the host response to *G. lamblia*. Thus, the in vivo interaction between antitrophozoite antibodies and the effector cells that traffic through the mucosa or are present in the intestinal lumen may constitute an important host defense mechnism to prevent or minimize penetration by *G. lamblia* at the mucosal surface.

The role of antibodies in defense against *Giardia* has been investigated in a murine model of giardiasis. Using this model, investigators have demonstrated that *Giardia* previously incubated with neutrophils or macrophages and IgG or IgA antitrophozoite antibodies are less able to infect weanling mice (89). Thus, the opsonizing or possibly lethal effect in vitro of antitrophozoite antibodies described above actually may contribute in vivo to limiting infection with *Giardia*. The murine model of immunoglobulin deficiency also has been used for investigating the role of immunoglobulins in infection with *Giardia*. In this model, mice treated with rabbit anti-IgM antisera develop deficiencies in all classes of immunoglobulins in serum and intestinal fluid (92). Following inoculation with *Giardia muris*, the animals do not develop antiparasite antibodies but do develop prolonged infection with a high parasite burden, in contrast to control mice, which develop parasite-specific antibody and clear their infection. The clearance of the parasite appears to correlate with both the appearance and the increase in levels of secretory IgA anti-*G. muris* antibody, the only detectable anti-*G. muris* isotype in intestinal fluid during infection (93). In contrast to the presence of only IgA antiparasite antibodies in intestinal secretions, both IgG and IgA antiparasite antibodies are present in the serum of the nonsuppressed animals. These studies provide evidence for a relationship between the presence of *Giardia*-specific antibody and the ability of the host to clear the infection. Studies of murine giardiasis also have shown that mice suckling milk containing anti-*Giardia* antibodies do not acquire infection upon challenge with *G. muris* during the suckling period (94,95). Thus, observations from a murine model of giardiasis implicate important roles for both circulating and secretory antiparasite antibodies in parasite clearance mechanisms.

2. Cellular Immune Responses

The presence of high titers of antitrophozoite antibodies in some, but not all, patients with recurrent giardiasis (81) suggests that circulating antibodies alone are not protective against the parasite. Indeed, recent investigations in the mouse indicate that cellular immune responses also may participate in host protective mechanisms against *Giardia*. The role of T lymphocytes in these responses has been examined in congenitally thymus-less (nude) mice, which are deficient in circulating total T lymphocytes and Peyer's patch helper T lymphocytes (96). In contrast to immunocompetent mice that, following inoculation with *G. muris*, clear the parasite and develop resistance to reinfection (97,98), nude mice develop chronic infection with large numbers of *G. muris* (99–101). Moreover, thymus implantation or reconstitution with syngeneic lymphoid cells from thymus-intact mice causes a progressive reduction in the number of *Giardia* in the infected animals (99,100). This reduction is accelerated when the lymphoid cells are from thymus-intact mice previously infected with *G. muris* (100). Mononuclear effector cells within the intestinal lumen may play a less important role in clearance of the parasites in these animals (96).

The mechanism of T-cell involvement in the murine response to *Giardia* is currently under investigation. Preliminary evidence indicates that *G. muris* induces an increase in the total number of Peyer's patch leukocytes but not a change in the relative percentages of total, helper, and suppressor Peyer's patch T lymphocytes (102). In addition, mice selectively depleted of helper/inducer T cells develop prolonged infection with *Giardia*, suggesting that this subset of T lymphocytes is required for parasite clearance (246). The ability of the parasite to induce a sequential shift in the percentage of Peyer's patch B cells bearing surface IgA (103) and secretion of antitrophozoite IgA antibody into the intestine (92,93) may relate to these T-cell changes. In other settings, the switch to IgA-bearing B cells involves regulation by T cells (104,105). Thus, cellular responses, in particular those involving T helper/inducer cells, likely play an important role in the ability of the mouse to clear infection with *G. muris*, possibly by facilitating secretion of parasite-specific antibody.

A poorly understood, and fortunately infrequent, form of infection with *G. lamblia* is chronic giardiasis. Recently, the mechanism of chronic infection was examined in C3H/He mice, a strain of mice that develop a prolonged, high-load infection following inoculation with *G. muris* (100,106). C3H/He mice are capable, however, of clearing a challenge infection after drug cure, and infected C3H/He nursing mothers are capable of protecting their suckling infants from challenge infection. The mechanism for the chronicity of infection in this strain was shown not to be due to the level of serum IgA or to the emergence of a more infective strain of trophozoites. However, altered cellular defense mechanisms were not investigated. This may be relevant, since macrophages from a related strain that is LPS-unresponsive (C3H/HeJ) exhibit markedly reduced spontaneous, although normal antibody-dependent, cytotoxicity for *Giardia* (107). In genetic studies of BALB/c (H-2^d) and C3H/He (H-2^k) mice, there appears to be no association between parasite clearance and the k/k or k/d haplotypes, indicating that histocompatibility genes are likely not involved in clearance of *G. muris* (108). The inability of protective mechanisms to clear the parasite in C3H/He mice awaits further investigation.

Although epidemiological studies suggest that persons repeatedly exposed to *G. lamblia* have a lower incidence of symptomatic giardiasis (see above), the ability of individual patients to acquire resistance to reinfection has not been reported. In fact, patients frequently describe more than one episode of giardiasis. Thus, some of the factors involved in the acquisition of resistance to infection in the mouse may not apply to infection with *G. lamblia* in humans. In particular, an association between T-cell abnormalities and giardiasis has not been reported in humans, suggesting that T-cell responses may not be as important in protective mechanisms against *Giardia* in humans. The exception to this generalization was originally thought to be AIDS, a disease characterized by quantitative and functional defects in helper/inducer T lymphcoytes and a 10–15% incidence of giardiasis (109,110). However, the recent observations of monocyte–macrophage (111–114) and B-cell (86,115) dysfunction in AIDS patients indicates that this disease is not the manifestation of an isolated T-cell abnormality but the result of dysfunction of several cell types involved in immunological function and host defense. Moreover, the incidence of giardiasis in AIDS patients may not be substantially higher than in healthy homosexuals (116). Thus, the incidence of giardiasis in AIDS patients, which awaits confirmation by additional studies, is likely the result of multiple factors, including exposure, the array of immunological defects, and probably other host factors.

Recent studies have focused on the interaction between monocytes and macrophages and *Giardia*. Macrophage involvement in the response to *Giardia* was originally suggested by Owen et al., who showed that murine macrophages in Peyer's patch epithelium were capable of phagocytizing *G. muris* trophozoites (117). Additional evidence supporting a role for macrophage effector activity toward the parasite was provided by the observation that the opsonizing activity of hyperimmune serum increased rabbit macrophage phagocytosis of *G. lamblia* trophozoites (87,88). Human macrophages also are capable of interacting with *Giardia*, exhibiting cytotoxic and phagocytic activity for trophozoites in vitro (118–120). In this regard, the ability of trophozoites to elicit an oxidative burst by human mononuclear phagocytes (119) and the correlation between superoxide anion production and trophozoite killing (121) suggest an intracellular killing mechanism involving the production of reactive oxygen intermediates. Elucidating the contribution of macrophages to the host response to *Giardia* in vivo will require additional investigation.

Although the inflammatory cell response in the intestinal mucosa during giardiasis is variable, both mononuclear and polymorphonuclear cell infiltration into the mucosa frequently occurs during infection (see Section III.C). These cells traffic through the mucosa and may mediate the human host response to *G. lamblia* as follows. After excystation, trophozoites in the intestinal lumen adhere to the epithelium and may begin to invade the mucosa, whereupon they encounter tissue macrophages, which are spontaneously cytotoxic for the parasite. This first level of defense, together with nonimmune host defense mechanisms, is usually sufficient for clearing the parasite. However, if the trophozoites overwhelm or escape this defense mechanism, the antitrophozoite antibody response elicited during infection comes into play. After the antibody reaches a sufficient titer, granulocyte effector cells interact with trophozoites via an antibody-dependent cytotoxic mechanism, possibly involving complement. This response represents a second level of host defense against the parasite and may be particularly important in prolonged infection. In this regard, material from *G. lamblia* trophozoites, possibly excretory-secretory products (67), has been shown to be chemotactic for inflammatory cells (111). Thus, as organisms at the epithelium are killed by cytotoxic effector cells, released material could attract additional effector cells, thereby augmenting these mechanisms for clearing *Giardia*. This chemotactic material may also attract effector cells into the intestinal lumen to interact with organisms that have not invaded the mucosa. Although other factors such as antigenic differences likely contribute to the variation in host susceptibility to infection (see Section II.C), in most individuals the humoral and cellular immune responses to *G. lamblia* successfully prevent tissue invasion.

Nonimmune mechanisms of protection also may participate in the host response to *G. lamblia*. The ability of human milk to kill *Giardia* (123), apparently through the giardicidal effect of free fatty acids released during the hydrolysis of milk triglycerides (124), may contribute to the protection of nursing infants. The role of gastric acidity in protecting the host against *G. lamblia* is unclear. Although the low pH of the stomach is toxic to trophozoites, it nevertheless may initiate excystation, leading to colonization of the proximal small intestine (see Section II.A). The first report of an association between reduced gastric acidity and infection was a study of 50 patients with giardiasis, 42% of whom were hypochlorhydric and 12% achlorydric (125). Subsequently, a patient with life-threatening giardiasis following gastric surgery was reported (126). However, that there may be a causal relationship between hypochorhydria or achlordydria and increase susceptibility to and severity of giardiasis has not been proved.

B. Pathogenesis

A number of possible mechanisms have been suggested to account for the diarrhea and malabsorption that occur during giardiasis.

1. Physical Occlusion of the Mucosa

The ability of trophozoites to adhere to the intestinal mucosa and physically occlude the surface, thereby preventing absorption of nutrients, was one of the earliest suggested mechanisms (127). However, as noted below (Section III.C), G. lamblia trophozoites attach preferentially at the bases of intestinal villi and less frequently at the distal villus where absorption of nutrients occurs across the more differentiated epithelial cells. Even where large numbers of trophozoites are attached to the mucosa, a substantial amount of surface is not occluded. Finally, since trophozoites inhabit the proximal portion of the small intestine, the remainder of the intestine is available for normal absorption. Thus, mechanical occlusion of the mucosal surface is an unlikely explanation for either the diarrhea or the malabsorption associated with giardiasis.

2. Bile Salt Deconjugation

Persons with giardiasis and steatorrhea have been reported to have free bile acids in their intestinal lumens (128), raising the possibility that G. lamblia could deconjugate bile salts and thereby lead to steatorrhea. However, many of the patients in this study also had intestinal bacterial overgrowth, complicating the conclusions that bile salt deconjugation was due to the Giardia. In a follow-up in vitro study (129), we examined the capacity of G. lamblia to deconjugate bile acids. Giardia lamblia trophozoites and Bacteroides fragilis were cultured in media with physiological concentrations of glycine- or taurine-conjugated cholic acid, deoxycholic acid, or chenodeoxycholic acid, after which the media were assayed for free bile salts. Thin-layer chromatography revealed that media in which G. lamblia had been cultured contained no detectable free bile salts, whereas media in which B. fragilis had been cultured contained substantial amounts of free bile salts, indicating that G. lamblia does not conjugate bile acids and that the diarrhea and steatorrhea of giardiasis are caused by one or more mechanisms other than the deconjugation of bile salts.

3. Bacterial Overgrowth

Persons with giardiasis and malabsorption also have been reported to have unusually high counts of three species of enterobacteria (Klebsiella pneumoniae,

Enterobacter cloacae, and *Enterobacter hafniae*) in their proximal small intestines, suggesting that infection with *G. lamblia* is associated with bacterial overgrowth (130). Eradication of the bacteria in most of these patients occurred after the *G. lamblia* were eliminated with a course of metronidazole. However, the possibility that the antibiotic acted directly to eliminate the bacteria cannot be excluded. Also, the study subjects had returned recently from Asia or Africa, regions where persons may exhibit qualitative and quantitative alterations in intestinal bacterial flora (131). Moreover, the presence of intestinal bacterial overgrowth in persons with giardiasis and malabsorption has not been reported by other investigators (132).

4. Enterotoxin Secretion

We examined the possibility that trophozoites produce an enterotoxin capable of stimulating the secretion of water and electrolyte (133). Viable trophozoites and culture medium from four different isolates of *G. lamblia* were tested for the ability to induce intestinal fluid secretion in animals and for the presence of cholera toxin–like antigen. By means of the rabbit ileal-loop assay, the infant mouse assay, the rabbit skin permeability factor assay, and a ganglioside Gm1 enzyme-linked immunosorbent assay, it was found that isolates from widely differing geographical locations did not produce an enterotoxin resembling either cholera toxin or *Escherichia coli* heat-labile or heat-stable classes of toxin (Table 1). The inactivity of the isolates in these three animal models of diarrheagenic activity and their inability to produce cholera toxin–like antigen suggests that the diarrhea induced by *G. lamblia* is caused by a mechanism other than stimulation by currently recognized enterotoxins.

5. Prostaglandin Release

Prostaglandins have been implicated in the pathogenesis of some diarrhea syndromes through the stimulation of intestinal mucosal adenyl cyclase (134,135) or by direct effect on intestinal motility (136). We have demonstrated that *G. lamblia* trophozoites activate human monocytes, causing them to generate and release substantial amounts of prostaglandin E_2 (120). In addition, increased prostaglandin E_2 levels have been found in the intestinal mucosa of mice infected with *G. lamblia* (137). That parasite-induced prostaglandin release from monocytes or mucosal tissue or both may contribute to the pathophysiology of the diarrhea associated with *G. lamblia* infection awaits further investigation.

6. Villous Atrophy

Giardia lamblia may induce a spectrum of morphological changes in mucosal architecture (see Section III.C), ranging from ultrastructural alterations detectable only by electron microscopy at one end of the spectrum to intense inflammatory cell infiltration with complete villous atrophy at the other end of the spectrum. That *G. lamblia* may induce these changes is supported by the

Table 1 Activity of *Giardia lamblia* Trophozoites and Culture Filtrates in Selected Enterotoxin Assays

G. *lamblia* isolates or controls	Test material	Fluid accumulation (FA) ratio		Permeability factor[c]	GMI ELISA[d]
		Ileal loop[a]	Infant mouse[b]		
W.B., P.O., L.T., R.S.	Viable trophozoites	0.0–0.1	0.061–0.068	0	0
W.B., P.O., L.T., R.S.	Culture filtrate	0.0–0.1	0.060–0.069	0	0
Cholera toxin (100 ng/ml)	Toxin	2.0	0.069	11–14 mm	+
Escherichia coli (heat-stable toxin only)	Culture filtrate	0.4	0.130	0	0

[a]FA ratio [volume of fluid in loop (ml)/length of loop (cm)] $\geq$ 0.2 at 18 hr is positive.

[b]FA ratio (weight of intestine/remaining body wt) $\geq$ 0.083 at 4 hr is positive.

[c]A zone of bluing $\geq$ 4 mm in diameter is positive.

[d]An $A_{410} \geq 0.15$ with a P/N ration (A test/A negative congrol) $\geq$ 2 is positive. Cholera toxin yielded $A_{410} = 2.0$ with PN = 100.

Reproduced with permission from *Gastroenterology 83*:797 (1982).

observations that restoration of mucosal architecture to normal follows eradication of the parasite (138-140). In addition, the severity of the mucosal changes (141-143) and the level of parasite load (144) in some persons with giardiasis appear to correlate with the degree of diarrhea and/or malabsorption. Thus, the reduction in the absorptive surface area associated with the mucosal changes, in particular villous atrophy, likely contributes to the pathogenesis of the diarrhea and malabsorption in these patients. However, minimal or absent morphological alterations in the intestinal mucosa of many persons with symptomatic giardiasis strongly implicate additional mechanisms in the pathogenesis of *G. lamblia*-induced diarrhea and malabsorption

7. Increased Epithelial Cell Turnover

A marked increase in enterocyte production and migration from crypt to villous tip occurs in mice infected with *G. muris* (145,146). This accelerated cell turnover appears to cause an increase in the number of less-differentiated epithelial cells in the distal absorptive region of the villus, thereby providing another possible mechanism for the malabsorption associated with giardiasis. These changes may be accompanied by an accumulation of lymphocytes in the epithelium, suggesting that the kinetic changes are mediated in part by a local immune response. An increased number of mucosal intraepithelial lymphocytes during giardiasis also has been observed in humans (138,141,143,144).

8. Brush Border Injury

Giardiasis may be associated with reduced mucosal levels of the disaccharidase enzymes lactase, sucrase, and leucyl-naphthylamidase (140). This reduction has been attributed to *Giardia*-induced morphological alterations in the mucosal brush border of which the glycocalyx and associated disaccharidase enzymes are a component (146). That *G. lamblia* causes brush border injury and a reduction in disaccharidase levels is supported further by the observation that eradication of the parasite reverses the morphological and functional brush border changes (140). In addition, transport studies in the rat (147) and mouse (148) indicate that trophozoites interfere with the active transport of D-glucose, L-alanine, and glycine but not with the passive diffusion of potassium. These findings are consistent with *G. lamblia*-induced injury of the microvillous membrane where transport mechanisms are located or alteration in the functional capacity of the substrate carriers.

In conclusion, the diarrhea and malabsorption caused by *G. lamblia* is likely multifacorial. Although mucosal occlusion, bile salt deconjugation, associated bacterial overgrowth, and secretion of known enterotoxins seem unlikely mechanisms, several possible mechanisms including prostaglandin secretion, villous atrophy, increased epithelial cell turnover, and brush border injury are intriguing explanations for some aspects of *G. lamblia*-induced diarrhea and malabsorption and warrant further investigation.

C. Pathology

1. Colonization and Attachment

In the mouse, G. muris trophozoites colonize the proximal 25% of the small intestine (149), with the largest number of organisms present in the region of the mid-jejunum (146). A similar distribution likely occurs in humans infected with G. lamblia. Colonization of the small intestine is facilitated by trophozoite attachment to the microvilli on mucosal epithelial cells. Morphological, biochemical, and immunofluorescence studies have demonstrated that trophozoite attachment appears to be regulated by contractile proteins including actin and myosin, which control the morphology of the ventral adhesive disc (150,151). Attachment to the intestinal mucosa occurs preferentially near the bases of villi, on the edges of Peyer's patch follicles, and considerably less frequently on the villous tips or the M cells that transport luminal antigen through the epithelium to lymphocytes in the underlying follicles (149).

2. Mucosal Histology

Light microscopy of the mucosa of the proximal small intestine of infected individuals frequently reveals normal histology. However, varying degrees of histological change may occur including infiltration of polymorphonuclear leukocytes and lymphocytes into the epithelium, accumulation of mononuclear leukocytes in the lamina propria, the development of shortened villi, loss of the brush border, damage to epithelial cells, and an increase in epithelial cell mitosis (138, 141–143). Extensive histological damage due to G. lamblia with total villous atrophy, flattening of the epithelial cells, and dense mononuclear cell infiltration (139,152,153) may resemble the changes associated with celiac sprue.

The controversy over whether G. lamblia can invade the intestinal mucosa has been resolved by histological studies (154–156) that clearly demonstrate the presence of trophozoites within the mucosa. In some patients the presence of trophozoite invasion actually correlated with gastrointestinal symptoms and/or steatorrhea (155,156). However, the actual frequency of mucosal invasion is unknown, since most persons with giardiasis do not undergo intestinal biopsy. Furthermore, special staining procedures (154,155) and meticulous examination of adjacent sections for distorted or sectioned organisms (154) may be required to identify trophozoites within the mucosa.

Histological changes also have been documented by electron microscopy. Scanning electron microscopy of the intestinal mucosa of mice infected with G. muris has revealed circular indentations on the epithelial surface where trophozoites had been attached to the mucosa (149). Transmission electron microscopy of the epithelium of jejunal mucosa from persons with giardiasis has shown that ultrastructural changes in epithelial cells including swelling of membrane-bound cytoplasmic structures, distortion of nuclei, and reduction of the height and number of epithelial cell microvilli may accompany inflamed as well as non-inflamed regions of the mucosa (153).

In addition to these observations, cell kinetic studies (145,146) have revealed an alteration in epithelial cell turnover during infection. In mice chronically infected with *G. muris* and the protozoan *Hexamita muris*, the metaphase-arresting agent colchicine was used to show that protozoal infection caused the production of epithelial cells to increase approximately 100% in the crypt and 50–80% in the villus. In the same study, radioautographic identification of cells along the surface of the villus revealed that enterocyte migration from crypt to villous tip was increased in the infected mice. Thus, noninvasive protozoal infection of the small intestine induces increased epithelial cell turnover and migration.

IV. THE DISEASE

A. Clinical Features

The most benign manifestation of infection with *G. lamblia* is asymptomatic cyst passage. In the original studies of experimental giardiasis in humans (157, 158) this form of infection occurred in all 21 experimentally infected subjects, the majority of whom spontaneously cleared the organism. In a more recent study (247), 5 of 10 subjects inoculated with one isolate of *G. lamblia* and none of five inoculated with another isolate developed symptomatic giardiasis, illustrating the potential role that strain differences (see Section II.C) may play in clinical manifestation of infection. In persons who develop symptomatic giardiasis, symptoms usually begin at the time cysts and/or trophozoites appear in the stool. In this regard, the reported prepatency period of 7–13 days in experimentally infected persons (157,158,246) closely corresponds to the incubation period of 9 days observed in tourists returning from Leningrad with symptomatic giardiasis (47). In contrast to the brief duration of infection that characterizes bacterial and viral gastroenteritis, the duration of infection with *G. lamblia* usually exceeds 1 week (157,158). In one epidemic, all reported cases lasted at least 7 days, and well over half lasted more than 10 days (45).

The symptoms associated with infection are primarily gastrointestinal in nature. In this regard, diarrhea is by far the most common symptom. It may be recurrent, as in 57% of cases in the Camas, Washington epidemic (45), or alternate with constipation (157,158). In addition to diarrhea, symptoms include fatigue, abdominal cramps, bloating, malodorous stool, flatulence, weight loss, and, less frequently, vomiting (Table 2). The passage of blood with the diarrhea has been described in only two cases (159,160), and its presence should suggest infection with an invasive organism, in contrast to *G. lamblia*, which is usually noninvasive. Constitutional symptoms including malaise and anorexia may be present during infection, but fever occurs infrequently (161).

Infrequently, syndromes related to the biliary system may accompany giardiasis. These syndromes include nonopacification of the gall bladder on oral cholecystography (162) and cholecystitis (163). The presence of trophozoites

Table 2 Symptoms of 183 Patients with Stool-Positive *Giardia lamblia* Infection

Symptoms	No. of cases	%
Diarrhea	169	92
Cramps	128	70
Nausea	107	58
Fever	51	28
Vomiting	42	23
Fatigue	36	20
Headache	35	19
Weight loss	23	13
Bloating	17	9
Flatus	11	6
Anorexia	4	2
Constipation	1	1

Source: Reproduced with permission from *Ann. Intern. Med. 87*:426–432 (1977).

in the gall bladder and biliary passages, which was reported over 50 years ago (164), may contribute to these conditions. Russian and Polish clinicians also have reported cholecystitis (165-167) as well as pancreatitis (168) in association with giardiasis. A case of granulomatous heptatitis has been attributed to infection with *G. lamblia* (169). The mechanism for the association of these biliary tract, pancreatic, and hepatic conditions with giardiasis may involve trophozoites ascending the common bile duct and then inducing an inflammatory reaction in the end organs. In contrast, the identification of *G. lamblia* trophozoites in the hepatic vessels of rodents (170) suggests that the parasite also could gain access to the liver via the portal venous system after penetrating the intestinal mucosa. However, this route of access to the liver seems exceedingly unlikely, since in humans trophozoites do not enter the vascular system.

Extraintestinal conditions that have been reported to accompany giardiasis include urticaria (160,171-173), erythema multiforme (167), and arthralgia (174,175). Although very uncommon, their presence in association with giardiasis raises the intriguing possibility of immune complex phenomena induced by circulating parasite antigen. A genetic predisposition for the extraintestinal syndromes has not been reported.

In addition to asymptomatic cyst passage and acute symptomatic infection,

Giardia lamblia

361

giardiasis also may present as chronic symptomatic infection. In contrast to the majority of experimentally infected (157,158) and naturally infected persons treated with antibiotics (176), the chronic form of giardiasis has been reported to last for months or longer (133,177-182). Chronic or persistent infection usually occurs in immunologically normal persons, although one patient with symptomatic giardiasis for 10 years was immunoglobulin-deficient (183). The cause of chronic giardiasis is unclear, although emerging drug resistance has been suggested as one possibility. In this regard, we documented a case of giardiasis in a young man that lasted 18 months despite seven courses of either metronidazole or quinacrine (133). The patient was cured eventually by a combination of both drugs, and in vitro studies showed his organisms to be more sensitive to a combination of both drugs than to either drug alone.

Malabsorption often accompanies symptomatic giardiasis (Table 3). The frequency of the associated malabsorption varies widely depending on the study population and the nutrient (184). The nutrient most frequently reported to be malabsorbed during giardiasis is fat (72,140,154,185-189). The steatorrhea is generally mild, with fecal fat determinations ranging between 5 and 20 g/day, and clears following eradication of the parasite. Clinical giardiasis also may cause the malabsorption of certain carbohydrates. Malabsorbed carbohydrates include the nonmetabolizable monosaccharide D-xylose and the disaccharides lactose and sucrose (140,188-192). The inability to absorb these carbohydrates is reflected in the reduced excretion of xylose in the D-xylose absorption test (190) and flat glucose curves during the oral lactose tolerance test (73,75,191). Lactose intolerance contributes to the diarrhea by the osmotic efeect of the nonabsorbed lactose. Although the symptoms of lactose intolerance will abate in most cases after the infection has cleared, I have seen several patients whose intolerance for lactose persisted for up to 4 weeks following eradication of the infection.

Table 3 Nutrients Malabsorbed During Giardiasis

Nutrient	Reference
Fat	72,140,154,185-189
Carbohydrates: D-xylose, lactose sucruse	73,75,140,188-191
Vitamins: A	192-194
B_{12}	188,195
Folate	195
Protein	69,199
Iron	200

In addition to fat and carbohydrates, certain vitamins may be malabsorbed in patients with giardiasis. Both children and adults with symptomatic infection have been shown to have impaired absorption of oil-based vitamin A (192,193). Moreover, the malabsorption of water-miscible vitamin A in a group of children with giardiasis (194) suggests that the impaired absorption of this vitamin is not related to fat malabsorption. Although none of these patients were reported to have visual changes, the possibility that severe, prolonged giardiasis could contribute to impaired vision due to vitamin A deficiency is unlikely. Giardiasis also may be accompanied by vitamin B_{12} (188,195,196) and folate (195) deficiencies. In the case of vitamin B_{12}, Schilling test studies have shown that the B_{12} malabsorption is corrected by eradication of the parasite (195,196). Despite the well-documented presence of G. lamblia-induced malabsorption of vitamin B_{12} and folate, megaloblastic anemia has been reported only in giardiasis patients with immunoglobulin deficiency and features of pernicious anemia (197,198). Thus, in an otherwise healthy person with giardiasis, the duration and severity of vitamin B_{12} and folate malabsorption appears to be insufficient to induce megaloblastic anemia.

Two additional nutrients that also may be malabsorbed during giardiasis are protein and iron. Protein-losing enteropathy, previously observed in patients with giardiasis who also had an underlying immunoglobulin deficiency (75), also has been reported in an immunologically normal person with symptomatic giardiasis (199). The impaired absorption of protein due to giardiasis occurs infrequently. Recently, the malabsorption of iron with secondary iron deficiency was shown to be a feature of giardiasis in children (200). The iron deficiency anemia was corrected by eradication of the parasite. In contrast to the absence of anemia in G. lamblia-induced vitamin B_{12} and folate deficiency, G. lamblia-induced malabsorption of iron and the consequent iron deficiency has led to anemia in some cases (200).

The malabsorption associated with giardiasis may have harmful consequences for the delicately balanced or marginal protein energy nutrition of certain persons. Those shown to be particularly affected are infants (179), children (140), persons with immunoglobulin deficiencies (74), and elderly persons (201). In this regard, one study revealed that children with giardiasis and either marasmus or kwashiorkor who were treated for their giardiasis experienced resolution of their diarrhea and greater weight gain than children whose giardiasis was not treated (202). Another population of persons whose nutritional status may be particularly affected by the adverse consequences of giardiasis are patients with AIDS. As the disease progresses, patients frequently develop extreme wasting and weight loss associated with intractable diarrhea (110,203,204). This wasting–chronic diarrhea syndrome may be exacerbated by infection with G. lamblia. Patients with AIDS may develop progressive wasting in the absence of diarrhea. In these patients as well, the development of giardiasis with malabsorption exacerbates their catabolic state.

B. Diagnosis

The most commonly used method for diagnosing giardiasis is the identification of *G. lamblia* cysts or trophozoites in stool. The initial step in identification is accomplished by examing small quantities of feces mixed with saline (Fig. 2*A*) and with iodine (Lugol's solution) or merthiodate-iodine-formaldehyde (MIF) under separate coverslips on a glass slide (205). Saline permits visualization of trophozoite motility, whereas iodine and MIF facilitate visualization of cyst and trophozoite structures. Concentrating a specimen will increase the recovery of cysts severalfold (Fig. 2*B*) over that of a direct smear (206). A commercially available device first described in 1978 provides an efficient method for concentrating cysts by the formalin-ether technique (207), after which the cysts may be stained with Lugol's solution (Fig. 2*C*) or MIF (Fig. 2*D*). Additionally, a fresh, polyvinyl alcohol-fixed specimen is stained with trichrome (Fig. 3*A*, *B*) in order to have a permanently stained specimen for reference and for detailed examination of parasite structures (208).

Despite the use of the above techniques, there is considerable variation in the recovery and identification of *G. lamblia* cysts and trophozoites in stool specimens from infected persons. When three or more specimens are examined, identification may range between 0 and 67% (Table 4). Factors contributing to such a wide range in identification include fluctuations in the passage of cysts and/or trophozoites, variation in the competence of persons performing the examination, and variation in the methodology used for parasite detection.

Persons suspected of harboring *G. lamblia* who have negative stool examinations may require more invasive diagnostic procedures. Particularly helpful in this regard is examination of duodenal fluid. Fluid may be obtained with either a duodenal gelatin capsule to which a retrievable nylon string is attached (Entero-Test, Hedeco corp., Palo Alto, CA) (209-211) or by intubation with a nasogastric tube. In several studies (210-213), identification of cysts or trophozoites in duodenal fluid was 80% or greater among patients with giardiasis (Table 4). Although used less frequently, duodenal biopsy with or without mucosal smears may aid in the diagnosis of infection. In two studies (212,214), parasites were identified in biopsy and/or mucosal smears in 100% of infected patients. Technical difficulty and patient acceptance, however, account for biopsy being used less frequently than examination of stool or duodenal fluid in the detection of *G. lamblia*.

To circumvent the problems associated with diagnostic microscopy, immunodiagnostic methods are currently being developed to facilitate rapid and accurate diagnosis of infection with *G. lamblia*. Preliminary data indicate that a double

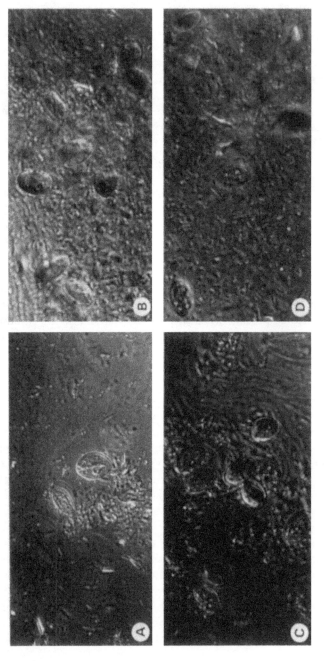

Figure 2 Identification of *G. lamblia* in stool. (*A*) *G. lamblia* cysts in a stool specimen mixed with saline under low (×100) magnification. (*B*) Increased numbers of cysts recovered from a concentrated specimen (×100). (*C,D*) *G. lamblia* cysts in a stool specimen mixed (*C*) with iodine (Lugol's solution) and (*D*) with merthiolate-iodine-formaldehyde (MIF) (×100). The bluish color is due to Nomarski interference contrast optics used to enhance photographic visualization. (Courtesy of W. S. Zeirdt, Microbiology Service, Clinical Pathology Department, NIH.)

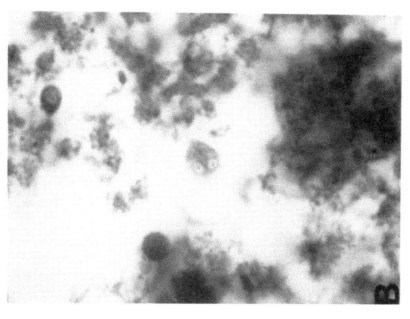

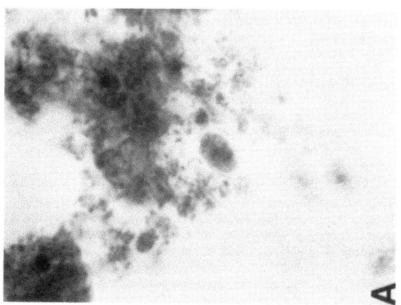

Figure 3 Trichrome mount of a polyvinyl alcohol-fixed stool specimen showing (*A*) a *G. lamblia* cyst and (*B*) a trophozoite (×100). (Courtesy of W. S. Zierdt, Microbiology Service, Clinical Pathology Department, NIH.)

Table 4 Standard Methods for Diagnosing *G. lamblia*

Test (No. positive/No. tested)				
Stool	Entero-Test	Aspiration	Biopsy	Ref.
–	40/49	37/45	–	210
4/6	5/6	4/7	0/6	211
6/12	–	10/12	12/12	212
0/5	5/5	5/5	–	213
2/5	–	–	4/4	214
43%	83%	81%	73%	% positive

antibody ELISA is sensitive and specific in the hands of experienced investigators in detecting *G. lamblia* in stool samples from infected persons (215). Adapted for direct visual interpretation, the sensitivity of the assay may exceed 98%, and its specificity 100% (216).

Based on the ability of *G. lamblia* to elicit an antibody response (see Section III.A), serological assays also are being developed for the diagnosis of giardiasis. Indirect immunofluorescence and ELISA assays, which have been used for the detection of antiparasite IgG antibodies in immunological studies (79-85), may eventually be useful adjuncts in the diagnosis of infection. The recent detection of serum anti-*Giardia* IgM and IgA antibodies in symptomatic patients by ELISA offers the potential advantage of distinguishing current from previous infection (83-85). However, problems in maintaining a ready source of antigen, standardization of results, apparent insensitivity of the assays in asymptomatic carriers, and difficulty in performing the assays in less developed countries limit the diagnostic usefulness of these assays.

C. Treatment and Prevention

The indications for the treatment of giardiasis are influenced by the clinical and epidemiological features of the infection and the potential side effects of the drug therapy. Therapy is indicated for most symptomatic patients since the infection usually is quickly and easily cured by the appropriate antibiotic. Persons with immunoglobulin deficiency and giardiasis appear to respond well to antibiotic therapy, although some investigators recommend follow-up parasitological examination to confirm eradication of the organism in this subset of patients. Patients with AIDS and giardiasis who have been evaluated at the

National Institutes of Health and Colorado have uniformly cleared their infection following antibiotic therapy (85,110). For the pregnant patient, the benefits of eradication of the parasite should be weighed against the potential drug-related risks to the fetus (see below). Treatment of persons in highly endemic regions such as some third world countries is controversial because of the high incidence of reinfection (248).

In addition to persons with symptomatic giardiasis, individuals with asymptomatic infection are treated by many clinicians, since the symptoms and associated malabsorption may be intermittent. Asymptomatic food handlers who have been implicated in the transmission of *G. lamblia* (36) should be treated. Similarly, asymptomatic children have been shown in several day care center epidemics to pose a potential risk for transmission (25-28); therapy for these subjects is controversial because of drug toxicity, rapid reinfection, and the absence of sequelae from asymptomatic infection.

Since first recognized as a pathogen, various therapeutic agents have been used to treat *G. lamblia*. These agents include the acridine derivative quinacrine, the imidazole derivatives metronidazole and tinidazole, and the nitrofuran derivative furazolidone. Although these agents have been evaluated in comparative studies, the studies have varied considerably in important parameters including the drugs tested, dosage schedules, follow-up parasitological evaluation, presence of a placebo control group, and evaluation of compliance. Taking into consideration the limitations of these studies, the efficacy and related features of each drug are discussed below.

Quinacrine, formerly used as an antimalarial agent, is currently recommended as the drug of choice for infection with *G. lamblia* (217). This agent is generally effective in more than 90% of infected persons (218-220). However, children treated with quinacrine may experience vomiting, a side effect that can lead to a reduced (68%) cure rate (221). In contrast, 95% of children treated with quinacrine who do not experience vomiting are cured (220).

The previous use of quinacrine as an antimalarial agent has provided considerable information on the drug's side effects and toxicity. Adverse side effects are infrequent but may include gastrointestinal symptoms such as nausea, vomiting, abdominal cramps, and diarrhea; dermatological changes including rashes and skin discoloration; and constitutional symptoms such as malaise, myalgia, headache, and fever. Toxic reactions to the drug are even less frequent and include exacerbation of preexisting psoriasis or its progression to exfoliative dermatitis and the development of acute toxic psychosis. For these reasons the drug is contraindicated in persons with psoriasis or a history of psychosis. Quinacrine also should not be given to persons receiving primaquine for malaria prophylaxis, because it may induce an increase in the serum primaquine concentration to a toxic level. The currently recommended dosage for adults is 100 mg three times per day for 5 days and for children 2 mg/kg in three divided doses per day for 5 days (217).

The imidazole derivatives metronidazole and tinidazole became available in the 1960s and also are very effective therapy for giardiasis. Cure rates between 88 and 100% have been reported with metronidazole (222–228), the derivative available in the United States. European investigators have used tinidazole with equivalent success (224–226) and have emphasized its efficacy in a single 1.5- or 2-g dose (226). Single-dose tinidazole offers the advantages of reduced cost and enhanced compliance. Recently, metronidazole also was shown to be effective as a single dose, although the currently recommmended schedule is 5 mg/kg in three doses for 5 days (217).

Side effects and toxicity associated with imidazole drugs occur infrequently and appear to be more common with high-dose therapy. The most common side effects are gastrointestinal and include nausea, abdominal cramps, vomiting, and diarrhea. Constitutional symptoms including anorexia and headache and dermatological side effects, in particular, urticaria, flushing, and pruritis, also have been reported. Metronidazole should be used with caution in persons with central nervous system disease, since dizziness, vertigo, incoordination, and ataxia may be associated with the drug. Because neutropenia has been reported in some patients receiving the drug, metronidazole is contraindicated in persons with a history of blood dyscrasia. Imidazole derivatives also are contraindicated in persons consuming alcohol, since they can induce a disulfiram-like reaction with alcohol.

Furazolidone was first recognized to be effective in the treatment of giardiasis in 1960 (229). This has since been confirmed in comparative studies (218,220, 223,228–230), although the effectiveness of this agent (80–95%) is generally less than that of quinacrine or the imidazole derivatives. In pediatric cases, furazolidone offers advantages of availability in suspension form and possibly fewer side effects. The side effects of furzolidone are rare and include brown discoloration of the urine, mild gastrointestinal symptoms, rash, hypersensitivity reactions, a disulfiram-like reaction during concurrent therapy with alcohol-containing medications, and possible induction of intravascular hemolysis in children with glucose 6-phosphate deficiency. In contrast to the bitter and metallic tastes of quinacrine and metronidazole, respectively, the acceptable taste of furazolidone facilitates compliance in pediatric cases.

The pregnant patient with giardiasis deserves special consideration since the safety of the above agents during pregnancy has not been established. Both quinacrine and metronidazole are known to pass through the placenta into the fetal circulation. Metronidazole has been shown to be carcinogenic in rodents and mutagenic in bacteria, although a tumorigenic effect in humans has not been demonstrated (231). Furazolidone has induced hemolysis in newborns with glucose 6-phosphate deficiency, and its potential for fetal toxicity is unknown. Thus, the use of quinacrine and metronidazole is discouraged during the first trimester, and therapy with furazolidone during pregnancy is contraindicated (232). After the first trimester, quinacrine rather than metronidazole is used by many clinicians, but the benefits of therapy must be weighed carefully against potential effects on the fetus. A poorly absorbed aminoglycoside with antiprotozoal effects, paramomycin, has been used successfully in two pregnant patients with giardiasis (233), but the effectiveness of this agent awaits confirmation.

The prevention of infection with *G. lamblia* is gaining wider appreciation as an important topic of investigation. Convincing evidence has established contaminated drinking water to be the principal mode of transmission in several epidemics of giardiasis (234-236). Indeed, for the past decade contaminated municipal water has led to *G. lamblia*'s status as one of the most frequent causes of waterborne diarrheal disease in the United States (237,238). The key factors contributing to contaminated municipal water include cross-contamination of drinking water supplies with sewage (43) and ineffective water treatment (45, 46). As discussed above, the ineffective treatment of drinking water by chlorination has been a common feature of many epidemics. The ability of chlorine to kill *G. lamblia* cysts appears to depend on a number of factors including pH, temperature, contact time, the level of chlorine, and the presence of other organic material (239). Thus, routine chlorination, as in the Rome, New York, epidemic, may be inadequate for killing *G. lamblia* cysts. In contrast, granular media filtration and diatomaceous earth filtration, both of which are capable of effectively removing *Entamoeba histolytica* cysts from water, and slow sand filtration appear equally effective in removing *G. lamblia* cysts (240). The use of both properly functioning filtration and disinfection should eliminate contaminated municipal water as a vehicle of transmission in epidemic giardiasis.

The disinfection of small quantities of water is particularly relevant for individuals who visit endemic regions. Recently, the chemical disinfectants Halazone ($C_7H_5Cl_2NO_4S$), bleach (NaOCl, 5.28%), Globaline [$(NH_2CH_2COOH)_4HI$: $1.25I_2$], Emergency Drinking Water Germicidal Tablet [EDWGT, $(NH_2CH_2COOH)_4HI$:1.24 I_2], and I_2 (I_2-HOI, saturated or 2% tincture) were tested for their ability to kill *G. lamblia* cysts under various conditions (241). At 20°C these disinfectants in their recommended application killed 99.8% cysts in clear and cloudy water. However, at 3°C in cloudy water all disinfectants except saturated I_2 were effective against the cysts, whereas at 3°C in clear water only Halazone and EDWGT were completely effective in inactivating the cysts. Thus, conveniently transported chemicals are available for disinfecting small quantities of drinking water, but both water temperature and clarity affect halogen inactivation of *G. lamblia* cysts and should be taken into account during disinfection procedures.

V. CONCLUSION

Regarded until recently as a nonpathogenic commensal, *G. lamblia* now has become the most frequently identified intestinal parasite of humans in the

United States. Firm clinical data summarized in this chapter indicate that the organism causes significant gastrointestinal morbidity, including malabsorption, and occasionally extraintestinal symptoms. However, despite new information on the biology of *G. lamblia*, the pathophysiological mechanisms responsible for the clinical features of infection are still unknown. Convincing evidence also indicates that *G. lamblia* induces a host immune response, although the contribution of this response to protection against the parasite is unclear. Elucidation of these and other issues related to infection with *G. lamblia* should be forthcoming as investigation of this intriguing organism continues.

REFERENCES

1. Dobeld, C. The discovery of the intestinal protozoa of man. *Proc. R. Soc. Med. 13*:1–15 (1969.
2. Bingham, A. R., and Meyer, E. A. *Giardia* excystation can be induced in vitro in active solutions. *Nature 277*:301–302 (1979).
3. Rice, E. W., and Schaefer, F. W., III. Improved in vitro excystation procedure for *Giardia lamblia* cysts. *J. Clin. Microbiol. 14*:709–710 (1981).
4. Farthing, M. J. G., Varon, S. R., and Keusch, G. T. Mammalian bile promotes growth of *Giardia lamblia* in axenic culture. *Trans. R. Soc. Trop. Med. Hyg. 77*:467–469 (1983).
5. Gillin, F. D., Gault, M. J., Hofmann, A. F., Gurantz, D., and Sauch, J. F. Biliary lipids support serum-free growth of *Giardia lamblia. Infect. Immun. 53*:641–645 (1986).
6. Farthing, M. J. G., Keusch, G. T., and Carey, M. C. Effects of bile and bile salts on growth and membrane lipid uptake by *Giardia lamblia*. Possible implications for pathogenesis of intestinal disease. *J. Clin. Invest. 76*:1727–1732 (1985).
7. Lev, B., Ward, H., Keusch, G. T., and Pereira, M. E. A. Lectin activation in *Giardia lamblia* by host protease. A novel host-parasite interaction. *Science 232*:71–73 (1986).
8. Vinyak, V. K., Sharma, G. L., and Naik, S. R. Experimental *Giardia lamblia* infection in Swiss mice—a preliminary report. *Indian J. Res. 70*:195–198 (1979).
9. Hill, D. R., Guerrant, R. L., Pearson, R. D., and Hewlett, H. L. *Giardia lamblia* infection in suckling mice. *J. Infect Dis. 167*:217–221 (1983).
10. Belosevic, M., Faubert, G. M., Maclean, J. D., Law, C., and Croll, N. A. *Giardia lamblia* infections in mongolian gerbils: an animal model. *J. Infect. Dis. 167*:222–226 (1983).
11. Sehgal, A. K., Grewal, M. S., Chakravarti, R. N., Broar, S. L., Deka, N. C., and Chhuttani, P. N. Experimental giardiasis in albino rats. *Indian J. Med. Res. 64*:1015–1018 (1976).
12. Craft, J. C. Experimental infection with *Giardia lamblia* in rats. *J. Infect. Dis. 156*:495–498 (1982).

13. Schleiuitz, P., Justus, P., Stenzel, P., Owen, R., and Meyer, E. Successful introduction of culture adapted *Giardia* into a rabbit model: ultrastructural features. *Gastroenterology 84*:1301 (1983).

14. Hewlett, E. L., Andrews, J. S., Ruffier, J., and Schaefer, F. W. Experimental infection of mongrel dogs with *Giardia lamblia* cysts and cultured trophozoites. *J. Infect. Dis. 156*:89–93 (1982).

15. Padchenko, I. K., and Stolyarchuk, N. C. On the possible circulation of *lamblia* in nature. *Prog. Protozool. 3*:311–312 (1969).

16. Nieschulz, O. Uber den Bau von *Giardia caprae* mihi. *Arch. Protistenkd. 49*: 278–286 (1924).

17. Ansari, M. A. R. Contribution a l'etude du genre *Giardia* kunstler. 1982. (Mastigophore: Octomitidae). *Ann. Parasitol. Hum. Comp. 27*:461–479 (1952).

18. Filice, F. P. Studies on the cytology and life history of a *Giardia* from the laboratory rat. *Univ. Calif. Publ. Zool. 57*:53–163 (1952).

19. Grant, D. R., and Woo, P. T. K. Comparative studies of *Giardia* spp. in small animals in southern Ontario. I. Prevalence and identity of the parasites with a taxonomic discussion of the genus. *Can. J. Zool. 56*:1348–1359 (1978).

20. Bertram, M. A., Meyer, E. A., Anderson, D. L., and Jones, C. T. A morphometric comparison of five axenic *Giardia* isolates. *J. Parasitol. 70*:530–535 (1984).

21. Bertram, M. A., Meyer, E. A., Lile, J. D., and Morse, S. A. A comparison of isozymes of five axenic *Giardia* isolates. *J. Parasitol. 69*:793–801 (1983).

22. Nash, T.E., McCutchan, T., Keister, D., Dame, J. B., Conrad, J. D., and Gillin, F. D. Restriction-endonuclease analysis of DNA from 15 *Giardia* isolates obtained from humans and animals. *J. Infect. Dis. 172*:64–73 (1985).

23. Edlind, T. D., and Chakraborty, P. R. Novel ribosomal RNA of the intestinal parasite *Giardia lamblia. Nucleic Acids Res. 12*:7889–7901 (1987).

24. Faust, E. C., Russell, P. F., and Jung, C. R. The flagellated protozoa. Flagellates of the digestive tract and genitalia. In *Clinical Parasitology* (E. C. Faust, P. F. Russell, and R. C. Jung, eds.). Lea and Febiger, Philadelphia, 1970, p. 66.

25. Black, R. E., Dykes, A. C., Sinclair, S. P., and Wells, J. G. Giardiasis in daycare centers. Evidence of person-to-person transmission. *Pediatrics 60*:468–491 (1977).

26. Pickering, L. K., Evasn, D. S., DuPont, H. L., Vollet, J. J., and Evans, D. J., Jr. Diarrhea caused by shigella, rotavirus, and *Giardia* in day-care centers: Prospective study. *J. Pediatr. 99*:51–56 (1981).

27. Sealy, D. P., and Schuman, S. H. Endemic giardiasis and day care. *Pediatrics 72*:174–158 (1983).

28. Polis, M. A., Tuazon, C. U., Alling, D. W., and Talmanis, E. Transmission of *Giardia lamblia* from a day care center to the community. *Am. J. Public Health 76*:1142–1144 (1986).

29. Meyers, J. D., Kuharic, H. A., and Holmes, K. K. *Giardia lamblia* infection in homosexual men. *Br. J. Vener. Dis. 55*:54–55 (1977).
30. Schemerin, M. J., Jones, T. C., and Klein, H. Giardiasis: association with homosexuality. *Ann. Intern. Med. 88*:801–804 (1978).
31. Hurwitz, A. L., and Owen, R. L. Venereal transmission of intestinal parasites. *West. J. Med. 128*:89–91 (1978).
32. Yoeli, M., Most, H., Hammond, J., and Scheinesson, G. P. Parasitic infections in a closed community. results of a 10-year survey in Willowbrook State School. *Trans. R. Soc. Trop. Med. Hyg. 66*:764–776 (1972).
33. Thacker, S. B., Simpson, S., Gordon, T. J., Wolf, M., and Kimball, A. M. Parasitic disease control in a residential facility for the mentally retarded. *Am. J. Public Health 69*:1279–1281 (1979).
34. Hossain, M. M., Ljungstrom, I., Glass, R. I., Lundin, L., Stoll, B. J., and Huldt, G. Amoebiasis and giardiasis in Bangladesh: parasitological and serological studies. *Trans. R. Soc. Trop. Med. Hyg. 77*:552–554 (1983).
35. Goldsmid, J. M. Intestinal parasitic infections of man in Tasmania. *Trans. R. Soc. Trop. Med. Hyg. 75*:110–112 (1981).
36. Osterholm, M. T., Forgang, J. C., Ristinen, T. C., Dean, A. G., Washburn, J.W., Godes, J. R., Rude, R. A., and McCullough, J. R. An outbreak of food-borne giardiasis. *New Engl. J. Med. 304*:24–28 (1981).
37. Petersen, L. R., Cartter, M. L., and Hadler, J. L. A food-borne outbreak of *Giardia lamblia. J. Infect. Dis. 157*:846–848 (1988).
38. Centers for Disease Control. Intestinal surveillance–United States 1976. *Morb. Mortal. Wkly. Rep. 27*:167 (1978).
39. Wright, R. A., Spencer, H. C., Brodsky, R. E., and Vernon, T. M. Giardiasis in Colorado: an epidemiologic study. *Am. J. Epidem. 105*:330–336 (1977).
40. Veazie, L. Epidemic giardiasis. *New Engl. J. Med. 281*:853 (1969).
41. Centers for Disease Control. Waterborne giardiasis–California, Colorado, Oregon, Pennsylvania. *Morb. Mortal. Wkly. Rept. 29*:121–123 (1980).
42. Hopkins, R. S., Shillam, P., Gaspard, B., Eisnach, L., and Karlin, R. J. Waterborne disease in Colorado: three year's surveillance and 18 outbreaks. *Am. J. Public Health 75*:254–257 (1985).
43. Moore, G. T., Cross, W. M., McGuire, D., Mollohan, C. S., Gleason, N. N., Healy, G. R., and Newton, L. H. Epidemic giardiasis at a ski resort. *New Engl. J. Med. 281*:402–407 (1969).
44. Barbour, A. G., Nichols, C. R., and Fukushima, T. An outbreak of giardiasis in a group of campers. *Am. J. Trop. Med. Hyg. 25*:384–389 (1976).
45. Shaw, P. K., Brodsky, R. E., Lyman, D. O., Wood, B. T., Hiller, C. P., Healy, G. R., MacLeod, K. I. E., Stahl, W., and Schultz, M. G. A community outbreak of giardiasis with evidence of transmission by a municipal water supply. *Ann. Intern. Med. 87*:426–432 (1977).
46. Dykes, A. C., Juranek, D. D., Lorenz, R. A., Sinclair, S., Jakubowski, W., and Davies, R. Municipal waterborne giardiasis: an epidemiologic investigation. Beavers implicated as a possible reservoir. *Ann. Intern. Med. 92*:165–170 (1980).

47. Walzer, P. D., Wolfe, M. S., and Schultz, M. G. Giardiasis in travelers. *J. Infect. Dis. 124*:235–237 (1971).
48. Brodsky, R. E., Spencer, H. C., Jr., and Schultz, M. G. Giardiasis in American travelers to the Soviet Union. *J. Infect. Dis. 130*:319–323 (1974).
49. Karapetyan, A. E. A method of cultivation of *Giardia. Tsitologiia 2*:379–384 (1960).
50. Karapetyan, A. E. In vitro cultivation of *Giardia duodenalis. J. Parasitol. 48*:337–340 (1962).
51. Meyer, E. A. Isolation and axenic cultivation of *Giardia* trophozoites from the rabbit, chinchilla, and cat. *Exp. Parasitol. 27*:179–183 (1970).
52. Meyer, E. A. *Giardia lamblia.* Isolation and axenic cultivation. *Exp. Parasitol. 39*:101–105 (1976).
53. Visvesvara, G. S. Axenic growth of *Giardia lamblia* in Diamonds' TP-S-1 medium. *Trans. R. Soc. Trop. Med. Hyg. 74*:213–215 (1980).
54. Diamond, L. S. Techniques of axenic cultivation of *Entamoeba histolytica* Schaudinn, 1903 and *E. histolytica*-like amoeba. *J. Parasitol. 54*:1047–1056 (1968).
55. Keister, D. B. Axenic culture of *Giardia lamblia* in TYI-S-33 medium supplemented with bile. *Trans. R. Soc. Trop. Med. Hyg. 77*:487–488 (1983).
56. Gillin, F. D., and Diamond, L. S. *Entamoeba histolytica* and *Giardia lamblia*: growth responses to reducing agents. *Exp. Parasitol. 51*:382–391 (1981).
57. Gillin, F. D., and Diamond, L. S. *Entamoeba histolytica* and *Giardia lamblia*: effects of cysteine and oxygen tension on trophozoite attachment to glass and survival in culture media. *Exp. Parasitol. 52*:9–17 (1981).
58. Gillin, F. D., and Reiner, D. S. Attachment of the flagellate *Giardia lamblia*: role of reducing agents, serum, temperature and ionic composition. *Mol. Cell. Biol. 2*:369–377 (1982).
59. Wiesehahn, G. P., Jarroll, E. L., Lindmark, D. G., Meyer, E. A., and Hallick, L. M. *Giardia lamblia*: autoradiographic analysis of nuclear replication. *Exp. Parasitol. 58*:94–100 (1984).
60. Kasprzak, W., and Majewska, A. C. Improvement in isolation and axenic growth of *Giardia intestinalis* strains. *Trans. R. Soc. Trop. Med. Hyg. 79*:551–557 (1985).
61. Friend, D. S. The fine structure of *Giardia muris. J. Cell. Biol. 29*:317–331 (1966).
62. Weinbach, E. C., Claggett, C. E., Keister, D. B., Diamond, L. S., and Kon, H. Respiratory metabolism of *Giardia lamblia. J. Parasitol. 66*:347–350 (1980).
63. Lindmark, D. G. Energy metabolism of the anaerobic protozoan *Giardia lamblia. Mol. Biochem. Parasitol. 1*:1–12 (1980).
64. Jarroll, E. L., Muller, P. J., Meyer, E. A., and Morse, S. A. Lipid and carbohydrate metabolism of *Giardia lamblia. Mol. Biochem. Parasitol. 2*:187–196 (1981).
65. Aldritt, S. M., Tien, P., and Wang, C. C. Pyimidine salvage in *Giardia lamblia. J. Exp. Med. 161*:437–445 (1985).

66. Smith, P. D., Gillin, F. D., Kaushal, N. A., and Nash, T. E. Antigenic analysis of *Giardia lamblia* from Afghanistan, Puerto Rico, Ecuador and Oregon. *Infect. Immun. 36*:71–719 (1982).
67. Nash, T. E., Gillin, F. D., and Smith, P. D. Excretory-secretory products of *Giardia lamblia. J. Immunol. 131*:2004–2010 (1983).
68. Nash, T. E., and Keister, D. B. Differences in excretory-secretory products and surface antigens among 19 isolates of *Giardia. J. Infect. Dis. 172*:1166–1171 (1985).
69. Einfeld, D. A., and Stibbes, H. H. Identification and characterization of a major surface antigen of *Giardia lamblia. Infect. Immun. 46*:377–383 (1984).
70. Tarian, B. E., Barnes, R. C., Stephens, R. S., and Stibbs, H. H. Tubulin and high-molecular-weight polypeptides as *Giardia lamblia* antigens. *Infect. Immun. 46*:152–158 (1984).
71. Istre, G. R., Dunlop, T. S., Gaspard, G. B., and Hopkins, R. S. Waterborne giardiasis at a mountain resort: evidence for acquired immunity. *Am. J. Public Health 74*:602–604 (1984).
72. Hughes, W. S., Cerda, J. J., Holtzapple, P., and Brooks, F. P. Primary hypogammaglobulinemia and malabsorption. *Ann. Intern. Med. 74*:903–910 (1971).
73. Brown, W. R., Butterfield, D., Savage, D., and Tada, T. Clinical, microbiological, and immunological studies in patients with immunoglobulin deficiencies and gastrointestinal disorders. *Gut 13*:589–595 (1972).
74. Ajdukiewicz, A. B., Youngs, G. R., and Bouchier, I. A. D. Nodular lymphoid hyperplasia with hypogammaglobulinemia. *Gut 13*:589–595 (1972).
75. Ament, M. E., Ochs, H. D., and Davis, D. D. Structure and function of the gastrointestinal tract in primary immunodeficiency syndrome: a study of 39 patients. *Medicine 52*:227–248 (1973).
76. Hermans, P. E., Diaz-Buxo, J. A., and Stobo, J. D. Idiopathic late-onset immunoglobulin deficiency. Clinical observations in 50 patients. *Am. J. Med. 61*:221–237 (1976).
77. LoGalbo, P. R., Sampson, H. A., and Buckley, R. H. Symptomatic giardiasis in three patients with X-linked agammaglobulinemia. *J. Pediatr. 101*:78–80 (1982).
78. Ridley, M. J., and Ridley, D. S. Serum antibodies and jejunal histology in giardiasis associated with malabsorption. *J. Clin. Pathol. 29*:30–34 (1976).
79. Vinayak, V. K., Jain, P., and Naik, S. R. Demonstration of antibodies in giardiasis using the immunodiffusion technique with *Giardia* cysts as antigen. *Ann. Trop. Med. Parasitol. 72*:581–582 (1978).
80. Visvesvara, G. S., Smith, P. D., Healy, G. R., and Brown, W. R. An immunofluorescence test to detect serum antibodies to *Giardia lamblia. Ann. Intern. Med. 93*:802–805 (1980).
81. Smith, P. D., Gillin, F. D., Brown, W. R., and Nash, T. E. IgG antibody to *Giardia lamblia* detected by enzyme-linked immunosorbent assay. *Gastroenterology 80*:1676–1680 (1981).

82. Wittner, M., Maayan, S., Farrer, W., and Tanowitz, H. B. Diagnosis of giardiasis by two methods. Immunofluorescence and enzyme-linked immunosorbent assay. *Arch. Pathol. Lab. Med. 107*:524–527 (1983).

83. Miotti, P. G., Gilman, R. H., Pickering, L. K., Ruiz-Palacios, G., Park, H. S., and Yolken, R. H. Prevalence of serum and milk antibodies to *Giardia lamblia* in different populations of lactating women. *J. Infect. Dis. 152*: 1025–1031 (1985).

84. Goka, A. K., Rolston, D. D. K., Mathan, V. I., and Farthing, M. J. G. Diagnosis of giardiasis by specific IgM antibody enzyme-linked immunosorbent assay. *Lancet 2*:184–186 (1986).

85. Janoff, E. N., Smith, P. D., and Blaser, M. J. Acute antibody responses to *Giardia lamblia* are depressed in patients with AIDS. *J. Infect. Dis. 157*: 798–804 (1988).

86. Lane, H. C., Masur, H., Edgar, L. C., Whalen, G., Rook, A. H., and Fauci, A. S. Abnormalities of B-cell activation and immunoregulation in patients with the acquired immunodeficiency syndrome. *New Engl. Med. J. 309*: 453–458 (1983).

87. Islam, A., Stoll, B. J., Ljungstroem, I., Biswas, J., Nazrul, H., and Huldt, G. G. lamblia infections in a cohort of Bangladeshi mothers and infants followed for one year. *J. Pediatr. 103*:996–1000 (1983).

88. Radulescu, S., and Meyer, E. A. Opsonization in vitro of *Giardia lamblia* trophozoites. *Infect. Immun. 32*:852–856 (1981).

89. Kapalan, B. S., Uni, S., Aikawa, M., and Mahmoud, A. A. F. Effector mechanisms of host resistance in murine giardiasis: specific IgG and IgA cell-modulated toxicity. *J. Immunol. 32*:1975–1981 (1985).

90. Smith, P. D., Keister, D. B., and Elson, C. O. Human host response to *Giardia lamblia*. II. Antibody-dependent killing by granulocytes in vitro. *Cell. Immunol. 82*:308–315 (1982).

91. Hill, D. R., Burge, J. J., and Pearson, R. D. Susceptibility of *Giardia lamblia* trophozoites to the lethal effect of human serum. *J. Immunol. 132*:2046–2052 (1984).

92. Snider, D. P., Gordon, J., McDermott, M. R., and Underdown, B. J. Chronic *Giardia muris* infection in anti-IgM-treated mice. I. Analysis of immunoglobulin and parasite-specific antibody in normal and immunoglobulin-deficient animals. *J. Immunol. 134*:4153–4162 (1985).

93. Snider, D. P., and Underdown, B. J. Quantitative and temporal analysis of murine antibody response in serum and gut secretions to infection with *Giardia muris*. *Infect. Immun. 52*:271–278 (1986).

94. Andrews, J. S., and Hewlett, E. L. Protection against infection with *Giardia muris* by milk containing antibody to *Giardia*. *J. Infect. Dis. 143*:242–246 (1981).

95. Hill, R. D., Guerrant, R. L., Pearson, R. D., and Hewlett, E. L. *Giardia lamblia* infection of suckling mice. *J. Infect. Dis. 147*:217–221 (1983).

96. Heyworth, M. F., Owen, R. L., and Jones, A. L. Comparison of leukocytes obtained from the intestinal lumen of *Giardia*-infected immunocompetent mice and nude mice. *Gastroenterology 89*:1360–1365 (1985).

97. Roberts-Thomson, I. C., Stevens, D. P., Mahmoud, A. A. F., and Stevens, K. S. Giardiasis in the mouse: an animal model. *Gastroenterology 71*:57–71 (1976).

98. Roberts-Thomson, I. C., Stevens, D. P., Mahmoud, A. A. F., and Warren, K. S. Acquired resistance to infection in an animal model of giardiasis. *J. Immunol. 117*:2036–2037 (1976).

99. Boorman, G. A., Lina, P. H. C., Zurcher, C., and Nieuwerkerk, H. T. M., *Hexamita* and *Giardia* as a cause of mortality in congenitally thymus-less (nude) mice. *Clin. Exp. Immunol. 15*:623–627 (1973).

100. Roberts-Thompson, I. C., and Mitchell, G. F. Giardiasis in mice. I. Prolonged infection in certain mouse strains and hypothymic (nude) mice. *Gastroenterology. 75*:42–46 (1978).

101. Stevens, D. A., Frank, D. P., and Mahmoud, A. A. F. Thymus dependency of host resistance to *Giardia muris* infection: studies in nude mice. *J. Immunol. 120*:680–682 (1978).

102. Carlson, J. R., Heyworth, M. F., and Owen, R. L. Response of Peyer's patch lymphocyte subsets to *Giardia muris* infection in BALB/c mice. I. T-cell subsets. *Cell. Immunol. 97*:44–50 (1986).

103. Carlson, J. R., Heyworth, M. F., and Owen, R. L. Response of Peyer's patch lymphocyte subsets to *Giardia muris* infection in BALB/c mice. II. B-cell subsets: enteric antigen exposure is associated with immunoglobulin isotype switching by Peyer's patch B cells. *Cell. Immunol. 97*:51–58 (1986).

104. Kawanishi, H., Saltzman, L. E., and Strober, W. Mechanisms regulating IgA class-specific immunoglobulin production in murine gut-associated lymphoid tissue. I. T cells derived from Peyer's patches that switch sIgM B cells to sIgA B cells in vitro. *J. Exp. Med. 157*:433–450 (1983).

105. Kawanishi, H., Saltzman, L. E., and Strober, W. Mechanisms regulating IgA class-specific immunoglobulin production in murine gut-associated lymphoid tissues. II. Terminal differentiation of postswitch sIgG-bearing Peyer's patch B cells. *J. Exp. Med. 158*:649–669 (1983).

106. Underdown, B. J., Roberts-Thomson, J. C., Anders, R. F., and Mitchell, G. F. Giardiasis in mice: studies on the characteristics of chronic infection in C3H/He mice. *J. Immunol. 126*:669–672 (1981).

107. Smith, P. D., Keister, D. B., Wahl, S. M., and Meltzer, M. S. Defective spontaneous but normal antibody-dependent cytotoxicity for an extracellular protozoan parasite. *Giardia lamblia*, by C3H/H3J mouse macrophages. *Cell. Immunol. 85*:244–251 (1984).

108. Roberts-Thomson, I. C., Mitchell, G. F., Anders, R. F., Tait, B. D., Kerlin, P., Kerr-Grant, A., and Cavanagh, P. Genetic studies in human and murine giardiasis. *Gut 21*:397–401 (1980).

109. Pitchenik, A. E., Fischl, M. A., Dickinson, G. M., Becker, D. M., Fournier, A. M., O'Connell, M. T., Colton, R. M., and Spira, T. J. Opportunistic infections and Kaposi's sarcoma among Haitians: evidence of a new acquired immunodeficiency state. *Ann. Intern. Med. 98*:277–284 (1983).

110. Smith, P. D., Lane, H. C., Gill, V. J. Manischewitz, J., Quinnan, G. V., Fauci, A. S., and Masur, H. Intestinal infections in the acquired immunodeficiency syndrome: etiology and response to therapy. *Ann. Inrern. Med.* *108*:328–333 (1988).

111. Smith, P. D., Ohura, K., Masur, H., Lane, H. C., Fauci, A. S., and Wahl, S. M. Monocyte function in the acquired immune deficiency syndrome. Defective chemotaxis. *J. Clin. Invest. 74*:2121–2128 (1984).

112. Smith, P. D., Wahl, L. M., Katona, I. M., Miyake, Y., and Wahl, S. M. Monocyte accessory cell function in the acquired immunodeficiency syndrome. Manuscript submitted.

113. Prince, H. E., Moody, D. J., Shubin, B. I., and Fahey, J. L. Defective monocyte function in acquired immune deficiency syndrome (AIDS): evidence from a monocyte-dependent T-cell proliferative system. *J. Clin. Immunol. 5*:21–25 (1985).

114. Shannon, K., Cowan, M. J., Ball, E., Abrams, D., Volberding, P., and Ammann, A. J. Impaired mononuclear-cell proliferation in patients with the acquired immune deficiency syndrome results from abnormalities of both T lymphocytes and adherent mononuclear cells. *J. Clin. Immunol. 5*:239–245 (1985).

115. Schnittman, S. M., Lane, H. C., Higgins, S. E., Folks, T., and Fauci, A. S. Direct polyclonal activation of human B lymphocytes by the acquired immune deficiency syndrome virus. *Science 233*:1084–1086 (1986).

116. Quinn, T. C., Stamm, W. E., Goodell, S. E., Mkrtichian, E., Benedetti, J., Corey, L., Schuffler, M. D., and Holmes, K. K. The polymicrobial origin of intestinal infections in homosexual men. *New Engl. J. Med. 309*:376–382 (1983).

117. Owen, R. L., Allen, C. L., and Stevens, D. P. Phagocytosis of *Giardia muris* by macrophages in Peyer's patch epithelium. *Infect Immun. 33*: 591–601 (1981).

118. Smith, P. D., Elson, C. O., Keister, D. B., and Nash, T. E. Human host response to *Giardia lamblia*. I. Spontaneous killing by mononuclear leukocytes in vitro. *J. Immunol. 128*:1575–1576 (1982).

119. Hill, D. R., and Pearson, R. D. Ingestion of *Giardia lamblia* trophozoites by human mononuclear phagocytes. *Infect. Immun. 55*:3155–3161 (1987).

120. Smith, P. D. Pathophysiology and immunology of giardiasis. *Ann. Rev. Med. 36*:295–307 (1985).

121. Wahl, S. M., McCartney-Francis, N., Hunt, D. A., Smith, P. D., Wahl, L. M., and Katona, I. M. Monocyte interleukin 2 receptor gene expression and interleukin 2 augmentation of microbiobicidal activity. *J. Immunol. 139*: 1342–1347 (1987).

122. Gately, C. L., Wahl, S. M., and Oppenheim, J. J. Characterization of hydrogen peroxide-potentiating factor, a lymphokine that increases the capacity of human monocytes and monocyte-like cell lines to produce hydrogen peroxide. *J. Immunol. 131*:2853–2858 (1983).

123. Gillin, F. D., and Reiner, D. S. Human milk kills parasitic intestinal protozoa. *Science 221*:1290–1291 (1983).

124. Hernell, O., Ward, H., Blackberg, L., and Pereira, M. E. A. Killing of *Giardia lamblia* by human milk lipases: an effect mediated by lipolysis of milk lipids. *J. Infect. Dis. 153*:715–720 (1986).

125. Haas, J., and Bucken, E. W. Zum Krankeitswert der Lamblien-Infection. *Dtsch. Med. Wochenschr. 92*:1869–1871 (1967).

126. Slonim, J. M., Ireton, H. J. C., and Smallwood, R. A. Giardiasis following gastric surgery. *Aust. N.Z. J. Med. 6*:479–480 (1976).

127. Veghelyi, P. Celiac disease initiated by giardiasis. *Am. J. Dis. Child. 57*: 894–899 (1939).

128. Tandon, B. N., Tandon, R. K., Satpathy, B. K., and Shrinwas. Mechanisms of malabsorption in giardiasis: a study of bacterial flora and bile salt deconjugation in upper jejunum. *Gut 18*:176–181 (1977).

129. Smith, P. D., Horsburgh, C. R., and Brown, W. R. In vitro studies on bile acid deconjugation and lipolysis inhibition by *Giardia lamblia. Dig. Dis. Sci. 26*:700–704 (1981).

130. Tomkins, A. M., Wright, S. G., Draser, B. S., and James, W. P. T. Bacterial colonization of jejunal mucosa in giardiasis. *Trans. R. Soc. Trop. Med. Hyg. 72*:33–36 (1978).

131. Gorbach, S. L., Banwell, J. G., Chatterjee, B. D., Jacobs, B., and Sack, R. B. Acute undifferentiated human diarrhea in the tropics. I. Alterations in intestinal microflora. *J. Clin. Invest. 50*:881–889 (1971).

132. Alp, M. H., and Hislop, I. G.. The effect of *G. lamblia* on the gastrointestinal tract. *Aust. Ann. Med. 18*:232–237 (1969).

133. Smith, P. D., Gillin, F. D., Spria, W. W., and Nash, T. E. Chronic giardiasis: studies on drug sensitivity, toxin production and host immune response. *Gastroenterology 83*:797–803 (1982).

134. Kimberg, D. V., Field, F. M., Johnson, J., Henderson, A., and Gershon, E. Stimulation of intestinal mucosal adenyl cyclase by cholera enterotoxin and prostaglandin. *J. Clin. Invest. 50*:1218–1230 (1971).

135. Jaffe, B. N., and Condon, S. Prostaglandin E and F in endocrine diarrheagenic syndromes. *Ann. Surg. 184*:516–524 (1976).

136. Benneet, A., and Flesher, B. Prostaglandins and the gastrointestinal tract. *Gastroenterology 59*:790–800 (1970).

137. Ganguly, N. K., Garg, S. K., Vasudev, V., Radhakrishna, V., Anand, B. S., and Mahajan, R. C. Prostaglandins E and F levels in mice infected with *Giardia lamblia. Indian J. Med. Res. 79*:755–759 (1984).

138. Hoskins, L. C., Winawer, S. J., Broitman, S. A., Gottlieb, L. S., and Zamcheck, N. Clinical giardiasis and intestinal malabsorption. *Gastroenterology 53*:265–279 (1967).

139. Levinson, J. D., and Nastro, L. J. Giardiasis with total villous atrophy. *Gastroenterology 74*:271–275 (1978).

140. Hartong, W. A., Gourley, W. K., and Arvanitakas, C. Giardiasis: clinical spectrum and functional structural abnormalities of the small intestinal mucosa. *Gastroenterology 77*:61–69 (1979).

141. Wright, S. G., and Tompkins, A. M. Quantification of the lymphocytic infiltration in jejunal epithelium in giardiasis. *Clin. Exp. Immunol. 29*: 408–412 (1977).

142. Duncombe, V. M., Bolin, T. D., Davis, A. E., Cummins, A. G., and Crouch, R. L. Histopathology in giardiasis: a correlation with diarrhea. *Aust. N.Z. J. Med. 8*:392–396 (1978).

143. Wright, S. G., and Tomkins, A. M. Quantitative histology in giardiasis. *J. Clin. Pathol. 31*:712–716 (1978).

144. Mauromichalis, M. F., Brueton, M. F., McNeish, A. S. Evaluation of the intraepithelial lymphocyte count in the jejunum in childhood enteropathies. *Gut 17*:600–603 (1976).

145. MacDonald, T. T., and Ferguson Small intestine epithelial cell kinetics and protozoal infection in mice. *Gastroenterology 74*:496–500 (1978).

146. Gillon, J., Thamery, A. L., and Ferguson, A. Features of small intestinal pathology (epithelial cell kinetics, intraepithelial lymphocytes, disaccharidases) in primary *Giardia muris* infection. *Gut 23*:498–506 (1982).

147. Anand, B. S., Kumar, M., Chakravarti, R. N., Sehgal, A. K., and Chhuttani, P. N. Pathogenesis of malabsorption in *Giardia* infection: an experimental study in rats. *Trans. R. Soc. Trop. Med. Hyg. 74*:565–569 (1980).

148. Anand, B. S., Mahmoud, A., Gangerly, N. K., Dilawari, M. M., and Mahajan, J. B. Transport studies and enzyme assays in mice infected with human *Giardia lamblia. Trans. R. Soc. Trop. Med. Hyg. 76*:616–619 (1982).

149. Owen, R. L., Nemanic, P. C., and Stevens, D. Ultrastructural observation in giardiasis in a murine model. I. Intestinal distribution, attachment, and relationship to the immune system of *Giardia muris. Gastroenterology 76*: 757–769 (1979).

150. Feely, D. E., Schollmeyer, J. V., and Erlandsen, S. L. *Giardia* spp.: distribution and contractile proteins in the attachment organelle. *Exp. Parasitol. 53*:145–154 (1982).

151. Feely, D. E., and Erlandsen, S. L. In vitro analysis of *Giardia* trophozoite attachment. *J. Parasitol. 68*:869–873 (1982).

152. Yardley, J. H., Takano, J., and Hendrix, T. R. Epithelial and other mucosal lesions of the jejunum in giardiasis. Jejunal biopsy studies. *Bull. Johns Hopkins Hosp. 115*:389–406 (1964).

153. Takano, J., and Yardley, J. H. Jejunal lesions in patients with giardiasis and malabsorption. An electron microscopy study. *Bull. Johns Hopkins Hosp. 116*:413–469 (1964).

154. Morecke, R., and Parker, J. G. Ultrastructural studies of the human *Giardia lamblia* and subjacent jejunal mucosa in a subject with steatorrhea. *Gastroenterology 52*:151–164 (1967).

155. Saha, T. K., and Gosh, T. K. Invasion of small intestinal mucosa by *Giardia lamblia. Gastroenterology 73*:402–405 (1977).

156. Brandborg, L. L., Tankersley, C. B., Gottlieb, S., and Barancik, M. Histological demonstration of mucosal invasion by *Giardia lamblia* in man. *Gastroenterology 52*:143–150 (1967).

157. Rendtorff, R. C. The experimental transmission of human intestinal protozoan parasites. II. *Giardia lamblia* cysts given in capsules. *Am. J. Hyg. 59*:209–220 (1954).
158. Rendtorff, R. C., and Holt, C. J. The experimental transmission of human intestinal protozoan parasites. IV. Attempts to transmit *Entamoeba coli* and *Giardia lamblia* cysts by water. *Am. J. Hyg. 60*:327–338 (1954).
159. Heap, T. Giardiasis: a common cause of prolonged diarrhoea in adults. *Med. J. Aust. 2*:592–595 (1974).
160. Dellamonica, P., LeFichoux, Y., Monnier, B., and Duplay, H. Dysenteria syndrome and urticaria in giardiasis. *Nouv. Presse. Med. 5*:30 (1976).
161. Wolfe, M. S. Current concepts in parasitology. Giardiasis. *New Engl. J. Med. 298*:319–320 (1978).
162. Goldstein, F., Thornton, J. J., and Szydlowski, T. Biliary tract dysfunction in giardiasis. *Am. J. Dig. Dis. 23*:559–560 (1978).
163. Soto, J. M., and Dreiling, D. A. *Giardia lamblia*. A case presentation of chronic cholecystitis and duodenitis. *Am. J. Gastroenterol. 67*:265–269 (1977).
164. Lyon, B. B. V., and Swalm, W. Giardiasis: its frequency, recognition, treatment and certain clinical factors. *Am. J. Med. Sci. 170*:348–364 (1925).
165. Turbin, B. N., and Ivascheukd, V. V. Lamblia-induced cholecystitis. *Vestn. Khir. 117*:20–22 (1976).
166. Dzys, E. P., Naurotskaia, G. A., and Ornelchenko, L. I. Lamblia invasion and chronic inflammatory diseases of the biliary tracts in children. *Pediatr. Akush. Ginekol. 2*:21–27 (1977).
167. Kononenko, V. M. Erythema multiforme exudativium in a child with lamblial cholecystitis. *Pediatr. Akush. Ginekol. 2*:30–31 (1976).
168. Koszarska, J., Gruszczynska, M., and Pilarska, K. Lambliasis as a cause of acute pancreatitis. *Wiad. Lek. 30*:875–877 (1977).
169. Roberts-Thomson, I. C., Anders, R. F., and Bhathol, P. S. Granulomatous hepatitis and cholonagitis associated with giardiasis. *Gastroenterology 83*: 480–483 (1982).
170. Radulescu, S., Lupascu, G., Ciplea, A. G., et al. Existence du flagella *Giardia muris* dans les tissues et organes des souris a infection spontanee. *Arch. Roum. Pathol. Exp. Microbiol. 30*:405–411 (1971).
171. Webster, B. H. Human infection with *Giardia lamblia*: an analysis of 32 cases. *Am. J. Dig. Dis. 3*:64–71 (1958).
172. Weisman, B. L. Urticaria and *Giardia lamblia* infection. *Ann. Allergy 46*: 23 (1979).
173. Hamrick, H. J., and Moore, G. W. Giardiasis causing urticaria in a child. *Am. J. Dis. Child. 157*:761–763 (1983).
174. Balastskii, A. V. Toxic-allergic reactions (rheumatism-like syndrome) in patients with lambliasis. *Vopr. Reum. 3*:61–65 (1976).
175. Goodbar, J. P. Joint symptoms in giardiasis (letter). *Lancet 1*:1010 (1977).
176. Kavousi, S. Giardiasis in infancy and childhood: a prospective study of 160 cases with comparison of quinacrine (Atabrine) and metronidazole (Flagyl). *Am. J. Trop. Med. Hyg. 28*:19–23 (1979).

177. Peterson, H. Giardiasis (lambliasis) *Scand. J. Gastroenterol. 7*(*Suppl. 14*): 1-44 (1972).

178. Visvesvara, G. S., and Healy, G. R. The possible use of an indirect immuno-fluorescent test using axenically grown *Giardia lamblia* antigens in diagnosing giardiasis. In *Proceedings, Symposium on Waterborne Transmission of Giardiasis* (W. Jakubowskii and J. C. Hoff, eds.). U.S. Environmental Protection Agency, Cincinnati, 1979, pp. 53-63.

179. Lo, C. W., and Walker, W. A. Chronic protracted diarrhea of infancy: a nutritional disease. *Pediatrics 72*:786-800 (1983).

180. Chester, A. C., MacMurray, F. G., Restifo, M. D., and Mann, O. Giardiasis as a chronic disease. *Dig. Dis. Sci. 30*:215-218 (1985).

181. Bolin, T. D., Davis, A. E., and Duncombe, V. M. A prospective study of persistent diarrhoea. *Aust. N.Z. J. Med. 12*:22-26 (1982).

182. Loftiness, T. J., Baillie, J., and Solitis, R. D. Malabsorption and protracted diarrhea associated with giardiasis. An unusual case. *Minn. Med. 67*:257-259 (1984).

183. Ament, M. E., and Rubin, C. E. Relation of giardiasis to abnormal intestinal structure and function in gastrointestinal immunodeficiency syndromes. *Gastroenterology 62*:216-226 (1972).

184. Khosla, S. N., Sharma, S. V., and Srivastava, S. C. Malabsorption in giardiasis. *Am. J. Gastroenterol. 69*:694-700 (1978).

185. Hoskins, L. C., Winawer, S. I., Broitman, S. A., Gottlieb, L. S., and Zamcheck, N. Clinical giardiasis and intestinal malabsorption. *Gastroenterology 53*:265-279 (1967).

186. Amini, F. Giardiasis and steatorrhea. *J. Trop. Med. Hyg. 66*:190-192 (1963).

187. Anita, F. P., Desai, H. G., Jeejeebhoy, K. N., Kane, M. P., and Borkar, A. V. Giardiasis in adults. Incidence, symptomatology, and absorption studies. *Indian J. Med. Sci. 20*:471-477 (1966).

188. Wright, S. G., Tomkins, A. M., and Ridley, D. S. Giardiasis: clinical and therapeutic aspects. *Gut 18*:343-350 (1977).

189. Barberi, D., De Brito, T., Hoshino, S., Nascimento, F. O. B., Martins-Campos, J. V., Quarentei, G., and Marcondes, E. Giardiasis in childhood. Absorption tests and biochemistry, histochemistry, light, and electron microscopy of jejunal mucosa. *Arch. Dis. Child. 45*:466-472 (1970).

190. Jacobson, E., Kubalska, I., and Zythiewicz, B. Assessment of intestinal absorption in children with giardiasis by means of the D-xylose test. *Pediatr. Pol. 47*:689-694 (1972).

191. Kluska, J. Carbohydrate absorption disorders in the course of lambliosis. *Wiad. Parazytol. 18*:43-45 (1972).

192. Cortner, J. A. Giardiasis, a cause of celiac syndrome. *Am. J. Dis. Child. 95*: 311-316 (1959).

193. Katsampes, C. P., McCoord, A. B., and Phillips, W. A. Vitamin A absorption test in cases of giardiasis. *Am. J. Dis. Child. 67*:189-193 (1944).

194. Mahalanabis, D., Simpson, T. W., Chakraborty, M. C., Ganguli, C., Bhatta-charjee, A. K. and Mukherjee, K. L. Malabsorption of water-miscible

vitamin A in children with giardiasis and ascariasis. *Am. J. Clin. Nutr. 32*: 313–318 (1979).

195. Cowen, A. E., and Campbell, C. B. Giardiasis a cause of vitamin B_{12} malabsorption. *Am. J. Dig. Dis. 18*:384–390 (1973).

196. Notis, W. M. Giardiasis and vitamin B_{12} malabsorption. *Gastroenterology 63*:1085 (1972).

197. Conn, H. O., Binder, H., and Burns, B. Pernicious anemia and immunologic deficiency. *Ann. Intern. Med. 68*:603–612 (1968).

198. Twomey, J. J., Jordan, P. H., Jarrold, T., Trubowitz, S., Ritz, N. D., and Conn, H. O. The syndrome of immunoglobulin deficiency and pernicious anemia. *Am. J. Med. 47*:232–237 (1969).

199. Sherman, P. Apparent protein losing enteropathy associated with giardiasis. *Am. J. Dis. Child. 134*:893–894 (1980).

200. DeVizia, B., Vincenzo, P., Vajro, P., Cucchiara, and Acampora, A. Iron malabsorption in giardiasis. *J. Pediatr. 107*:75–78 (1985).

201. Gebhard, R. L. Malabsorption—a cause of geriatric nutritional failure. *Geriatrics 38*:97–101 (1983).

202. Okeahialam, T. P. Giardiasis in protein energy malnutrition. *E. Afr. Med. J. 59*:765–770 (1982).

203. Kotler, D. P., Gaetz, H. P., Lange, M., Klein, E. B., and Holt, P. H. Enteropathy associated with the acquired immunodeficiency syndrome. *Ann. Intern. Med. 101*:461–468 (1984).

204. Gillin, J. S., Shike, M., Alcock, N., Urmacher, C., Krown, S., Kurtz, R. C., Lightdale, C., and Winawer, S. J. Malabsorption and mucosal abnormalities of the small intestine in the acquired immunodeficiency syndrome. *Ann. Intern. Med. 102*:619–622 (1985).

205. Markell, E. K., and Voge, M. Fixatives, stains, and preservatives. In *Medical Parasitology*. W. B. Saunders, Philadelphia, 1976, pp. 373–381.

206. McMillan, A., and McNeillage, A. J. C. Comparison of the sensitivity of microscopy and culture in the laboratory diagnosis of intestinal protozoal infection. *J. Clin. Pathol. 37*:809–811 (1984).

207. Zierdt, W. S. A simple device for concentration of parasite eggs, larvae and protozoa. *Am. J. Clin. Pathol. 70*:89–93 (1978).

208. Thornton, S. A., West, H., DuPont, H. L., and Pickering, L. K. Comparison of methods for identification of *Giardia lamblia. Am. J. Clin. Pathol. 80*: 858–860 (1983).

209. Beal, C. B., Viens, P., Grant, R. G. L., and Hughes, J. M. A new technique for sampling duodenal contents. *Am. J. Trop. Med. Hyg. 19*:349–352 (1970).

210. Bezjak, B. Evaluation of a new technic for sampling duodenal contents in parasitologic diagnosis. *Dig. Dis. 17*:848–850 (1972).

211. Thomas, G. E., Goldsmid, J. M., and Wicks, A. C. B. Use of the enterotest duodenal capsule in the diagnosis of giardiasis. *S. Afr. Med. J. 48*:2219–2220 (1974).

212. Kamath, K. R., and Murugasu, R. A comparative study of four methods

for detecting *Giardia lamblia* in children with diarrheal disease and malabsorption. *Gastroenterology 66*:16–21 (1974).

213. Rosenthal, P., and Liebman, W. M. Comparative study of stool examinations, duodenal aspiration, and pediatric entero-test for giardiasis in children. *J. Pediatr. 96*:278–279 (1980).

214. Ament, M. E. Diagnosis and treatment of giardiasis. *J. Pediatr. 80*:633–637 (1972).

215. Unger, B. L. P., Yolken, R. H., Nash, T. E., and Quinn, T. C. Enzyme-linked immunosorbent assay for the detection of *Giardia lamblia* in fecal specimens. *J. Infect. Dis. 149*:90–97 (1984).

216. Green, E. L., Miles, M. A., and Warhurst, D. C. Immunodiagnostic detection of *Giardia* antigen in faeces by a rapid visual enzyme-linked immunosorbent assay. *Lancet 2*:691–693 (1985).

217. Drugs for parasitic infections. *Med. Lett. 28*:9–18 (1986).

218. Bassily, S., Farid, Z., Mikhail, J. W., Dent, D. C., and Lehman, J. S. The treatment of *Giardia lamblia* infection with mepacrine, metronidazole and furazolidone. *J. Trop. Med. Hyg. 73*:15–18 (1970).

219. Wolf, M. S. Giardiasis. *J. Am. Med. Assoc. 233*:1362–1364 (1975).

220. Kavousi, S. Giardiasis in infancy and childhood: a prospective study of 160 cases with comparison of quinacrine and metronidazole. *Am. J. Trop. Med. Hyg. 28*:19–23 (1979).

221. Craft, J. C., Murphy, T., and Nelson, J. D. Furazolidone and quinacrine. Comparative study of therapy for giardiasis in children. *Am. J. Dis. Child. 135*:164–166 (1981).

222. Khambatta, R. B. Metronidazole in giardiasis. *Ann. Trop. Med. Parasitol. 65*:487–489 (1971).

223. Levi, G. C., de Avila, C. A., and Neto, V. A. Efficacy of various drugs for treatment of giardiasis. *Am. J. Trop. Med. Hyg. 26*:564–565 (1977).

224. Jokipii, A. M. M., and Jokipii, L. Comparative evaluation of two dosages of tinidazole in the treatment of giardiasis. *Am. J. Trop. Med. Hyg. 27*:758–761 (1978).

225. Masry, N. A. E., Farid, Z., and Miner, W. F. Treatment of giardiasis with tinidazole. *Am. J. Trop. Med. Hyg. 27*:201–202 (1978).

226. Jokipii, L., and Jokipii, A. M. M. Treatment of giardiasis: comparative evaluation of ornidazole and tinidazole as a single oral dose. *Gastroenterology 83*:399–404 (1982).

227. Guyta, S., and Srivastava, G. Drug therapy for giardia infestation. *Indian Pediatr. 15*:687 (1978).

228. Nair, K. V., Sharma, S. M., and Tandon, B. N. Success of metronidazole and furazolidone in the treatment of giardiasis. *J. Indian Med. Assoc. 72*:162 (1979).

229. Webster, B. H. Furazolidone in the treatment of giardiasis. *Am. J. Dig. Dis. 5*:618–622 (1960).

230. Murphy, T. V., and Nelson, J. D. Five vs. ten days' therapy with furazolidone for giardiasis. *Am. J. Dis. Child. 157*:267–270 (1983).

231. Beard, C. M., Noller, K. L., O'Fallon, W. M., Kurland, L. T., and Dockerty, M. B. Lack of evidence for cancer due to use of metronidazole. *New Engl. J. Med. 301*:519 (1979).
232. Safety of antimicrobial drugs in pregnancy. *Med. Lett. 27*:93–96 (1985).
233. Kreutner, A. K., del Bene, V. E., and Amstey, M. S. Giardiasis and pregnancy. *Am. J. Obstet. Gynecol. 160*:895–901 (1981).
234. Croun, G. F. Waterborne outbreaks. *J. Water Pollut. Control Fed. 49*: 1268–1279 (1977).
235. Lippy, E. F. Tracing a giardiasis outbreak at Berlin, New Hampshire. *J. Am. Water Works Assoc. 70*:512–520 (1978).
236. Kirner, J. C., Littler, J. D., and Angelo, L. A. A waterborne outbreak of giardiasis in Camas, Wash. *J. Am. Water Works Assoc. 70*:35–40 (1978).
237. Horwitz, M. A., and Hughes, J. M. Outbreaks of waterborne disease in the United States, 1974. *J. Infect. Dis. 133*:588 (1976).
238. Nelson, J. D. Etiology and epidemiology of diarrheal diseases in the United States. *Am. J. Med. 78*:76–80 (1985).
239. Jarroll, E. L., Jr., Bingham, A. K., and Meyer, E. A. Effect of chlorine on *Giardia lamblia* cyst viability. *Appl. Environ. Microbiol. 41*:483–487 (1981).
240. Logsdon, G. S., Dewalle, F. B., and Henricks, D. W. Filtration as a barrier to passage of cysts in drinking water. In *Giardia and Giardiasis* (S. L. Erlandsen and E. A. Meyer, eds.). Plenum Press, New York, 1984, pp. 287–308.
241. Jarroll, E. L., Jr., Bingham, A. K., and Meyer, E. A. *Giardia* cyst destruction: effectiveness of six small-quantity water disinfection methods. *Am. J. Trop. Med. Hyg. 29*:8–11 (1980).
242. Gillin, F. D., Reiner, D. S., Gault, M. J., Douglas, H., Das, S., Wunderlich, A., and Sauch, J. F. Encystation and expression of cyst antigens by *Giardia lamblia* in vitro. *Science 235*:1040–1043 (1987).
243. Adam, R. D., Aggarwal, A., Lal, A. A., de la Cruz, V. F., McCutcher, T., and Nash, T. E. Antigenic variation of a cysteine-rich protein in *Giardia lamblia*. *J. Exp. Med. 167*:109–118 (1988).
244. Nayak, N., Ganguly, N. K., Walia, B. N. S., Wahi, V., Kanwar, S. S., and Mahajan, R. C. Specific secretory IgA in the milk of *Giardia lamblia*-infected and uninfected women. *J. Infect. Dis. 155*:724–727 (1987).
245. Deguchi, M., Gillin, F. D., and Gigli, I. Mechanisms of killing of *Giardia lamblia* trophozoites by complement. *J. Clin. Invest. 79*:1296–1302 (1987).
246. Heyworth, M. F., Carlson, J. R., and Ermak, T. H. Clearance of *Giardia muris* infection requires helper/inducer T lymphocytes. *J. Exp. Med. 165*: 1743–1748 (1987).
247. Nash, T. E., Herrington, D. A., Losonsky, G. A., and Levine, M. M. Experimental infections with *Giardia lamblia*. *J. Infect. Dis. 156*:974–984 (1987).
248. Gilman, R. H., Marquis, G. S., Miranda, E., Vestegui, M., and Martinez, H. Rapid reinfection by *Giardia lamblia* after treatment in a hyperendemic third world community. *Lancet 1*:343–345 (1988).

7
Entamoeba histolytica

WILLIAM A. PETRI, JR., and JONATHAN I. RAVDIN
University of Virginia School of Medicine, Charlottesville, Virginia

I. INTRODUCTION

Amebiasis is a potentially invasive enteric disease caused by the protozoan parasite *Entamoeba histolytica*. The spectrum of human disease includes asymptomatic intestinal colonization, invasive colitis, liver abscess, intestinal perforation, and peritonitis. Appreciation of the global magnitude of amebic disease coupled with recognition of groups at high risk for amebic infection in the United States has recently stimulated research on a disease initially described over a century ago.

The relationship of dysentery to liver abscess may have first been observed by James Annesley in his two-volume monograph on prevalent diseases of India published in 1828 (1) (Table 1). Amebas were isolated from the stool of patients with cholera in 1869 by the British surgeon Timothy Lewis (2,3). F. Losch from St. Petersburg, Russia, made the association of amebas in the stool to dysentery. Losch studied a 24-year-old peasant with chronic diarrhea that persisted from 1871 until his death in 1874. Amebas seen in this patient's stool were noted to "exceptionally" contain ingested erythrocytes and leukocytes (1-3). Losch apparently succeeded in inducing amebiasis in one of four dogs inoculated orally and rectally with freshly passed ameba-containing stools from the peasant (1-3). In 1883 Robert Koch performed autopsies on five patients who had died of dysentery, two of whom had also had liver abscesses (1,3). Koch observed amebas in histological sections from the base of colonic ulcers and in capillaries near the liver abscesses (1,3).

Sir William Osler reported the first recognized North American case of amebiasis in 1890. The patient, a 29-year-old physician who had been a resident of Panama until 6 months prior to admission, presented with fever and six to eight daily mucoid stools containing traces of blood. Amebas were seen in fluid

Table 1   History of Amebiasis Research

Year	Finding	Investigators
1828	Dysentery complicated by liver abscess	Annesley (1)
1875	Amebas in stool of patients with dysentery	Losch (1–3)
1891	Amebic dysentery and liver abscess described	Councilman and Lafleur (6)
1893	Cyst is infective form of ameba	Quincke and Roos (1–3)
1903	*Entamoeba histolytica* named, distinguished from commensal *E. coli*	Scaudinn (1–3)
1912	Emetine therapy	Rogers (7)
1925	Description of life cycle	Dobell (10)
1961	Axenic culture	Diamond (11)

surgically drained from two large liver abscesses and subsequently in the patient's stools (4). That same year Simon described a second patient from Johns Hopkins who had an amebic liver abscess with extension to the lung (5). Councilman and Lafleur introduced the terms *amebic dysentery* and *amebic liver abscess* in a review of 14 cases diagnosed in Baltimore. They emphasized that amebas from the stool of patients with dysentery contained internalized red blood cells, noted that amebic liver abscess was often seen without concurrent dysentery, and described the flask-shaped intestinal ulcer of invasive amebiasis (6). Quincke and Roos, in 1893, described the cyst form of ameba and showed that the cyst but not the trophozoite would cause disease in kittens when inoculated orally (1–3). They were also the first investigators to distinguish a separate amebic species in human stool that was not associated with dysentery, which was most likely *Entamoeba coli* (1–3). Schaudinn named the ameba causing dysentery *Entamoeba histolytica* and distinguished it morphologically from the commensal *Entamoeba coli* (1–3).

Leonard Rogers reported successful treatment of three cases of amebiasis in Calcutta by injection with emetine (7). This marked the beginning of antiamebic chemotherapy, although the patients treated with emetine were later found to be prone to relapses with their infections (as emetine did not eliminate intraluminal infection). Cysts of *E. histolytica* but not of *E. coli* taken orally produced dysentery in human volunteer studies conducted in the Philippines by Walker and Sellards (8). Cultivation in vitro of *E. histolytica* was accomplished in 1925 by Boeck and Drbohlav; the cultured amebas caused dysentery in a kitten model of disease (9). Amebic trophozoites were found to encyst in Boeck's medium when rice starch was added by Dobell, who described the amebic life cycle (10). It was not until 1961 that the axenic (free of associated microorganisms) culture of *E. histolytica* was described by Diamond (11). Axenic culture of *E. histolytica* has directly contributed to the rapid increase in our knowledge of this parasite in the last 25 years.

II. THE ORGANISM

A. Life Cycle and Epidemiology

It is important to distinguish the potentially highly virulent *Entamoeba histolytica* from other enteric protozoans that are mostly nonpathogenic. There are eight species of amebas that have been shown to be enteric parasites in humans: *Entamoeba histolytica, E. hartmanni, E. coli, E. gingivalis, E. polecki, Endolimax nana, Dientamoeba fragilis,* and *Iodamoeba butschlii*. All of these organisms, except *E. gingivalis*, which inhabits the mouth, can be isolated from human stool. These parasitic protozoans are distinguished by morphological criteria and by their pathogenicity for humans (12,13) (Fig. 1).

Entamoeba gingivalis trophozoites have a cytoplasm full of dark staining bodies and food vacuoles. *E. gingivalis* is associated with poor dental hygiene and must be distinguished from *E. histolytica* in the sputum of patients with lung abscess. *Entamoeba histolytica* trophozoites are large (12-60 μm), exhibit unidirectional motility, and can contain ingested erythrocytes. The cysts of *E. histolytica* contain up to four nuclei. The *E. histolytica*-like Laredo strain is nonpathogenic and grows optimally at 24°C in vitro, as opposed to an optimal growth temperature of 35°C for *E. histolytica* (14). *Entamoeba hartmanni*, formerly called the small race of *E. histolytica*, is a nonpathogenic commensal of identical morphology, but its trophozoite or cyst forms are smaller than those of *E. histolytica* (<12μm) (15). *Entamoeba coli* is frequently isolated together with *E. histolytica* in endemic areas in the tropics but is nonpathogenic. The trophozoites of *E. coli* never contain ingested erythrocytes, and their motility is more sluggish and less directed than that of *E. histolytica*. *Entamoeba coli* cysts contain up to eight nuclei (12,13). *Entamoeba polecki* infects pigs and monkeys in the tropics and has recently been associated with human disease in Upper Volta (16) and in Papua New Guinea. It is identified by its characteristics uninucleate cyst with a large karysome in the nucleus.

Dientamoeba fragilis, named for its susceptibility to osmotic lysis, has not been recognized to have a cyst form. The trophozoites are small (5-12μm), have active motility, and characteristically have four to eight chromatin granules in the one or two nuclei present. Although originally thought not to be pathogenic, it is increasingly being recognized as a cause of prolonged (17) or inflammatory (18) diarrhea. *Endolimax nana* and *Iodamoeba butschlii* are both nonpathogenic commensals. *Endolimax nana* trophozoites are small (6-15μm), move sluggishly,

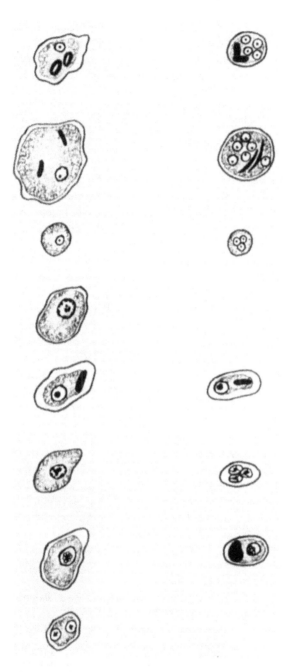

Figure 1　Amebas that infect the human gastrointestinal tract. [Described, top to bottom, in chart on p. 389.]

Figure 1 (Continued)

	Human pathogen	Est. frequency	Trophozoite (μm)	Cyst (μm)	Characteristic features
Entamoeba histolytica	+	1–10%	10–20 (10–60)	5–20	Central punctate karyosome, erythrophagocytosis
E. coli	–	3–30%	15–25 (10–50)	10–30	Larger to 8 nuclei, splinter-like chromatoid bodies
E. hartmanni	–		10	4–10	"Small race"
E. gingivalis	–	10–90%	15 (3–35)	–	Mouth trophozoite only
E. polecki	±	–	16–8	2–14	Uninucleate cyst with large karyosome
Endolimax nana	–	10–33%	8–12	6–10	
Iodamoeba butschlii	–	5–8%	9–13	6–15	"I" cyst
Dientamoeba fragilis	+	5	5–12	–	Binucleate trophs with connecting thread

Source: Reprinted from Ravdin, J. I., and Guerrant, Current Problems in Diagnosis and Treatment of Amebic Infections," Remington & Swartz, 1986.

and have a single nucleus containing a large central karyosome; the cyst form contains four nuclei (12,13). *Iodamoeba butschlii* trophozoites are small (6-20 μm), with sluggish movement; the cyst form is easily identified by its large glycogen vacuole, which stains with iodine (12,13).

The life cycle of *Entamoeba histolytica* is relatively simple. The infective form of the parasite is the quadrinucleate cyst, which is resistant to gastric acidity and can survive outside the host in a moist environment for several weeks (12). Infection with *E. histolytica* occurs when cysts are ingested from fecally contaminated material and excystation occurs in the small or large bowel. The cyst's nuclei divide to form eight nuclei (metacyst) followed by cytoplasmic division to form eight trophozoites (19). The trophozoites reside in the large bowel, where tissue invasion or encystation can occur. It is the trophozoite that has the potential to invade the host; cysts are never found in tissues but are excreted in stool to start a new round of infection (12). Because it has not yet been possible to induce encystation of axenic cultures of *E. histolytica*, investigations into the factors that control cyst formation have been severely limited.

There is no known significant anthropod vector of amebiasis although the common housefly and cockroach can retain viable *E. histolytica* cysts for several hours to days and potentially could contaminate food (20). Primates appear to be infected with *E. histolytica*, as amebas indistinguishable from *E. histolytica* have been isolated from Old and New World monkeys, apes, and gibbons (20).

Amebiasis is one of the most common parasitic infections worldwide: The prevalence of infection is estimated to be 480 million people (21) (Table 2). The annual incidence of infection is much higher; in endemic areas it approaches 100% of the population with the continual loss and reacquisition of the parasite

Table 2 Global Prevalence and Incidence of Amebiasis—1984

Continent	Infections (millions)	Disease (abscess and colitis) (millions)	Deaths (thousands)
North and South America	95	10	10–30
Asia	300	20–30	20–50
Africa	85	10	10–30
Europe	20	0.1	–
Total	500	40–50.1	40–110

Source: Reprinted from Walsh, J. A. Prevalence of *Entamoeba histolytica* infection. In *Amebiasis: Human Infection by Entabmoeba Histolytica* (J. I. Ravdin, ed.). Wiley New York, 1988.

(21,22). The vast majority of patients infected with *E. histolytica* are asymptomatic, but approximately 1% of those infected are disabled by dysentery or amebic liver abscess, resulting in 40 thousand to 110 thousand deaths annually. Groups at increased risk include the very young , the very old, and pregnant women (21,23). Amebic colitis was the leading medical cause of maternal mortality in one report from Tanzania (23). The parasite has a worldwide distribution, but the incidence of infection is greater in Central and South America, Africa, and India. The preponderance of morbidity and mortality in the developing world is likely a result of the complex socioeconomic problems in these countries, which tend to allow fecal-oral spread of the cyst (20,21).

A serological survey of 20,000 individuals in 46 communities distributed throughout Mexico found 6% of people surveyed had serum antiamebic antibodies, with the range in individual communities from 0.25 to 21%. There was no correlation of climate to prevalence of amebic infection, but areas with poorer sanitation had a higher percentage of individuals with antiamebic antibodies (24). In Mexico City, amebiasis was diagnosed in 2-15% of patients admitted with an acute diarrheal illness (25) and in 1.6-2.1% of all patients admitted to general hospitals (26) and was the fourth leading cause of death in a series of 7914 autopsies (27).

1. High-Risk Groups in Developed Nations

Epidemiological studies have not only demonstrated the global magnitude of infections with *E. histolytica* but have also identified groups at increased risk for amebic infection in developed nations where amebiasis is uncommon (Table 3). Physicians should be alerted to the possible diagnosis of amebiasis when treating a member of a high-risk group.

Immigrants from areas endemic for amebiasis constitute a large percentage of the cases of amebic liver abscess reported from North America and Europe. In Chicago, 32 of 35 cases of amebic liver abscess reported were in immigrants (28), and 37% of 392 patients with amebiasis diagnosed in Stockholm over a 10-year period were immigrants (29). Two of seven cases of invasive amebiasis admitted to the University of Virginia Hospital in the period 1975–1984 were also immigrants.

Residents of developed countries who travel to endemic areas are also at risk for acquiring amebiasis. Amebiasis is more common in long-term visitors to an endemic area, although a short stay is not without risk. Of 216 German travelers who developed amebic liver abscess, one-third had been in an endemic area less than 6 weeks, while 36% had been exposed from 6 weeks to 10 years, and 30%, for longer than 10 years (30). These German citizens had acquired their infection in the Far East (45%), tropical Africa (42%), the Mideast (17%), South America (8%), subtropical Africa (4%), and Europe (4%) (30). Travelers with amebiasis diagnosed at the Roslagslitt Hospital in Stockholm over a 10-year

Table 3   Risk Factors for Acquisition and Increased Severity of Amebiasis

Factors predisposing to acquisition	Factors predisposing to increased severity
Residence in or travel to endemic areas (especially Mexico, India, South Africa)	Pediatric age group
Recent immigration from an endemic area	Pregnancy
Lower socioeconomic status and crowding	Corticosteroid use
Poor sanitation	Malnutrition
Institutionalization, especially for mental retardation	
Promiscuous male homosexual practices	
Communal living with poor sanitation	

Source: Reprinted from Ravdin, J. I. Diagnosis and management of infection by *Entamoeba histolytica, Infections in Medicine, 4*:155–165, 1987.

period were predominantly long-term visitors (177/215 patients); 26% acquired their infection in Central and South America, 37% in Asia, and 25% in Africa (28). Travelers will usually manifest symptoms of liver invasion within a half year of their return. Of 103 travelers who returned initially symptom free, 95% developed symptoms of a liver abscess within 8–20 weeks (29). Traveler's diarrhea is usually caused by enterotoxigenic *Escherichia coli* and is rarely due to amebiasis (31,32).

Infection with *E. histolytica* has been a recognized problem in institutions for the mentally retarded for over 40 years, with outbreaks reported in the literature as recently as 1981 (40). In one midwestern United States institution where three patients had died of invasive amebiasis, 14% of the residents were found to have serum antiamebic antibodies as assayed by indirect hemagglutination (IHA) (33). A Mississippi institution with a 20-year history of 127 deaths from invasive amebiasis (67 of 127 confirmed by premortem biopsy or autopsy) had 17% of a sample group of residents actively excreting *E. histolytica* in their stools and 28% with positive IHA titers (34). Clustering of cases in buildings housing the most severely mentally retarded patients with the poorest personal hygiene supported a person-to-person mode of transmission (34–36); drinking water supplies and health care personnel were not implicated (36,37).

Attempts to eliminate amebiasis from institutions have been met with frustration. Mass treatment has been effective for the initial control of symptomatic outbreaks of amebiasis but has been followed by a return to a pretreatment level of prevalence by 6–12 months (35,36,38,39). Treatment combined with the segregation of infected from noninfected residents has also been unsuccessful at decreasing the prevalence of amebiasis (38,40). However, improved facilities coupled with a tripling of the staff caring for the residents was thought to be responsible for a decline in the prevalence of amebiasis from 35% to 7% in a Kansas mental institution (41). Mortality from invasive amebiasis may be higher in mentally retarded patients: Juniper, in reporting 149 consecutive cases of invasive amebiasis over 14 years, noted a 15% overall mortality for institutionalized mental patients, perhaps due to a delay in recognizing the disease in these individuals (42). Two of seven patients admitted to the University of Virginia Hospital with invasive amebiasis were chronically institutionalized.

Members of communal groups may also be at greater risk of infection (43, 44). *Entamoeba histolytica* infected 146 of 563 residents of a kibbutz in Israel, with the highest incidence in the 0-9-year-old age group (36%). The epidemic was linked to the poor personal hygiene of the food handlers and was controlled by chemotherapy and improved sanitation. Disease prevalence 5 years later, however, was back almost to pretreatment levels (43).

Sexually active male homosexuals in New York and San Francisco have been found to be commonly infected with *E. histolytica* (45–48). Most studies conducted at venereal disease clinics have reported 20-30% of homosexual males to be infected with *E. histolytica* (45–52). Prevalence of infection correlated with multiple sexual partners, a history of syphilis or gonorrhea, and the practice of oral-anal sex (48–52). The majority of homosexual males in these studies complained of gastrointestinal symptoms, making it difficult to ascertain if infection with *E. histolytica* was symptomatic. Phillips et al. noted that homosexual males infected with *E. histolytica* were more likely to give a history of blood or mucus in their stool (49), but all other series have been unable to find an association of prevalence of *E. histolytica* infection with gastrointestinal symptoms (48,50–52). There are a few case reports of invasive amebiasis or amebic liver abscesses in homosexual males (53,54). The reason for such a low incidence of invasive disease could be that the infecting strains of *E. histolytica* are nonpathogenic, as indicated by zymodeme studies of 52 isolates from homosexual males (55), or because of as yet undefined host–parasite interactions.

There are several other epidemiological risk factors worthy of mention. Amebiasis may be fulminant during pregnancy; in one series of patients with amebic colitis in Nigeria, 48 of 155 patients were pregnant, a rate that was much higher than by chance alone (56), and as mentioned previously amebic colitis was the leading medical cause of maternal mortality in series from the

Kilimanjaro Christian Medical Center in Tanzania (23). Invasive amebiasis and liver abscess in children is not uncommon (57), and delays in diagnosis due to a low index of suspicion have led to more serious disease (58,59). In a series of 11 children with invasive amebiasis seen at the Children's Hospital of Los Angeles, the majority had an atypical presentation. Four children had hematochezia without diarrhea, and two were initially thought to have an exacerbation of ulcerative colitis. An important historical point was that 10 of the 11 children were of Hispanic background (59). In children with persistent rectal bleeding and/or diarrhea and negative routine stool exams, sigmoidoscopy or colonoscopy with tissue biopsy are invaluable aids in making the diagnosis of invasive amebiasis (60). Serological surveys of native Americans living on reservations have shown higher rates of positive IHA than the general population (61). A recent outbreak of amebiasis was caused by colonic irrigation at a chiropractic clinic in Colorado. Perhaps because of the means of acquisition of infection, the disease was unusually severe, with six deaths and 10 of 36 patients requiring colectomy (62). Finally, there are numerous case reports of amebic colitis being misdiagnosed as inflammatory colitis. Seven of 18 patients with amebic colitis seen in central Virginia were misdiagnosed as having inflammatory bowel disease initially, and five of those patients were treated with sulfasalazine or corticosteroids before the correct diagnosis was made. The use of corticosteroids in patients with amebic colitis can result in life-threatening complications (63–65). Colonic biopsy specimens from patients thought to have inflammatory bowel disease should be examined for amebic trophozoites with special stains (66), and stool and serological studies should be performed to rule out amebic colitis prior to making a diagnosis of inflammatory bowel disease.

B. Growth and Metabolism

The culture of *E. histolytica* is separated into xenic, monoxenic, or axenic systems. In xenic culture the amebas are grown in the presence of several unknown associates, while in monoxenic culture there is one known associated microorganism to support amebic growth. In axenic culture there are not other metabolizing organisms. The reader is referred to an excellent and practical review of *Entamoeba* culture by Diamond (68). Clinical isolates from fresh stool or rectal biopsies are initially cultured in xenic media such as Robinson's (69) or Locke-Egg medium (9). One of the difficulties with xenic culture is that of preventing overgrowth of the associated bacteria with antibiotics added to the medium (67).

Amebas from clinical isolates can be maintained in long-term culture by adapting them to monoxenic culture with a single bacterial or trypanosomatid associate. *Entamoeba coli* and *E. hartmanni* must be maintained in monoxenic culture, as they have never been grown successfully in axenic culture (68).

Axenic culture is the ideal medium in which to maintain *E. histolytica* for scientific study. Diamond, in 1961, first described axenic cultivation of *E. histolytica* (11). The medium currently in use is TYI-S-33 (trypticase-yeast extract-iron-serum) (68,70). The source of the trypticase, which is a pancreatic digest of casein, is essential for success in cultivation, as most commercial casein digests will not support the growth of *Entamoeba* (68). The digest currently used in TYI-S-33 is casein digest peptone (catalog #97023, BBL Microbiology Systems, Cockeysville, MD). A major disadvantage of axenic culture is the inability of the parasite to encyst (68).

Virulent strains of *E. histolytica* trophozoites in axenic culture may become attenuated upon prolonged passage. The ability to form cecal ulcers in animal models upon intracecal inoculation is lost for some (71,72) but not all (73,74) virulent strains in axenic culture. All virulent isolates should retain the ability to form hepatic abscesses upon intrahepatic inoculation (75,76). Serial passage of axenic strains in animals by intrahepatic injection increases the virulence of axenic *E. histolytica* (77,78). *Entamoeba histolytica* can be cloned in soft agar (79) or by micromanipulation (68), which gives one the ability to produce and compare mutants from a single cloned population. For biochemical studies, *E. histolytica* can be grown in plastic tissue culture flasks with a yield of 2×10^5 trophozoites per milliliter of medium (79). Trophozoites in culture reproduce by binary fission; there is no known sexual stage of reproduction.

The biochemistry of *E. histolytica* has recently been reviewed (80). The end products of carbohydrate metabolism are ethanol and carbon dioxide when the organism is growing anaerobically; acetate is also formed in the presence of oxygen (80). Glucose uptake by trophozoites is via a specific receptor; uptake via this receptor is several orders of magnitude greater than glucose uptake via pinocytosis and is the rate-limiting step in glycolysis (81). The conversion of fructose-6-phosphate to fructose-1,6-diphosphate is via a unique enzyme that utilizes inorganic pyrophosphate (82). Amebas do not contain mitochondria or cytochromes; however, ferredoxin-like iron-containing proteins are present and are likely involved in electron transport (83). *Entamoeba histolytica* has been the only eukaryote found not to produce the enzymes of glutathione metabolism (84). Hydrolyzed nucleic acids promote the in vitro growth of *E. histolytica*. The organism is incapable of de novo purine nucleotide synthesis (85); it is not known if amebas can synthesize pyrimidine nucleotides or if salvage pathways exist (80,85).

The trophozoite's cell ultrastructure is notable for a lack of mitochondria and the presence of a large number of intracellular vacuoles (86) (Fig. 2). There are no membrane-associated or free ribosomes; all the ribosomes are collected in microcrystalline ribonucleoprotein bodies (87). A Golgi-like apparatus has been described by some (88,89) but not all (90,91) investigators. Cytoplasmic microfilaments are present and appear to be involved in cell surface capping, motility,

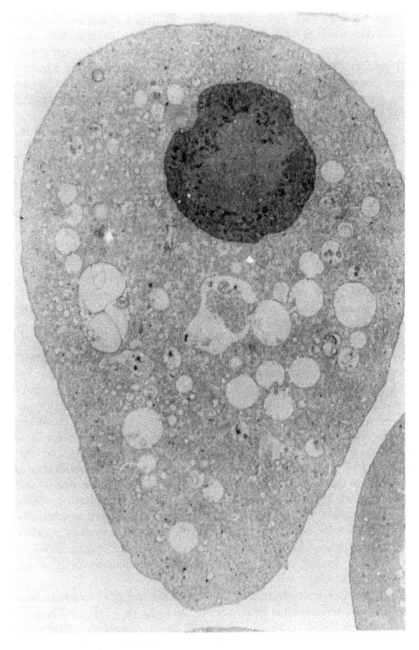

Figure 2   Electron micrograph of *Entamoeba histolytica* demonstrating numerous intracellular vacuoles.

endocystis, and amebic extracellular killing (93). A fuzzy surface coat or glyco-calyx is more prominent on trophozoites from in vivo isolates but is also present on axencially cultivated amebas (89,94).

C. Immunology and Virulence

The major antigenic components of *E. histolytica* remain to be well defined. Animal models have been used to show protection against intracecal infection (95) and intrahepatic infection (96) by immunization with whole trophozoites. Amebic fractions that have been shown to be protective include ribosomal and lysosomal fractions (97), an RNA-protein preparation (98), and the void (high molecular weight) fraction from column chromatography of solubilized amebas on Sephadex G-150 (99,100) or G-200 (101).

Peripheral blood lymphocytes from patients treated for liver abscess but not healthy controls underwent blast transformation when exposed to a crude soluble preparation of amebic antigen (102–104). A soluble amebic protein preparation stimulated monocyte-derived macrophages from uninfected patients to kill amebas in vitro (105). This soluble protein preparation contained amebic galactose (Gal) and *N*-acetylgalactosamine (GalNAc) inhibitable lectin (106) (see below) that is mitogenic for human lymphocytes (107). It remains to be demon-strated which of the proteins from these crude mixtures of amebic proteins, including the amebic Gal/GalNAc lectin, are responsible for the induction of cell-mediated immunity in invasive amebiasis. Another approach to identify amebic antigens is the use of Western blots to identify amebic proteins recog-nized by antibody from patients treated for amebic abscess. This approach has identified several amebic proteins that are consistently recognized by patient's sera (108).

Entamoeba histolytica may have several mechanisms to evade host defenses. Resistance to complement-mediated lysis (by activation of the alternate or classical complement pathways) has been correlated with amebic virulence in animal models (109). Trophozoites cap, shed, or ingest antibody directed to their surface components (92). Amebas lyse human neutrophils (110) and unstimulated macrophages (105) in vitro, and the release of toxic products from lysed neturophils likely contributes to the pathogenesis of invasive disease (76, 111,112). The sera from patients with amebic liver abscess have been shown to depress the response of immune T lymphocytes to amebic antigen (113), sug-gesting that the depression of cell-mediated immune mechanisms seen with acute amebic liver abscess may be due to serum suppressive factors.

1. Organism Virulence Factors

Strains of *E. histolytica* in monoxenic or axenic culture are not of equal viru-lence when tested in animal models. Prolonged axenic culture may attentuate virulence (71,72), while passage through animals generally increases virulence

(77,78). The association of bacteria with amebas has been shown by many investigators to increase amebic virulence (71,72,114,115), but the effect is a relative one, as some axenic (bacteria-free) amebic strains retain the ability to form cecal ulcers and liver abscesses in animal models (73,74). The addition of cholesterol to axenic cultures increases virulence (116,117); the increase is not due to incorporation of exogenous cholesterol into the amebic membrane, as the increased pathogenicity persisted for several culture passages after removal of cholesterol from the culture medium (117). Viruses have been detected in axenic amebic strains (118), but attempts to show lysogenic conversion of virulence have not been successful (119).

Amebas isolated from patients with amebic dysentery had much higher rates of erythrophagocytosis than strains isolated from healthy human carriers (120, 121). Phagocytic-deficient clones were avirulent as measured by liver abscess formation (122), giving further evidence of the importance of phagocytosis for virulence. Cell lysis is also a virulence factor: The ability of E. histolytica to lyse cell monolayers in vitro has been directly correlated to amebic virulence as measured by liver abscess formation in newborn hamsters (122-124). Analysis of amebic isoenzyme patterns from clinical isolates has shown an association of a phosphoglucomutase isoenzyme ("β band") and hexokinase isoenzyme with invasive strains: All 38 isolates from aspirated human liver abscess but only 3 of 67 isolates from asymptomatic cyst passers had the β band of phosphogluco-mutase ("pathogenic zymodeme") (125). Whether or not the phosphoglucomu-tase isoenzyme pattern remains stable over time and the relationship between the isoenzyme and pathogenicity remain to be established.

III. THE HOST

A. Host Defense Mechanisms

That immunity against repeated infection with E. histolytica exists in humans has not yet been adequately established. In animal models, protective immunity has been shown to exist: Vaccination with amebic antigen protects against subsequent intracecal or intrahepatic inoculation of amebas in a variety of rodent species (95-101). In humans, amebic liver abscess rarely recurs; of 1021 patients with amebic liver abscess in Mexico City followed for 5 years, only three (0.29%) developed a second abscess (126). There are rare case reports of recurrent invasive intestinal amebiasis despite the presence of antiamebic serum antibodies (127), but invasive disease is generally thought to provide immunity against reinvasion (128). Repeated intestinal colonization after treatment of asymptomatic cyst passers in the endemic situation is the rule rather than the exception (21,22,40,43). Coproantibodies have been detected in stool of patients with invasive amebiasis (129,130) but apparently do not protect against repeated colonization.

Between 81 and 100% of patients with invasive amebic infections will have serum antibodies to *E. histolytica* detectable by indirect hemagglutination (IHA) (127,128,131–134). Asymptomatic carriers of *E. histolytica* have a positive IHA (≥1/128) between 0 and 8% of the time, which probably reflects prior invasive disease in these currently asymptomatic carriers (131,132). The serum anti-amebic antibody titer in invasive disease as measured by indirect hemagglutination is detectable within a week of the onset of symptoms (128), is highest immediately prior to treatment, and persists at least 6 months and up to 3 years after infection (127,132,134). The role of serum antibody in protecting against infection is not clear, as antibody titers do not correlate with clinical outcome or with protection against repeat disease. Circulating antigen-antibody complexes have been detected without evidence of the complications of immune complex-related disease in patients with amebic liver abscess (135).

Entamoeba histolytica trophozoites activate both the alternative and classical complement pathway and are lysed when incubated with nonimmune human sera (136,137). Classical pathway activation by *E. histolytica* trophozoites can occur without the participation of specific antiamebic antibodies, and the magnitude of activation is greater than that induced by the alternative pathway (137). Resistance to complement-mediated lysis is associated with greater amebic virulence (109). Depletion of complement with cobra venom factor in a hamster model of amebiasis resulted in larger liver abscesses and metastatic foci (138).

Polymorphonuclear neutrophils are killed and phagocytized by virulent strains of *E. histolytica* (106,110,139). Neutrophils were the predominant cell type present in the early inflammatory response to experimentally induced amebic liver abscess in the hamster (111) and gerbil (76). The release of toxic nonoxidative intracellular products from neutrophils lysed by amebas may contribute to the tissue destruction seen with liver abscess (76,111,112) (Fig. 3).

The importance of cell-mediated immunity in limiting the extent of invasive disease has been best demonstrated in animal models. Manipulations that depressed cell-mediated immunity such as steroid treatment, neonatal thymectomy, splenectomy, radiation, silica injections, and antimacrophage globulin enhanced the formation of amebic liver abscesses and extraintestinal foci of infection (140–143).

There is a depression of cell-mediated immunity specific for amebic antigens in acutely infected patients with liver abscess and invasive amebiasis lasting from 10 days to 4 weeks after treatment (144–146). The ratio of T4 helper to T8 suppressor cells was also lower in patients with amebic liver abscess (146). Peripheral lymphocytes from patients with amebic liver abscess had a blastogenic response specific for amebic antigens (102,103,146).

Evidence of the effectiveness of the cell-mediated immune response has come from in vitro studies of the interactions of trophozoites and human mononuclear cells. Human peripheral blood neutrophils, lymphocytes, monocytes, and non-activated monocyte-derived macrophages were readily killed by virulent axenic

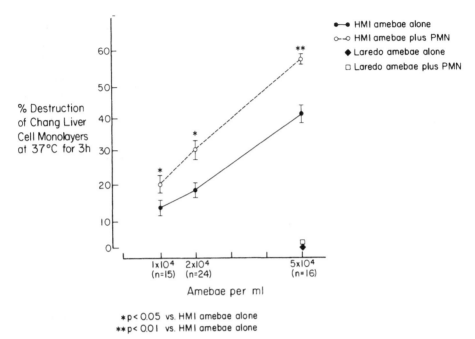

Figure 3 The effect on Chang liver cell monolayers due to the interaction of neutrophils with axenic amebas. Monolayer destruction was measured by [^{3}H] thymidine release from radiolabeled Chang cells at 37°C over 3 hrs. Axenic amebas (●) strain HM1:IMSS progressively destroyed Chang liver cell monolayers as the percent destruction of monolayers increased to 37% at 5 × 10^4 amebas/ml ($p <$ .001). PMN (2 × 10^6/ml) had no effect on Chang cells but when added to amebas (o--o) monolayer destruction disgnificantly increased at all concentrations of amebas studied ($p <$ 0.05 at 1 × 10^4 and 2 × 10^4 amebas/ml and $p <$ .01 at 5 × 10^4 amebas/ml). Nonpathogenic Laredo amebas (5 × 10^4/ ml) alone (♦) or with PMN present (□) had no effect on Chang liver cell monolayers. (Reprinted from *Journal of Infectious Diseases, 154*:19–26, 1986.)

E. histolytica trophozoites. However, monocyte-derived macrophages activated with mitogen- or amebic antigen-elicited lymphokines were capable of killing amebic trophozoites (Fig. 4) (105). Partially purified or recombinant gamma-interferon is sufficient to activate human macrophages to kill amebas; monoclonal antibody to gamma-interferon significantly but not completely inhibited activation of macrophage amebicidal activity by amebic antigen elicited lymphokine (Salata et al. submitted) (Table 4). In contrast to the lysis of peripheral blood lymphocytes by *E. histolytica*, immune T lymphocytes (146,147), upon activation by preincubation with a soluble preparation of amebic antigen, were capable of killing trophozoites in vitro. Salata et al. (113) recently demonstrated

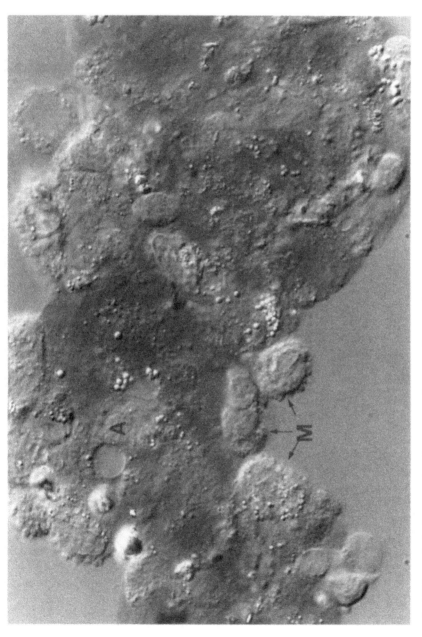

Figure 4 Killing of virulent amebas by activated macrophages. Monocyte-derived macrophages, activated with lymphokine elicited by mitogens or an amebic soluble protein preparation, killed 55% of amebas within 3 hr in a trypan blue exclusion assay. (Reprinted from *Reviews of Infectious Diseases 8*:261–271, 1986.)

Table 4 Effect of Specific Antibody to Gamma-Interferon on the Ability of Con A or Amebic Antigen Elicited Lymphokines to Activate Monocyte-Derived Macrophages to Kill Virulent Amebic Trophozoites[a]

Macrophages incubated previously with:	Viability, % controls at 37°C for 6 hr	
	Ameba	Macrophage
Con A elicited lymphokine	41.7 ± 9.9	58.3 ± 3.7
Con A elicited lymphokine + ANTI–IFN-γ antibody	73.3 ± 8.9[b]	26.7 ± 2.3[b]
Amebic antigen elicited lymphokine	45.6 ± 3.9	55.8 ± 4.3
Amebic antigen elicited lymphokine + ANTI–IFN-γ antibody	82.0 ± 4.8[b]	31.1 ± 2.4[b]

[a]Lymphokines were elicited by incubation of nonimmune lymphocytes for 3 days with concanavalin A (Con A) (20 μg/ml) or immune lymphocytes for 5 days with an amebic antigen preparation from strain HM1:IMSS (100 μg/ml). Lymphokines were then added as 10–15% of total volume to normal human monocyte-derived macrophages, which were incubated for 13 days in suspension in Teflon-coated vials with or without a specific monoclonal antibody to gamma-interferon (IFN-γ) (at two neutralizing units per unit of measured IFN-γ activity). Macrophages and amebas were incubated at a ratio of 100:1 for 6 hr at 37°C, and cell viability was determined by trypan blue exclusion criteria.
[b]$p \leqslant 0.05$ vs. respective lymphokines without added anti-IFN-γ antibody.
Source: Reprinted with permission from *Amer. J. Trop. Med. Hygiene 37*:72–78, 1987.

that sera from patients treated for amebic liver abscess suppressed the antigen-specific T-cell blastogenic response to amebic proteins; this may contribute to the depression of cell-mediated immunity during acute disease and the lack of spontaneous resolution of liver abscess.

A nonimmunological factor that may be very important in protection against amebic invasion is colonic mucus. In humans, amebic trophozoites can be found in the lumen or trapped in mucus, with the underlying colonic mucosa appearing normal (148,149). Depletion of the mucus layer is noted at sites of microulceration and attachment of amebas (150). Lysis of the epithelium and ulceration then progresses (151). In a gerbil model, the earliest morphological response to *E. histolytica* trophozoites was release of goblet cell mucin (76). Amebas appeared trapped in luminal mucus or adherent to the surface epithelium. Edema of the lamina propria was followed by focal epithelial erosion and an inflammatory response. Recent studies in hamsters and guinea pigs support the focal nature of amebic ulcerations (74). Amebas injected into rat colonic loops became motile, were absorbed by mucus, aggregated, and sloughed into the lumen within 3 hr (152). Crude rat colonic mucus inhibited in vitro trophozoite motility at >2 mg/ml. A trypsin- and glutareldehyde-sensitive component on rat colonic mucosa could bind fixed or live amebic trophozoites in vitro (153) (Fig. 5). Rabbit colonic mucus inhibited attachment of trophozoites to mammalian cells (154); mucin also inhibited the cytopathogenicity of a soluble amebic enterotoxin (155). Purified rat colonic mucus inhibited *E. histolytica* adherence to and destruction of Chinese hamster ovary cells in vitro.

Conditions that predispose individuals to more serious infection with *E.histolytica* include treatment with corticosteroids (63–65), pregnancy (23,56), extreme youth (children, especially neonates, are highly susceptible) (57–59), and malnutrition (157–158). A retrospective review of 89 patients admitted with invasive amebiasis to the Dhaka Bangladesh Diarrheal Diseases Research Hospital, of whom 86% were moderately to severely malnourished, had an overall mortality of 31% (158) compared to an expected mortality of 0.5% for uncomplicated amebic dysentery from one series in South Africa (65). Malnutrition was also shown to predispose to amebic infection and increased mortality in a series of 295 cases of amebic colitis in Nigeria (159).

Homosexual men do not commonly have complications from intestinal infection with *E. histolytica*, with only a few reports of invasive amebiasis or amebic liver abscess (53,54). Patients with the acquired immune deficiency syndrome (AIDS) who are infected with *E. histolytica* have not had more severe disease than homosexual men without AIDS (160,161). Whether this lack of severe disease is due to infection with avirulent strains of amebas (55) and/or because of the selective nature of the immune defects in AIDS (161) remains a matter of speculation. An equally interesting question has to do with what role chronic parasitic infections such as amebiasis may play in determining the latency of HIV infection. The expression of HIV virus in HIV-infected T cells in culture occurs only after immunological activation of the T cells with a mitogen such as phytohemagglutinin (PHA) (162). PHA stimulation of the T4 cells causes interleukin 2 release, which is followed by expression of the previously latent HIV virus and then cell death. Unstimulated HIV-infected T cells can be maintained in cell culture without cell death for 50–60 days in the absence of PHA stimulation. The *E. histolytica*, Gal/GalNAc-binding lectin, like PHA, is a lymphocyte mitogen (107). The epidemic of amebiasis preceded the epidemic of AIDS in San Francisco by several years, and approximately 80% of individuals diagnosed with AIDS in San Francisco currently have at least one intestinal parasite (160). AIDS cases from Haiti and Africa have shown high levels of parasitic infection: Of 18 African patients with AIDS residing in Belgium, nine had parasitic infections, four with *E. histolytica* (163); 14 of 46 Haitians with AIDS had parasitic infections, and 3 of 14 were infected with *E. histolytica* (164). Mitogenic stimulation of HIV latently infected T cells by the amebic Gal/ GalNAc lectin or mitogens from other parasitic infections potentially could result in HIV expression and AIDS.

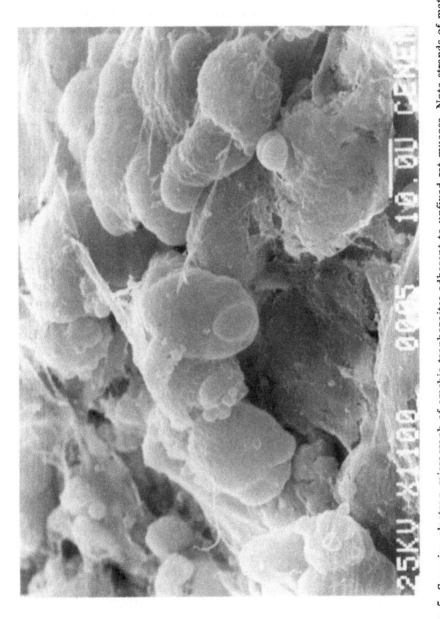

Figure 5 Scanning electron micrograph of amebic trophozoites adherent to unfixed rat mucosa. Note strands of material, possibly mucus, adherent to amebas. (Reprinted from *Infection and Immunity*, 4:292–297, 1985.)

B. Pathogenesis

The pathogenesis of invasive colonic amebiasis is due to (1) colonization of the gut by an ameba with virulent capabilities, (2) disruption of intestinal mucosal barriers by amebic enzymes or toxins, (3) establishment of adherence to the colonic epithelium by the amebic Gal/GalNAc surface lectin, and (4) lysis of intestinal and host inflammatory cells by adherent amebas. Colonization and virulence may be influenced by parasite strain specificity ["pathogenic zymodemes" (125)], interactions with the colonic bacterial flora (71,72,114,115), and incompletely defined host factors such as nutrition (165). Disruption of the colonic mucus layer and interruption of cell-to-cell adhesion may be accomplished by one of the numerous proteolytic activities isolated from *E. histolytica* (166–169), including major acid (166) and neutral (167) proteases and a collagenase (169). Amebic secretion of a cytotoxin or enterotoxin could cause the diffuse superficial mucosal inflammation in the absence of ulceration seen prior to attachment of amebas in animal models (170) and human colonic biopsy specimens (90,150). Enterotoxic activity has been described for amebic homogenates using rabbit ileal loops (171) and by pretreating rats and rabbits with indomethacin to impair prostaglandin-mediated mucosal cytoprotection (172, 173). Lysates of *E. histolytica* contain serotonin, which may be partly responsible for the enterotoxic effect (174). Enterotoxins or cytotoxins have not been demonstrated to be released from trophozoites under normal conditions. The development of toxin-negative amebic mutants or monoclonal antibodies specific for the different enterotoxins and cytotoxins will be necessary to ascribe a role in pathogenesis to these activities.

Human pathology, animal models, and in vitro organ culture systems have demonstrated that ulceration of the intestinal surface occur only at sites of adherent trophozoites (73,74,148,150,153,170,175). In vitro, *E. histolytica* trophozoites kill target cells only upon direct contact (93,110,176,177) following establishment of a specific adherence event inhibitable by galactose (Gal) or *N*-acetyl-D-galactosamine (GalNAc) (106,107,177) (Fig. 6). This amebic Gal/GalNAc-inhibitable surface lectin that mediates adherence has been recently isolated (106,107,178). The lysis of the target cell by the adherent ameba in vitro is dependent on calcium and amebic phospholipase A activity (179,180), amebic microfilament function (93), and maintenance of an acid pH in intracellular vesicles (181). Cytolytic activity is enhanced by phorbol esters (182) and may involve an amebic ionophore protein (183,184). Axenic *E. histolytica* trophozoites are chemoattractant for (112) and can kill human neutrophils in vitro (110–112). Amebic lysis of host neutrophils appears to contribute significantly to tissue destruction (76,111,112) (Fig. 3).

The migration of amebas from intestinal lesions to the liver is thought to occur hematogenously (148). Axenic strains of *E. histolytica* inoculated into the

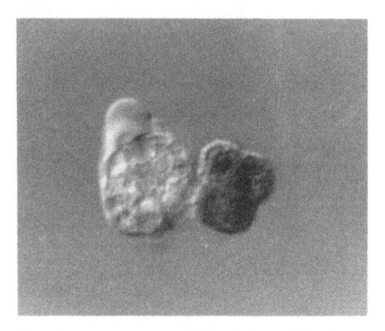

Figure 6 *Entamoeba histolytica* killing of adherent Chinese hamster ovary cells.

portal vein of hamsters resulted in extensive liver parenchymal necrosis and abscess formation (111). As with intestinal lesions, lysis of polymorphonuclear neutrophils by amebas is thought to be responsible for the zone of necrotic and lysed tissue surrounding the amebas (76,111). The use of in vitro (185) and animal (186) models of amebic pathogenesis has recently been reviewed.

C. Pathology

The lytic effect of amebic trophozoites in tissue is evidenced by the amorphous eosinophilic debris found in areas of amebic invasion (148,150,187,188) (Fig. 7). Individual trophozoites are frequently surrounded by a clear halo, apparently a fixation artifact (150), and are 15-60 μm in diameter with numerous vacuoles and a distinctive nucleus with a central karyosome (12,13,150,187). Trophozoites can be distinguished from other mononuclear cells with the Gridley stain, which intensely stains ingested red blood cells (189). Amebas have also been visualized in sputum and cervical smears and from paracecal abscess with the Papanicolaou stain (190,191). A lack of exuberant inflammation is characteristic of invasive amebiasis (148,150,187,188) and may be a reflection of the trophozoite's ability to lyse neutrophils (76,110-112). Electron microscopy has demonstrated the presence of ingested neutrophils within trophozoites from invasive disease (192).

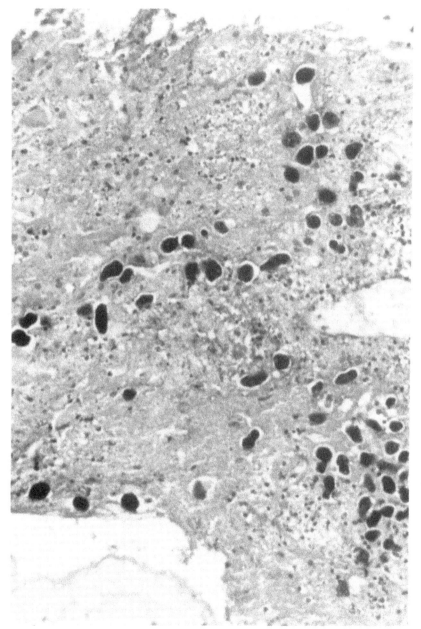

Figure 7 Periodic acid Schiff stain of amebic trophozoites from liver abscess. (Courtesy of Dr. Sharon Reed.)

There is a spectrum of colonic lesions observed in patients with amebic dysentery. Prathap and Gilman reviewed the histopathology of 53 patients with acute intestinal amebiasis (defined by the presence of motile erythrophagous *E. histolytica* trophozoites in patients with bloody dysentery) (150). Nonspecific thickening of the mucosa with edema of the lamina propria and mild to moderate neutrophilic infiltration was seen in 22 patients, with amebic trophozoites demonstrable in the surface exudate of only three. Microulceration of the surface epithelium was seen in 17 patients, with adherent amebas adjacent to sites of epithelial lysis in 15 of 17 patients. Superficial ulceration in 10 patients was characterized by the presence of large numbers of amebas and infiltrating neutrophils with pronounced mucus depletion. Deep ulceration in 10 patients resembled the classic flask-shaped ulcer described by Councilman and Lafleur (6) which extended to the submucosa with numerous amebas and rare inflammatory cells. No bacteria were seen within the ulcers (150). Granulating ulcers were seen in three patients. Invasion of trophozoites is not via mucosal crypts as originally thought (90,193) but directly through the surface epithelium (148,150). Male homosexuals colonized with *E. histolytica* have been shown to have diffuse nonspecific mucosal damage on biopsy (194).

Amebic liver abscesses are composed of acellular bacteriologically sterile necrotic debris, with trophozoites seen only on the periphery (148,187,195, 196). Liver abscesses result from hematogenous dissemination via the portal vein (148). Periportal fibrosis without trophozoites is also observed in patients with amebic colitis (196,197), which may represent past trophozoite invasion or host reaction to amebic antigens or toxins.

IV. THE DISEASE

A. Clinical Features

The clinical syndromes due to human infection with *E. histolytica* are listed in Table 5. The varied clinical presentations of this infection coupled with physicians' lack of familiarity with the disease have led to frequent misdiagnoses in developed countries.

1. Intestinal Disease

The majority of patients infected with *E. histolytica* are colonized without symptoms or with occasional abdominal colic and alteration in bowel habits (198). A prospective study of 184 patients referred for sigmoidoscopy to a clinic in India showed no difference in rectal biopsy histological findings or symptoms between patients who were stool culture positive and those negative for *E. histolytica*. Fifteen culture-positive patients were followed for a mean of 8.6 months; none developed symptoms of invasive amebiasis, and spontaneous elimination of the parasites occurred in all (198). In endemic areas such loss and reacquisition

Table 5 Clinical Syndromes

Intestinal disease

  Colonization

  Acute rectocolitis

  Chronic nondysenteric colitis

  Intestinal perforation with peritonitis

Extraintestinal disease

  Liver abscess

    Uncomplicated
    Extension to thorax or peritoneum

  Brain abscess

  Cutaneous

  Venereal infection

---

of the parasite is common, with up to 100% of the population being infected during the course of a year (22).

Acute amebic rectocolitis is characterized by the gradual onset over 1-3 weeks of frequent grossly bloody diarrheal bowel movements with abdominal pain and tenderness (65,199) (Table 6). Only one-third of the patients are febrile, and weight loss is common. Virtually all patients will have heme-positive stools (65,199) although fecal leukocytes may be absent, presumably due to the ameba's ability to lyse human neutrophils (110). Sigmoidoscopy reveals a hemorrhagic or normal mucosa with shallow ulcers having raised edges (199) or, in one case report, necrotizing lesions with grayish pseudomembrane formation (200). The classical flask-shaped ulceration with extension into the submucosa (Fig. 8) is found in only a minority of patients (150). Mortality from uncomplicated invasive amebiasis in one 20-year series of 3013 adults hospitalized in South Africa was 0.5% (65); however, mortality may be as high as 26-31% in series containing individuals at increased risk due to pregnancy, malnutrition, or underlying disease (153-159).

Chronic nondysenteric intestinal amebiasis can be confused with inflammatory bowel disease, with disastrous consequences if steroids are mistakenly administered. Of a series of 159 patients from Pakistan with chronic amebiasis, only 17% were symptomatic for less than a year, with 37% having greater than 5 years of intermittent diarrhea, mucus in stools, abdominal pain, flatulence, and/ or weight loss (201). All patients with chronic amebiasis had *E. histolytica* present in the stool, with 89% of patients having positive serology for antiamebic

Table 6   Clinical Manifestations of Invasive Intestinal Amebiasis

---

Symptoms

  Bloody mucoid diarrhea, usually for 1–4 weeks

  Abdominal pain

  Weight loss common

  Bloating, tenesmus, cramps

Signs

  Fever in only one-third

  Diffuse abdominal tenderness

  Tender liver

  All have heme (+) stools

Source: Reprinted from Ravdin, J. I. Diagnosis and management of infection by *Entamoeba histolytica, Infections in Medicine 4*:155–165, 1987.

antibody and 77% having ulcers seen on colonoscopy (201). Chronic presentations of amebic colitis are not confined to highly endemic areas; in 17 patients with symptomatic amebic colitis seen in central Virginia, 56% gave a history of longer than 4 weeks, and 29% more than 1 year, of gastrointestinal symptoms that responded to antiamebic therapy. Small mucosal lesions containing amebas, and not large flask-shaped ulcers, were seen in chronic amebiasis (201).

An ameboma is a segmented mass of granulation tissue that can present as a tender palpable mass in the cecum or ascending colon. Concurrent amebic dysentery is present in two-thirds of patients with amebomas (65,202). In contrast, only 0.5–1.5% of patients with amebic dysentery have been found to have amebomas (65), which can be confused with carcinoma on barium enema, appearing as single or multiple apple-core lesions (202,203). Colonoscopy with biopsy will establish the diagnosis (204), and patients respond to antiamebic chemotherapy.

Toxic megacolon is a severe but fortunately unusual complication of amebic colitis and has been associated with inappropriate administration of corticosteroids (63). The colon is markedly distended, and intramural gas may be present (202,205). These patients often require colectomy and have a much higher mortality than patients with uncomplicated intestinal amebiasis.

Amebic peritonitis from intestinal perforation causes a mortality as high as 40–75% (206,207). The onset of peritonitis may be acute but is more commonly insidious from slow leakage through a severely diseased colon (65,206,207). Early recognition and treatment of amebic peritonitis may decrease mortality:

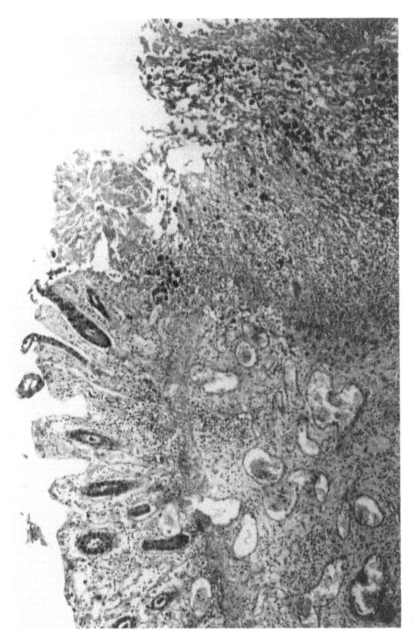

Figure 8 Light micrograph demonstrating a flssk-shaped ulceration in a pathological specimen from a patient with severe colonic amebiasis (periodic acid Schiff stain). (Reprinted from *Reviews of Infectious Diseases* 6:1185–1207, 1982.)

Patients who developed peritonitis while hospitalized and receiving antiamebic chemotherapy had a much lower mortality (12.5%) (206). Amebic peritonitis due to intestinal perforation has a higher mortality because of the coexistent bacterial infection that results from colonic perforation (207). It is unclear whether these patients benefit from surgical exploration as opposed to conservative management with antiamebic and antibacterial therapy (65,206-208).

2. Extraintestinal Disease

Liver Abscess. Approximately 10% of patients who have had invasive amebiasis will develop liver abscess, although only a minority of patients will have amebic dysentery or even have *E. histolytica* isolated from their stools at the time they present with an amebic liver abscess (210-212) (Table 7). A history of dysentery, which can be obtained in a large number of patients (210,211,213,214), is critical for arriving at a correct admitting diagnosis so that antiamebic chemotherapy can be rapidly started. In one series a correct admitting diagnosis was arrived at for only 16% of 48 patients subsequently found to have amebic liver abscesses (215).

Liver abscess can occur at any age and be fulminant in the very young (57, 59,216). It may be more prevalent in patients with underlying diseases or receiving corticosteroids (217) and occurs predominantly in males (212,215).

Patients may have either an acute or chronic presentation with amebic liver abscess (Table 7). Of patients with less than 10 days of symptoms, 85% had fever and abdominal pain, while of patients with 2-12 weeks of symptoms, only one-third had fever and abdominal pain but two-thirds had hepatomegaly and weight loss (212). Multiple amebic abscesses were more common in the group that presented acutely (212).

Table 7 Clinical Manifestations of Amebic Liver Abscess

Symptoms
   History of bloody diarrhea within last year
   Right upper quadrant abdominal pain
   Fever
   Weight loss
   Right chest or shoulder pain
Signs
   Fever in up to 75% patients
   Liver palpable and tender in 80%
   Localized intercostal tenderness
   Rales, rhonchi right base of lung

On physical exam there is exquisite point tenderness over the liver (218,211), hepatomegaly is present in less than half of patients, dullness and rales at the right base are common, and peritoneal signs or jaundice are unusual (211,212). Laboratory findings include a leukocytosis in 80%, mild anemia in more than 50%, elevated alkaline phosphatase in 80%, and a high erythrocyte sedimentation rate (211,212). Bilirubinemia is present only in the setting of severe disease or peritonitis (211,212).

Complications of Liver Abscess. Extension of an amebic liver abscess to the thorax or peritoneum results in more severe disease with increased mortality. Serous pleural effusion, elevation of the right hemidiaphragm, and atelectasis, which occur in up to 75% of patients with amebic liver abscess (215,218,219), do not represent direct extension of disease but can lead to the misimpression that the patient has primary pulmonary disease (215). Empyema due to rupture of the abscess into the pleural cavity presents with sudden respiratory distress and pain. In addition to antiamebic chemotherapy, these patients require adequate drainage either by repeated aspiration (220) or thoracotomy (221). The lung parenchyma is usually infected by direct extension from the liver, with hematogenous infection uncommon (222). Hepatobronchial fistulas occur and have been associated with spontaneous cure (211,222).

Peritonitis from rupture of an amebic abscess into the peritoneum has a lower mortality (18–33%) (207,211) than peritonitis from a perforated colon. Left-lobe amebic liver abscesses more commonly rupture into the peritoneum or pericardium than right-lobe abscesses (222). Left-lobe abscesses are much less common than right-lobe abscesses (211,212,219), are more difficult to diagnose, and can present with gastric compression or abscess perforation (222).

Amebic pericarditis resulting from extension of an amebic liver abscess (almost invariably in the left lobe) to the pericardium results in 30–40% mortality despite antiamebic chemotherapy and pericardiocentesis (211,223). Only 10 of 25 patients with amebic pericarditis in one series had diffusely elevated ST segments on EKG characteristic of pericarditis (223). Pericardial disease may be manifest initially by a friction rub and serous effusion or with acute cardiac tamponade. Pericardiocentesis can be diagnostic as well as therapeutic, but amebic trophozoites will be found only in the minority of aspirates (223).

Other Extraintestinal Syndromes. Cutaneous amebiasis is rare but may be found perianally in patients with amebic dysentery (224,225) or from enterocutaneous fistules (148). Amebic brain abscesses are seen in less than 2% of autopsies of patients who have died of amebiasis and are associated with concurrent liver abscess (226,227). Patients with brain abscess present with meningoencephalitis, altered mental status, and focal neurological signs and can progress rapidly (227,228). Computerized tomography reveals irregular lesions predominantly in the left hemisphere that contrast enhance (229). The diagnosis is made by examining tissue for amebic trophozoites; the combination of surgical decompression and metronidazole has improved the clinical outcome (229,230). Venereal amebiasis, with the exception of the epidemic colonization of male homosexuals, is unusual, with case reports of amebic ulceration of the penis (231,232) and cervix (233). The diagnosis is made by biopsy, and medical therapy is adequate (231–233).

B. Diagnosis

1. Intestinal Infection

The diagnosis of intestinal infection by *E. histolytica* rests on the demonstration in stool or mucosal scrapings of amebic trophozoites and cysts (Table 8). The morphological identification of *E. histolytica* requires high skill, and individual laboratories vary greatly in their ability to correctly identify the parasite (33). A single stool exam will miss one-third to one-half of all cases of amebiases detected by three or more consecutive exams (37,234). Substances that interfere with the stool examination for parasites and that should be avoided until all three specimens are obtained include bismuth, kaolin compounds, hypertonic or soap suds enemas, barium, magnesium hydroxide, castor oil, antibiotics (including tetracycline and sulfonamides), and antiparasitic drugs (235).

Ideally, stools should be examined within 30 min, before the trophozoites have disintegrated (235). The initial microscopic exam should be a saline wet mount of stool to search for *E. histolytica* trophozoites, which have a characteristic linear motility and may contain ingested red blood cells. Stool that cannot be examined immediately or fixed should be stored at 4°C. Fixation of stool should be in separate vials of 10% formalin and polyvinyl alcohol (PVA) at a

---

Table 8 Diagnostic Evaluation of Intestinal Amebiasis

---

1. Test stool for blood (should be positive), fecal leukocytes (often negative), and Charcot-Leyden crystals.
2. Perform three separate stool examinations for ova and parasites, including wet saline mount, iodine stain for cysts, permanent trichrome stain for trophozoites.
3. Perform lower gastrointestinal endoscopy with scraping or biopsy of ulcers if stool exam is negative or immediate tissue diagnosis is indicated.
4. Perform serum antibody test.
5. Avoid barium studies or other materials that interfere with examination of stool for parasites.

Source: Reprinted from Ravdin, J. I. Diagnosis and management of infection by *Entamoeba histolytica*, *Infections in Medicine* 4:155–165, 1987.

ratio of one part stool to five parts fixative, with the stool broken up and the vial shaken vigorously (235).

Iron hematoxylin or Wheatly trichrome stains (235,236) are performed on fresh or PVA-fixed specimens, and *E. histolytica* trophozoites are identified by their characteristic size (10–60 μm), centrally located karyosome, and fine peripheral chromatin structure (12,13). A formalin–ethyl acetate solution (9 ml 10% formalin, 3 ml ethyl acetate) is used to look for amebic cysts, which are concentrated at the bottom of the tube upon centrifugation (237). Amebic cysts are identified by their number of nuclei and their nuclear morphology (12,13).

Recently a monoclonal antibody to *E. histolytica* has been used to detect trophozoites and cysts in stool specimens by an enzyme-linked immunosorbent (ELISA) assay (238). The lack of cross-reaction of the monoclonal antibody with other enteric commensal protozoans such as *Endolimax nana* or *Entamoeba coli* makes this a promising future tool for identification of *E. histolytica* in stool specimens.

Culture of *E. histolytica* from stool has never gained wide acceptance in clinical practice. This is partly because there is no medium completely selective for *E. histolytica* so that identification still depends on skilled microscopic identification of the trophozoites in culture. The culture itself involves careful manipulation of antibiotics in the medium to prevent overgrowth of the associated bacteria (68). Cultivation of *E. histolytica* from stool has been shown to be more sensitive than microscopy alone (237,239) and may be helpful in cases where there are low levels of cyst passage, such as chronic nondysenteric amebiases or as a test of cure.

Gastrointestinal endoscopy with biopsies or scrapings plays an important role in the diagnosis of intestinal amebiasis (204,240,241). Patients should not be prepared for colonoscopy with cathartics or enemas, since these will interfere with identification of the parasite. The colonic mucosa characteristically has small ulcers or punctate hemorrhagic areas. Sigmoidoscopy alone is inadequate to rule out invasive amebiasis, because disease may be localized to the cecum or ascending colon (202). A cotton swab should not be used to obtain stool specimens; amebas will adhere to the fibers and be missed. Biopsies should be taken from the edge of ulcers and stool specimens aspirated with a pipette. Special stains such as periodic acid Schiff (PAS) should be used to highlight the amebas in the biopsy specimen. Clinical settings in which endoscopy with biopsy is especially useful are indicated in Table 9.

Serological tests for antiamebic humoral antibody are a valuable aid in the diagnosis of amebiasis. The most widely used test is an indirect hemagglutination assay (IHA), which is positive in up to 88% of patients with confirmed amebic dysentery, 99% of patients with amebic liver abscess, and only 5% of the general population in developed countries (131). IHA titers remain elevated (≥128) for

Table 9 Diagnostic Evaluation of Amebic Abscess[a]

1. Laboratory studies including amebic serology, white count, and liver function tests
2. Chest X-ray looking for elevation of right hemidiaphragm with or without effusion and atelectasis, and KUB for cholelithiasis which is associated with cholecystitis and pyogenic liver abscess
3. Ultrasound or computerized tomography of hepatobiliary system to differentiate liver abscess for cholecystitis

[a]Stool exam is useful to identify *E. histolytica* only in a minority of patients with amebic liver abscess. Aspiration is rarely required to establish a diagnosis.

years after treatment of invasive colitis; other serological tests that distinguish IgM and IgG antibodies may be useful in differentiating acute from prior infection (242).

Radiological studies such as a barium enema not only interfere with the examination of stool for parasites but also cannot distinguish amebiasis from any other process causing colonic ulceration (202,203) and should therefore be avoided.

2. Extraintestinal Infection

The diagnosis of extraintestinal amebiasis is a challenge for physicians in developed countires who rarely encounter the disease (Table 9). Only a minority of patients will have concurrent diarrhea or *E. histolytica* isolated from their stool. When encountering a febrile patient with right upper quadrant abdominal pain, one should suspect an amebic liver abscess when the patient is from a group at high risk for amebic infection (such as an immigrant or a traveler from an endemic area) and can give a history of prior dysentery. Amebic serology is the key for confirming the diagnosis of extraintestinal amebiasis but is not always immediately available. Noninvasive imaging techniques of the hepatobiliary system should be used the first day of hospitalization to distinguish liver abscess from acute cholecystitis. A series of 75 patients admitted with fever, right upper quadrant pain, nausea, and vomiting from an area in Texas endemic for amebiasis were evaluated within 24 hr by hepatobiliary radionuclide and ultrasound scans (243). These scans identified nine patients with liver abscess subsequently proven to be amebic by serology and clinical response to therapy with metronidazole. Clinically these patients were indistinguishable from the patients with cholecystitis except for being in a younger age group. Patients with cholecystitis may present in a more acute manner, be more likely to give a history of prior abdominal complaints, and not have hepatomegaly on physical examination as often seen in amebic abscess.

An amebic liver abscess has been described on ultrasound in 40% of cases as being round or oval, having no wall echoes, with echogenicity less than normal liver, being contiguous to the liver capsule, and having distal sonic enhancement (216) (Fig. 9). Ultrasound has the advantages of providing simultaneous evaluation of the gallbladder, being a rapid procedure, and not entailing radiation exposure. The resolution of an amebic liver abscess following therapy has been determined by ultrasound to average 7 months. Radionuclide scans of the liver have generally been replaced by computerized tomography (CT) (Fig. 10). Both techniques are sensitive but not specific for amebic liver abscess (215,244).

Serological tests, such as the IHA, will be positive for antiamebic antibodies in up to 99% of patients with an amebic liver abscess (131,244). Disadvantages to serological testing include the time delay in getting results back and the fact that serology may be initially negative with an acute (less than 7-day) presentation (244).

The differential diagnosis of a cystic lesion in the liver accompanied by the signs, symptoms, and laboratory abnormalities seen in amebic liver abscess must also include pyogenic abscess, echinococcal cysts, and tumor. Classically, amebic liver abscesses were thought to be single and to predominate in the right lobe of the liver, but it is now appreciated that up to 50% of patients who present acutely will have multiple abscesses. Helpful studies to rule out echinococcal disease include serology, absence of epidemiological risk factors, and lack of calcium in the cyst. Patients with bacterial liver abscess are more likely to be elderly and to have had recent abdominal surgery or abdominal malignancy and lack the epidemiological risk factors associated with amebic disease. Other than serological studies, there are no laboratory findings that distinguish pyogenic from amebic liver abscess. As an amebic abscess is in fact devoid of neutrophils and contains only necrotic debris, it appears as a cold defect on gallium-67 scans, in contrast to bacterial etiology, which causes a "true" abscess containing pus cells and is enhanced on gallium scanning. Although a time delay is necessary, a gallium study may be useful in such a clinical setting. However, in an unstable patient where one cannot clinically differentiate pyogenic from amebic liver abscess, aspiration of the abscess under CT or ultrasound guidance can be diagnostic. Aspiration of an amebic liver abscess yields a sterile odorless brown or yellow liquid. Trophozoites are demonstrated in the minority of cases, as most amebas are in the wall of the abscess. Percutaneous drainage of a pyogenic liver abscess is therapeutic as well as diagnostic (245). Aspiration of an echinococcal cyst is to be avoided because of the risk of anaphylaxis and seeding for new cysts if scolices spill into the peritoneum. The majority of patients with amebic liver abscess can be diagnosed and treated without aspiration. When amebic and pyogenic liver abscesses cannot be initially distinguished clinically, it is reasonable to add metronidazole to antibiotic coverage for facultative gram-negative rods and microaerophilic streptococci pending the results of serological studies.

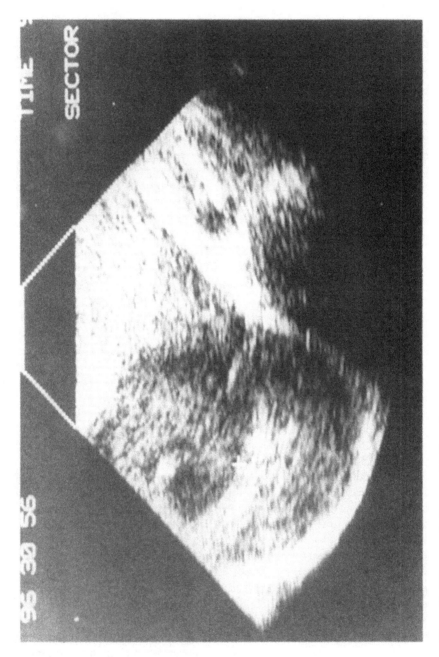

Figure 9   Ultrasound of an amebic liver abscess.

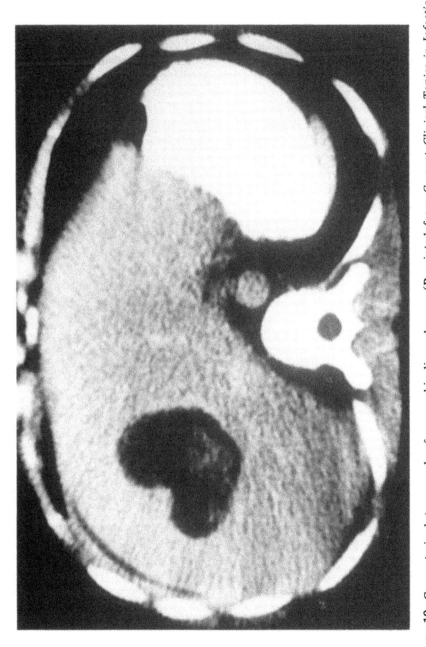

Figure 10 Computerized tomograph of an amebic liver abscess. (Reprinted from *Current Clinical Topics in Infectious Diseases*, J. S. Remington and M. N. Swartz, eds., 7:82–111, 1986.)

C. Treatment and Prevention

The drugs used to treat amebic infections, and their dosages, side effects, and preferred treatment regimens, have been recently reviewed (246-248) (Table 10). The therapy of amebiasis differs for asymptomatic and invasive disease. For an asymptomatic cyst passer, the initial question has to do with whether or not therapy is required. In highly endemic areas where the incidence of reinfection approaches 100%, little is to be accomplished by treating an asymptomatic carrier. In developed countries with little risk of reinfection, treatment eliminates the risk of future invasive disease and prevents the spread of infection. Asymptomatic carriers are treated with a poorly absorbed luminal agent such as diloxanide furoate, iodoquinol, or the aminoglycoside paromomycin. The poor absorption of these agents minimizes systemic side effects while maximizing drug delivery to the amebic cysts and trophozoites in the lumen of the colon. Metronidazole, one of the best drugs to treat invasive disease, is well absorbed and requires prolonged administration (10 days) to be highly effective in eliminating amebas from the large bowel (247).

Treatment of invasive amebiasis requires a combination of a well-absorbed drug to treat disease in the wall of the intestine and extraintestinally and a luminal drug to eliminate carriage of the amebas. Systemically absorbed anti-amebic drugs include metronidazole, tinidazole (unavailable in the United States), emetine, and dehydroemetine (administered intramuscularly only), and chloroquine. Chloroquine has not been shown to be effective at treating intestinal disease and is reserved for amebic liver abscess not responding to

Table 10 Therapeutic Regimens for the Treatment of Amebiasis

1. Luminal infection but negative serology and proctoscopy
   a. Diloxanide furoate 500 mg PO tid $\times$ 10 days
   b. Paromomycin 30 mg/kg/day in three divided doses PO $\times$ 5-10 days
   c. Iodoquinol 650 mg PO tid $\times$ 20 days
   d. Metronidazole 750 mg PO tid $\times$ 10 days

2. Invasive colonic disease or liver abscess[a]
   a. Metronidazole 750 mg PO or IV tid $\times$ 5-10 days plus a luminal agent
   b. Dehydroemetine 1-1.5 mg/kg/day IM $\times$ 5 days plus a luminal agent

[a]Chloroquine (base) 600 mg PO qd $\times$ 2 days, 300 mg base PO qd $\times$ 2-3 weeks can be added to metronidazole or dehydroemetine if an initial clinical response is not seen, but is usually unnecessary.
Source: Reprinted from Ravdin, J. I. Diagnosis and management of infection by *Entamoeba histolytica, Infections in Medicine* 4:155-165, 1987.

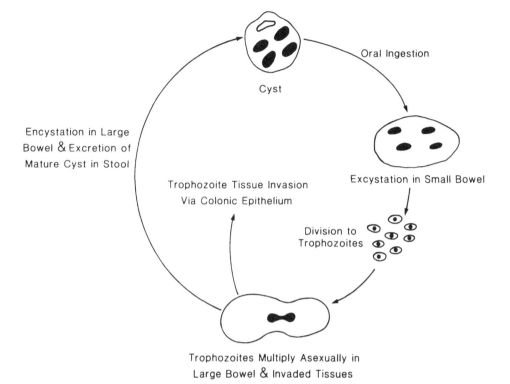

Figure 11 Life cycle of *Entamoeba histolytica*. Amebiasis results from the oral ingestion of *E. histolytica* cysts. Excystation and division of the quadrinucleate cyst to eight trophozoites occurs in the small bowel. The trophozoites reproduce asexually in the large bowel and either remain commensally in the bowel lumen or invade the intestinal epithelium, resulting in local and hematogenously disseminated disease. Encystment occurs in the bowel lumen only; cysts are never found within invaded tissue. Excretion of cysts from the large bowel completes the life cycle.

metronidazole. Emetine and dehydroemetine are ipecac alkaloids that are not tolerated when given orally, have frequent cardiovascular side effects, and are also second-line drugs. Metronidazole is the drug of choice for invasive infection with *E. histolytica*. A poorly absorbed antiamebic agent should be added to therapy with metronidazole (especially if the course is less than 10 days) to eliminate luminal *E. histolytica*; amebic liver abscess has occurred 1–3 months after treatment of amebic colitis with metronidazole alone (249). It is not clear when other agents should be added to metronidazole; patients with amebic liver abscess who fail metronidazole will usually respond to emetines plus chloroquine or require drainage (248). Metronidazole has been shown to be potentially both mutagenic and carcinogenic (250,251), and while the benefits of this drug outweigh the risks in treating invasive amebiasis, the ideal drug to treat amebiasis has yet to be found.

Needle aspiration of an amebic liver abscess is a safe procedure under experienced hands but is usually unnecessary, since the majority of patients will respond to chemotherapy alone within 3–5 days (212). Surgical resection in intestinal disease is extremely difficult because of the friability of the infected tissue, and it is not generally recommended except when unavoidable, such as with toxic megacolon (208).

Prevention of disease due to *E. histolytica* requires interruption of the fecal-oral spread of the cyst. Patients should be advised of the risks of travel to endemic areas, sexual activity that promotes fecal-oral contamination, and the lack of any measure short of boiling water as being effective in eradicating *E. histolytica* cysts (which are resistant to chlorination). Current research efforts directed at elucidating the molecular basis of disease pathogenesis, encystment, host intestinal factors, and host immunity may provide a means for future pharmacological or immunological prophylaxis. Pending the development of an effective vaccine or the availability of financial resources to improve public sanitation, amebiasis will remain a serious endemic disease in the population of the developing world as well as within high risk groups in developed countries.

ACKNOWLEDGMENTS

William A. Petri, Jr. is a Lucille P. Markey Scholar; Jonathan I. Ravdin was a Hartford Foundation Fellow. We thank Mutsuko Kennerly and Cynthia Kogut for excellent secretarial assistance.

REFERENCES

1. Bloomfield, A. L. A bibliography of internal medicine: amebic dysentery. *J. Chronic Dis. 5*:235–252 (1957).
2. Stilwell, G. G. Amebiasis: its early history. *Gastroenterology 28*:606–622 (1955).
3. Kean, B. H., Mott, K. E., and Russel, A. J. *Tropical Medicine and Parasitology: Classic Investigations.* Cornell University Press, Ithaca, NY, 1978, pp. 71–168.
4. Osler, W. On the amoeba coli in dysentery and in dysenteric liver abscess. *Johns Hopkins Hosp. Bull. 1*:53–54 (1890).
5. Simon, F. Abscess of the liver, perforation into the lung; amoeba coli in sputum. *Johns Hopkins Hosp. Bull. 1*:97 (1890).
6. Councilman, W. T., and Lafleur, H. A. Amoebic dysentery. *Johns Hopkins Hosp. Rep. 2*:395–548 (1891).

7. Rogers, L. The rapid cure of amoebic dysentery and hepatitis by hypodermic injections of soluble salts of Emetime. *Br. Med. J. 1*:1424-1425 (1912).
8. Walker, E. L., and Sellards, A. W. Experimental entamoebic dysentery. *Phillip. J. Sci. B. Trop. Med. 8*:253-331 (1913).
9. Boeck, W. C., and Drbohlav, J. The cultivation of *Entamoeba histolytica. Am. J. Hyg. 5*:371-407 (1925).
10. Dobell, C. Researches on the intestinal protozoa of monkey and man. *Parasitology 20*:357-412 (1928).
11. Diamond, L. S. Axenic cultivation of *Entamoeba histolytica. Science 134*: 336-337 (1961).
12. Brown, H. W. *Basic Clinical Parasitology*, 3rd ed. Appleton-Century-Crofts, New York, 1969, pp. 17-44.
13. Koneman, E. W., Allen, S. D., Dowell, V. R., and Sommers, H. M. *Color Atlas and Textbook of Diagnostic Microbiology*. Lippincott, Philadelphia, Pa., 1983, pp. 578-581.
14. Edelman, M. H., and Spingarn, C. L. Cultivation of *Entamoeba histolytica* as a diagnostic procedure: a brief review. *Mount Sinai J. Med. 43*:27-32 (1976).
15. Goldman, M., Carver, R. K., and Gleason, N. N. Antigenic analysis of *Entamoeba histolytica* by means of fluorescent antibody. II. *E. histolytica* and *E. hartmanni. Exp. Parasitol. 10*:366-388 (1960).
16. Salaki, J. S., Shirley, J. L., and Strickland, G. T. Successful treatment of symptomatic *Entamoeba polecki* infection. *Am. J. Trop. Med. Hyg. 28*: 190-193 (1979).
17. Dardick, K. R. Tetracycline treatment of *Dientamoeba fragilis. Conn. Med. 47*:69-70 (1983).
18. Shein, R., and Gelb, A. Colitis due to *Dientamoeba fragilis. Am. J. Gastroenterol. 78*:634-636 (1983).
19. Barker, D. C., and Swales, L. S. Characteristics of ribosomes during differentiation from trophozoite to cyst in axenic *Entamoeba* sp. *Cell Differ. 1*: 297-306 (1972).
20. WHO Expert Committee on Amebiasis. *World Health Org. Technol. Rep. Ser. 421*:1-52 (1969).
21. Walsh, J. A. In *Estimating the Burden of Illness in the Tropics in Tropical and Geographic Medicine* (K. S. Warren and A. A. F. Mahmoud, eds.). McGraw-Hill, New York, 1984.
22. Bray, R. S., and Harris, W. G. The epidemiology of infection with *Entamoeba histolytica* in the Gambia, West Africa. *Trans. R. Soc. Trop. Med. Hyg. 71*:401-407 (1977).
23. Armon, P. J. Ameobiasis in pregnancy and the puerperium. *Br. J. Obst. Gynecol. 85*:264-269 (1978).
24. Gutierrez, G. National serologic survey II. Search for antibodies against *Entamoeba histolytica* in Mexico. In *Proceedings of the International Conference on Amebiasis* (B. Sepulveda and L. S. Diamond, eds.). Instituto Mexicano del Seguro Social, Mexico, 1976, pp. 609-618.

25. Gutierrez-Trujillo, G., Ludlow, A., Espinosa, G., Herrera, S., Munoz, O., Rattoni, N., and Sepulveda, B. Caracteristicas principales de la amibiasis invasora en el nino. Actualizacion de algunos conceptos clinicos y epidemiologicos. *Arch. Invest. Med. (Mex.) 11 (Suppl. 1)*:281–286 (1980).

26. Alvarez-Alva, R., and de la Loza-Saldfuar, A. Frecuencia del absceso hepatico amibiano en hospitales del Instituto Mexicano del Seguro Social de la Republica Mexicana. *Arch. Invest. Med. (Mex.) 2*:327 (1971).

27. Perez-Tamayo, R., and Brandt, H. Amebiasis. In *Pathology of Protozoal and Helminthic Diseases*. (R. A. Marcial-Rojas, ed.) Robert E. Krieger, Huntington, NY, 1971, 145–187.

28. Abuabara, S. F., Barrett, J. A., Hau, T., and Jonasson, O. Amebic liver abscess. *Arch. Surg. 117*:239–244 (1982).

29. Pehrson, P. O. Amoebiasis in a non-endemic country. Epidemiology, presenting symptoms and diagnostic methods. *Scand. J. Infect. Dis. 15*:207–214 (1983).

30. Knoblock, J., and Mannweiler, E. Development and persistence of antibodies to *Entamoeba histolytica* in patients with amebic liver abscess. Analysis of 216 cases. *Am. J. Trop. Med. Hyg. 32*:727–732 (1983).

31. Guerrant, R. L., Rouse, J. D., Hughes, J. M., and Rowe, B. Turista among members of the Yale Glee Club in Latin America. *Am. J. Trop. Med. Hyg. 29*:895–900 (1980).

32. Heath, H. Chemotherapy and chemoprophylaxis of travelers diarrhea. *Ann. Int. Med. 102*:260–261 (1985).

33. Krogstad, D. J., Spencer, H. C., Healy, G. R., Gleason, N. N., Sexton, D. J., and Herron, C. A. Amebiasis: epidemiologic studies in the United States 1971–1974. *Ann. Int. Med. 88*:89–97 (1978).

34. Sexton, D. J., Krogstad, D. J., Spencer, H. C., Healy, G. R., Sinclair, S., Sledge, C. E., and Schultz, M. G. Amebiasis in a mental institution: serologic and epidemiologic studies. *Am. J. Epidemiol. 100*:414–423 (1974).

35. Brooke, M. M. Epidemiology and control of amebiasis in institutions for the mentally retarded. *Am. J. Mental Def. 68*:187–192 (1963).

36. Thacker, S. B., Simpson, S., Gordon, T. J., Wolfe, M., and Kimball, A. M. Parasitic disease control in a residential facility for the mentally retarded. *Am. J. Public Health 69*:1279–1281 (1979).

37. Birnkrant, W. B., Greenberg, M., and Most, H. Amebiasis in a hospital for the insane. *Am. J. Public Health 35*:805–814 (1945).

38. Nelson, T. L., and Brunetti, R. Control of diarrheal diseases in California state hospitals for retarded children. *Calif Med. 86*:22–24 (1957).

39. Sanders, D. F., and Bianchi, G. N. Amebiasis in Australia. 2. An epidemic in an institution for mental defectives and observations on the therapeutic effectiveness of "intestopan" and "humatin." *Med. J. Aust. 6*:261–266 (1970).

40. Thacker, S. B., Kimball, A. M., Wolfe, M., Choi, K., and Gilmore, L. Parasitic disease control in a residential facility for the mentally retarded: failure of selected isolation procedures. *Am J. Public Health 71*:303–305 (1981).

41. Brooke, M. M., Wilcox, D. E., Kaiser, R. L., and Melvin, D. M. Investigation of factors associated with the decline of intestinal protozoa in a Kansas mental institution. *Am. J. Hyg. 76*:52-60 (1962).

42. Juniper, K. Amebiasis in the United States. *Bull. NY Acad. Med. 47*:448-461 (1971).

43. Hart, J., Spirman, U., and Shattach, J. An outbreak of amebic infection in a kibbutz population. *Trans. R. Soc. Trop. Med. Hyg. 78*:346-348 (1984).

44. Millet, V. E., Spencer, M. J., Chapin, M. C., Garcia, L. S., Yatabe, J. H., and Stewart, M. E. Intestinal protozoan infection in a semicommunal group. *Am. J. Trop. Med. Hyg. 32*:54-60 (1983).

45. Sohn, N., and Robilotti, J. G. The gay bowel syndrome. *Am. J. Gastroenterol. 67*:478-484 (1977).

46. Schmerin, M. J., Gelston, A., and Jones, T. C. Amebiasis, an increasing problem among homosexuals in New York City. *JAMA 238*:1386-1387 (1977).

47. Hurwitz, A. L., and Owen, R. L. Venereal transmission of intestinal parasites. *West. J. Med. 128*:89-90 (1978).

48. William, D. C., Shookhoff, H. B., Felman, Y. M., and DeRamos, S. W. High rates of enteric protozoan infections in selected homosexual men attending a venereal disease clinic. *Sex Trans. Dis. 5*:155 (1978).

49. Phillips, S. C., Mildvan, D., William D. C., Gelb, A. M., and White, M. C. Sexual transmission of enteric protozoa and helminths in a venereal disease clinic population. *New Engl. J. Med. 305*:603-606 (1981).

50. Quinn, T. C., Stamm, W. E., Goodell, S. E., Krtichian, E. M., Benedetti, J., Corey, L., Schuffler, M., and Holmes, K. K. The polymicrobial origin of intestinal infections in homosexual men. *New Engl. J. Med. 309*:576-582 (1983).

51. Hakansson, C., Thoren, K., Norkrans, G., and Johannisson, G. Intestinal parasitic infection and other sexually transmitted diseases in asymptomatic homosexual men. *Scan. J. Infect. Dis. 16*:199-202 (1984).

52. Markell, E. K., Havens, R. F., Kuritsubo, R. A., and Wingeral, J. Intestinal protozoa in homosexual men of the San Francisco Bay area: prevalence and correlates of infection. *Am. J. Trop. Med. Hyg. 33*:239-245 (1984).

53. Thompson, J. E., Freischlag, J., and Thomas, D. S. Amebic liver abscess in a homosexual man. *Sex. Trans. Dis. 10*:153-155 (1983).

54. Ylvisaker, J. T., and McDonald, G. B. Sexually acquired amebic colitis and liver abscess. *West. J. Med. 132*:153-157 (1980).

55. Sargeaunt, P. G., Oates, J. K., Maclenna, I., Oriel, J. D., and Goldmeier, D. *Entamoeba histolytica* in male homosexuals. *Br. J. Vener. Dis. 59*:193-195 (1983).

56. Lewis, E. A., and Anita, A. U. Amoebic colitis: review of 295 cases. *Trans R. Soc. Trop. Med. Hyg. 63*:633 (1969).

57. Martinez-Palomo, A., and Martinez-Baez, M. Selective primary health care: strategies for control of disease in the developing world. X. Amebiasis. *Rev. Infect. Dis. 5*:1093-1102 (1983).

58. Dykes, A. C., Ruebush, T. K., Gorelkin, L., Lushbaugh, W. B., Upshur, J. K., and Cherry, J. D. Extraintestinal amebiasis in infancy: report of three patients and epidemiologic investigations of their families. *Pediatrics 65*: 799–803 (1980).
59. Merritt, R. J., Coughlin, E., Thomas, D. W., Jariwala, L., Swanson, V., and Sinatra, F. R. Spectrum of amebiasis in children. *Am. J. Dis. Child. 136*: 785–789 (1982).
60. Jammal, M. A., Cox, K., and Ruebner, B. Amebiasis presenting as rectal bleeding without diarrhea in childhood. *J. Pediatr. Gastroenterol. Nutr. 4*: 294–296 (1985).
61. Healy, G. R. The status of invasive amebiasis in the United States as determined by studies with the indirect hemagglutinin test. In *Proceedings of the International Conference on Amebiasis* (B. Sepulveda and L. S. Diamond, eds.). Instituto Mexicano del Seguro Social Mexico, 1976.
62. Istre, G. R., Kreiss, K., Hopkins, R. S., Healy, G. R., Benziger, M., Canfield, T. M., Dickinson, P., Englert, T. R., Compton, R. C., Mathews, H. M., and Simmons, R. A. An outbreak of amebiasis spread by colonic irrigation at a chiropractic clinic. *New Engl. J. Med. 307*:339–342 (1982).
63. Eisert, J., Hannibal, J. E., and Sanders, S. L. Fatal amebiasis complicating corticosteroid management of pemphigus vulgaris. *New Engl. J. Med. 261*: 843–845 (1959).
64. Tucker, P. C., et al. Amebic colitis mistaken for inflammatory bowel disease. *Arch. Intern. Med. 135*:681 (1975).
65. Adams, E. B., and MacLeod, I. N. Invasive amebiasis. I. Amebic dysentery and its complications. *Medicine 56*:315–323 (1977).
66. McAllister, T. A. Diagnosis of amoebic colitis on routine biopsies from rectum and sigmoid colon. *Br. Med. J. 1*:362–364 (1962).
67. Dougherty, E. C. Introduction to axenic cultivation of invertebrate metazoa: a goal. *Ann. NY Acad. Sci. 77*:27 (1959).
68. Diamond, L. S. Cultivation of *Entamoeba histolytica* in vitro. In *Amebiasis: Human Infection by Entamoeba histolytica* (J. I. Ravdin, ed.). Wiley, New York, 1988, pp. 27–40.
69. Robinson, G. L. The laboratory diagnosis of human parasitic amoeba. *Trans. R. Soc. Trop. Med. Hyg. 62*:283 (1968).
70. Diamond, L. S., Harlow, D. R., and Cunnick, C. A new medium for axenic cultivation of *Entamoeba histolytica* and other Entamoeba. *Trans. R. Soc. Trop. Med. Hyg. 72*:431 (1978).
71. Phillips, B. R., Diamond, L. S., Bartgis, I. L., and Stuppler, S. A. Results of intracecal inoculations of germfree and conventional guinea pigs and germfree rats with axenically cultivated *Entamoeba histolytica*. *J. Protozool. 19*: 498–499 (1972).
72. Wittner, M., and Rosenbaum, R. M. Role of bacteria in modifying virulence of *Entamoeba histolytica*. *Am. J. Trop. Med. Hyg. 19*:755–761 (1970).
73. Chadee, K., and Meerovitch, E. The mongolian gerbil (*Meriones unguiculatus*) as an experimental host for *Entamoeba histolytica*. *Am. J. Trop. Med. Hyg. 33*:47–54 (1984).

74. Anaya-Velazquez, F., Martinez-Palomo, A., Tsutsumi, V., and Gonzalez-Robles, A. Intestinal invasive amebiasis: an experimental model in rodents using axenic or monoxenic strains of *Entamoeba histolytica. Am. J. Trop. Med. Hyg. 34*:723–730 (1985).

75. Mattern, C. F. T., Keister, D. B., and Casper, P. A. Experimental amebiasis. III. A rapid in vitro assay for virulence of *Entamoeba histolytica. Am. J. Trop. Med. Hyg. 27*:882–887 (1978).

76. Chadee, K., and Meerovitch, E. The pathogenesis of experimentally induced amebic liver abscess in the gerbil *(Meriones unguiculatus). Am. J. Pathol. 117*:71–80 (1984).

77. Lushbaugh, W. B., Kairalla, A. B., Loadolt, C. B., and Pittman, F. E. Effect of hamster liver passage on the virulence of axenically cultivated *Entamoeba histolytica. Am. J. Trop. Med. Hyg. 28*:248–254 (1978).

78. Gold, D., and Norman, L. Studies on the preservation and enhancement of the virulence of some strains of *Entamoeba histolytica* in axenic and monoxenic cultures. *J. Parasitol. 65*:970–972 (1979).

79. Gold, D., Bos, H. J., Diamantstein, T., and Hahn, H. On culture of *Entamoeba histolytica* in plastic tissue culture flasks. *Z. Parasitenkd. 67*:341–344 (1982).

80. McLaughlin, J., and Aley, S. The biochemistry and functional morphology of the *Entamoeba. J. Protozool. 32*:221–240 (1985).

81. Serrano, R., and Reeves, R. E. Physiologic significance of glucose transport in *Entamoeba histolytica. Exp. Parasitol. 37*:411–416 (1975).

82. Reeves, R. E., Serrano, R., and South, D. J. 6-Phospho-fructokinase (pyrophospate) properties of the enzyme from *Entamoeba histolytica* and its reaction mechanism. *J. Biol. Chem. 251*:2958–2962 (1976).

83. Muller, M. The hydrogenosome. *Symp. Soc. Gen. Microbiol. 30*:127–142 (1980).

84. Fahey, R. C., Newton, G. L., Arrick, B., Overdank-Bogart, T., and Aley, S. B. *Entamoeba histolytica*: a eukaryote without glutathione metabolism. *Science 224*:70–72 (1984).

85. Lo, H. S., and Wang, C. C. Purine salvage in *Entamoeba histolytica. J. Parasitol. 71*:662–669 (1985).

86. Rosenbaum, R. M., and Wittner, M. Ultrastructure of bacterized and axenic trophozoites of *Entamoeba histolytica* with particular reference to helical bodies. *J. Cell. Biol. 45*:367–382 (1970).

87. Kress, Y., Wittner, M., and Rosenbaum, R. M. Sites of cytoplasmic ribonucleoprotein-filament assembly in relation to helical body formation in axenic trophozoites of *Entamoeba histolytica. J. Cell. Biol. 49*:773–784 (1971).

88. Eaton, R. D. P., Meerovitch, E., and Costerton, J. W. The functional morphology of pathogenicity in *Entamoeba histolytica. Ann. Trop. Med. Parasitol. 64*:299–304 (1970).

89. Proctor, E. M. Studies of ultrastructure of various strains of *Entamoeba histolytica* and of *Entamoeba coli*. In *Proceedings of International Conference*

on Amebiasis (B. Sepulveda and L. S. Diamond, eds.). Mexico City, 1977, pp. 311–323.

90. Griffin, J. L., and Juniper, K. Ultrastructure of *Entamoeba histolytica* from human amoebic dysentery. *Arch. Pathol. 91*:271–280 (1971).

91. Knight, R., Bird, R. G., and McCaul, T. F. Fine structural changes at *Entamoeba histolytica* rabbit kidney cell (RK13) interface. *Am. Trop. Med. Parasitol. 69*:197–202 (1975).

92. Aust-Kettis, A., and Sundqvist, K. G. Dynamics of the interaction between *Entamoeba histolytica* and components of the immune response. I. Capping and endocytosis: influence of inhibiting and accelerating factors; variation of the expression of surface antigens. *Scand. J. Immunol. 35*:44 (1978).

93. Ravdin, J. I., Croft, B. Y., and Guerrant, R. L. Cytopathogenic mechanisms of *Entamoeba histolytica*. *J. Exp. Med. 152*:377–390 (1980).

94. Lushbaugh, W. B., and Miller, J. H. Fine structural topochemistry of *Entamoeba histolytica* Schuadinn, 1903. *J. Parasitol. 60*: 421–433 (1974).

95. Swartzwelder, J. C., and Muller, G. R. A comparison of the infection rate and gross pathology of amebic infection in normal and antigen-injected rats. *Am. J. Trop. Med. Hyg. 30*:181–183 (1950).

96. Ghadirian, E., and Meerovitch, E. Vaccination against hepatic amebiasis in hamsters. *J. Parasitol. 64*:742–743 (1978).

97. Sepulveda, B., Arroyo-Begovich, A., Tanimoto-Weki, M., Martinez-Palomo, A., and Ortiz-Ortiz, L. Simposio: induccion de inmunidad protectora antiamibiana con "nuevos" antigenos en el hamster lactante. *Arch. Invest. Med. (Mex.) 9(Suppl. 1)*:309 (1978).

98. Sharma, A., Hag, A., Ahmed, S., and Lederer, E. Vaccination of rabbits against *Entamoeba histolytica* with aqueous suspensins of trehelose-dimycolate as the adjuvant. *Infect. Immun. 48*:634–637 (1985).

99. Krupp, I. M. Protective immunity to amebic infection demonstrated in guinea pigs *Am. J. Trop. Med. Hyg. 23*:355–360 (1974).

100. Ghadirian, E., Meerovitch, E., and Hartman, D. P. Protection against amebic liver abscess in hamsters by means of immunization with amebic antigens and some of its fractions. *Am. J. Trop. Med. Hyg. 29*:779–784 (1980).

101. Vinayak, V., Sawhney, S., Jain, P., and Chakravarti, R. N. Protective effects of crude and chromatographic fractions of axenic *Entamoeba histolytica* in guinea pigs. *Trans. R. Soc. Trop. Med. Hyg. 74*:483–437 (1980).

102. Savanet, T., Viriyanond, P., and Nimitmongkol, N. Blast transformation of lymphocytes in amebiasis. *Am. J. Trop. Med. Hyg. 22*:705–710 (1973).

103. Harris, W. G., and Bray, R. S. Cellular sensitivity in amebiasis—preliminary results of lymphocytic transformation in response to specific antigen and to mitogen in carrier and disease states. *Trans. R. Soc. Trop. Med. Hyg. 70*: 340–343 (1976).

104. Ganguly, N. K., Mahajan, R. C., Sharma, S., Chandanani, R. E., Sharma,

R. R., and Mohan, C. Isolation of antigen fraction responsible for delayed hypersensitivity in amoebiasis. *Indian J. Med. Res. 70*:17–21 (1979).

105. Salata, R. A., Pearson, R. D., and Ravdin, J. I. Interaction of human leukocytes and *Entamoeba histolytica*. Killing of virulent amebae by the activated macrophage. *J. Clin. Invest. 76*:491–499 (1985).

106. Ravdin, J. I., Murphy, C. F., Salata, R. A., Guerrant, R. L., and Hewlett, E. L. The *N*-acetyl-D-galactosamine inhibitable adherence lectin of *Entamoeba histolytica*. I. Partial purification and relationship to amebic in vitro virulence. *J. Infect. Dis. 151*:804–815 (1985).

107. Salata, R. A., and Ravdin, J. I. The *N*-acetyl-D-galactosamine inhibitable adherence lectin of *Entamoeba histolytica*. II. Mitogenic activity for human lymphocytes. *J. Infect. Dis. 151*:816–822 (1985).

108. Joyce, M. P., and Ravdin, J. I. Antigens of *Entamoeba histolytica* recognized by immune sera from liver abscess patients. *Am. J. Trop. Med. Hyg. 38*:74–80 (1988).

109. Reed, S. L., Sargeaunt, P. G., and Braude, A. I. Resistance to lysis by human complement of pathogenic *Entamoeba histolytica*. *Trans. R. Soc. Trop. Med. Hyg. 77*:248–253 (1983).

110. Guerrant, R. L., Brush, J., Ravdin, J. I., Sullivan, J. A., and Mandell, G. L. Interaction between *Entamoeba histolytica* and human polymorphonuclear neutrophils. *J. Infect. Dis. 143*:83–93 (1981).

111. Tsutumi, V., Mena-Lopez, R., Anaya-Velazquez, F., and Martinez-Palomo, A. Cellular basis of experimental amebic liver abscess formation. *Am. J. Pathol. 117*:81–91 (1984).

112. Salata, R. A., John, J. E., Ahmed, P., and Ravdin, J. I. The interaction of human neutrophils and *Entamoeba histolytica* increases cytopathogenicity for liver cell monolayers. *J. Infect. Dis. 154*:19–26 (1986).

113. Salata, R. A., Conales, L., Martinez-Palomo, A., Trevino, N., and Ravdin, J. I. Immune sera suppresses the antigen specific response in T lymphocytes from patients cured of amebic liver abscess. Meeting of the American Society of Tropical Medicine and Hygiene, 1985, abstract 87.

114. Phillips, B. P., and Gorstein, F. Effects of different species of bacteria on the pathology of enteric amebiasis in monocontaminated guinea pigs. *Am. J. Trop. Med. Hyg. 15*:863–868 (1966).

115. Bracha, R., and Mirelman, D. Virulence of *Entamoeba histolytica* trophozoites. Effects of bacteria, microaerobic conditions and metronidazole. *J. Exp. Med. 160*:353–368 (1984).

116. Das, S. R., and Ghoshal, S. Restoration of virulence to rat of axenically grown *Entamoeba histolytica* by cholesterol and hamster liver passage. *Ann. Trop. Med. Parasitol. 70*:439–443 (1976).

117. Meerovitch, E., and Ghadirian, E. Restoration of virulence of axenically cultivated *Entamoeba histolytica* by cholesterol. *Can. J. Microbiol. 24*: 63–65 (1978).

118. Diamond, L. S., Mattern, C. F. T., and Bargis, I. L. Viruses of *Entamoeba*

histolytica. I. Identification of transmissable virus-like agents. *J. Virol. 9*: 326–341 (1972).

119. Mattern, C. F. T., Keister, D. B., and Diamond, L. S. Experimental amebiasis. IV. Amebal viruses and the virulence of *Entamoeba histolytica. Am. J. Trop. Med. Hyg. 28*:653–657 (1979).

120. Trissl, D., Martinez-Palomo, A., Torre, M., Hoz, R., and Surez, E. P. Surface properties of *Entamoeba*: increased rates of human erythrocyte phagocytosis in pathogenic strains. *J. Exp. Med. 148*:1137–1145 (1978).

121. Bhatia, V. N., Parmar, U., Subramanian, C., Sharma, S., and Singh, D. S. Virulence, haemolysis pattern and haemophagocytosis index of *Entamoeba histolytica. Indian J. Med. Res. 76*:545–551 (1982).

122. Orozco, E., Guarneros, G., Martinez-Palomo, A., and Sanchez, T. *Entamoeba histolytica*: phagocytosis as a virulence factor. *J. Exp. Med. 158*: 1511–1522 (1983).

123. Mattern, C. F. T., Keister, D. B., and Caspar, P. A. Experimental amebiasis. III. A rapid in vitro assay for virulence of *Entamoeba histolytica. Am. J. Trop. Med. Hyg. 27*:882–887 (1978).

124. Bos, H. J., Leijendekker, W. J., and van den Eijk, A. A. Cytopathogenicity including serum effects on contact-dependent and toxin-induced lysis of hamster kidney cell monolayers. *Exp. Parasitol. 50*:342–348 (1980).

125. Sargeaunt, P. G., Jackson, T. F. H. G., and Simjee, A. E. Biochemical homogeneity of *Entamoeba histolytica* isolates, especially those from liver abscess. *Lancet 1*:1386–1388 (1982).

126. De Leon, A. Prognostico tardio en el absceso hepatico amibiano. *Arch. Invest. Med. (Mex.) 1 (Suppl. 1)*:205–206 (1970).

127. Krupp, I. M. Antibody response in intestinal and extraintestinal amebiasis. *Am. J. Trop. Med. Hyg. 19*:57–62 (1970).

128. Sepulveda, B. Amebiasis: host-pathogen biology. *Rev. Infect. Dis. 4*:1247–1253 (1982).

129. Shealan, M., and Baker, R. P. Detection of coproantibodies in amebiasis of the colon: a preliminary report. *Am. J. Clin. Pathol. 54*:615–617 (1970).

130. Mahajan, R. C., Agarwal, S. C., Chittani, P. N., and Chitkara, N. L. Coproantibodies in intestinal amebiasis. *Indian J. Med. Res. 60*:547–550 (1972).

131. Kagan, I. G. Serologic diagnosis of parasitic diseases. *New Engl. J. Med. 282*:685–686 (1970).

132. Patterson, M., Healy, G., and Shabot, J. M. Serologic testing for amoebiasis. *Gastroenterology 78*:136–141 (1980).

133. Elsdon-Dew, R. The serology of amoebiasis. *Trans R. Soc. Trop. Med. 64*: 18 (1970).

134. Krupp, I. M., and Powell, S. J. Comparative study of the antibody response in amebiasis. Persistence after successful treatment. *Am. J. Trop. Med. Hyg. 20*:421–424 (1971).

135. Onyemelukwe, G. C., and Onyewotu, I. I. Amoebic liver abscess-serum anticomplementary screening for immune complexes. *Trans. R. Soc. Trop. Med. Hyg. 75*:613–614 (1981).

136. Ortiz-Ortiz, L., Capin, R., Sepulveda, B., and Zamacona, G. Activation of the alternate pathway of complement by *Entamoeba histolytica. Clin. Exp. Immunol. 34*:10–18 (1978).

137. Calderon, J., and Schreiber, R. D. Activation of the alternative and classical complement pathways by *Entamoeba histolytica. Infect. Immun. 50*:560–565 (1985).

138. Ghadirian, E., and Meerovitch, E. Effect of complement depletion on hepatic amoebiasis in hamsters. *Clin. Immunol. Immunopath. 24*:315–319 (1982).

139. Jarumilinta, R., and Kradolfer, F. The toxic effect of *Entamoeba histolytica* on leukocytes. *Ann. Trop. Med. Parasitol. 58*:375–381 (1964).

140. Ghadirian, E., and Meerovitch, E. Effect of splenectomy on the size of amoebic liver abscesses and metastatic foci in hamsters. *Infect. Immun. 31*:571–573 (1981).

141. Ghadirian, E., and Meerovitch, E. Effect of immunosuppression on the size and metastasis of amoebic liver abscesses in hamster. *Parasite Immunol. 3*: 329–338 (1981).

142. Ghadirian, E., Meerovitch, E., and Kongshain, P. A. L. Role of macrophages in host defense against hepatic amoebiasis in hamsters. *Infect. Immun. 42*:1017–1019 (1983).

143. Ghadirian, E., and Meerovitch, E. Macrophage requirement for host defense against experimental hepatic amoebiasis in the hamster. *Parasite Immunol. 4*:219–225 (1982).

144. Kretschmer, R. R., Sepulveda, B., Almazan, A., and Gamboa, F. Intradermal reactions to an antigen (histolyticin) obtained from axenically cultivated *Entamoeba histolytica. Trop. Geo. Med. 24*:275–281 (1972).

145. Ortiz-Ortiz, L., Zamacona, G., Sepulveda, B., and Capin, N. R. Cell-mediated immunity in patients with amebic abscess of the liver. *Clin. Immunol. Immunopathol. 4*:127–134 (1975).

146. Salata, R. A., Martinez-Palomo, A., Murray, H. W., Conales, L., Trevino, N., Segovia, E., Murphy, C. F., and Ravdin, J. I. Patients treated for amebic liver abscess develop cell-mediated immune responses effective in vitro against *Entamoeba histolytica. J. Immunol. 136*:2633–2639 (1986).

147. Salata, R. A., and Ravdin, J. I. Review of human immune mechanisms directed against *Entamoeba histolytica. Rev. Infect. Dis. 8*:261–272 (1986).

148. Brandt, H., and Perez-Tamayo, R. The pathology of human amebiasis. *Hum. Pathol. 1*:351 (1970).

149. Juniper, K., Steele, V. W., and Chester, C. L. Rectal biopsy in the diagnosis of amebic colitis. *South. Med. J. 51*:545 (1958).

150. Prathap, K., and Gilman, R. The histopathology of acute intestinal amebiasis. *Am. J. Pathol. 60*:229–239 (1970).

151. Pittman, F. E., El-Hashimi, W. K., and Pittman, J. C. Studies in human amebiasis. II. Light and electron-microscopic observations of colonic mucosa and exudate in acute amebic colitis. *Gastroenterology 65*:588–603 (1973).

152. Leitch, G. J., Dickey, A. D., Udezula, I. A., and Bailey, G. B. *Entamoeba histolytica* trophozoites in the lumen and mucus blanket of rat colons studied in vivo. *Infect. Immun.* 47:68–73 (1985).

153. Ravdin, J. I., John, J. E., Johnston, L. I., Innes, D. J., and Guerrant, R. L. Adherence of *Entamoeba histolytica* trophozoites to rat and human colonic mucosa. *Infect. Immun.* 48:292–297 (1985).

154. Mirelman, D., Feingold, C., Wexler, A., and Bracha, R. Interaction between *Entamoeba histolytica* bacteria and intestinal cells. *Ciba Found. Symp. 99*: 2–30 (1983).

155. Feingold, C., Bracha, R., Wexler, A., and Mirelman, D. Isolation, purification and partial characterization of an enterotoxin from extracts of *Entamoeba histolytica* trophozoites. *Infect. Immun.* 48:211–218 (1985).

156. Chadee, K., Petri, W. A., Innes, D. J., and Ravdin, J. I. Rat and human colonic mucins bind to and inhibit the adherence lectin of *Entamoeba histolytica. J. Clin. Invest.* 80:1245–1254 (1987).

157. Rode, H., Davies, M. R. Q., and Cywes, S. Amoebic liver abscesses in infancy and childhood. *S. Afr. J. Surg.* 16:131–138 (1978).

158. Wanke, C. A., and Butler, T. Intestinal amoebiasis in a hospital population in Bangladesh. Program and Abstracts of the 25th Interscience Conference on Antimicrobial Agents and Chemotherapy, 1985, abstract No. 65.

159. Lewis, E. A., and Antia, A. U. Amoebic colitis: review of 295 cases. *Trans. R. Soc. Trop.Med. Hyg.* 63:633–638 (1969).

160. Druckman, D. A., and Quinn, T. C. *Entamoeba histolytica* infections in homosexual men. In *Amebiasis: Human Infection by Entamoeba histohistolytica* (J. I. Ravdin, ed.). Wiley, New York, 1988, pp. 563–575.

161. Fauci, A. S., Masur, H., Gelmann, E. P., Markham, P. D., Hahn, B. H., and Lane, H. C. The acquired immunodeficiency syndrome: an update. *Ann. Intern. Med.* 102:800–813 (1985).

162. Zagury, D., Bernard, J., Leonard, R., Cheynier, R., Feldman, M., Sarin, P. S., and Gallo, R. C. Long term culture of HTLV–III–infected T cells: a model of cytopathology of T cell depletion in AIDS. *Science* 231:850–853 (1986).

163. Cluneck, N., et al. Acquired immunodeficiency syndrome in African patients. *New Engl. J. Med.* 310:492–497 (1984).

164. Pape, J. W., et al. Characteristics of the acquired immunodeficinecy syndrome (AIDS) in Haiti. *New Engl. J. Med.* 309:945–950 (1983).

165. Diamond, L. S. Amebiasis: nutritional implications. *Rev. Infect. Dis. 4*: 843–850 (1982).

166. Scholze, H., and Werries, E. A weakly acidic protease has a powerful proteolytic activity in *Entamoeba histolytica. Mol. Biochem. Parasitol. 11*: 293–300 (1984).

167. Keene, W. E., Pettit, M. G., Allen, S., and McKerrow, J. H. The major neutral proteinase of *Entamoeba histolytica. J. Exp. Med.* 163:536–549 (1986).

168. Neal, R. A. Enzymic proteolysis of *Entamoeba histolytica*; biochemical characteristics and relationship with invasiveness. *Parasitology* 50:531–550 (1960).

169. Munoz, M. D. L., Calderon, J., and Rojkind, M. The collagenase of *Entamoeba histolytica. J. Exp. Med. 155*:42–51 (1982).

170. Chadee, K., and Merrovitch, E. *Entamoeba histolytica*: early progressive pathology in the cecum of the gerbil (*Meriones unguiculatus*). *Am. J. Trop. Med. Hyg. 34*:283–291 (1985).

171. Lushbaugh, W. B., Kairalla, A. B., Cantey, J. R., Hofbauer, A. F., and Pittman, F. E. Isolation of a cytotoxin-enterotoxin from *Entamoeba histolytica. J. Infect. Dis. 139*:9–17 (1979).

172. Udezula, I. A., Leitch, G. J., and Bailey, G. B. Use of indomethacin to demonstrate enterotoxic activity in extracts of *Entamoeba histolytica* trophozoites. *Infect. Immun. 36*:795–801 (1982).

173. Feingold, C., Bracha, R., Wexler, A., and Mirelman, D. Isolation, purification and partial characterization of an enterotoxin from extracts of *Entamoeba histolytica* trophozoites. *Infect. Immun. 48*:211–218 (1985).

174. McGowan, K., Kane, A., Asarkof, N., Wicks, J., Guerina, V., Kellum, J., Baron, S., Gintzler, A. R., and Donowitz, M. *Entamoeba histolytica* causes intestinal secretion: role of serotonin. *Science 221*:762–764 (1983).

175. Takeuchi, A., and Phillips, B. R. Electron microscope studies of experimental *Entamoeba histolytica* infection in the guinea pig. I. Penetration of the intestinal epithelium by trophozoites. *Am. J. Trop. Med. Hyg. 24*:34–48 (1975).

176. Knight, R., Bird, R. G., and McCaul, T. F. Fine structural changes at *Entamoeba histolytica* rabbit kidney cell (RK13) interface. *Ann. Trop. Med. Parasitol. 69*:197–202 (1975).

177. Ravdin, J. I., and Guerrant, R. L. Role of adherence in cytopathogenic mechanisms of *Entamoeba histolytica*. Study with mammalian tissue culture cells and human erythrocytes. *J. Clin. Invest. 68*:1305–1313 (1981).

178. Petri, W. A., Jr., Smith, R. D., Schlesinger, P. H., and Ravdin, J. I. Isolation of the galactose-binding lectin of *Entamoeba histolytica* which mediates amebic adherence. *J. Clin. Invest. 80*:1238–1244 (1987).

179. Long-Krug, S. A., Fischer, K. J., Hysmith, R. M., and Ravdin, J. I. Phospholipase A enzymes of *Entamoeba histolytica*: description and subcellular localization. *J. Infect. Dis. 152*:536–541 (1985).

180. Ravdin, J. I., Murphy, C. F., Guerrant, R. L., and Long-Krug, S. A. Effects of antagonists of calcium and phospholipase A on the cytopathogenicity of *Entamoeba histolytica. J. Infect. Dis. 152*:542–549 (1985).

181. Ravdin, J. I., Murphy, C. F., Schlesinger, P. H., Gluzman, I. Y., and Krogstad, D. J. The cellular regulation of vesicle exocytosis by *Entamoeba histolytica. J. Protozool. 35*:159–163 (1988).

182. Weikel, C. S., Murphy, C. F., Orozco, M. E., and Ravdin, J. I. Phorbol esters specifically enhance the cytolytic activity of *Entamoeba histolytica. Infect. Immun. 56*:1485–1491 (1988).

183. Young, JD-E., Young, T. M., Lu, L. P., Unkeless, J. C., and Cohn, Z. A. Characterization of a membrane pore-forming protein from *Entamoeba histolytica. J. Exp. Med. 156*:1677–1690 (1982).

184. Lynch, E. C., Rosenberg, I. M., and Gitler, C. An ion-channel forming protein produced by *Entamoeba histolytica*. *EMBO J. 1*:801–804 (1982).
185. Petri, W. A., Jr., and Ravdin, J. I. In vitro models of amebic pathogenesis. In *Amebiasis: Human Infection by Entamoeba histolytica* (J. I. Ravdin, ed.). Wiley, New York, 1988, pp. 191–204.
186. Meerovitch, E., and Chadee, K. In vivo models for pathogenicity in amebiasis. In *Amebiasis: Human Infection by Entamoeba Histolytica* (J. I. Ravdin, ed.). Wiley, 1988, pp. 177–190.
187. Joyce, M. P., and Ravdin, J. I. Pathology of human amebiasis. In *Amebiasis: Human Infection by Entamoeba Histolytica* (J. I. Ravdin, ed.). Wiley, New York, 1988, pp. 129–146.
188. Castro, H. F. Anatomic and pathological findings in amebiasis. Report of 320 cases. In *Amebiasis in Man* (C. A. Padilla and G. M. Padilla, eds.). Charles C. Thomas, Springfield, Ill. 1974, p. 44.
189. Gridley, M. F. A stain for *Entamoeba histolytica* in tissue sections. *Am. J. Clin. Pathol. 24*:243–244 (1954).
190. Walsh, T. J., Berkman, W., Brown, N. L., Padleckas, R., Jao, W., and Mond, E. Cytopathologic diagnosis of extracolonic amebiasis. *Acta Cytol. 27*: 671–675 (1983).
191. Munguia, H., Franco, E., and Valenzuela, P. Diagnosis of genital amebiasis in women by the standard Papanicolaou technique. *Am. J. Obstet. Gynecol. 94*:181–188 (1966).
192. Griffin, J. L. Human amebic dysentery. Electron microscopy of *Entamoeba histolytica* contacting, ingesting and digesting inflammatory cells. *Am. J. Trop. Med. Hyg. 21*:895–906 (1972).
193. McAllister, T. A. Diagnosis of amoebic colitis on routine biopsies from rectum and sigmoid colon. *Br. Med. J. 1*:362–364 (1962).
194. McMillan, A., Gilmour, H. M., McNeillage, G., and Scott, G. R. Amoebiasis in homosexual men. *Gut 25*:356–360 (1984).
195. Chatgidakis, C. B. The pathology of hepatic amoebiasis as seen on the Witwatersand. *S. Afr. J. Clin. Sci. 4*:230–245 (1953).
196. Powell, S. J., Wilmot, A. J., and Elsdon-Dew, R. Hepatic amoebiasis. *Trans. R. Soc. Trop. Med. Hyg. 53*:190–195 (159).
197. Palmer, R. B. Changes in the liver in amebic dysentery. *Arch. Pathol. 25*: 327–335 (1959).
198. Nanda, R., Anand, B. S., and Baveja, U. *Entamoeba histolytica* cyst passers: clinical features and outcome in untreated subjects. *Lancet 2*: 301–303 (1984).
199. Juniper, K. Acute amebic colitis. *Am. J. Med. 33*:377–386 (1962).
200. Friedrick, I. A., Korstein, M. A., and Gottfried, E. B. Necrotizing amebic colitis with pseudomembrane formation. *Am. J. Gastroenterol. 74*:529–531 (1980).
201. Haider, Z., and Rasul, A. Chronic non-dysenteric intestinal amoebiasis. A review of 159 cases. *J. Pakistan Med. Assoc. 25*:75–78 (1975).
202. Cardoso, J. M., Kimura, K., Stoopen, M., Cervantes, L. F., Elizondo, L.,

Churchill, R., and Moncada, R. Radiology of invasive amebiasis of the colon. *Am. J. Roentgenol. 128*:935–941 (1977).

203. Messersmith, R. N., and Chase, G. J. Amebiasis presenting as multiple apple core lesions. *Am. J. Gastroenterol. 79*:238–241 (1984).
204. Blumencranz, H., Kasen, L., Romeu, J., Waye, J. D., and Leleiko, N. S. The role of endoscopy in suspected amebiasis. *Am. J. Gastroenterol. 78*: 15–22 (1983).
205. Frengenburg, D., Chiat, H., Mandel, P. R., and Ross, S. T. Toxic megacolon in amebic colitis. *Am. J. Roentgenol. 99*:74–76 (1967).
206. Powell, S. J., and Wilmot, A. J. Prognosis of peritonitis complicating severe amoebic dysentery. *Trans. R. Soc. Trop. Med. Hyg. 60*:544–548 (1966).
207. Monga, N. K., Sood, S., Kaushik, S. P., Sachdeva, H. S., Sood, K. S., and Datta, D. V. Amebic peritonitis. *Am. J. Gastroenterol. 66*:366–373 (1976).
208. Grigsby, W. P. Surgical treatment of amebiasis. *Surg. Gynecol. Obstet. 128*:609–627 (1969).
209. Barker, E. M. Colonic perforations in amoebiasis. *S. Afr. Med. J. 32*:634–638 (1958).
210. Peters, R. S., Gitlin, N., and Libke, R. D. Amebic liver abscess. *Ann. Rev. Med. 32*:161–174 (1981).
211. Adams, E. B., and MacLeod, I. N. Invasive amebiasis. II. Amebic liver abscess and its complications. *Medicine 56*:325–334 (1977).
212. Katzenstein, D., Rickerson, V., and Braude, A. New concepts of amebic liver abscess derived from hepatic imaging, serodiagnosis, and hepatic enzymes in 67 consecutive cases in San Diego. *Medicine 61*:237–246 (1982).
213. Barbour, G. L., and Juniper, K. A clinical comparison of amebic and pyogenic abscess of the liver in sixty six patients. *Am. J. Med. 53*:323–334 (1972).
214. Boom, R. A., Fonseca, L., Yanez, C., Gil, D., and Karson, T. Differential diagnosis between amoebic liver abscess and acute cholecystitis. *J. Med. Syst. 7*:205–212 (1983).
215. Thompson, J. E., Forlenza, S., and Verma, R. Amebic liver abscess: a therapeutic approach. *Rev. Infect. Dis. 7*:171–179 (1985).
216. Ralls, P. W., Mikity, V. G., Colleti, P., Boger, D., Halls, J., and Quinn, M. F. Sonography in the diagnosis and management of hepatic amebic abscess in children. *Pediatr. Radiol. 12*:239–243 (1982).
217. Overbosch, D., Stuiver, P. C., and van der Kaay, H. J. Hepatic amoebiasis. Current concepts and a report of 25 cases in the Netherlands. *Acta Leidensia 51*:3–17 (1983).
218. Nwafo, D. C., and Egbue, M. O. Intrathoracic manifestations of amoebiasis. *Ann. R. Coll. Surg. Engl. 63*:126–128 (1981).
219. Ognibene, A. J., and Wells, R. F. Amebiasis. In *Internal Medicine in Vietnam*, Vol. II. *General Medicine and Infectious Diseases* (A. J. Ognibene and O. Barrett, eds.). U. S. Army, Washington, D.C., 1982.

220. Ibarra-Perez, C., and Selman-Lama, M. Diagnosis and treatment of amebic empyema. *Am. J. Surg. 134*:283–287 (1977).
221. Verghese, M., Eggleston, F. C., Handa, A. K., and Singh, C. M. Management of thoracic amebiasis. *J. Thor. Cardiovasc. Surg. 78*:757–760 (1979).
222. Rasaretnam, R., and Wijetilaka, S. E. Left lobe amoebic liver abscess. *Postgrad. Med. J. 52*:269–274 (1976).
223. MacLeod, I. N., Wilmot, A. J., and Powell, S. J. Amoebic pericarditis. *Q. J. Med. 138*:293–311 (1966).
224. Ruiz-Moreno, F. Perianal skin amebiasis. *Dis. Colon Rectum 10*:65–69 (1967).
225. Poltera, A. A. Pseudomalignant cutaneous amoebiasis in Uganda. *Trop. Geog. Med. 25*:139–146 (1973).
226. Kean, B. H., Gilmore, H. R., and Van Stone, W. W. Fatal amebiasis: report of 148 fatal cases from the Armed Forces Institute of Pathology. *Ann. Intern. Med. 44*:831–845 (1956).
227. Orbison, J. A., Reeves, N., Leedham, C. L., and Blumberg, J. M. Amebic brain abscess—review of the literature and report of five additional cases. *Medicine 30*:247–282 (1951).
228. Lombardo, L., Alonso, P., Arroyo, L. S., Brandt, H., and Mateos, J. H. Cerebral amebiasis: report of 17 cases. *J. Neurosurg. 21*:704–709 (1964).
229. Becker, G. L., Knep, S., Lance, K. P., and Kaufman, L. Amebic abscess of the brain. *Neurosurgery, 6*:192–194 (1980).
230. Hughes, F. B., and Falhnie, S. T. Multiple cerebral abscesses complicating hepatopulmonary amebiasis. *J. Pediatr. 86*:95–96 (1975).
231. Thomas, J. A., and Antony, A. J. Amoebiasis of the penis. *Br. J. Urology 48*:269–273 (1976).
232. Gupta, S., Mehrota, M. L., and Ambasta, S. S. Penile amoebiasis: an unusual presentation. *Br. J. Urology 47*:690 (1975).
233. Jayaweera, F. R. B. Amoebic ulceration of the cervix uteri and penis. Two case reports. *Ceylon Med. J. 20*:117–121 (1975).
234. Thacker, S. B., Simpson, S., Gordon, T. J., Wolfe, M., and Kimball, A. M. Parasitic disease control in a residential facility for the mentally retarded. *Am. J. Public. Health 69*:1279–1281 (1979).
235. Healy, G. R. Laboratory diagnosis of amebiasis. *Bull. NY Acad. Med. 47*: 478–493 (1971).
236. Wheatley, W. B. A rapid staining procedure for intestinal amoebae and flagellates. *Am. J. Clin. Path. 21*:990–991 (1951).
237. Young, K. H., Bullock, S., Melvin, D. M., and Sprull, C. L. Ethyl acetate as a substitute for diethylether in the ether-formalin sedimentation technique. *J. Clin. Microbiol. 10*:852–853 (1979).
238. Ungar, B. L. P., Yolken, R. H., and Quinn, T. C. Use of monoclonal antibody in an enzyme immunoassay for the detection of *Entamoeba histolytica* in fecal specimens. *Am. J. Trop. Med. Hyg. 34*:465–472 (1985).
239. Edelman, M. H., and Spingarn, C. L. Cultivation of *Entamoeba histolytica* as a diagnostic procedure: a brief review. *Mt. Sinai J. Med. 43*:27–32 (1976).

240. Crowson, T. D., and Hines, C. Amebiasis diagnosed by colonoscopy. *Gastrointest. Endosc. 24*:254–255 (1978).
241. McAllister, T. A. Diagnosis of amoebic colitis on routine biopsies from rectum and sigmoid colon. *Br. Med. J. 1*:362–364 (1962).
242. Jackson, T. F. H. G., Anderson, C. B., and Simjee, A. E. Serologic differentiation between past and present infection in hepatic amoebiasis. *Trans. R. Soc. Trop. Med. Hyg. 78*:342–345 (1984).
243. Schorlemmer, R. N., Saltzstein, E. C., Peacock, J. B., Mercer, L. C., and Dougherty, S. H. Amebic liver abscess. Differential diagnosis of cholecystitis. *Am. J. Surg. 46*:827–829 (1983).
244. Kessel, J. F., Lewis, W. P., Pasquel, C. M., and Turner, J. A. Indirect hemagglutination and complement fixation tests in amebiasis. *Am. J. Trop. Med. Hyg. 14*:540–550 (1965).
245. McDonald, M. I., Corey, G. R., Gallis, H. A., and Durack, D. T. Single and multiple pyogenic liver abscesses. *Medicine 63*:291–302 (1984).
246. Anonymous. Drugs for parasitic infections. *Med. Lett. 28*:9–16 (1986).
247. Wolfe, M. S. The treatment of intestinal protozoan infections. *Med. Clin. N. Am. 66*:707–720 (1982).
248. Norris, S. M., and Ravdin, J. I. The pharmacology of antiamebic drugs. In *Amebiasis: Human Infection with Entamoeba Histolytica* (J. I. Ravdin, ed.). Wiley, New York, 1988, pp. 734–740.
249. Weber, D. C. Amebic abscess of liver following metronidazole therapy. *JAMA 216*:1339–1340 (1971).
250. Rustia, M., and Shubik, P. Induction of lung tumors and malignant lymphomas in mice by metronidazole. *J. Natl. Cancer Inst. 48*:721–729 (1972).
251. Speck, W. T., Stein, A. B., and Rosenkranz, H. S. Mutagenicity of metronidazole: presence of several active metabolites in human urine. *J. Natl. Cancer Inst. 56*:283–284 (1976).

8

The Host Immune Response Against Parasitic Helminth Infection

THOMAS B. NUTMAN

Laboratory of Parasitic Diseases, National Institutes of Health, Bethesda, Maryland

I. INTRODUCTION

Although major strides have been made in controlling certain helminth parasitic infections, either through transmission control schemes or new chemotherapeutic agents, some of these diseases continue to cause considerable morbidity and mortality throughout the developing world. Indeed, filariasis and schistosomiasis have each been estimated to affect over 100 million people worldwide. The reason for the high prevalence and continued transmission of these infections is in part due to the inability to find methods for inducing protective immunity to parasites. As the impact of parasitic infections is significant in terms of both their effects on individual health and the socioeconomic status of communities at large, methods for combatting them have focused increasingly on finding means to induce protective immune responses. As a consequence, great emphasis has been placed on investigating the unique relationship that exists between the parasite and the hose immune system.

The focus of this chapter is on delineating the various aspects of the host immune response to parasitic helminth infection in an attempt to understand how or whether an effective immune response occurs in response to infection and how helminth parasites induce disease. While many of the recent developments in knowledge have been made possible by the large body of work done using animal models, this chapter will largely center on studies in humans.

II. THE PARASITES

Parasitic helminths have evolved mechanisms for avoiding rejection by the immune system in their evolutionary adaptation to life within the human host.

Because these parasites must survive within the definitive host for a period of time that is sufficiently long to ensure continued transmission of the infective stages to their intermediate hosts, it is not suprprising that chronic infections are required to maintain the life cycle.

Several pertinent aspects of these diseases occur precisely because of chronicity. First, chronic infections by helminth parasites cause the release of large quantities of parasite antigens during their life span. These antigens have profound immunopathological consequences; they may be deposited in host tissue as immune complexes, or they may induce by themselves both immediate and delayed type hypersensitivity reactions. In addition, chronic stimulation by parasite antigens may result in immunosuppression, either of parasite-specific immune responses [as in human filariasis (1)]—a mechanism that probably promotes survival of the parasite—or of a more general, nonspecific type that has been implicated in diminished resistance to infection with other pathogens (2).

Second, because the parasites' survival is dependent on their ability not to overwhelm the host, the clinical outcome of infection with helminth organisms is not usually mortality but morbidity. Essentially, these parasites have been able to develop a relationship with the host that is in reasonable equilibrium. Most illustrative of this situation is the concept of *concomitant immunity*, which occurs in schistosome-infected individuals (3). This is a state in which adult worms are well established in the host, at the same time inducing an immune response that limits further infection by the infective stages of the parasite.

Third, if parasites reside in anatomical sites secluded from the host immune response, chronic infections can occur. This appears to be the case in intestinal helminthiases in which organisms such as hookworms, *Ascaris lumbricoides*, and *Strongyloides stercoralis* appear to exist for extremely long periods of time despite immune responsiveness (both humoral and cellular) on the part of the host (4).

III. GENETIC AND ENVIRONMENTAL DETERMINANTS OF SUSCEPTIBILITY TO INFECTION

While rapid progress has been made in defining the genetic basis of susceptibility to protozoal infection (5), largely by the use of inbred strains of mice, relatively less work has been done in infections due to helminth parasites. Nevertheless, there has been a growing interest in this field, as epidemiological studies in endemic areas have revealed differential susceptibilities to infection within the entire population as well as within families studied (6). Since disease seems to develop only in the presence of immune responsiveness on the part of the host, factors modulating or affecting this responsiveness have been sought both experimentally and clinically. Some of these data have been reviewed elsewhere (7).

Although the cause of differential susceptibility to clinical expression of helminth infections has been addressed in only a few human studies, the data have implicated, in part, the major histocompatibility complex (MHC). In Sri Lankians and southern Indians with elephantiasis due to *Wuchereria bancrofti* infection, there was an association between HLA-B15 and the pesence of chronic lymphatic obstruction (8). Further, when a large Polynesian population living in an endemic area for bancroftian filariasis was studied, familial clustering of patients was seen, suggesting genetic transmission of the disease susecptibility (9). However, the "genetics" of this familial susceptibility was linked to neither their HLA-A nor HLA-B loci. More recently, work done in mice (10) and with human filarial-specific T-cell clones (11) has implicated the immune response (IR) genes as necessary for the induction or development of an immune response to the filarial parasites.

In Japanese patients with schistosomiasis, the HLA Bw52-Dw12-DR2 haplotype was strongly associated with low T-cell responsiveness to *Schistosoma japonicum* antigen (12,13). This low level of responsiveness was associated with $CD8^+CD4^-$ suppressor cells found in the peripheral blood lymphocytes of these individuals. In contrast, subjects with postschistosomal cirrhosis of the liver were significantly less likely to have this haplotype than patients without *Schistosoma*-induced liver disease (14). More important, those patients who did develop liver disease were very much more likely to have the HLA haplotype Bw44-DEn, which is felt to be a putative marker for schistosome antigen-specific immune responsiveness (and thus for the development of liver disease).

While environmental factors have been felt to be less important than genetic ones in determining how the host responds to the parasite, the phenomenon of sensitization in utero has been studied in areas endemic for filariasis. This work has shown that antifilarial antibodies of isotypes that do not cross the placenta (e.g., IgE of IgM) were present in the cord blood of approximately one-half of the babies of infected mothers (15) and in the sera of babies born in a region endemic for *W. bancrofti* (16). Thus, for at least certain groups of individuals, the environmental factors surrounding their birth may be important in determining how they subsequently respond to this helminthic infection.

IV. EVASION OF THE IMMUNE RESPONSE BY THE PARASITES

For reasons of survival, invasive helminth parasites have evolved mechanisms to avoid the consequences of the host immune responses. In every instance where parasite-infected individuals have been studied immunologically, evidence of both cell-mediated and humoral immune responsiveness has been demonstrated. However, despite this immune reactivity, there is little evidence of immunologicaly mediated resistance to the parasite. The reasons for the host's inability to mount protective responses are unclear, but a likely explanation may involve the parasites' ability to disguise antigens that might be targets of the immune response. Other possibilities include antigenic variation, rapid antigen turnover, stage specificity of the immune response, or blocking of specific effector functions (17).

A. Antigenic Variation, Surface Antigen Turnover, and Stage-Specific Antigens

Antigenic variation, a mechanism whereby the host immune response appears to provide a selective pressure for the parasite to switch from one surface antigen to another—thereby avoiding the lethal effects of the parasite-host interaction—has been well established for African trypanosomes (18) and experimental infections with certain *Plasmodium* and *Babesia* spp. (19,20). To date, however, there is no evidence that this mechanism of immune evasion occurs in multicellular helminths. However, another mechanism that must be considered is that of rapid surface antigen turnover, which has been shown to occur in schistosomula (21). As the surface molecules appear to be in a constant state of movement across the parasite membranes, the mere rapidity of this movement could easily allow for avoidance of antibody- and/or cell-dependent attack.

Another way by which the invasive helminths may avoid the host responses may depend on their ability to change from one developmental stage to another within their host. Stage-specific surface antigens have been identified in almost all the helminth parasites studied [schistosomes (22) and filariae (23,24) most notably]; this change in surface antigens might allow the parasite to escape the effects of the host immune response.

B. Antigenic Disguise

Perhaps the best-documented mechanism of immune evasion in helminths is that of immunological disguise, whereby the parasite is able to acquire host molecules on its surface and thus appear to the host immune system as "self" rather than foreign. This concept has been delineated quite completely for schistosomes by several investigators (25-27); host molecules such as major histocompatibility antigen glycoproteins (26) and blood group glycolipids (27) have been demonstrated on the surface of these parasites. In addition, extensive immunochemical characterization and hybridization experiments using recombinant DNA probes specific for MHC genes against schistosomes DNA have shown that the MHC molecules on the surface of the schistosome are not produced by the parasite but rather are acquired from the host (28). Another example of parasite acquisition of host antigen is the case of microfilariae of the filarial parasite *W. bancrofti*: human serum albumin was found to be a major surface component of the microfilarial form of the parasite that circulates in the bloodstream (29).

Another concept that has emerged in an attempt to understand how these parasites have adapted to the host is that of molecular mimicry, whereby some antigens of parasite origin appear to mimic host molecules. This has been verified experimentally by finding a parasite-derived molecule able to cross-react with host alpha$_2$-macroglobulin (30).

V. IMMUNOLOGICAL CONSEQUENCES OF PARASITIC INFECTION

A. Immunopathology

There is strong evidence to suggest that the consequences and intensity of the immune response are central to understanding the immunopathology associated with helminth infections (31). While certain factors that regulate this immune response—antibody, cellular factors, circulating immune complexes, and free parasite antigen—have been identified, they must be understood to a far greater degree than at present before they can be modulated in a manner that will benefit the human host. However, as the immune response bears directly on the diversity of pathological reactions associated with parasitic infections, its determinants and the factors that regulate it need to be addressed.

1. Immune Complexes and Circulating Parasite Antigen

As immune complexes are potent initiators of inflammatory reactions, their role and the role of parasite antigens must be taken into account when the pathology associated with parasitic infections is considered. Circulating parasite antigens have now been identified in the serum of patients infected with schistosomiasis (32) or filariasis (33–36). Although work on the chemical nature of these circulating antigens is in a preliminary stage, there have been some recent suggestions that they have immunomodulatory effects on various immune responses, particularly on mitogen-driven immune responses in vitro (B. K. L. Sim and Hussain, R. unpublished observations). Furthermore, several studies have indicated that components of laboratory-derived soluble parasite antigens have mitogenic activity (37). Also, using fast protein liquid chromatography (FPLC) fractionation of parasite antigen derived from *Brugia malayi*, antigens involved in T- and B-cell activation have been identified and isolated (37).

Circulating immune complexes have been identified in both experimental (38) and human filarial (39) and schistosomal (40) infections. These complexes have been shown to induce lymphatic inflammation and vasculitis in at least one filarial infection as a result of their deposition (41). Furthermore, observations of immune-complex glomerulonephritis have been made in patients with hepatosplenic schistosomiasis (42), loiasis (43), and onchocerciasis (44). Further, the clinical syndrome of acute schistosomiasis has also been attributed to the presence of immune complexes (40).

2. Delayed Type Hypersensitivity Reactions

T-cell-mediated immune responses are found commonly in helminth infections, the pathological consequences of which are most often reflected in granuloma formation. Such granulomata have been best studied in *Schistosoma mansoni* infections, where T-cell control of their size and development has been documented (45,46). Indeed, work with T cells from patients with recent *S. mansoni* infections has indicated that $CD3^+CD4^+$ T cells mediate granulomatous hypersensitivity (47). Furthermore, work done with murine schistosome antigen-reactive T-cell clones has indicated not only that these "helper/inducer" cells regulate the formation of granulomas but also that they produce lymphokines such as eosinophil stimulation promoter and macrophage-activating factor. These products may contribute to the recruitment of cells to the area of granulomatous inflammation (48). While granulomas presumably act to isolate and thereby eradicate the parasite, often these local areas of immunological activity actually damage normal tissue. For example, in schistosomiasis, scarring of the portal tracts resulting from the fibrosis following granuloma formation (46) can lead to cirrhosis and portal hypertension. In lymphatic filariasis, similar fibrotic reactions have been found surrounding adult parasites in the lymphatic channels and lymph nodes (1); this "scarring" is felt to be in part responsible for the lymphedema, elephantiasis, hydrocele, and chyluria found in this condition.

3. Antiidiotypes and Autoantibodies

Autoantibodies have also been implicated as causing disease in certain helminthic infections, presumably reflecting the polyclonal B-cell activation that often accompanies these infections (17). While this immunopathological mechanism has been formally demonstrated in some of the protozoal diseases, the evidence for its existence in helminthic infections is less clear. Nevertheless, autoantibodies against nuclear material [the RNAse-resistant part of the extractable nuclear antigen (ENA), the SM antigen] were found in a vast majority of patients with chronic schistosomiasis, and much more frequently than in patients with diseases such as systemic lupus erythematosus or rheumatoid arthritis (49).

The role of antiidiotypic antibodies in modulating the pathology associated with chronic schistosomiasis has recently been established (50). These naturally occurring antibodies bound antibodies against schistosome egg antigens and were able to modulate the granulomatous inflammation around parasite eggs in vivo.

4. Immediate Hypersensitivity

Classic IgE-mediated immediate hypersensitivity reactions are rarely found in chronic helminthiases. However, during the acute phase of infections with *invasive* helminth parasites such as *Ascaris* spp., hookworms, schistosomes, or filariae, patients may manifest symptoms suggestive of allergic reactivity, such as wheezing or urticaria (51). Furthermore, in the clinical syndromes associated with *Loa loa* infection [with its angioedematous Calabar swellings (52)], with tropical pulmonary eosinophilia (53), and with larva currens in strongyloidiasis (54), IgE-mediated reactions are felt to reflect the underlying mechanism of these signs and symptoms.

Eosinophil-associated pathology, unlike IgE-mediated hypersensitivity, is found frequently in helminth infections. The eosinophil's cationic proteins are toxic to a variety of normal tissues and cells both in vitro and in vivo (55,56). Furthermore, the eosinophil, when activated, releases proinlammatory reactants such as leukotrienes [most notably, LTC4 (57)] and PAF-acether (58), and these molecules must be taken into account in the localized pathology found in tissue-invading helminth infections. In parasitic diseases associated with extreme hypereosinophilia, such as the endomyocardial fibrosis found in loiasis in expatriates (52,59) or the tropical (filarial) pulmonary eosinophilia syndrome (53), evidence has been accumulating that the major source for the tissue destruction appears to be the eosinophil and its toxic molecules.

B. Immunomodulation

While suppression of immune responsiveness has been widely studied in experimental systems utilizing a large number of helminth parasites, work addressing this issue in humans has focused primarily on filariasis and schistosomiasis. Two generalizations that have emerged from human studies on these two quite distinct sets of organisms are that (a) the immunosuppression, except in the face of overwhelming infections, tends to be parasite-specific and not, therefore, generalized; and (b) effective treatment tends to reverse the immunologically suppressed responses.

Although T-cell responses to parasite antigen occur early inthe course of helminth infections in both humans and experimental animals (60,61), as the infection becomes more chronic these responses become suppressed and are manifested by a *hypo*responsiveness specific for parasite antigens and not to other antigens (1). It has been shown, for example, that lymphocytes from patients with microfilaremia from either *B. malayi* or *W. bancrofti* infections failed to respond to filarial antigens while maintaining their reactivity to mitogens and nonparasite antigens (62,63). Serum suppressor factors (64), suppressor adherent cells (assumed to be moncytes) (64), and T-lymphocyte suppressor cells (65) have been implicated as mediators of this parasite-specific immunosuppression. More recently, when T helper/T suppressor ratios have been examined (66) in filaria-infected populations along with absolute quantitation of the suppressor T cells, abnormally low values were obtained; these T-cell abnormalities appeared to return to normal after successful treatment with diethylcarbamazine (67), the drug of choice for those infections. Indeed recent work done to examine directly the mechanism of the immune unresponsiveness to filarial antigens has shown that lymphocytes from patients with microfilaremia are unable to produce lymphokines (either IL-2 or gamma-interferon) in response to parasite antigen while retaining their ability to respond to non-parasite stimuli; further, this presumed immunological tolerance to parasite antigen could not be overcome by the removal of monocytes or CD8$^+$ cells or by the addition of CD4$^+$ helper/inducer cells (68).

Modulation of the humoral immune response has also been demonstrated in both schistosomiasis and filariasis. When levels of antischistosome antibodies of both the IgM and IgG isotypes were followed longitudinally as acute infections became chronic, a profound and progressive drop in these levels was seen (61). Further, in the microfilaremic form of filariasis, the level of parasite-specific antibodies is extremely low (1). When this phenomenon was studied more extensively in these patients using in vitro models of parasite antigen-driven antibody production, a profound inability to produce antifilarial antibody was seen (69).

While both the humoral and cellular responses appear to be diminished and modulated in a parasite-specific manner, it should be noted that the mediators of this suppression are not necessarily antigen-specific. Thus, it appears that while there is exquisite specificity between the parasite and the host's immune system, the resultant effector mechanisms act in a non-specific fashion; for example, histamine is specifically released by sensitized basophils and/or mast cells but acts to suppress any H-2 receptor-bearing T cell (70).

VI. UNIQUE FEATURES OF THE IMMUNE
RESPONSES TO HELMINTH PARASITES

A. Immediate Hypersensitivity Responses

Helminth parasitic infections are frequently accompanied by immune responses characteristic of immediate type hypersensitivity reactions. In these infections, such responses are most often characterized by the presence of eosinophils, mast cells, and IgE. While the accumulation of these cells and this antibody isotype are found in other disorders, especially those associated with atopy, both their quantity and their invariable presence make these reactions in helminth infections rather distinctive.

1. IgE
Although in most individuals IgE antibody responses are tightly regulated both quantitatively and qualitatively (71), the presence of helminth infection appears

to overcome these regulatory mechanisms so that high levels of IgE are consistently produced in vivo (1). Furthermore, most of the IgE produced is not parasitic-specific and is therefore felt to represent nonspecific potentiation of a normally well-controlled immune response (72-74). This potentiating effect seems to be selective for the IgE isotype and has been shown to be T-cell-dependent (75).

Elevated total serum IgE levels in parasitized patients have been documented by many studies (76,77). Characteristically, patients with invasive helminth infections have serum IgE levels approaching 100 times those of normal individuals (51). The factors responsible for this degree of elevation are not well defined; however, there seem to be not only quantitative differences in these parasitized individuals but qualitative differences as well.

Although atopic individuals have moderate elevations of IgE, characteristically their IgE responses are restricted to a small number of antigens. In marked contrast, patients with invasive helminth infection produce IgE antibodies with specificity against a broad range of antigens (78), suggesting a markedly deregulated state. The mechanism of this deregulation is still unclear, although T-cell-derived helper factors controlling IgE production have been described in patients with hyper IgE states associated with both allergic conditions and parasite infection (79-81).

More recently, in both animals and humans, lymphocytes bearing the Fcε receptor have been shown capable of making molecules known as IgE binding factors [IgE-BF (82)], which have a role in the regulation of IgE. When these IgE-BFs have been quantitated in patients with extreme elevations of IgE due to tropical pulmonary eosinophilia, a condition manifested by an unusual immunological hypersensitivity to filarial parasites, there were marked increases compared to noninfected individuals (T. B. Nutman, unpublished observations). This suggests that these IgE-BF levels may correlate with the serum level of IgE and may provide clues to the regulation of this reaginic antibody.

The importance of the IgE response in helminth parasitic diseases remains ill-defined, though in some cases IgE production has correlated with resistance to helminth infection (83,84) and protective immunity. While the mechanisms for this IgE-mediated resistance are still being investigated, evidence has been accumulating that suggests that IgE may (a) allow release from eosinophils, mast cells, macrophages, or lymphocytes of inflammatory mediators that could be toxic to the parasite (55,56); (b) activate macrophages by interaction with their Fc epsilon receptors (85); and (c) incite local inflammation allowing for recruitment of effector cells such as eosinophils (86).

2. Eosinophils

Although eosinophil levels vary to a great degree among patients with helminth infections, their elevation is virtually a constant finding.

The idea that eosinophils are cytotoxic is not novel, but the clearest demonstration of eosinophil cytotoxicity has come from investigations on the role of the cells in the immunity to parasitic helminth infections. Many parasites, including schistosomes (87) and their eggs (88), *Fasciola hepatica, Trichinella spiralis* (89), *Onchocerca volvulus* (90), *Dipetalonema vitae* (90), and *Brugia malayi* (91), have been shown to be damaged or killed by the eosinophil's cytotoxic mechanisms. The cytotoxicity is clearly a result of the deposition of eosinophil degranulation products, although the exact nature of the mechanisms involved that lead to eosinophil-parasite interaction and degranulation are less well defined. Complement receptors (CR1 and CR3) and Fc receptors (IgG, IgE) appear to be the most important ligands mediating binding between the eosinophil and the parasite target cell (87,90), but lectins have also been implicated in this cell-target interaction (90). Although occasionally adherence alone can cause release of the eosinophil granular contents, usually this process is dependent on the presence of parasite-specific antibody. By whatever mechanism the degranulation occurs, however, the result is such that the adherence of the eosinophil to the parasite is strengthened, thereby allowing a more prolonged interaction and presumably a more potent cytotoxic capacity (92).

The eosinophil granule-associated proteins—major basic protein, eosinophil cationic protein, and the eosinophil-derived neurotoxin—are each directly cytotoxic to parasites in vitro as is eosinophil peroxidase either in conjunction with H_2O_2 and halide, or directly through its phospholipid-cleaving enzymes (55,56). Furthermore, several factors enhance the eosinophil's helminthotoxic capacity. Mast cell-associated mediators have been shown to enhance both antibody- and complement-dependent eosinophil-mediated cytotoxicity (93). Factors derived from T cells, such as eosinophil stimulation promoter (94), eosinophil differentiation factor (EDF) (95), and GM-CSF (96), have also been implicated in the enhancement of eosinophil-mediated killing. Furthermore, factors derived from monocytes also enhance eosinophil-mediated cytotoxicity. In particular, both tumor necrosis factor (97) and a 40-kD protein termed eosinophil activating factor (98) have each been used successfully in this regard.

More recently, much attention has been drawn to the heterogeneity of eosinophils in terms of both their density (99,100) and their metabolic activity (101). An eosinophil subset, termed "hypodense" eosinophils, is felt to reflect a state associated with cellular activation. These activated cells, found most commonly in patients with parasitic or other diseases associated with hypereosinophilia (56), have increased numbers of surface Fc receptors (100) and are metabolically much more active than "normodense" eosinophils (101-103). More important, these cells are extremely cytotoxic for helminth larvae in vitro (104).

While most of the evidence for eosinophil cytotoxicity is based on in vitro experimentation, evidence that this occurs in vivo has been accumulating. First, eosinophils from immune animals have been shown to confer a high degree of resistance to Schistosoma mansoni when adoptively transferred to naive animals (105). Second, in studies involving humans undergoing the Mazzotti reaction (onchocerciasis), there was clear-cut evidence of eosinophil attachment to and eosinophil-mediated degradation of the dying filarial parasite in biopsy material (106).

Thus, the evidence continues to accumulate showing that the eosinophil, on an evolutionary basis, has been selected for its capacity to be cytotoxic for helminth parasites and is thereby a major defense in the host's protective immune response against these organisms.

3. Basophils and Mast Cells

Although the evidence is less clear-cut than with the eosinophil, basophils and mast cells are felt to play a role in the inflammatory reactions against invasive helminth parasites. Both these cell types have large numbers of high affinity receptors for IgE, large amounts of easily triggered mediators, and (at least for the basophil) major basic protein associated with their granules.

Basophils, which on average constitute less than 1% of the normal peripheral blood leukocyte pool, have been found in increased numbers in patients with parasitic helminth infections (107). As these cells appear to be under T-cell control for their production and recruitment (108), it is likely that a complex network of interaction between the parasite and the host immune reactants is called into play in the presence of tissue-invading parasites. Further, in vivo experiments with guinea pigs vaccinated against schistosomiasis have provided evidence that basophils, in some way, mediate resistance to S. mansoni (109).

Tissue-dwelling mast cells are felt to be of two types, those derived from bone marrow or fetal liver, found in connective tissue, and those regulated and recruited by T cells, found in the intestinal mucosa. The latter appear to participate in the host defense against parasite infection, as their numbers increase greatly in the small intestine after helminth infectipn. Furthermore, there is evidence that these cells are responsible for expulsion of these gastrointestinal parasites (110) and the prevention of reinfection (111). Mast cells, together with eosinophils, have been seen surrounding schistosumla in the epidermis of primates (112) and some egg-induced granulomas of schistosome-infected livers (113). Depletion of mast cells has been shown to abrogate inflammatory responses against schistosomula (114). Most recently, mast cells, in concert with peroxidase and iodide, have been shown to be capable of mediating cytotoxicity to schistosomula (115). However, whether these cells play a significant role in the host defense against parasites remains to be determined.

4. Modulation of Immediate Hypersensitivity

Characteristically, patients with filariasis or schistsomiasis have all the components that contribute to immediate hypersensitivity (i.e., high levels of parasite-specific and polyclonal IgE, eosinophilia, and tissue-dwelling mast cells sensitized to parasite antigens), though they rarely show any clinically evident immediate type hypersensitivity reactions to the parasite antigens (51). Work done by several investigators has suggested that this immediate hypersensitivity responsiveness is modulated in helminth infections. Several mechanisms such as competition for the FceR by "irrelevant" (non-parasite-specific) IgE (116) or inhibition of mast cell mediator release by shed parasite antigens (117) have been proposed; however, the most likely mechanism—and the only one that has been found to be operative in humans—to account for this modulation is the presence of so-called blocking antibodies, that is, IgG antibodies directed against the same antigens that are being recognized by antibodies of the IgE isotype (118). Recently, in a qualitative study of the immune responses (both IgG and IgE) to filarial parasite antigens using Western blotting techniques (119), dual recognition of antigens by IgG and IgE antibodies has been shown. Furthermore, the relative magnitude of IgG to IgE could be used to give a plausible explanation of why patients with invasive helminth infections have so little allergic reactivity in the face of IgE elevations. While the nature of these blocking antibodies and their relationship to the regulation of the IgE response to parasite antigens are still being delineated, antifilarial IgG4 subclass antibody which is present at high levels in filaria-infected individuals (120) and which shows parallel antigen recognition to IgE may provide the link necessary to explain the presence of blocking antibodies.

B. Hypergammaglobulinemia and Polyclonal Activation

Hypergammaglobulinemia with elevated levels of parasite-specific antibodies of most (if not all) isotypes has been recognized in many helminthiases, particularly in filarial infections (1). Indeed, in a study of patients with tropical (filarial) pulmonary eosinophilia (53) and in one on individuals with loiasis (52), hypergammaglobulinemia was a common finding. While presumably reflecting a polyclonal expansion of B cells, the mechanism for this polyclonal activation is not well defined. Work examining the interaction between parasite antigen and B-cell responses in vitro has indicated that polyclonal immunoglobulin responses occur as a result of this interaction almost without exception (121); furthermore, this polyclonal activation occurs in a broad range of helminth parasite infections. In addition, several investigators have isolated antigens from various helminths that appear to have mitogenic activity (17). These mitogenic factors, however, seem to act indirectly on B cells in that their primary effect is directed at the T-cell arm, which then mediates helper function (122).

Whatever the mechanism, it is clear that the resultant polyclonal activation may participate in the immunosuppression seen in these infections or in the development of autoantibodies.

VII. EFFECTOR MECHANISMS MEDIATING HOST IMMUNITY TO HELMINTH PARASITES

A. Acquired Protective Immunity to Helminth Parasites

As discussed initially, invasive helminths characteristically produce chronic infections and have adopted mechansisms that seem to prevent the host from developing protective immune responses. The phenomenon of concomitant immunity in schistosomiasis is a particularly good example where protection against reinfection is only partial (123). Furthermore, this type of immunity usually wanes after therapy, so that individuals at risk for reexposure to the parasite continue to be susceptible. Nevertheless, recent evidence on a population in a heavily endemic area for schistosomiasis in Kenya has indicated that so-called resistance to reinfection is dependent on the production of an IgG antibody response to a particular 27-kD molecule and the absence of an IgM "blocking" antibody directed against the same molecule (A. E. Butterworth, unpublished).

Effective acquired immunity must also be directed against the appropriate stages of the parasite, as has been demonstrated in human malaria against the infective sporozoite (124). While stage-specific immune responses have been demonstrated against infective larval stages in helminth infections in humans, there is little to suggest that they are protective. However, using animal vaccine models employing attenuated or irradiated infective stages of both *S. mansoni* and *B. malayi*, a great deal of evidence has accumulated to suggest that protection, either partial or complete, can be induced by the induction of stage-specific responses.

Immunity against parasites, as mentioned previously, is also influenced by the genetic background of the host. In murine models of immunity to schistosomiasis, a single gene controlling this immunity has been identified (5). In humans, however, while the major histocompatibility loci are clearly important in immune responsiveness to parasites, it is presently unknown whether protective immunity is under the same kinds of genetic influences.

B. Effector Mechanisms in Parasite Immunity

While humoral responses have been considered the hallmark of an effective immune reaction, there is considerable evidence that protective immunity is not mediated by antibodies alone. Thus, passive transfer of antibody in experimental systems (including schistosomiasis, intestinal helminth infections, and filariasis) has not been able to completely protect against challenge infection. Indeed, in helminth infections, antibodies must act in concert with cellular components of the immune network in order to eliminate these parasites. For example, the in vitro killing of schistosomula does not occur in the presence of antischistosome antibody alone; instead it requires the presence of either complement (125) or effector cells such as eosinophils (87), neutrophils (126), macrophages (127), monocytes (128), mast cells (115), or platelets (129). Neither is this phenomenon limited to schistosomes, as microfilariae have also been shown to require effector cells along with specific antibodies.

An important set of effector mechanisms that in some way aid in the induction of parasite immunity are those resulting from the production of soluble mediators, such as cytokines derived from parasite antigen-sensitized T lymphocytes or from monocytes and macrophages. In general, these substances serve to activate macrophages, eosinophils, and presumably cytotoxic T cells to kill helminth parasites. In particular, eosinophil-mediated killing of schistosomula has been shown to be enhanced by factors released from antigen-stimulated lymphocytes (130) and more recently by a number of recombinant or purified molecules such as GM–CSF (96), tumor necrosis factor (97), EDF (95), and the monocyte-derived eosinophil activating factor (98). In addition, in the situations where activated macrophages have been able to mediate antibody-dependent killing, gamma interferon has been implicated as a mediator of the macrophage activation as have IgE immune complexes (17).

Finally, molecules that have been elicited by these activated effector cells, such as eosinophil-derived platelet activating factor, arachidonic acid metabolites, and a large number of other factors, have been shown to recruit or chemoattract effector cells [and eosinophils in particular (56)].

Thus, the nature of the effector mechanisms as they act in vivo is still not elucidated entirely, as many of the data pertaining to these are based on in vitro studies. However,what is clear is that the immune interactions that are called into play to eradicate invasive helminth parasites are extremely complex and require antibodies of particular isotypes and specificities as well as the recruitment of appropriately activated effector cells.

REFERENCES

1. Ottesen, E. A. Immunological aspects of lymphatic filariasis and onchocerciasis in man. *Trans. R. Soc. Trop. Med. Hyg. 78 (Suppl.)*:9 (1984).
2. Weidanz, W. P. Malaria and alterations in immune reactivity. *Br. Med. Bull. 38*:167 (1982).
3. Smithers, S. R., and Terry, R. J. Immunity in schistosomiasis. *Ann. N.Y. Acad. Sci. 160*:826 (1969).

4. Cohen, S. Survival of parasites in the immunocompetent host. In *Immunology of Parasitic Infections*, 2nd ed. (S. Cohen and K. S. Warren, eds.). Blackwells, Oxford, 1982, p. 431.
5. Sher, A., and Scott, P. A. Genetic factors influencing the interaction of parasites with the immune system. *Clin. Immunol. Allergy 2*:489 (1982).
6. Subrahmanyan, D., Mehta, K., Nelson, D. S., Rao, Y. V. B. G., and Rao, C. K. Immune reactions in human filariasis. *J. Clin. Microbiol. 8*:228 (1978).
7. Mitchell, G. F., Anders, R. F., Brown, G. V., Handman, E., Roberts-Thomason, I. C., Chapman, B., Forsyth, K. P., Kahl, L. P., and Cruse, K. M. Analysis of infection characteristics and antiparasite immune responses in resistant compared to susceptible hosts. *Immunol. Rev. 61*:135 (1980).
8. Chan, S. H., Dissanayake, S., Mak, J. W., Ismail, M. M., Wee, G. B., Srinivasan, N., Soo, B. H., and Zaman, V. HLA and filariasis in Sri Lankins and Indians. *Southeast Asian J. Trop. Med. Public Health 15*:218 (1984).
9. Ottesen, E. A., Mendell, N. R., MacQueen, J. M., Weller, P. F., Amos, D. B., and Ward, F. E. Familial predisposition to filarial infection—not linked to HLA–A or –B locus specificities. *Acta Tropica 38*:205 (1981).
10. Fanning, M., and Kazura, J. Genetic association of murine susceptibility to *Brugia malayi* microfilaremia. *Parasite Immunol. 5*:305 (1983).
11. Nutman, T. B., Ottesen, E. A., Fauci, A. S., and Volkman, D. J. Parasite antigen-specific T cell lines and clones: major histocompatibility complex restriction and B cell helper function. *J. Clin. Invest. 73*:1754 (1984).
12. Sasazuki, T., Nishinwia, Y., Mito, M., and Onta, N. HLA-linked genes controlling immune response and disease susceptibility. *Immunol. Rev. 70*:51 (1983).
13. Kaji, R., Kanyo, R., Yaro, A., and Kojima, S. Genetic control of immune responses to *Schistosoma japonicum* antigen. *Parasite Immunol. 5*:25 (1983).
14. Ohta, N., Nishimura, Y. K., Iuchi, M., and Sasazuki, T. Immunogenetic analysis of patients with post-schistosomal liver cirrhosis in man. *Clin Exp. Immunol. 49*:493 (1982).
15. Weil, G. J., Hussain, R., Kumaraswami, V., Tripathy, S. P., Phillips, K. S., and Ottesen, E. A. Prenatal allergic sensitizatin to helminth antigens in offspring of parasite-infected mothers. *J. Clin. Invest. 71*:1124 (1983).
16. Dissanayake, S., DeSilva, L. V. K., and Isamil, M. M. IgM antibodies to filarial antigens in human cord blood: possibility of transplacental infection. *Trans. R. Soc. Trop. Med. Hyg. 74*:541 (1980).
17. Sher, A., and Ottesen, E. Parasites. In *Immunologic Diseases* 4th ed. (M. Samter, ed.) (in press).
18. Cross, G. A. M. Antigenic variation in trypanosomes. *Proc. R. Soc. B 202*: 55 (1978).
19. Brown, K. N., and Brown, I. N. Immunity to malaria: antigenic variation in chronic infection of *Plasmodium knowlesi*. *Nature 208*:1286 (1965).

20. Howard, R. J., and Barnwell, J. W. Roles of surface antigens on malaria-infected red blood cells in evasion of immunity. In *Contemporary Topics in Immunobiology*, Vol. 12 (J. Marchalonis, ed.). Plenum, New York, 1984.
21. Samuelson, J. C., Sher, A., and Caulfield, J. P. Newly transformed schistosomula spontaneously lose surface antigen and C3 acceptor sites during culture. *J. Immunol. 130*:242 (1983).
22. Harn, D. A., Mitsuyama, M., and David, J. R. *Schistosoma mansoni*: anti-egg monoclonal antibodies protect against cercarial challenge in vivo. *J. Exp. Med. 159*:1371 (1984).
23. Canlas, M., Wadee, A., and Piessens, W. A monoclonal antibody to surface antigens on microfilariae of *Brugia malayi* reduces microfilariae in infected birds. *Am. J. Trop. Med. Hyg. 33*:420 (1984).
24. Lal, R. B., and Ottesen, E. A. Characterization of stage specific antigens on infective stage larvae of the filarial parasite *Brugia malayi*. *J. Immunol. 140*: 2032 (1988).
25. Smithers, S. R., Terry, R. J., and Hockley, D. H. Host antigens in schistosomiasis. *Proc. R. Soc. Lond.* (*Biol.*) *171*:483 (1969).
26. Goldring, O. L., Kusel, J. R., and Smithers, S. R. *Schistosoma mansoni* origin in vitro of host-like surface antigens. *Exp. Parasitol. 43*:82 (1977).
27. Sher, A., Hall, B. F., and Vadas, M. A. Acquisition of murine major histocompatibility complex gene products by schistosomula of *S. mansoni*. *J. Exp. Med. 148*:46 (1978).
28. Simpson, A. J. G., Singer, D., McCutchan, T. F., Sacks, D. L., and Sher, A. Evidence that schistosome MHC antigens are not synthesized by the parasite but are acquired from the host as intact glycoproteins. *J. Immunol. 131*:962 (1983).
29. Maizels, R. M., Philipp, M., Dasgupta, A., and Partono, F. Human serum albumin is a major component on the surface of microfilariae of *Wuchereria bancrofti*. *Parasite Immunol. 6*:185 (1984).
30. Damian, R. T., Greene, N. D., and Hubbard, W. J. Occurrence of mouse a^2-macroglobulin antigen determinants on *S. mansoni* adults with evidence of their nature. *J. Parasitol. 59*:64 (1973).
31. Ottesen, E. A. Immunopathology of lymphatic filariasis in man. *Springer Semin. Immunopathol. 2*:372 (1980).
32. Santoro, F., Prater, M., Castro, C. N., and Capron, A. Circulating antigen, immune complexes, and C3D levels in human schistosomiasis. Relationship with *Schistosoma mansoni* egg output. *Clin. Exp. Immunol. 42*:219 (1980).
33. Forsyth, K. P., Spark, R., Kazura, J., Brown, G.V., Peters, P., Heywood, P., Dissanayake, S., and Mitchell, G. F. A monoclonal antibody-based immunoradiometric assay for detection of circulating antigen in bancroftian filariasis. *J. Immunol. 134*:1172 (1985).
34. Dissanayake, S., Forsyth, K. P., Ismail, M. M., and Mitchell, G. F. Detection of circulating antigen in bancroftian filariasis by using a monoclonal antibody. *Am. J. Trop. Med. Hyg. 33*:1130 (1984).
35. Reddy, M. V., Malhotra, A., and Harinath, B. C. Detection of circulating antigen in bancroftian filariasis by sandwich ELISA using filarial serum IgG. *J. Helminthol. 58*:259 (1984).

36. Hamilton, R. G., Hussain, R., and Ottesen, E. A. Immunoradiometric assay for detection of filarial antigens in human serum. *J. Immunol. 13*:2237 (1984).
37. Lal, R. B., Lynch, T., and Nutman, T. B. *Brugia malayi* antigens associated with lymphocyte activation in filariasis. *J. Immunol. 139*:1652 (1987).
38. Karavodin, L. M., and Ash, L. R. Circulating immune complexes in experimental filariasis. *Clin. Exp. Immunol. 40*:312 (1980).
39. Prasad, G. B. K. S., Reddy, M. V. R., and Harinath, B. C. Immune complexes and immunoglobulins involved in human filariasis. *Indian J. Med. Res. 77*:813 (1977).
40. Lawley, T. J., Ottesen, E. A., Hiatt, R. A., and Gazze, L.A. Circulating immune complexes in acute schistosomiasis. *Clin. Exp. Immunol. 37*:221 (1979).
41. Henson, P. M., Mackenzie, C. D., and Spector, W. D. Inflammatory reactions in onchocerciasis. *Bull. WHO 57*:667 (1979).
42. Andrade, Z. A., and Van Marck, E. Schistosomal glomerular disease (a review). *Mem. Inst. Oswaldo Cruz 79*:499 (1984).
43. Zuidema, P. J. Renal changes in loiasis. *Folia Med. Nederl. 14*:168 (1971).
44. Ngu, J. L., Chatelanat, F., Leke, R., Ndumbe, P., and Yombissi, J. Nephropathy in Cameroon: evidence for filarial derived immune complex pathogenesis in some cases. *Clin. Nephrol. 24*:128 (1985).
45. Colley, D. G. Adoptive suppression of granuloma formation. *J. Exp. Med. 14*:696 (1976).
46. Phillips, S. M., and Fox, E. G. The immunopathology of parasitic disease. *Clin. Immunol. Allergy 2*:667 (1982).
47. Doughty, B. L., Ottesen, E. A., Nash, T. E., and Phillips, S. M. Delayed hypersensitivity granuloma formation around *Schistosoma mansoni* eggs in vitro. III. Granuloma formation and modulation in human schistosomiasis mansoni. *J. Immunol. 133*:993 (1984).
48. Lammie, P. J., Linette, G. P., and Phillips, S. M. Characterization of *Schistosoma mansoni* antigen-reactive T cell clones that form granulomas in vitro. *J. Immunol. 134*:4170 (1985).
49. Bendixen, G., Hadidi, T., Manthorpe, T., Permin, H., and Struckmann, J. Antibodies against nuclear components in schistosomiasis. Results compared to values in patients with rheumatoid arthritis, systemic lupus erythematosis, and osteoarthritis. *Allergy 39*:107 (1984).
50. Olds, G. R., and Kresina, T. F. Network interactions in *Schistosoma japonicum* infection. Identification and characterization of a serologically distinct immunoregulatory auto-antiidiotypic antibody population. *J. Clin. Invest. 76*:2338 (1985).
51. Ottesen, E. A. Parasite infections and allergic reaction—how each affects the other. In *Bronchial Asthma: Mechanisms and Therapeutics* 2nd ed. (E. B. Weiss, M. S. Segal, and M. Stein eds.). Little, Brown, New York, pp. 522, 1985.
52. Nutman, T. B., Miller, K. D., Mulligan, M., and Ottesen, E. A. *Loa loa* infection among temporary residents of an endemic area: identification of

a hyperresponsive syndrome with unique clinical manifestations. *J. Infect. Dis.* *154*:10 (1986).

53. Neva, F. A., and Ottesen, E. A. Tropical (filarial) eosinophilia. *New Engl. J. Med.* *298*:1129 (1978).

54. Neva, F. A. Biology and immunology of human strongyloidiasis. *J. Infect. Dis.* *153*:397 (1986).

55. Gleich, G. J. Immunobiology of the eosinophil. *Ann. Rev. Immunol.* *2*:429 (1984).

56. Kay, A. B. Eosinophils as effector cells in immunity and hypersensitivity disorders. *Clin. Exp. Immunol. 62*: (1985).

57. Shaw, R. J., Cromwell, D., and Kay, A. B. Preferential generation of leukotriene C4 by human eosinophils. *Clin. Exp. Immunol. 56*:716 (1984).

58. Moqbel, R., MacDonald, A. J., and Kay, A. B. Platelet activating factor (PAF-acether) enhances eosinophil cytotoxicity in vitro. *Proc. 6th International Congress Immunology*, 1986, p. 650.

59. Brockington, I. G., Olsen, E. G. F., and Goodwin, J. F. Endomyocardial fibrosis in Europeans resident in tropical Africa. *Lancet 1*:583 (1976).

60. Weiss, N. *Dipetalonema viteae*: in vitro blastogenesis of hamster spleen and lymph node cells to phytohemagglutinin and filarial antigens. *Exp. Parasitol. 146*:282 (1978).

61. Ottesen, E. A., Hiatt, R. A., Cheever, A. W., Sotomayor, Z. R., and Neva, F. A. The acquisition and loss of antigen-specific cellular immune responsiveness in acute and chronic schistosomiasis in man. *Clin. Exp. Immunol. 33*:38 (1978).

62. Ottesen, E. A., Weller, P. F., and Heck, L. Specific cellular immune unresponsiveness in human filariasis. *Immunology 33*:413 (1977).

63. Piessens, W. F., McGreevey, P. B., Piessens, P. S., McGreevey, M., Koiman, I., Saroso, J. S., and Dennis, D. T. Immune responses in human infections with *Brugia malayi*. Specific cellular unresponsiveness to filarial antigens. *J. Clin. Invest. 65*:172 (1980).

64. Piessens, W. F., Ratuwaytano, S., Tuti, S., Palmieri, J. H., Piessens, P. W., Koiman, I., and Dennis, D. T. Antigen-specific suppressor cells and suppressor factors in human filariasis with *Brugia malayi*. *New Engl. J. Med. 302*:833 (1980).

65. Piessens, W. F., Partono, F., Hoffman, S. L., Ratiwayanto, S., Piessens, P. W., Palmieri, J. R., Koiman, I., Dennis, D. T. and Carney, W. P. Antigen-specific suppressor T lymphocytes in human lymphatic filariasis. *New Engl. J. Med. 307*:144 (1982).

66. Piessens, W. F., Hoffman, S. L., Ratiwayanto, S., Piessens, P. W., Parono, F., Kurniawan, L., and Marwoto, H. A. Opposing effects of filariasis and chronic malaria on immunoregulatory T lymphocytes. *Diag. Immunol. 1*: 257 (1983).

67. Piessens, W. F. Ratiwayanto, S., Piessens, P. W., Tuti, S., McGreevey, P. B., Darcis, F., Palmieri, J. R., Koiman, I., and Dennis, D. T. Effect of treatment with diethylcarbamazine on immune responses to filarial antigens in patients infected with *Brugia malayi*. *Acta Tropica 38*:227 (1981).

68. Nutman, T. B., Kumaraswami, V., and Ottesen, E. A. Parasite-specific immune unresponsiveness in lymphatic filariasis: insights after analysis of parasite antigen-driven lymphokine production. *J. Clin. Invest. 79*:1516 (1987).

69. Nutman, T. B., Kumaraswami, V., Pao, L., Narayanan, P. K., and Ottesen, E. A. An analysis of in vitro B cell immune responsiveness in human lymphatic filariasis. *J. Immunol. 138*:3954 (1987).

70. Hofstetter, M., Fasano, M. B., and Ottesen, E. A. Modulation of the host response in human schistosomiasis. IV. Parasite antigen induces release of histamine that inhibits lymphocyte responsiveness in vitro. *J. Immunol. 130*:1376 (1983).

71. Marsh, D. G., Bico, W. B., and Ishizaka, K. Genetic control of basal serum IgE level and its effect on specific reagin sensitivity. *Proc. Natl. Acad. Sci. USA 71*:3588 (1974).

72. Jarrett, E. E. E., and Stewart, D. C. Potentiation of rat reaginic (IgE) antibody by helminth infection. Simultaneous potentiation of separate reagins. *Immunology 23*:749 (1972).

73. Jarrett, E. E. E., and Bazin, H. Elevation of total serum IgE in rats following helminth parasite infection. *Nature 251*:541 (1974).

74. Turner, K., Fedde, A. L., and Quinn, E. H. Non-specific potentiation of IgE by parasite infections in man. *Int. Arch. Allergy Appl. Immunol. 58*: 232 (1979).

75. Jarrett, E. E. E. Stimuli for the production and control of IgE in rats. *Immunol. Rev. 41*:52 (1978).

76. Kojima, S., Yokagawa, M., and Tada, T. Raised levels of serum IgE levels in human helminthiasis. *Am. J. Trop. Med. Hyg. 21*:913 (1972).

77. Hussain, R., Hamilton, R., Kumarawami, V., Adkinson, N. F., Jr., and Ottesen, E. A. IgE responses in human filariasis: I. Quantitation of filaria-specific IgE. *J. Immunol. 127*:1623 (1981).

78. Hussain, R., and Ottesen, E. A., IgE responses in human filariasis. III. Specificities of IgE and IgG antibodies compared by immunoblot analysis. *J. Immunol. 135*:1415 (1985).

79. Nutman, T. B., Volkman, D. J., Hussain, R., Fauci, A. S., and Ottesen, E. A. Filarial parasite-specific T cell lines: induction of IgE synthesis. *J. Immunol. 134*:1178 (1985).

80. Romagnani, S., Maggi, E., Del Prete, G. F., and Ricci, M. IgE synthesis in vitro induced by T cell factors from patients with elevated serum IgE levels. *Clin. Exp. Immunol. 52*:85 (1983).

81. Sarayan, J., Leung, D. Y. M., and Geha, R. Induction of human IgE synthesis by a factor derived from T cells of patients with hyperIgE states. *J. Immunol. 130*:242 (1983).

82. Sarfati, M., Nutman, T. B., Fonteyn, C., and Delespesse, G. Presence of antigenic determinants common to Fc IgE receptors on human macrophages, T and B lymphocytes and IgE-binding factors. *Immunology 59*: 569 (1986).

83. Dessein, A. J., Parker, W. L., James, S. L., and David, J. R. IgE antibody

and resistance to infection. I. Selective suppression and eosinophil response to *Trichinella spiralis* infection. *J. Exp. Med. 153*:423 (1981).

84. Gusmao, R. D., Stanley, A. M., and Ottesen, E. A. *Brugia pahangi*: immunologic evaluation of the differential susceptibility of filarial infection in inbred Lewis rats. *Exp. Parasitol. 52*:147 (1981).

85. Capron, A., Dessaint, J. P., Joseph, M., Rousseaux, R., Capron, M., and Bazin, H. Interaction between IgE complexes and macrophages in the rat: a new mechanism of macrophage activation. *Eur. J. Immunol. 1*:315 (1977).

86. Kay, A. B., and Austen, K. F. The IgE-mediated release of eosinophil leukocyte chemotactic factor from human lung. *J. Immunol. 107*:899 (1977).

87. Butterworth, A. E., Sturrock, R., Houba, V., et al. Eosinophils as mediators of antibody-dependent damage to schistosomula. *Nature 256*:727 (1975).

88. James, S. L., and Colley, D. G. Eosinophil mediated destruction of *Schistosoma mansoni* eggs. *J. Reticulonedothel. Soc. 20*:359 (1976).

89. Kazura, J. W., and Aichawa, M. Host defense mechanisms against *Trichinella spiralis* infection in the mouse: eosinophil-mediated destruction of newborn larvae in vitro. *J. Immunol. 124*:355 (1980).

90. McLaren, D. J. Ultrastructural studies of eosinophils and their interaction with parasites. *Trans. R. Soc. Trop. Med. Hyg. 74(Suppl)*:28 (1980).

91. Sim, B. K., Kwa, B. H., and Mak, J. J. The presence of blocking factors in *Brugia malayi* microfilaremic patients. *Immunology 2*:411 (1984).

92. Butterworth, A. E. Eosinophils and immunity to parasites. *Trans. R. Soc. Trop. Med. Hyg. 74 (Suppl)*:38 (1980).

93. Capron, M., Capron, A., Dessaint, J. P., Tropier, G., Johanson, S. G. O., and Prin, L. Fc receptors for IgE on human and rat eosinophils. *J. Immunol. 126*:2987 (1981).

94. Colley, D. G. Eosinophils and immune mechanisms I. Eosinophil stimulation promotor (ESP): a lymphokine induced by specific antigen of phytohemagglutinin. *J. Immunol. 110*:1419 (1973).

95. Sanderson, C. J., Warren, D. J., and Strath, M. Identification of a lymphokine that stimulates eosinophils in vitro. Its relationship to interleukin 3, and functional properties of eosinophils produced in cultures. *J. Exp. Med. 162*:60 (1985).

96. Silverstein, D. W., Bina, J. C., Soberman, R., Austen, K. F., and David, J. R. Enhancement of human eosinophil cytotoxicity and leukotriene synthesis by biosynthetic (recombinant) granulocyte-macrophage colony-stimulating factor. *J. Immunol. 137*:3290 (1986).

97. Silverstein, D. S., and David, J. R. Tumor necrosis factor enhances eosinophil toxicity to *Schistosoma mansoni* larvae. *Proc. Natl. Acad. Sci. USA 82*: 8667 (1985).

98. Thorne, K. J., Richardson, B. A., Veith, M. C., Tai, P. C., Spry, C. J., and Butterworth, A. E. Partial purification and biological properties of eosinophil activating factor. *Eur. J. Immunol. 15*:1083 (1985).

99. DeSimone, C., Donelli, G., Meli, D., Rosati, F., and Sorice, F. Human eosinophils and parasitic diseases. II. Characterization of two cell fractions isolated at different densities. *Clin. Exp. Immunol. 48*:289 (1982).

100. Winquist, I., Olofsson, T., Olsson, I., Persson, A. M., and Hallberg, T. Altered density, metabolism and surface receptors of eosinophils in eosinophilia. *Immunology 47*:531 (1982).

101. Bass, D. A., Grover, W. H., Lewis, J., Szeida, P., DeChatelet, L. R., and McCall, C. E. Comparison of human eosinophils from normals and patients with eosinophilia. *J. Clin. Invest. 64*:1558 (1980).

102. Shaw, R. J., Walsh, G. M., Cromwell, O., Moqbbel, R., Spry, C. J. F., and Kay, A. B. Activated eosinophils generate SRS–A leukotrienes after physiological (IgG-dependent) stimulation. *Nature 316*:150 (1985).

103. Prin, L., Charon, J., Capron, M., Gosset, P., Taelman, H., Tonnel, A. B., and Capron, A. Heterogeneity of human eosinophils. II. Variability of respiratory burst activity related to cell density. *Clin. Exp. Immunol. 57*: 735 (1984).

104. Capron, M., Spiegelberg, H. L., Prin, L., Bennich, H., Butterworth, A. E., Pierce, R. J., Aliqouaissi, M., and Capron, A. Role of IgE receptors in effector function of human eosinophils. *J. Immunol. 132*:462 (1984).

105. Capron, M., Nogueira-Quieroz, J. A., Papin, J. P., and Capron, A. Interactions between eosinophils and antibodies: in vivo protective role against rat schistosomiasis. *Cell. Immunol. 83*:60 (1984).

106. Kephart, G. M., Gleich, G. J., Connor, D. H., Gibson, D. W., and Ackerman, S. J. Deposition of eosinophil granule major basic protein onto microfilariae of *Onchocerca volvulus* in the skin of patients treated with diethylcarbamazine. *Lab. Invest. 50*:51 (1984).

107. Parawesch, M. R. *The Human Blood Basophil: Morphology, Origin, Kinetics, Function, and Pathology.* Springer-Verlag, New York, 1976, p. 235.

108. Askenase, P. W. Immunology of parasitic diseases: involvement of basophils. *Springer Semin. Immunopathol. 2*:417 (1980).

109. Pearce, E. J., Galli, S. J., Brown, S. J., Askenase, P. W., Gleich, G. J., and McLaren, D. J. *Schistosoma mansoni*: the effect of eosinophil and basophil depletion on resistance to infection in guinea pigs vaccinated with irradiated cercariae. *Parasitology 87*:455 (1983).

110. Kojima, S., Kitamura, Y., and Takatsu, K. Prolonged infection of *Nippostrongylus brasiliensis* in genetically mast cell-depleted w/w^V mice. *Immunol. Lett. 2*:159 (1980).

111. Rothwell, T. L. W., and Dineen, J. K. Cellular reactions in guinea pigs following primary and secondary challenge with *Trichostrongylus colubriformis*, with special reference to the roles played by eosinophils and basophils in the rejection of the parasite. *Immunology 22*:733 (1972).

112. Hsu, Y. L., Hsu, H. F., Pennick, G. D., Hanson, H. O., Schiller, H. J., and Cheng, H. F. Immunoglobulin E, mast cells and eosinophils in the skin of rhesus monkeys immunized with X-irradiated cercariae of *Schistosoma japinicum. Int. Arch. Allergy Appl. Immunol. 59*:383 (1979).

113. Epstein, W. K., Fukuyama, K. F., Danno, K., and Kwan-Wong, E. Granulo-matous inflammation in normal and athymic mice infected with *Schisto-soma mansoni* schistosomula: an ultrastructural study. *J. Pathol. 127*:207 (1979).

114. Capron, M., Rousseaux, J., Mazingue, C., Bazin, H., and Capron, A. Rat mast cell-eosinophil interactions in antibody-dependent eosinophil cyto-toxicity to *Schistosoma mansoni* schistosomula. *J. Immunol. 126*:468 (1978).

115. Henderson, W. R., Chi, E. Y., Jong, E. C., and Klebanoff, S. J. Mast cell mediated toxicity to schistosomula of *Schistosoma mansoni*: potentiated by exogenase peroxidase. *J. Immunol. 137*:2695 (1986).

116. Godfred, R. C., and Gradidgfe, C. F. Allergic sensitisation of human lung fragments prevented by saturation of IgE binding sits. *Nature 259*:484 (1976).

117. Mazinque, C., Camus, D., Dessaint, J. P., Capron, M., and Capron, A. In vitro and in vivo inhibition of mast cell degranulation by a factor from *Schistosoma mansoni*. *Int. Arch. Allergy Appl. Immunol. 63*:178 (1980).

118. Ottesen, E. A., Kumaraswami, B., Paranjape, R., Poindexter, R. W., and Tripathy, S. P. Naturally occurring blocking antibodies modulate immedi-ate hypersensitivity response in human filariasis. *J. Immunol. 127*:2014 (1981).

119. Hussain, R., and Ottesen, E. A. IgE responses in human filariasis. III. Specificities of IgE and IgG antibodies compared by immunoblot analysis. *J. Immunol. 135*:1415 (1985).

120. Ottesen, E. A., Skvaril, F., Tripathy, S. P., Poindexter, R. W., and Hussain, R. Prominence of IgG4 in the IgG antibody response to human filariasis. *J. Immunol. 134*:2707 (1985).

121. Nutman, T. B., Withers, A. S., and Ottesen, E. A. In vitro parasite-antigen induced antibody responses in human helminth infections. *J. Immunol. 135*:2794 (1985).

122. Rosenberg, Y. J. The ability of non-specific T-cell stimulators to induce helper cell-dependent increases in either polyclonal or isotype-restricted Ig production in vitro. *Cell. Immunol. 130*:242 (1983).

123. Smithers, S. R., and Doenhoff, M. Schistosomiasis. In. *Immunology of Parasitic Infection*, 2nd ed. (S. Cohen and K. S. Warren, eds.). Blackwell, Oxford, 1982, p. 527.

124. Cochrane, A. H., Nussenzweig, R. S., and Nardin, E. H. Immunization against sporozoites. In. *Malaria* (J. P. Kreir, ed.). Academic Press, New York, 1980, p. 163.

125. Clegg, J. A., and Smithers, S. R. The effects of immune rhesus monkey serum on schistosomula of *Schistosoma mansoni* during activation in vitro. *Int. J. Parasitol. 2*:79 (1972).

126. Dean, D. A., Wistar, T., and Murell, K. D. Combined in vitro effects of rat antibody and neutrophilic leukocytes on schistosomula of *Schistosoma mansoni*. *Am. J. Trop. Med. Hyg. 23*:420 (1974).

127. James, S. L., Lazdins, J. K., Meltzer, M., and Sher, A. Macrophages as effector cells of protective immunity in murine schistosomiasis I. Activation of peritoneal macrophages during natural infection. *Cell. Immunol.* *67*:255 (1982).
128. Ellner, J. J., and Mahmoud, A. A. F. Killing of schistosomula of *Schistosoma mansoni* by normal human monocytes. *J. Immunol. 123*:949 (1979).
129. Joseph, M., Auriault, C., Capron, A., Vorng, H., and Viens, P. A. New function for platelets: IgE-dependent killing of schistosomes. *Nature 303*: 810 (1983).
130. James, S. L., and Colley, D. G. Eosinophil-mediated destruction of *Schistosoma mansoni* eggs III. Lymphokine involvement in the induction of eosinophil functional abilities. *Cell. Immunol. 38*:48 (1978).

9
Strongyloidiasis

ROBERT M. GENTA and PETER D. WALZER
Cincinnati Veterans Administration Medical Center and University of Cincinnati College of Medicine, Cincinnati, Ohio

I. INTRODUCTION

Strongyloides stercoralis, first identified as the etiological agent of the "Cochin China diarrhea" by Normand in 1876 (1), has been long regarded as an exotic parasite, found only in tropical regions, or in troops, travelers, and immigrants from developing countries. This view can no longer be held. Endemic foci of strongyloidiasis have been identified in Europe and North America (2,3), and sporadic indigenous cases are being reported with increasing frequency from industrialized countries.

Because of its peculiar ability to recycle and multiply within its host, *S. stercoralis* may persist indefinitely in infected individuals, usually producing few significant signs and symptoms (4). In immunocompromised patients, the apparent balance between host and parasite may be disrupted. The intestinal worm population increases dramatically, and migrating larvae may disseminate to distant organs, an event that is frequently fatal (5). The increased use of immunosuppressive and cytotoxic therapies over the past two decades and the appearance of the acquired immune deficiency syndrome (AIDS) have rekindled the interest of biomedical researchers in the relationship between *S. stercoralis* and its hosts. Although a century after its discovery many basic questions remain unanswered, the development of animal models and the study of infected patients have resulted in a better understanding of the immunobiology of *S. stercoralis*.

II. TAXONOMY

The family Stongyloididae (class secernentasida, order Rhabditorida) is formed by only one genus, *Strongyloides* Grassi, 1879. The members of this genus, also

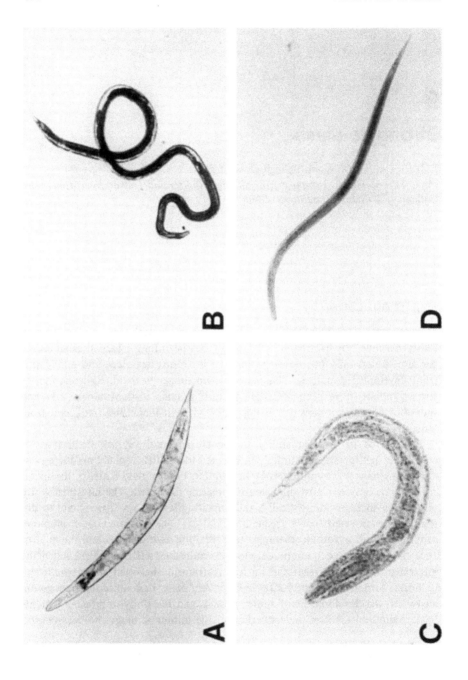

called threadworms, are heterogenetic, with free-living and parasitic generations, and comprise 38 named species. Most of these are parasites of mammals, but some can be found in birds, reptiles, and amphibians. The only species to be dealt with in this chapter is *Strongyloides stercoralis* Bavay, 1876 (synonyms: *Anguillula stercoralis, S. intestinalis, S. canis, S. felis*) (6), but several other species are important either because they may cause disease in humans and livestock or because they are used as animal models of human strongyloidiasis.

Strongyloides fulleborni von Listow, 1905 is a parasite of a variety of primates, but it may also infect humans. It was found in 34% of 76 infants in a village in Zaire, in 10% of 131 patients with strongyloidiasis in Zambia (7), and in 15–25% of villagers of the New Guinea highlands (8). Because of its high prevalence in primates in research facilities and zoos in the United States, *S. fulleborni* may represent an occupational hazard of animal caretakers (9).

Strongyloides ransomi Schwartz and Alicata, 1930 is a parasite of swine of considerable economic importance in North America (10). *Strongyloides westeri* Ihle, 1917 is a worldwide parasite of horses and other equines and is considered an important pathogen in horse farms in Kentucky (11). *Strongyloides papillosus* Wedl, 1856 is found in sheep, goats, and ruminants on the American continent and in swine in Europe. Although it can be transmitted to laboratory rabbits, it has not been widely used as a model of human strongyloidiasis.

The rat threadworm *S. ratti* Sandground, 1925 has been found in rodents throughout the world (13). It is easily maintained in laboratory rats and has been one of the most studied intestinal nematodes. Its importance as a model of human strongyloidiasis will be extensively discussed later in this chapter.

III. LIFE CYCLE

A. Free-Living Generation

A natural reservoir for infection is provided by free-living *S. stercoralis*, which can be found in moist soil in warm climates (14). The free-living males are

---

Figure 1 (A) Free-living *S. stercoralis* female obtained from fecal cultures of an infected patient. Note the large uterus packed with eggs. The length of these forms is approximately 1 mm. (B) Parasitic female recovered from the intestine of an experimentally infected dog. The length varies between 1.5 and 2.2 mm. (C) Rhabditiform larva. This is the form most commonly seen in the stools of infected patients. They measure between 0.2 and 0.35 mm and have a distinctive bulbar esophagus which occupies less than a third of the larva. (D) Filariform larva. This is the infective stage. These swiftly moving larvae measure up to 0.6 mm and have a long tubular esophagus that continues indistinctly with the intestine.

fusiform worms measuring approximately 0.7 mm in length by 0.04–0.05 mm in diameter. They have a characteristically pointed ventrally coiled tail, where the ejaculatory duct can be easily visualized. Free-living females (Fig. 1A) are larger (1 mm × 0.06–0.07 mm), do not have a coiled tail, and often contain visible eggs in their uterus, which occupies most of the body space and are considerably smaller than the parasitic females (Fig. 1B). When embryonated eggs are deposited, they soon liberate rhabditiform larvae (Fig. 1C), which feed on bacteria and other organic debris. These larvae may mature along two distinct lines. They can either undergo several molts, continue to feed, and gradually develop into sexually mature adults, or they can molt and metamorphose into nonfeeding filariform larvae (Fig. 1D). This actively motile form has the capacity to penetrate mammalian skin and to initiate the parasitic generation. Although it is generally believed that unfavorable external conditions prompt the switch from the free-living to the parasitic cyle, no specific factors capable of changing the direction of a given worm population have yet been identified.

B. Parasitic Generation

When filariform larvae come into contact with mammalian skin, they readily penetrate it and enter small dermal blood or lymphatic vessels. They are then passively carried to the lungs by the venous circulation, where they break out of the capillaries into the alveolar spaces. Here the filariform larvae mature to reach the adolescent stage, copulate, and start their upward migration to trachea and epiglottis, from where they are swallowed. Male worms, apparently incapable of tissue penetration, pass out with the feces, whereas females establish themselves just underneath the small intestinal mucosa (Fig. 2) and complete their maturation to adults. The prepatent period in humans is believed to last between 12 and 20 days (14,15). Parasitic adult females are considerably longer than their free-living counterparts (measuring up to 2.2 mm) (Fig. 1B), and their comparatively shorter uterus contains fewer eggs. The eggs, passed into the lamina propria, hatch liberating rhabditiform larvae that reach the intestinal lumen. As they proceed in the alimentary tract with the intestinal contents, these larvae face a developmental choice. The majority remain rhabditiform, grow in size, and are passed with the feces into the external environment, where they either molt to filariform larvae or initiate a free-living generation. Some of the rhabditiform larvae molt into the tissue-penetrating filariform stage while still in the host's intestine, burrow through the colonic wall or the perianal skin, reach the venous system, and start an endogenous parasitic cycle known as autoinfection (Fig. 3).

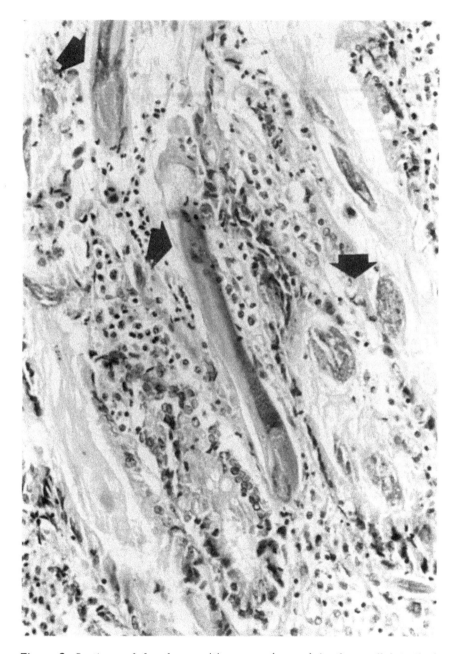

Figure 2 Sections of female parasitic worms (arrows) in the small intestinal mucosa of a heavily infected dog.

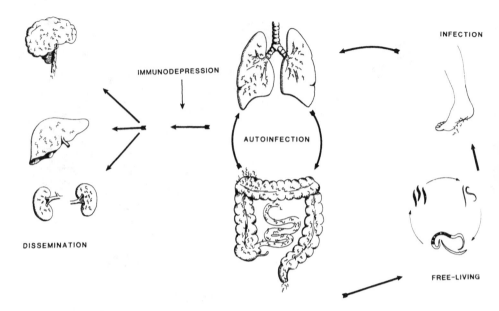

Figure 3   The life-cycle of *S. stercoralis*.

C. Autoinfection

The developmental destiny of a luminal rhabditiform larva is regulated by still unknown factors. Local and systemic host responses as well as inherent characteristics of the parasite population may be interacting to maintain an optimal worm load by means of this continuous internal recycling (16,17). It remains unclear whether this self-replicating cycle occurs in all infected subjects or only in certain patients. However, the frequent finding of *S. stercoralis* infections in persons who have been away from endemic areas for decades suggests that autoinfection may indeed be a widespread phenomenon (18).

D. Hyperinfection

Under certain circumstances of decreased host resistance, the apparent equilibrium between infected host and parasite may be disrupted. In the absence of immune regulation, more larvae undergo intraluminal molting and successfully complete the autoinfectious cycle, thus increasing the number of intestinal worms. This enhanced autoinfection may result in the migration of larvae into virtually every organ, a catastrophic event known as dissemination (5). It is this unique ability to develop hyperinfection (or dissemination) that makes *S. stercoralis* a potentially fatal opportunistic parasite.

IV. MORPHOLOGY AND PHYSIOLOGY

Strongyloides stercoralis is but one of the over 500,000 species of nematodes existing in the world (14). Before reliable animal models became available, only minimal numbers of larvae and adult worms could be obtained exclusively from infected patients. It is therefore hardly surprising that, while the morphological characteristics of its various stages have been accurately described, virtually no work has been done on the physiology and metabolism of this important human parasite.

A detailed account of the general anatomy and physiology of nematodes is beyond the scope of this chapter and can be found in several excellent monographs on the subject (13,14,19). We shall, however, provide the information that may be useful to understand the diagnostic criteria, the adaptation of the parasite to its host, and the immune responses directed against it.

A. Morphology

1. Cuticle
The cuticle is a noncellular structure secreted by the cellular layer immediately beneath it, the hypodermis (20) (Fig. 4). As the cuticle is the part of the parasite that comes into contact with the host, the delineation of its antigenic characteristics is of the utmost importance. Unfortunately, no information is available on the composition of *S. stercoralis* cuticle. In the species where it has been studied, the cuticle of both adult worms and larvae may consist of as many as 10 structurally different layers (20,21). Its composition is probably different in every nematode, but in general it is formed of approximately 75% water, the remainder consisting of proteins with various amounts of lipids and carbohydrates. It has been shown in several parasitic nematodes that the cuticle of the third-stage larva is a dynamic structure of constant renovation. This, if confirmed for *S. stercoralis*, may have important implications related to the ability of the parasite to shed antisurface antibodies that may be produced by the host.

Recently, Grove et al. have shown that free-living *S. ratti* filariform larvae have a faint, electron-dense surface coat external to the epicuticle (22). This surface coat, 12 nm thick, is shed during skin penetration and is believed to provide some degree of protection when the larvae are in the external environment.

2. Muscles
Somatic muscles, responsible for the worm's movement, consist of elongated cells attached to the hypodermis with their external end and lining the celomatic cavity with their internal surface. Specialized muscle cells are found in the genital areas (copulatory and vulvar muscles), in the esophagus and intestine (esophagointestinal muscles), and in other locations where specialized functions exist (14,23).

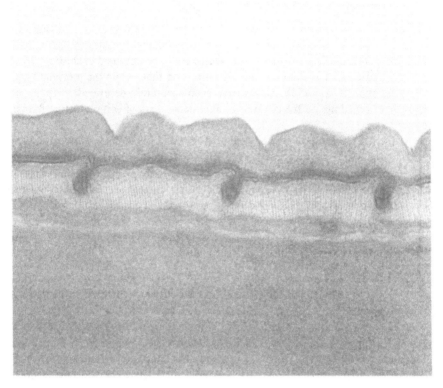

Figure 4 Transmission electron micrograph of the cuticle of an *S. stercoralis* filariform larva. Several electron-dense layers are alternated with lamellar structures and layers of less dense amorphous material. The composition of this cuticle remains completely unknown. (Original magnification X 6,400.)

3. Digestive Tract

In *S. stercoralis*, the digestive tract is a long, straight tube with a stellar cross section formed by esophagointestinal muscle lined by specialized cells and glands able to secrete a variety of enzymes. It is likely that some of the proteases produced by the esophageal glands of filariform larvae may be involved in the skin penetration process. Several characteristics of the digestive tract of *S. stercoralis* larvae are of practical importance for its identification. Rhabditiform larvae (the form most commonly found in the feces of infected patients) have a very prominent esophagus, which occupies the proximal third of the larval body (13). When observed under high power, the esophageal bulb (a pear-shaped structure at the distal end of the esophagus) can be seen contracting rhythmically as the larva feeds. Filariform larvae have a short buccal cavity, which helps to differentiate them from hookworm larvae (which have a long cavity), and a slender esophagus that occupies almost the entire proximal half of the body.The transition between esophagus and intestine can be seen as a small stricture. In contrast, the hookworm esophagus does not extend beyond one-third of the larval length.

B. Physiology

1. Nutrition

Very little is known about where *Strongyloides* spp. derive their nutrients. Rhabditiform larvae are believed to feed on bacteria and other organic debris, whereas filariform larvae are classically known as the "nonfeeding stage." Adult females lodged in the intestinal lamina propria may feed on mucosal products or even on mucosal cells (14). This unresolved question is of practical importance because of the yet unclear relationship between strongyloidiasis, intestinal pathology, and malnutrition.

2. Respiration

Nematodes with ready access to oxygen, such as microfilariae and other blood- and tissue-inhabiting parasites, may have aerobic metabolism. Those like *Ascaris* spp. and *Enterobius* spp., which live in the intestinal lumen where the oxygen tension is very low, are anaerobic. The oxygen tension in the paraluminal region of the mucosa, where *S. stercoralis* females dwell, is relatively high. No data are available for *Strongyloides* spp.; it may be noted, however, that *Trichostrongylus* spp. and *Nematodius* spp., which also live in paramucosal locations, have a much more aerobic metabolism than intraluminal worms (20,23).

3. Excretion

The practical importance of identifying the excretory products of *Strongyloides* spp. is related to the so-called excretory-secretory antigens produced by filariform larvae. These yet uncharacterized products are highly antigenic and appear to be very species-specific (24). It is not known, however, whether they are indeed excreted substances or cuticular components shed as part of the active metabolism of the larval cuticle (22).

4. Locomotion

All nematodes move by undulation. They form waves in their bodies by flexion, and these propel them (14). The rhabditiform larvae of *S. stercoralis*, when observed in fecal material or in culture, move rather slowly. Parasitic females obtained from infected animals also move slowly, but nothing is known about their locomotion within the host. The most active forms are the filariform larvae, which move extremely fast both in vitro and in vivo. This is demonstrated by their ability to penetrate the host's skin in a matter of seconds and by the clinical phenomenon known as "larva currens" (running larva) (see Section X).

5. Reproduction

Strongyloides stercoralis appears to have the ability to behave both as a dioecious nematode (two sexes involved in the fertilization process) and as parthenogenetic females (15–17). The free-living and the first parasitic generations appear to be sexual, whereas the autoinfectious generations seem to be parthenogenetic. The evolutionary advantages of this flexible reproductive manner are invaluable. The gene pooling of the sexual generations ensures species adaptability, while the parthenogenetic generation within a host guarantees that the genotypes best adapted to each particular host are perpetuated unchanged (25).

V. VIRULENCE AND ANTIGENICITY

The wide spectrum of clinical manifestations found in human strongyloidiasis, as well as the wide geographical distribution of the parasite, suggest the possibility of the existence of different strains of *S. stercoralis*.

As early as 1930, Faust speculated on the existence of a separate Central American strain of *S. stercoralis* found in Panama (26). Later, Gaillard, in a series of papers published between 1939 and 1951 (27–29), considered three distinct geographical races of *S. stercoralis*, which differed in their ability to infect different hosts besides humans. An Indochinese form easily infected dogs and was prone to heterogonic (free-living and sexual) development; a second strain, found in the region of Calcutta, India, infected cats but not dogs. Strains obtained from patients from Africa and the West Indies neither developed heterogonically nor infected other species.

While we have not studied this problem systematically, some of our observatins tend to support Gaillard's findings. Larvae obtained from the stools of one North American and one Puerto Rican patient failed to produce patent infections when inoculated into *Erythrocebus patas* monkeys; when the same monkeys were later inoculated with larvae grown heterogonically from the feces of a patient from Thailand, patent infections developed in all animals (30). Larvae recovered from these monkeys were later successfully used to infect dogs.

A further indirect suggestion of some geographical strain variation is provided by our finding that pooled sera from patients with infections acquired in different parts of the world (Southeast Asia, Europe, South America, and North America) appear to recognize different *S. stercoralis* antigens in an immunoblotting system (31). Also, a group of Thai patients had significantly higher parasite-specific IgE responses than patients from Latin America, when measured by a radioallergosorbent test prepared with *S. stercoralis* antigens of Southeast Asian origin (32). Infections acquired in this area are often associated with a characteristic dermatitis (larva currens) caused by the intradermal migration of filariform larvae, a manifestation only rarely observed in patients with European or American strongyloidiasis (33).

The antigenic makeup of *S. stercoralis* has not been extensively studied. The surface of filariform larvae has antigenic determinants that are recognized by serum IgG and IgA antibodies of infected patients (34–36) and by serum IgG and IgM antibodies of experimentally infected dogs (37). These determinants are, at least in part, shared by filariform larvae of *S. ratti*, which can be used in an indirect immunofluorescence diagnostic test (38). In preliminary experiments we have shown that *S. stercoralis* filariform larvae rapidly promote complement conversion in vitro, through both the classic and alternative pathways, in a dose-related fashion (31).

The composition of the larval surface has not been analyzed, but preliminary work indicates that no carbohydrate moieties are present (31).

Extracts of whole larvae are rich in collagenase and other proteolytic enzymes (39). This finding is consistent with the ability of these larvae to penetrate intact mammalian skin and proceed swiftly within the tissues during their migration (40). However, more work is needed to evaluate the role of these enzymes in the pathogenesis of the infection.

VI. EPIDEMIOLOGY AND TRANSMISSION

A. Epidemiology

Information about the prevalence of intestinal parasites is usually based on the detection of diagnostic forms (cysts, trophozoites, eggs, or larvae) in single stool samples obtained from the subjects studied. The shortcomings of this procedure, which can lead to serious underestimates of the true prevalence of any parasitosis (41), are especially evident in the case of strongyloidiasis. This infection is diagnosed by a single stool examination in only 30–60% of the cases (see Section XI). Therefore, *S. stercoralis* is likely to be more common than some of the reported prevalence rates would indicate.

In the United States, endemic foci of strongyloidiasis have been known to exist in many areas of the southeast, with the highest prevalence being reported from states with warm and humid climates, such as Louisiana (42,43), and extending as far north as Kentucky. In this state, a recent study based on the examination of a single stool specimen revealed that 3% of school-age children were infected (3). Large series of cases reported from Kentucky (4), Tennessee (44), and North Carolina (45), while not providing prevalence rates, suggest that the parasite may still be quite common in those areas. In addition to the autochthonous, mostly rural cases, a high prevalence of strongyloidiasis is found in areas where large segments of the population are formed of immigrants from developing countries, such as in southern California, southern Florida, and some large cities. In a major hospital in New York City, *S. stercoralis* was recently found to be the most commonly diagnosed intestinal helminth (46).

Southeast Asian refugees have high rates of infection in the United States (47, 48), Canada (49), France (50), and Australia (51). In Europe, autochthonous strongyloidiasis has been reported from the Iberian Peninsula (52-54), France (55-57), Italy (2,58), Greece (59), Yugoslavia (60,61), Rumania (62,63), Poland (64-66), and the Soviet Union (67). Recently, one apparently indigenous case was diagnosed in Nottingham, England (68). Imported cases have been reported mostly from countries with large immigrant populations, such as France (69-72) and Great Britain (73,74), but also from Switzerland (75), the Scandinavian countries (76,77), and Finland (78).

In addition to these possibly limited foci in temperate parts of the world, *S. stercoralis* is widespread throughout the tropics. Exceptionally high infection rates (up to 60%) have been reported from certain areas of Brazil (79-81), and indigenous cases have occurred in Argentina (82,83), Colombia (84), Venezuela (85), and Central America (86). The infection is common also in other parts of Latin America, and even in Andean populations living at altitudes of over 4500 m above sea level, *S. stercoralis* has been found in 1-3% of the stools examined (87). Cases of strongyloidiasis have been reported from virtually every island of the Caribbean basin (88,89), and many immigrants from that area living in the United States and the United Kingdom have been found to carry the infection (90-92). Numerous reports indicate that the parasite is highly prevalent in many parts of Africa (93-95), southeast Asia (96-98), and the Pacific region (99).

Although individuals from endemic areas undoubtedly constitute the majority of the infected patients seen in industrialized nations, it is important to remember another group of people at risk for strongyloidiasis: the veterans of wars. Some of these individuals have spent years in highly endemic areas of southeast Asia, the South Pacific, and Africa, usually under extremely unsanitary conditions. Numerous members of these groups, particularly former prisoners of war, have been found to harbor long-standing unrecognized infections. Case-finding studies have now been conducted in Great Britain (100), Australia (101), the United States (102,103), and Canada (104), and sporadic cases of infected legionnaires have been reported from France (72). While the overall prevalence rates of strongyloidiasis in these veterans may not be very high, any patient with a history of long permanence in endemic areas should be considered at risk.

B. Transmission

Cutaneous penetration of filariform larvae found in contaminated soil is the most common way by which human strongyloidiasis is acquired. The ingestion of infective larvae is not believed to be a common mode of transmission in humans, although coprophagia may play an important role in dogs. In some reported cases, *S. stercoralis* has been transmitted in unusual manners, such as through renal transplantation (105) or apparently from immersion in a swimming pool (106), but these events represent little more than medical curiosities. Transmammary transmission during breast feeding, a well-documented mode of infection for *S. ratti* in rodents (107), appears to occur occasionally in human *S. fulleborni* infections (108) but has not been observed for *S. stercoralis*.

The peculiar autoinfectious cycle of *S. stercoralis* is of fundamental importance in determining its continuing persistence in the so-called imported cases, particularly in those individuals who, having come from an endemic area, reside in highly sanitized cities where transmission through contaminated soil does not normally occur.

Intimately connected with the autoinfectious cycle and the long persistence of the parasite in its host is the still unanswered question of interhuman transmission. This is thought to take place because of the high prevalence of strongyloidiasis found in some mental institutions (109–111). A recent study by Grove, however, does not support this possibility (112). This author examined the wives of 18 Australian former prisoners of war who had harbored chronic infections for over 30 years and found that none of them were infected or had antibodies indicating exposure to the parasite. The low rates of infection found in homosexual males with high prevalence of other fecally transmitted intestinal parasites (*Giardia lamblia* and *Entamoeba* spp.) (113) provides further indirect evidence that direct interhuman infection is not frequent. Thus, the high prevalence of strongyloidiasis found in some mental institutions may be related to poor sanitary conditions, coprophagia, and fecal-oral contamination taking place among the residents.

Primates and dogs may harbor *S. stercoralis*, and the importance of this animal reservoir in the transmission of human strongyloidiasis in southeast Asia has been emphasized (114). In industrialized countries, human infections contracted from dogs have been reported (115) but do not seem to be very frequent. However, animal caretakers, veterinarians, and zoo keepers should be aware of the possibility of acquiring the infection from the stools of infected animals and should treat all such specimens as potentially infective.

VII. PATHOLOGY AND PATHOGENESIS

The pathological lesions specifically associated with chronic, uncomplicated *S. stercoralis* infections in otherwise healthy hosts are little known, because only rarely have such cases come to autopsy. However, a few patients in whom strongyloidiasis was an incidental finding have been reported, and the pathological descriptions of these cases indicate that the worms can exist within the intestinal mucosa without causing significant inflammatory responses or other tissue damage. The examination of two such cases as early as 1886 led Golgi and Monti to declare that the *Anguillula intestinalis* (as *S. stercoralis* was known then) was an "innocent inhabitant of the human intestine" (116). This concept became so well established that in some European countries strongyloidiasis is still known by the deceptive term "benign ancylostomiasis."

The classic descriptions of the pathology of strongyloidiasis were made by DePaola and co-workers in 1962 (117,118) and later by Caymmi-Gomes (119). Based on the histopathological examination of a large number of autopsied cases and on the anatomopathological descriptions found in the literature, these authors proposed the subdivision of the intestinal lesions in three distinct forms. In "catarrhal enteritis" (mild strongyloidiasis), the small intestine is congested, the mucosa is covered with abundant mucous secretions, and scattered petechial hemorrhages may be found. The most remarkable histological features is an increased mononuclear infiltrate in the submucosa. Parasites are found only in the glandular cryptae (Fig. 5a). In the more severe "edematous enteritis," the intestinal wall is grossly thickened, the mucosal folds are flattened, and the affected tracts of intestine assume a rubbery consistency. Microscopically, there is edema of the submucosa, flattening of the villi, and parasites are scattered throughout all the intestinal layers. In the most severe form ("ulcerative enteritis"), the intestinal walls are rigid because of edema and fibrosis, the mucosa is grossly atrophic, and large ulcers can be seen throughout the affected areas. An abundant inflammatory infiltrate, most often consisting of neutrophils, as well as all stages of *S. stercoralis*, are found throughout the intestinal walls (Fig. 5b).

As convenient as this classification may be from a didactic viewpoint, in practice the three forms of enteritis may overlap and be found simulatneously in different segments of the intestine of the same patient. Moreover, it is important to point out that this classification was conceived in an endemic country (Brazil) at a time when medical facilities were less than optimal and specific drugs for strongyloidiasis were not readily available.

In a small number of patients with infections limited to the gastrointestinal tract, the inflammatory responses may cause a significant alteration of the duodenal and jejunal mucosa, with heavy lymphocytic infiltration and flattening of the villi, resulting in a spruelike malabsorption (120–122). Uncommonly, the mucosal damage occurs predominantly in the large intestine, with clinical manifestations simulating ulcerative colitis (123). The asymptomatic presence of *S. stercoralis* larvae in the appendix has been frequently observed, and eosinophilic appendicitis caused by the parasite has been described (124).

In patients with disseminated strongyloidiasis, gut lesions reflect the large number of worms dwelling within the mucosa of the intestine and penetrating the colonic walls. In addition, the stomach (125) and the peritoneal cavity (126) may be invaded by migrating parasites. However, because most of these patients are immunocompromised, inflammatory responses may be less prominent than the extent of tissue damage would suggest.

Particularly in patients who receive effective antihelminthic therapy before succumbing to disseminated strongyloidiasis, the gastrointestinal pathology is often overshadowed by the lesions directly and indirectly caused by the worm in other organs. The "direct" lesions are the result of the mechanical damage caused by the parasites migrating through the tissues and the inflammatory responses associated with the migration. The extraintestinal organ most affected by the mechanical damage is the lung. Upon passing from the vascular bed to the alveolar space, each larva breaks a capillary or a small vessel. During an initial infection or in the course of a well-controlled autoinfection, only a few parasites pass through the lungs at any given time, and the microhemorrhages are of no functional or clinical significance. In severe disseminated infection, when hundreds of thousands of adults may dwell in the intestine, the combined effects of innumerable alveolar microhemorrhages may result in massive pulmonary bleeding. This may manifest itself clinically with respiratory distress and hemopthysis and pathologically with a picture of diffuse intraalveolar hemorrhage (Fig. 5c). While the mechanical damage inflicted by the migrating larvae upon the alveolar capillaries provides a reasonable explanation for the pulmonary hemorrhages seen in some patients, other factors may be involved in the pathogenesis of pulmonary bleeding. Alveolar hemorrhages often occur several days after the parasites have been cleared by antihelminthic therapy, and careful histological examination of numerous specimens fails to reveal larvae in the pulmonary parenchyma. This suggests that vascular damage apparently following the infection may be mediated by immunological mechanisms.

As larvae penetrate the large intestine, they create small breaks in the mucosa that may result in the invasion of the bloodstream by enteric bacteria. It has also been suggested that the larvae themselves carry bacteria in a piggyback fashion on their cuticle (119). Whatever the mechanism, the widespread dissemination of larvae is frequently associated with gram-negative sepsis (127). A frequent consequence of this is the development of diffuse or patchy bronchopneumonia (128,129). In rare cases, abscesses containing parasites have been found in the pulmonary parenchyma (130).

A less common but well-documented occurrence is the development of meningitis in association with disseminated strongyloidiasis. In the majority of cases, gram-negative bacteria have been demonstrated in the CSF, whereas in other patients S. stercoralis larvae have been found in the meningeal spaces and, rarely, within the brain (131,132). The inflammatory responses associated with the parasites are variable and depend on the immune state of the individual patients. A purulent exudate is found most commonly, but cases of lymphocytic

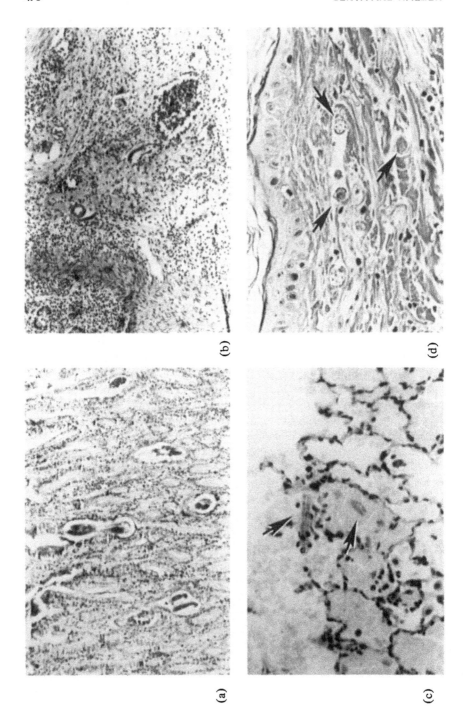

("aseptic") meningitis have been described. In one patient, several cerebral abscesses containing larvae were found at autopsy (133).

Filariform larvae, and occasionally rhabditiform larvae and adult worms, often reach other visceral organs, such as mesenteric lymph nodes, biliary tract, and liver (119). In these locations, probably because of an unfavorable environment, the parasites appear to die, and the inflammatory responses associated with them are frequently granulomatous (134). In some cases, larvae have been found in the pancreas, spleen, heart, endocrine glands, and ovaries (128–135), with various degrees of tissue reactions.

The pathological lesions with the cutaneous migration of larvae (larva currens) have been described as allergic (136), with dermal edema and a sparse eosinophilic exudate. It is remarkable, however, that no cases are reported in which the parasites have been identified in tissue sections. In some cases, multiple biopsies were taken from and around the tip of the progressing serpiginous lesion, but even serial sections failed to demonstrate larvae (136). In disseminated disease, *S. stercoralis* larvae have been found in the skin associated with purpura and a mononuclear infiltrate (137). Recently, we observed a patient with severe disseminated strongyloidiasis and bone marrow depression. Biopsies of serpiginous purpuric lesions on the abdomen revealed numerous filariform larvae in the dermis and within the vessels. No cellular responses were present in association with the parasites (Fig. 5d).

VIII. HOST RESPONSES

A. Parasite-Specific Immune Responses

Until recently, the study of humoral and cellular immune responses specifically directed against *Strongyloides* antigens was hampered by the lack of a readily available source of parasite products. The development of reproducible animal models has now enabled researchers to obtain adequate quantities of pure *Strongyloides* sp. larvae that can be used to prepare antigens. Initially, most efforts have been concentrated on the development of immunological tests for

---

Figure 5   (a) Adult worms, larvae, and eggs in the small intestinal mucosa of a patient with catarrhal enteritis. (b) In more severe infections the massive penetration of larvae through the colonic mucosa causes mucosal ulcerations and may be accompanied by inflammatory responses. (c) In the lungs (arrows), larvae cause intraalveolar hemorrhage, which may be fatal. (d) The migration of larvae into the skin (arrows) may be accompanied by intradermal hemorrhage, with or without cellular infiltration.

diagnostic applications. By using soluble antigens obtained from *S. fulleborni* and *S. ratti* filariform larvae, respectively, Crump-Brannon and Faust (138) and Pellegrino et al. (139) developed intradermal tests based on the detection of immediate sensitivity responses. An initial evaluation in infected patients and controls showed these tests to be both sensitive and specific, and other authors have used them for diagnostic studies and epidemiological surveys (140,141). However, the difficulty of obtaining antigenic materials satisfactory for human use, as well as the availability of in vitro assays for the determination of specific antibodies, apparently discouraged the further investigation of skin tests.

The development of enzyme-linked immunosorbent assays (ELISA) using soluble *S. stercoralis* or *S. ratti* filariform larval antigens (142–144) and of an indirect immunofluorescence test (IIFT) using fresh or formalin-fixed whole filariform larvae (34,35,38) resulted in the discovery that between 85 and 95% of the patients with chronic, uncomplicated strongyloidiasis had specific IgG antibodies against filariform larval antigens. ELISA was later adapted for the detection of circulating parasite-specific IgA antibodies, and approximately 85% of all infected patients had serum IgA against. *S. stercoralis* antigens. (36). When the recognition patterns of these antibodies were analyzed by immunoblotting techniques, it was found that a portion of the antigens reacting with IgA were different from those recognized by IgG (36).

By using an in vitro histamine release assay from peripheral basophils, it was shown that all of 18 infected patients studied had specific IgE antibodies directed against both *S. stercoralis* and *S. ratti* filariform larval somatic antigens (145). These patients also had specific IgE antibodies against a yet uncharacterized excretory/secretory (E/S) product of *S. stercoralis* filariform larvae but not against the E/S product of *S. ratti*. When the histamine-release assay was performed in the presence of the patients' own serum, the percentage of release was considerably lower than the release obtained when the assay was conducted in the presence of the serum of a noninfected donor. One possible interpretation of this finding is that infected patients develop "blocking antibodies" that protect them from continuous stimulation of IgE-bearing cells (mast cells and basophils) by the circulating parasite antigens. Such blocking factors have been demonstrated in patients with chronic schistosomiasis and bancroftian filariasis and consist of IgG4 antibodies whose presumed function is to prevent a chronic anaphylactoid state (146,147).

Because of technical difficulties, the histamine-release assay does not lend itself to the investigation of large numbers of patients. To examine the specific IgE responses in a larger population of infected people, we have recently developed a solid-phase radioallergosorbent assay (RAST) (32). Between 80 and 85% of patients with current *S. stercoralis* infections were found to have serum IgE antibodies reacting with parasite antigens.

The functional role of these responses remains unclear. During the past several years we have examined the parasite-specific immune responses in a number of immunosuppressed patients with severe or disseminated strongyloidiasis. The majority of these subjects had levels of parasite-specific IgG, IgA, and IgE antibodies similar to those of immunocompetent patients with chronic uncomplicated infections. A small subgroup of patients, however, who died of disseminated strongyloidiasis had no detectable parasite-specific IgE antibodies and no peripheral eosinophils (148). These data, based on the study of a limited number of patients, must be interpreted cautiously. However, they suggest that the role of the eosinophil-IgE axis in protecting from hyperinfection deserves further investigation.

In a small study conducted in Brazil, Carvhalho et al. (149) found that patients with severe strongyloidiasis (but without dissemination) had lower levels of total IgG antibodies and lower peripheral eosinophil counts than persons with asymptomatic or mild disease. However, when the titers of parasite-specific IgG abd IgE antibodies were measured in these three groups of patients, no significant differences were detected (150).

Cell-mediated immune responses have not been extensively studied. In a group of patients with chronic uncomplicated S. stercoralis infections, peripheral lymphocytes were found to exhibit proliferative responses in vitro only when cultured in the presence of serum from a noninfected donor (151). The patients' own serum exerted an inhibitory effect on the parasite-specific lymphoproliferative responses, suggesting that blocking factors similar to those identified in schistosomiasis (147) and filariasis (146) may be operative also in strongyloidiasis. The complete lack of lymphoproliferative responses found in a small group of immunocompromised patients with disseminated strongyloidiasis is difficult to interpret, because all these individuals were receiving immunosuppressive doses of corticosteroids (148).

B. Resistance

While surveying residents of endemic areas in Thailand (98) and Brazil (81), we have identified in each population a number of subjects who had circulating IgG and IgE antibodies against S. stercoralis antigens but no clinical or parasitological evidence of current infection. The limited sensitivity of stool examinations suggests that some of these individuals may have harbored occult infections (i.e., with a parasite load too small to be detected); it is also possible that some had been unknowingly treated with drugs that may have eradicated their infections. However, some of these seropositive subjects might represent a segment of the population capable of developing immune responses that effectively and specifically protect them from the infection.

Such a situation exists in other human parasitic diseases, as well as in animal models of strongyloidiasis. In areas endemic for filariasis, a large percentage of the population has antifilarial antibodies but neither circulating microfilariae nor signs or symptoms of occult filariasis (filarial fevers, tropical eosinophilia) (152). Persons with antibodies to *Schistosoma* antigens and no apparent infections are found in all endemic areas, and they are believed to represent a previously exposed group who developed protective responses against the parasite (153). Recently, analyses of individual posttreatment patterns of hookworm reinfection conducted in India have provided quantitative evidence of predisposition, possibly genetically determined, to heavy infection (154).

It has long been known that rats experimentally infected with large inocula of *S. ratti* larvae (2000–4000 larvae) expel the intestinal adult worms within 3 weeks, become increasingly resistant to subsequent challenges (155–157), and develop both serological and cellular parasite-specific responses (158–161). Less studied, however, are infections with small inocula. When we injected rats with as few as 100 larvae (a dose possibly closer to a natural infection than the large inocula normally used in this model), we found that these rats did not expel their worms during the 2-month observation period and did not mount detectable IgG and in vitro cellular responses to *S. ratti* antigens. Surprisingly, however, they responded to a large challenge infection with a rapid expulsion of the parasites, in a fashion similar to rats previously inoculated with 3000 larvae (162). The implication of these preliminary findings is that, at least in the rodent model of strongyloidiasis, the size of the inoculum may be important in determining the host response to the parasite. It is not known whether this occurs in human infections, but it is possible that the frequent exposure to *S. stercoralis* infective larvae experienced by residents of endemic areas may induce, at least in some subjects, the development of protective immune responses.

That individual resistance plays an important role in the modulation of *S. stercoralis* infection is apparent from studies conducted on both primates and dogs. When nine previousy unexposed young *Erythrocebus patas* monkeys were inoculated with 1000 live *S. stercoralis* filariform larvae of human origin, all animals developed patent infections. Some, however, progressed rapidly to lethal dissemination even in the absence of immunosuppressive therapy, while other monkeys survived for several months on high doses of oral prednisone (30). Even greater individual variation is observed in a canine model that we are currently maintaining in our laboratory (163). Most parasite-naive young beagles inoculated with 3000 live *S. stercoralis* filariform larvae develop a patent infection, which appears to last indefinitely in some dogs, while it is apparently self-cured in others. A smaller group of dogs, while mounting parasite-specific immune responses similar to those of the patently infected animals, never develop detectable infections. At present, the means of investigating the parasite-specific immune responses in these animals or in humans are limited. It is reasonable to assume that these groups of animals react to the parasite with different immune responses, but these differences are not yet apparent because of our present technical limitations.

Another concept that needs clarification is that of "self-cure." Apparently spontaneous cures have occurred in some of our experimentally infected dogs. While these animals maintained high titers of anti-*Strongyloides* IgG antibodies in their serum, baermanization of their stools performed three times weekly for over 2 months failed to reveal any parasitic forms. By all current standards, such an animal would be considered cured. At necropsy, however, some dogs were found to harbor small numbers of live and apparently fecund adult female worms in their intestine. We have not tested the resistance of these animals to subsequent inoculations, but these occult infections might conceivably exist in humans, providing the constant antigenic stimulus that maintains the immune system in a state of alert against further infections (concomitant immunity).

C. Risk Factors for Severe Strongyloidiasis

In highly endemic areas, strongyloidiasis has been found to be equally common in both sexes and in all age groups (18,98). A similar distribution was observed in a population of Cambodian refugees who recently immigrated to Australia (51).

In contrast, clinical studies from parts of the United States and Europe where this parasite is common but not highly endemic have emphasized the frequent association of strongyloidiasis with other conditions (Table 1). Rarely encountered in otherwise healthy adults, in these areas strongyloidiasis is more common in older men (over 50 years) with previous gastrointestinal surgery, a history of the use of antacids, and chronic obstructive pulmonary disease with intermittent use of corticosteroids (3,45,103,164). The possibility of higher prevalence in whites than in blacks has been suggested in one study (164), but it has not been conclusively documented.

The relationship with older age and concurrent disease suggests that even chronic, relatively benign *S. stercoralis* infections may be favored by the presence of predisposing host factors. The depression of the immune system found in older age and in individuals on low doses of steroids, although often clinically unappreciated, might favor the internal multiplication of parasites and allow their persistence. Protein-calorie malnutrition is one of the most common causes of immunodeficiency in the world (165). The ubiquitous presence of *S. stercoralis* in many populations of developing countries, where malnutrition is widespread, further suggests the possibility that this parasite needs an immunologically impaired host to survive. The nature of the predisposing factors that may favor strongyloidiasis is not known, but it is possible that local mechanisms at the intestinal level may be involved. In the tropics, malnourished as well as

Table 1   Risk Factors for Severe Strongyloidiasis

1. Age: very young and over 50
2. Concurrent conditions:
   Autoimmune diseases
   Malignancies (particularly hematological)
   Chronic infections (TB, leprosy)
   Previous gastric surgery
   Severe malnutrition
   Immune deficiency syndromes
   HTLV-1 infection
   HIV infection
3. Immunsuppression:
   Corticosteroid therapy
   Organ transplantation
   Irradiation
4. Miscellaneous:
   Alcoholism
   Antacid therapy (H_2 receptor inhibitors)
   Pregnancy

many apparently healthy persons have profound structural and functional alterations of the small intestinal mucosa (166). A depression of the responses at this level might facilitate the establishment of self-perpetuating colonies of *S. stercoralis*. A similar mechanism might be operative during steroid therapy. In rats, both short- and long-term corticosteroid administration affects the absorptive function and the cell kinetics of the duodenal and jejunal epithelium and quite likely decreases the effectiveness of the local immune responses (167). While the effects of corticosteroids on the intestinal responses of healthy subjects have not been investigated, data from patients with inflammatory bowel disease strongly suggest that local cell-mediated immunity is profoundly affected (168).

In contrast to the high prevalence of intestinal protozoal infections found in patients with the acquired immune deficiency syndrome (AIDS) (169), to date only a very few cases of disseminated strongyloidiasis have been reported in such patients. In Europe and North America this might only reflect the lack of epidemiological overlapping between these two infections. However, in countries like Haiti and Zaire, where both HIV and *S. Stercoralis* are highly prevalent, one would have expected to see the emergence of disseminated strongyloidiasis as an important opportunistic infection in AIDS patients. This lack of association is difficult to explain. At this time, we can only speculate that the immunological functions depressed by the HIV infection may not be those primarily responsible for the local and systemic control of *S. stercoralis*.

IX. ANIMAL MODELS

Three *Strongyloides* systems have been used in an attempt to elucidate the complex immunobiological interaction between this nematode and its hosts. Each of them has characteristic features that allow the investigation of some aspects of strongyloidiasis.

A. Rodents

The related species *S. ratti* (see Section II) has been extensively studied in both rat and mouse systems. This parasite is common in wild rodents throughout the world, in some areas the prevalence of natural infections being as high as 50% (170). Because of its ability to undergo a heterogonic (free-living, sexual) cycle in culture, *S. ratti* can be easily maintained in laboratory rats by repeated passage of the infection. To prepare the cultures, feces of experimentally infected rats are collected fresh and mixed with an approximately equal volume of activated charcoal and sterilized peat moss Enough tap water is added to make the mixture moist but not liquid. Several grams of this preparation are then placed in a Petri dish and incubated at room temperature in a humid environment. After 3–4 days, free-living male and female adults develop, which produce larvae that rapidly become filariform. Between day 7 and day 10, the cultures contain innumerable filariform larvae, which can be harvested, washed, and used to infect new rats.

The kinetics of experimental infections have been described (155–158). Rats are inoculated subcutaneously with 1000–3000 filariform larvae obtained from fecal cultures. Very rapidly, most larvae migrate through the tissues, and eventually between one-half and one-third of them reach the duodenum, where parasitic adult female worms establish themselves underneath the mucosal surface and produce eggs. About half of these eggs hatch in the intestinal lumen, so that in the feces of infected animals both eggs and rhabditiform larvae are found. These experimental infections become patent within 4 or 5 days, and rats so infected pass eggs and larvae in the feces for approximately 2 weeks. Infected rats mount systemic and local immune responses (155,158–162), and after approximately 10 days they effectively promote the expulsion of the intestinal worms, a process usually completed within 20 days. Rats become increasingly resistant to subsequent challenges. The acquired resistance to infection and reinfection may be induced in unexposed animals by transfer of serum (159, 161), IgG antibodies (160), and mesenteric lymph node cells (171). In female rats, the larval migration and the ability to expel intestinal worms depend on the estral cycle and the hormonal status (172,173). The administration of cortico-steroids or other immunosuppressive agents, including antilymphocytic serum, reduces the rats' ability to expel the parasites, and the infections may last for longer periods (174,175). The crucially important phenomenon of autoinfec-tion, however, has not been demonstrated in rodents. In addition, several investi-gators have recently challenged the accepted textbook accounts of the larval migratory routes (skin, lungs, intestine) and have showed that other areas, such as the soft tissues of the head, may be important migratory stations, at least under certain experimental circumstances (159,176).

Some strains of mice are susceptible to *S. ratti* infection, and the parasite has been successfully maintained in these rodents by several investigators (177–179). Infected mice have been used for immunological studies (161) as well as to assess the effectiveness of antihelminthic drugs against *Strongyloides* spp. (180–182). Attempts to induce infections in mice using *S. stercoralis* have been unsuccessful (183).

Important differences between the biological behavior of *S. ratti* and *S. stercoralis*, most notably the former's lack of an autoinfectious cycle, limit the use of the rodent systems as models of human strongyloidiasis. Nevertheless, several relevant applications can be found for these models. The pathological lesions and the tissue responses associated with intestinal worms and migrating larvae can be conveniently studied in rats and mice (184–186). The study of the immune-mediated intestinal expulsion, whose role in human infections is still unclear, may yield important information on the local interaction between intestinal mucosa and parasite. Because of their low cost and a lesser degree of humane concern, rats and mice lend themselves to the evaluation of new drugs to treat strongyloidiasis. In addition, the functional similarities between *S. ratti* and *S. stercoralis* larval antigens (38,143–145) make the rat model a simple and inexpensive source of antigens for the performance of diagnostic assays.

B. Primates

Primates have been known for a long time to be naturally infected with *S. fulle-borni*, but only recently have fatal disseminated *S. stercoralis* infections been reported, mostly from great apes in zoos (9,187–189). The parasitological aspects of experimental infections with *S. fulleborni* and *S. stercoralis* in apes were studied as early as 1929 (16,190), and a detailed study on the dynamics of experimental *S. stercoralis* infections in gibbons has been conducted by de Paoli (191). More recently other investigators have provided parasitological, pathological, and immunological information on a primate model (30,192,193). In this work, young *Erythrocebus patas* monkeys were infected with a human strain of *S. stercoralis*, and their infections were followed over a period of several months, both before and after administration of suppressive doses of corticosteroids. Several of the younger monkeys developed fatal disseminated infections even before immunosuppressive therapy was initiated. Other monkeys developed massive infections only after prolonged therapy with corticosteroids. All animals developed parasite-specific cellular and humoral responses; these, however, did not appear to correlate with the clinical and parasitological course of the infections. Pathological lesions found at postmortem examinations were similar to those characteristically seen in patients dying of disseminated strongyloidiasis (mucosal lesions in the small and large intestine and pulmonary hemorrhage).

The principal drawback of the primate model is the difficulty of acquiring and maintaining these animals. They are very expensive both to purchase and house, and they require special husbandry and the care of specifically trained animal technicians. In addition, humane concerns severely restrict the use of monkeys for the study of strongyloidiasis.

C. Canines

Dogs are naturally infected with a strain of *S. stercoralis* that cannot be distinguished on morphological or biological grounds from the human strain (27,29, 114,194,195). As early as 1928, the Japanese researcher Nishigori infected dogs with *S. stercoralis* of human origin and demonstrated the occurrence of the autoinfectious cycle in these animals (196). Since then, many other investigators have reproduced the features of human strongyloidiasis in dogs (197,198), and in more recent years the canine model has become better standardized (199-201).

In our laboratory, parasite-naive beagles are infected with known inocula of *S. stercoralis* filariform larvae originally obtained from a Southeast Asian patient (37,163). A patent infection develops in most animals between 12 and 20 days postinoculation. Most infected dogs continue to pass larvae for several months, when the infections become so light as to be undetectable by daily fecal examination. At this point, high doses of oral steroids (up to 10 mg/kg of prednisone per day) usually transform these occult infections into massive hyperinfections with dissemination, which may lead to the death of the animals. Interestingly, the behavior of these infections in dogs appears to parallel that of human infections in the sense that a great individual variability is present. Some animals never develop symptoms, even if they pass several thousands of larvae per gram of feces per day, whereas other dogs rapidly become sick and die with relatively light infections. Furthermore, the development of hyperinfection is not constant, and some animals seem to be able to continue to regulate their parasitic population even in the presence of prolonged high-dose steroid therapy.

Infected dogs develop transient parasite-specific cellular responses, as measured by in vitro lymphoproliferative responses of peripheral lymphocytes (37). Specific IgM antibody titers rise shortly after inoculation and become undetectable after 4–6 weeks (37,199). In contrast, anti-*Strongyloides* IgG antibodies develop within the first few weeks postinoculation and remain elevated throughout the infection (37,199).

From the study of both patients and animal models of *S. stercoralis* infection, it is apparent that the magnitude of the parasite-specific systemic immune responses does not correlate with the clinical manifestations, nor does it parallel parasitological events. Local responses at the mucosal level may play an important role in the regulation of the intestinal parasite population. Information in this area is completely lacking, and the study of the local defense mechanisms against intestinal helminths may represent one of the most viable areas of inquiry for future research in strongyloidiasis.

X. CLINICAL MANIFESTATIONS

One of the most puzzling aspects of chronic strongyloidiasis in immunocompetent hosts is the diversity of clinical manifestations reported among different groups of patients. In some series most infected persons were asymptomatic (32,55,202,203), whereas in others gastrointestinal complaints (4,44,45) or chronic dermatitis (100,102) were the most common presentations. There are several possible explanations for this unusual situation. One is the geographical variety of the populations studied. Large series of patients with proven infections have been reported from the United States (4,44,45,102,164), Europe (2,55,56,58,70,72,100), South America (81,84), and Australia (51,101). The wide spectrum of clinical manifestations observed in these patients may reflect a number of variables. The socioeconomic conditions of the patients in each group were widely different, and the infections had been acquired in such diverse areas as southeast Asia, North and South America, and Europe. Therefore, differences in individual resistance and parasite strain may have influenced the evolution of the parasitosis. The presence of concurrent factors (such as subclinical malnutrition or old age) may also have modulated the clinical aspects of the infections. Cultural diversity and the degree of patients' sophistication in reporting their symptoms may have affected the investigators' clinical impressions. In addition, the design of the studies and the different settings in which they were conducted may have introduced biases. A study based in an American Veterans Administration hospital is likely to show a prevalence of older men with concurrent conditions, whereas a survey carried out in a Brazilian prenatal care center will likely discover asymptomatic infections in young women.

Another important source of diversity is the characteristically intermittent

Table 2   Clinical Manifestations of Strongyloidiasis

Chronic strongyloidiasis
  1. Asymptomatic passage of larvae in the stools
  2. Gastrointestinal manifestations
      Epigastric pain
      Bloating
      Postprandial fullness
      Heartburn
      Abdominal tenderness
      Diarrhea
      Constipation
      Guaiac-positive stools
      Malabsorption
  3. Extraintestinal manifestations
      Larva currens
      Urticaria
      Arthritis
Disseminated Strongyloidiasis
  1. Gastrointestinal manifestations
      Diarrhea
      Abdominal pain
      Paralytic ileus
  2. Extraintestinal manifestations
      Pneumonia
      Pulmonary hemorrhage
      Meningitis
      Peritonitis
      Sepsis
      Shock
      Granulomatous hepatitis

nature of symptoms caused by *S. stercoralis*. The analysis of single-case reports shows that most infected persons experience symptoms in a very sporadic fashion, with long periods of well-being alternating with symptomatic phases. Thus, studies based on one-time observation of patients may be biased by the irregularity of the manifestations.

The discussion that follows reviews the clinical aspects of chronic strongyloidiasis in immunocompetent hosts as well as the manifestations of overwhelming infections in immunocompromised subjects. When approaching the individual patient, it is important to remember that only a few of these manifestations may occur over the course of their infections, and the absence of one or even all of them does not exclude strongyloidiasis.

When gastrointestinal manifestations are present, they are usually nonspecific. Vague abdominal pain, most often epigastric, a feeling of postprandial fullness or bloating, and heartburn are among the symptoms most commonly reported (4, 118,204). In some cases gastritis associated with the presence of larvae in the stomach has been demonstrated (205,206). Most patients report the occurrence of brief episodes of diarrhea alternating with constipation; these symptoms may last for a few weeks or months and then subside for long periods during which bowel function is apparently normal. When present, the diarrhea usually consists of semiformed stools, only rarely mixed with blood (202), although guaiac-positive stools have been occasionally found in persons with chronic infections (123). Physical examination in these patients may be normal or reveal mild abdominal tenderness on palpation. Less commonly, chronic strongyloidiasis may mimic inflammatory bowel disease, particularly ulcerative colitis. In a few instances, patients have undergone surgery for "chronic colitis," and the correct diagnosis was established only by the pathological examination of the resected colon (123). In one case, strongyloidiasis was associated with the typical histopathological findings of ulcerative colitis (207), but a cause-and-effect relationship was not established.

In patients who underwent gastric resection with the creation of a small intestinal blind loop, *S. stercoralis* worms have been localized in large numbers in the blind loop. Such infections have been found to be particularly difficult to eradicate (208).

Malabsorption has occasionally been described in patients with strongyloidiasis (120,121,209). The majority of these reports, however, have been from areas of the world where tropical sprue and spruelike conditions are exceedingly common among the local populations (88,90), and it has been difficult to establish a clear relationship of cause and effect between *S. stercoralis* infection and malabsorption. Indeed, the alterations of the small intestinal mucosa frequently found in residents of the tropics may result in an impairment of the local immune mechanisms, which may predispose to more severe forms of strongyloidiasis. In a group of Colombian patients, Garcia and his colleagues (84) have convincingly argued that malnutrition was the cause rather than the effect of severe strongyloidiasis.

Granulomatous hepatitis caused by *S. stercoralis* larvae in apparently immunocompetent patients has been reported (85,134), but it more commonly associated with severe, disseminated infections.

Two types of cutaneous manifestations have been described in patients with chronic strongyloidiasis. Urticarial rashes, possibly indicating a sensitization to parasite antigens, which subsided after successful antiparasitic treatment, have been found sporadically in patients from all parts of the world (2,3,81,101). In contrast, a characteristic dermatitis caused by the subcutaneous migration of filariform larvae (named larva currens, after the swift linear progression of the migrating larvae) has been reported almost exclusively in Caucasian patients who acquired the infection in southeast Asia (210–214). In many of these patients, larva currens was the only sign of strongyloidiasis, and the demonstration of parasites in the stools was not always possible (100,102). However, therapy with thiabendazole caused the permanent disappearance of the dermatitis, and this was interpreted as evidence *ex adjuvantibus* of the parasitic nature of this ailment.

In the absence of dissemination, other extraintestinal manifestations are infrequent. Asthma has been reported in a few patients, but the relationship with strongyloidiasis was not clear (215). Chronic obstructive pulmonary disease has been found to be frequently associated with strongyloidiasis in some series of American patients (3,164). A direct effect of the recycling parasites on the pulmonary parenchyma, although it cannot be excluded, appears unlikely. A more plausible explanation for this apparent association may be the fact that these patients are often on steroid therapy, a factor predisposing to strongyloidiasis.

Arthritis associated with the local deposition of immune complexes containing *S. stercoralis* antigens has been described (216,217). Cardiac arrhythmias and arrest have been ascribed to a direct myocardial damage caused by the migrating larvae (218) or to electrolyte imbalance precipitated by severe intestinal strongyloidiasis (219). Depression and neurosis apparently caused by chronic strongyloidiasis have been reported (173,220), but they likely represent reactive responses to the long-lasting symptoms (chronic diarrhea in one case and dermatitis in another).

In contrast to the usually mild and nonspecific manifestations of chronic infections, the severity of disseminated strongyloidiasis in compromised hosts becomes rapidly apparent. The ability of *S. stercoralis* to cause fatal systemic infections has been recognized since the beginning of the century. Before the introduction of immunosuppressive drugs into clinical practice, disseminated infections occurred mostly in patients with severe malnutrition or advanced malignant tumors. However, in a significant number of cases reported before 1950 there was no apparent associated disease (221-224).

With the widespread use of immunosuppressive and cytotoxic drugs, the typical patient seen in today's clinical practice is one in whom *S. stercoralis* infection had not been suspected prior to the initiation of immunsuppressive or antineoplastic therapy (5,127). Over the course of their underlying illness (most commonly autoimmune diseases, hematological malignancies, or organ transplantations), these patients may develop severe abdominal pain, diarrhea, or diffuse pulmonary infiltrates (225-232). Because of the effect of the immunosuppressive drugs that these patients usually receive, eosinophilia is rarely present, and the possibility of a parasitic infection is rarely entertained.

Dose and duration of immunosuppressive therapy necessary to precipitate disseminated infections vary greatly and are likely to be related to the magnitude of the preexisting infection, immune status, and invidividual resistance of each patient. Thus, the subconjunctival administration of corticosteroids (233) or short courses of oral prednisone prescribed for dermatitis (234) or asthma (235) have been sufficient to cause fatal disseminated infections. In other cases high doses of methylprednisone administered to prevent rejection of transplanted kidneys (236-239) or treat cerebral edema (135) have triggered rapidly progressive overwhelming infections. Most commonly, however, the development of hyperinfection and dissemination is associated with chronic steroid therapy for autoimmune or lymphoproliferative disease (128,226,240,241). In a small percentage of patients, cytotoxic therapy alone has caused disseminated infection (5,127,242). Rarely, chronic conditions such as leprosy (230) and tuberculosis (243) have been found in association with fatal strongyloidiasis; in one case the dissemination occurred in a patient with inappropriate ACTH secretion syndrome caused by a small-cell carcinoma of the lung (244).

Irrespective of the nature of the precipitating factors, the clinical course of disseminated infections is rather uniform. At the time when patients develop abdominal or pulmonary signs, stool examination usually reveals *S. stercoralis* larvae and sometimes even adult worms and eggs (5,127,232), but in some patients the rate of internal repenetration is so high that no parasites are found in routine fecal examinations (245). Occasionally, *S. stercoralis* larvae have been identified in sputum specimens collected to elucidate the nature of the pulmonary symptoms (82,221,232,246-248), in gastroenteric aspirates (249), and in skin biopsies (31,137). These methods may provide the diagnosis in unsuspected cases, but when the possibility of disseminated strongyloidiasis is considered, the accurate examination of multiple fecal samples collected at each evacuation is the most reliable procedure to establish the diagnosis.

Unless specific treatment is promptly administered, the evolution of these hyperinfections is invariably fatal. Severe diarrhea may lead to dehydration and electrolyte imbalance (219,241,250), but most commonly paralytic ileus develops (135,251), and the clinical picture is dominated by bacterial infections. Probably because of the large numbers of larvae migrating from the large intestine into the bloodstream, gram-negative sepsis occurs rapidly, with infections developing in virtually any organ. The most common form of pulmonary involvement is diffuse bronchopneumonia (5,128), but occasionally the formation of parenchymal abscesses has been observed (130,252). Intraalveolar hemorrhage, often so severe as to cause the patient's death, is a frequent event during the course of disseminated strongyloidiasis. In some cases, fatal pulmonary hemorrhages occur a few days after apparently successful treatment of the parasite, suggesting that an immunologically mediated mechanism of vascular damage may be operative in these circumstances (193).

Gram-negative meningitis is the most frequent central nervous system manifestation of disseminated strongyloidiasis, and larvae may be found in the cerebrospinal fluid. Rarely, larvae have been found in the absence of bacteria in patients with signs of meningeal involvement, thus raising the possibility of pure parasitic (aseptic) meningitis (131,132,253,254). A less common form of CNS involvement is the formation of cerebral and cerebellar abscesses containing *S. stercoralis* larvae (133).

Clinical signs of hepatitis are rare, but at autopsy the liver is often found to be affected by the larval dissemination. The pathological characteristics (granulomas forming around fragments of larvae) are suggestive of a chronic process (85,134). Peritonitis accompanied by the pesence of parasites in the peritoneal fluid has been described (126) but is not a common manifestation. Likewise, while the larval invasion of virtually every organ has been reported in pathological studies (119), the clinical picture of overwhelming *S. stercoralis* infections is usually dominated by the intestinal, pulmonary, and central nervous system involvement.

A special case is represented by patients with immune deficiency syndromes. Two such cases have been reported to date (255,256). Both patients had severe forms of acquired hypogammaglobulinemia associated with strongyloidiasis apparently resistant to treatment. While pulmonary involvement was documented by large numbers of parasites in the sputum, neither patient had the severe signs or symptoms commonly present in disseminated strongyloidiasis. The investigation of such patients, together with the study of the parasite-specific immune responses of AIDS patients with strongyloidiasis, may provide important information on the yet unknown mechanisms that control and modulate the dynamics of *S. stercoralis* infections.

XI. DIAGNOSIS

A. Radiology

Radiographic studies of the gastrointestinal tract are not sufficiently specific to be recommended as a diagnostic procedure for strongyloidiasis. However, the ability to recognize the various radiological patterns seen in this infection is often helpful to suggest the presence of this nematode in patients who undergo a gastrointestinal series as part of their workup (257).

The radiological aspect of the small intestine may be entirely normal in light infections, but in some cases the characteristic signs of gastritis and duodenitis may be seen (125). These changes consist of prominent mucosal folds in the antrum and a spastic duodenal bulb and C loop with thickened, prominent transverse folds (257-259). When malabsorption is present, the picture is similar to that of tropical sprue, with an increased diameter of the small intestinal lumen, generalized hypotonia, and various degrees of mucosal edema. With severe, long-standing infections, when edema and fibrosis are present, there may be rigidity of multiple segments of the small intestine (257). In cases of hyperinfection and dissemination, complete disruption of the mucosal patterns, ulcerations, and paralytic ileus have been observed (135,251,260).

Patients with uncomplicated intestinal strongyloidiasis have normal chest X-rays. In the presence of dissemination, pulmonary involvement may be heralded by bilateral edema and patchy, often rapidly changing infiltrates (128,235, 261).

B. Parasitology

1. Stool Examination

The most common stage of *S. stercoralis* identified in the feces is the rhabditiform larva (Fig. 1C), but in occasional patients filariform larvae, adult females, and even eggs have been visualized (262,263).

A number of factors, however, make the parasitological diagnosis of strongyloidiasis a uniquely challenging task. Although no human data are available, animal studies suggest that in chronic, asymptomatic infections (such as those found in most patients) the parasite load may be relatively small. Another factor that contributes to limit the number of fecal larvae is the low rate of egg production by the *S. stercoralis* female. It has been estimated that no more than 50 eggs per day are passed by each adult worm, in sharp contrast with other intestinal nematodes such as *Ascaris lumbricoides*, whose female may pass up to 1 million eggs a day (263). In addition, these few eggs are apparently produced rather irregularly (14), and this may result in the uneven distribution of larvae in the fecal matter. Because of this, the sampling error may be great, and the chances of finding larvae in the small quantity of feces usually examined in a clinical parasitology laboratory may be very slim. Finally, the peculiar ability of *S. stercoralis* larvae to repenetrate the intestinal mucosa may further reduce the number of fecal larvae. In fact, we have observed immunosuppressed monkeys with severe infections consisting of over 300,000 adult worms that on certain days would have negative stools (30). In those circumstances, it is possible that all larvae were repenetrating through the colonic mucosa and none were passed out with the feces. Necropsy findings confirmed the presence of heavy mucosal penetration in the colon.

Considering the above factors, it is hardly surprising that the sensitivity of a single stool examination as performed in clinical laboratories is low. The chances of finding *S. stercoralis* in an infected patient using one direct smear of stools have been reported to be between 30 and 60% (98,264).

Several methods have been proposed to improve the diagnostic efficiency of stool examination. According to some authors, formalin-ether concentration techniques significantly increase the sensitivity (203). Pelletier (102) found that the screening of larger amounts of fecal material by examining multiple microscopic slides for a period of up to 9 hr per specimen considerably increased the sensitivity of the test. Nielsen and Mojon (265) suggested that the collection and examination of seven stool specimens on seven consecutive days yields a much higher rate of positivity than one single specimen. Neither of these two methods, however, is easily applicable to the busy schedule of a diagnostic parasitology laboratory.

The method of Baermann (266) allows the examination of a larger volume of feces (up to several grams), and it is more sensitive than direct microscopy. In this technique, the test stools are placed on a sieve in a funnel filled with warm water (Fig. 6), and the larvae migrate through the sieve and fall to the bottom of the funnel, where they can be collected and counted. We use this method to perform larval quantitation in our experimental animals and whenever possible in our patients (103). The sensitivity does indeed appear to be high (264,267), but the method has several drawbacks. First of all, it can only be performed on fresh stools. Second, it requires a rather cumbersome apparatus, best placed under a hood, and requires careful washing and sterilization after each use. The whole procedure may take up to 2 hr to perform, and it may expose the laboratory personnel to infective larvae.

Fecal culture in Petri dishes after mixing with charcoal or peat moss also increases the sensitivity of fecal examination (268). However, the cultures need to be examined using the Baermann method described above. In addition, certain strains of *S. stercoralis*, particularly the so-called New Wolrd strain, do not go through the free-living cycle, a fact that may restrict the usefulness of cultures in dealing with infections acquired on the American continent. This

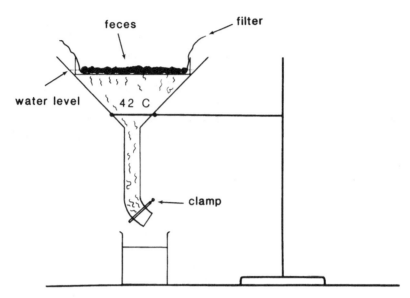

Figure 6 The Baermann apparatus. This system, originally designed to collect free-living nematodes from the soil, is adapted to the clinical laboratory. It provides a greater sensitivity than any other method for the recovery of *S. stercoralis* larvae from the stool of infected patients.

limitation also applies to the method of Harada-Mori (268), which is simpler than conventional fecal cultures and does not require subsequent baermanization. This technique, however, has not been extensively tested in strongyloidiasis.

In conclusion, while stool examination remains the primary technique for the diagnosis of strongyloidiasis, its limitations should not be overlooked. If no special techniques are available, when the diagnosis is strongly suspected on clinical grounds, the careful examination of several specimens collected on different days will be necessary before strongyloidiasis can be excluded with reasonable confidence.

2. Body Fluid and Tissue Examination

Strongyloides stercoralis larvae can also be demonstrated in the duodenal fluid, using small intestinal intubation, endoscopy with aspiration, or the "string test." The examination of duodenal aspirate is reportedly very sensitive (264,268). This is an excellent method when it is necessary to achieve a rapid demonstration of parasites, as in the case of an immunocompromised patient with suspected overwhelming infections and in patients unable to pass stools because of paralytic ileus. The string test consists of a gelatine capsule (marketed as Enterotest) containing 140 cm of coiled thread. The capsule is swallowed by the patient together with a glassful of water, it dissoves, and the thread reaches the duodenum. After approximately 4 hr the thread is pulled out and is squeezed between gloved fingers. The fluid is then examined for larvae under a dissecting microscope. Initial studies claimed a high sensitivity for this test (269), but other authors did not find it superior to stool examination (270). The procedure is cumbersome, it is not always well accepted by patients, and it should probably be used only in cases where the collection of repeated fecal samples is not possible.

Small intestinal biopsies have occasionally revealed unsuspected *S. stercoralis* infections (271). To our knowledge, no studies have been performed to compare the sensitivity of this procedure with that of less invasive methods for the diagnosis of human strongyloidiasis. In experimentally infected dogs, parasites were demonstrated in less than 50% of open duodenal and jejunal biopsies (with the surgical removal of a sample of mucosa measuring approximately 0.5 cm^2) obtained at various times during the course of the infection (31). The area of intestinal mucosa obtained by the biopsy capsules used in clinical practice rarely exceeds 10 mm^2. Thus the likelihood of finding worms in such samples is probably minimal, and other methods should be preferred for the diagnosis of this parasitosis. Intestinal biopsies, however, may have an important place in the evaluation of mucosal morphology and function during the course of *S. stercoralis* infections with prominent gastrointestinal manifestations.

In severe infections, larvae and adult parasites have been found in specimens of gastrointestinal fluid and sputum (Fig. 7), and larvae in tissue and bronchoalveolar lavage (221,246–249), ascitic fluid (272), pancreatic aspirates (273), and cerebrospinal fluid (131,253). Occasionally, larvae have been identified in specimens surgically removed from the small intestine, colon (123), appendix (124), and skin (31). In most of these cases, *S. stercoralis* represented an unexpected finding in specimens examined for other reasons. This emphasizes the importance of recognizing the various forms of this parasite not only in preparations where the organism remains intact (such as in fluids) but also in histological sections, where only small fragments of larvae or adult worms may be present (Fig. 7).

When hyperinfection or dissemination are suspected, it is important to examine sputum and bronchoalveolar lavage specimens for the presence of *S. stercoralis* larvae. With the Papanicolaou stain, the larval morphology is well preserved, but their light pinkish-purple color makes the larvae somewhat difficult to find, particularly on bloody specimens. In contrast, on a gram-stained preparation, larvae take a dark reddish color, which makes them readily visible; their structures, however, are altered by the high temperature used to prepare the slides. Thus, the combined use of these two staining techniques would allow both easy and accurate identification of the parasites.

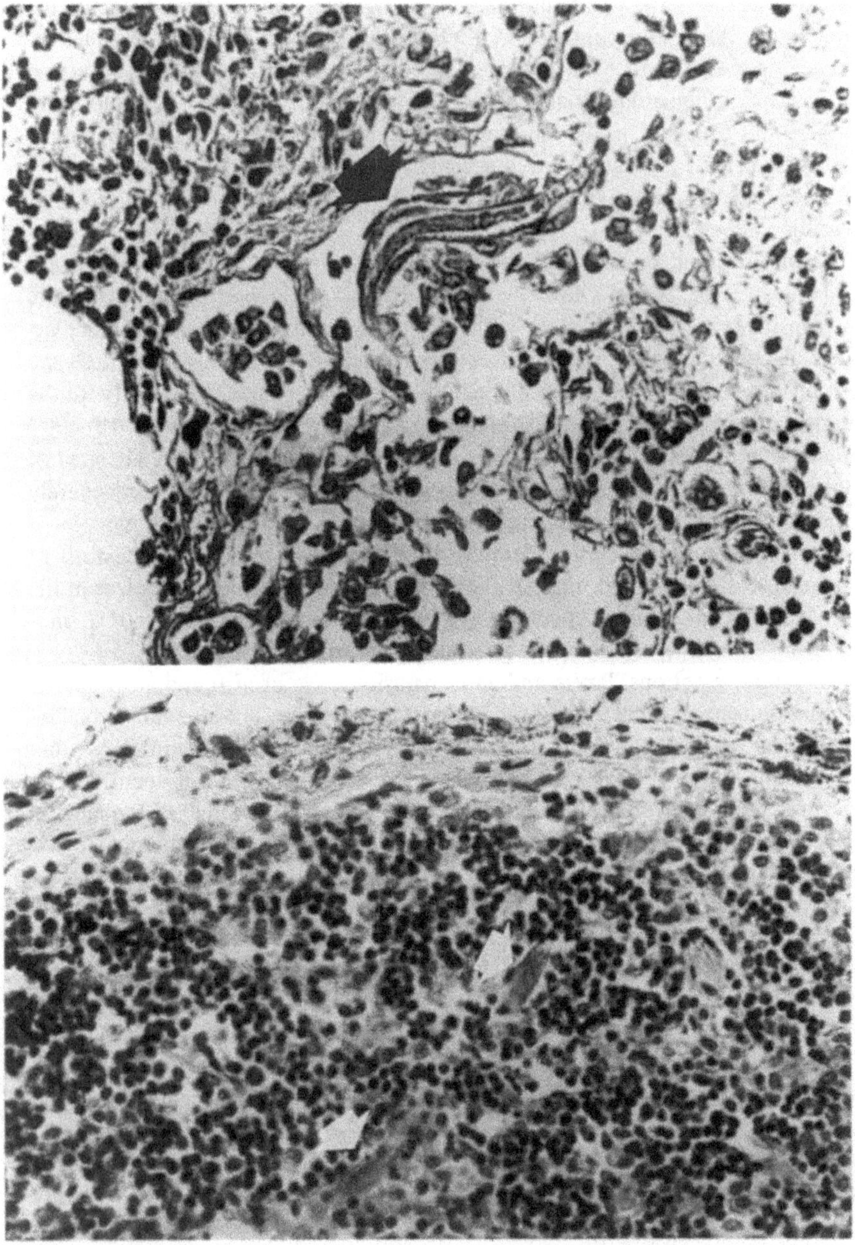

Figure 7

The examination of fluids of bronchial origin is especially useful to evaluate the response to treatment in known disseminated infections (Fig. 8). The rate of disappearance of larvae from the lungs may be a more accurate indicator of the systemic effectiveness of antihelminthic therapy than the examination of stools.

C. Hematology

The only hematological abnormality commonly found in patients with chronic, uncomplicated strongyloidiasis is a moderate elevation of the peripheral eosinophil count. While cases have been reported of persons with extreme elevation (more than 30% of the total white count) (274), in most series, between 70 and 80% of the patients had values between 6 and 15% (or between 500 and 1500 eosinophils/mm^3) (4,44,45,81,101). In patients whose eosinophil counts have been followed up for some time, there has been a considerable day-to-day variation in the degree of eosinophilia (103). In fact, it is not uncommon to find infected individuals who, on certain days, have normal eosinophil counts. This may explain why in many series, which are often based on only one time point, 20 or 30% of the parasitized persons have no increased eosinophilia.

Thus, the presence of unexplained eosinophilia in a patient should always be thoroughly investigated, and if the geographical history is consistent, repeated stool examinations should be performed to rule out parasitic infection. On the other hand, the absence of elevated eosinophilia in a person at risk for strongyloidiasis should suggest the need to obtain several blood counts on different days.

A special case is represented by patients with disseminated strongyloidiasis. As most of them have been receiving immunosuppressive drugs capable of reducing the eosinophilic response, their peripheral eosinophilia is more commonly normal or low than elevated (5,18). Futhermore, the review of over 100 published cases of disseminated strongyloidiasis has suggested that eosinopenia in these patients may be associated with a poorer outcome (127).

D. Immunology

Total serum IgE levels are elevated (>200 IU/ml) in 50-70% of the patients with strongyloidiasis (32,81,98,101,275,276). It is remarkable, however, that in one

---

Figure 7 Fragments of filariform larvae may be difficult to see in the histological sections of highly cellular tissues, such as lymph nodes (left), whereas they may be quite apparent in the lungs (right). Definite identification of the parasites is rarely possible in these cases, but the presence of fragments of nematode in extraintestinal tissues should alert the pathologist about the possibility of disseminated strongyloidiasis.

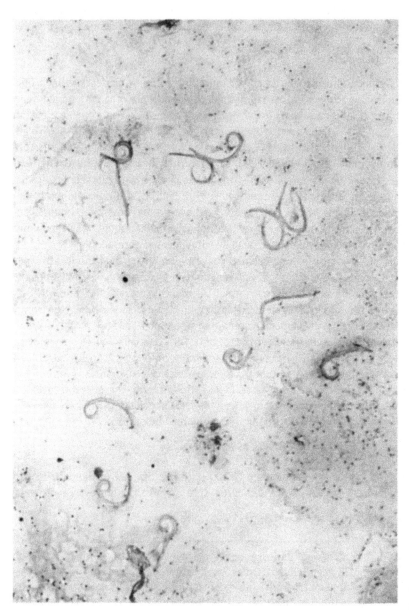

Figure 8 Sputum of an immunosuppressed patient who died of respiratory failure caused by disseminated strongyloidiasis. Filariform larvae were also present in the ascitic fluid, urine, and skin.

study involving former British prisoners of war with chronic infections, less than 10% of the subjects examined had significant elevation of total serum IgE (227).

The diagnostic relevance of such an elevation is similar to that of eosinophilia: If present, it should be investigated, but its absence does not necessarily rule out strongyloidiasis.

The other classes of immunoglobulins do not appear to be affected by the presence of this parasite. However, in a small study conducted in Brazil, Carvalho and his colleagues found that patients with severe manifestations of strongyloidiasis had lower levels of total serum IgG and IgM than patients with asymptomatic infections (149).

E. Serology

Although still in the early phases of its development, immunoserology appears to be a promising tool in the diagnosis of strongyloidiasis. Several immunoassays have now been developed, all hinged on the demonstration of serum antibodies against filariform larvae or their antigenic products (Table 3).

1. Indirect Immunofluorescence Test (IIFT)
This test is based on the detection of serum IgG antibodies directed against the surface of fresh or formalin-fixed filariform larvae (34,35,38,278). A known number of larvae are incubated with the test sera at appropirate dilutions, and after several washings and the incubation with fluorescein-labeled anti-human IgG, the fluorescence present on the surface of each larva is evaluated using a standard fluorescence microscope. The sensitivity of this test is between 85 and 95%, and its specificity is highly satisfactory. Occasional weak cross-reactivity has been noted in patients with filarial infections (35).

2. Enzyme-Linked Immunosorbent Assay (ELISA)
For the performance of this test, a soluble antigen prepared by sonication and subsequent saline extraction of filariform larvae is used to coat standard ELISA plates (142-144). The assay, based on the detection of parasite-specific IgG antibodies, may be carried out by using serial serum dilutions (144) or by comparing the net absorbance of a single serum dilution with that of positive and negative reference sera tested simultaneously on each plate (36,148,278). When evaluated in 268 patients with *S. stercoralis* and in over 600 controls, the single-dilution ELISA exhibited an index of positive accuracy of 97% and an index of negative accuracy of 95% (279). Rare apparent false positives are found in patients with *Filaria* sp. and *Ascaris lumbricoides* infections

3. Solid-Phase Radioallergosorbent Test (RAST)
The majority of patients with strongyloidasis have elevated total serum IgE antibodies, a portion of which are specific for parasite antigens (145). To exploit

Table 3 Immunodiagnosis of Strongyloidiasis

Test	Sensitivity	Comments	References
Skin test	95%	Not approved for diagnostic use in humans. Antigens may contain impurities.	138–141
IIFT	85–95%	Detects IgG. Filariform larvae (fresh or fixed) are used. Cross-reactivity found rarely with *Filaria* sp.	32,35,38
ELISA	85–95%	Detects IgG. Soluble antigens prepared from filariform larvae are used. Cross-reactivity found rarely with *Filaria* sp.	142–144,148,279
IHA	80%	Detects IgG. Specificity is not satisfactory.	301
RAST	85%	Detects IgE. Soluble filariform antigens used. Needs ^{131}I. Rare false positives in patients with ascariasis and in allergic subjects with total IgE > 2500 IU.	32

this immunological response for diagnostic purposes, we have developed a solid-phase radioallergosorbent test that allows the detection of parasite-specific IgE antibodies in the patient's serum (32). This RAST appears to be as specific as ELISA, but it is less sensitive: only between 80 and 85% of infected patients have specific-IgE levels measurable by this method. For this reason, and because of the need for nuclear medicine facilities for its performance, RAST is not advocated as a diagnostic test. Nevertheless, because of the reported association between low IgE responses and poor prognosis (148), it may have a useful part in the immunological evaluation of patients with strongyloidiasis.

4. Uses and Interpretation of Serology

The detection of *S. stercoralis* is particularly important in patients who are likely to become immunocompromised, such as candidates for organ transplants, individuals about to receive chemotherapy for cancer, or persons infected with HIV. The diagnosis and treatment of strongyloidiasis in these patients before they are immunosuppressed will prevent the development of potentially fatal hyperinfection and dissemination. However, even in a relatively endemic area (such as the southeastern United States), only a small percentage of the population is infected, and most infected people are asymptomatic. In these circumstances the screening for strongyloidiasis by stool examination would not be cost-effective. Also, it would be very impractical to ask asymptomatic patients to provide repeated fresh stool samples and to process such a large volume of specimens in the clinical parasitology laboratory.

Conversely, the application of serology as a screening method is simple and cost-effective. With ELISA, large numbers of serum specimens may be tested at one time and at a minimal cost. When a seropositive patient is identified, a careful search for the parasite is likely to yield positive results. In a recent study conducted at the Cincinnati VA Medical Center, we have tested 700 veterans of the Vietnam and other wars (103). Seropositive patients were then requested to provide several samples of fresh stools, and parasites were searched for by using direct smears, concentration techniques, baermanization, and culture. In most cases several stool samples had to be examined before *S. stercoralis* larvae were identified. Most of the patients in whom the diagnosis was established were older men with other ailments. Many of them had been on low intermittent regimens of steroids for several years, usually for chronic obstructive pulmonary disease, and some of their infections might have progressed to dissemination if left untreated.

The scope of screening may vary depending on the local epidemiological conditions. In endemic areas in the United States or in tropical countries, it would be advisable to test all individuals who may eventually become immuno-compromised. In nonendemic areas, a patient's geographical history should help to make the decision. In general, natives of endemic areas (even if they have left those areas years before), persons with a history of travel to endemic areas, and veterans of foreign wars should be considered at high risk for strongyloidiasis.

Immunocompromised patients with hyperinfection and dissemination present special diagnostic challenges. The presence of immune deficiency or long-standing immunosuppression may have profound effects on the responses against parasitic infections. A case in point is the frequent absence of eosinophilia in these patients (18). In our experience with ELISA, most patients with dissemination had elevated IgG antibodies against *S. stercoralis* antigens (31,36,148). This suggests that IgG serology may have a useful place in the serodiagnosis of immunocompromised patients with opportunistic infections.

Presently, we have studied only two patients with AIDS and strongyloidiasis, and both showed a complete absence of detectable parasite-specific humoral responses (18,31). In these and other immunodeficient patients, tests aimed at the detection of circulating parasite antigens could provide a rapid and reliable laboratory diagnosis. Such assays, however, are still at the experimental stage in some other helminthic diseases and are not presently available for strongyloidiasis.

Serology can also be usefully applied for the performance of epidemiological studies. Although it is not yet clear whether the presence of parasite-specific IgG or IgE antibodies reflects only current or also past infection, the prevalence of these antibodies in a population may provide useful information about the endemicity of *S. stercoralis*. We have conducted several small sereoepidemiological studies in various parts of the world. The highest prevalence of anti-*Strongyloides* antibodies was found in a Thai village, where 45% of 187 subjects tested were positive (98). A similarly high prevalence of seropositivity was reported in southeast Asian refugees living in Australia (51). In a rural area of southern Brazil, 27% of the individuals tested had a positive ELISA (81), supporting the high prevalence of strongyloidiasis found in that region by earlier parasitological surveys (79,80). Conversely, we found no positives in a randomly selected sample of 50 sera from South Korean adults (31). We also tested 200 sera obtained from Qatar (Arabian Peninsula) and found that the only persons with anti-*Strongyloides* antibodies were workers of Indian or Pakistani origin (31); this indicates that *S. stercoralis* may not be prevalent in arid desert zones.

XII. TREATMENT

Treatment of *S. stercoralis* infection is indicated both in symptomatic and asymptomatic infection. Thiabendazole (Mintezol), a broad-spectrum benzimidazole antihelminthic drug, has long been considered the agent of choice (280). Although its precise mode of action is unclear, thiabendazole may inhibit the parasite enzyme fumarate reductase and also suppress egg or larval development (281). Thiabendazole is administered orally as a chewable tablet or liquid suspension in the dose of 50 mg/kg per day (maximum 3.0 g) in two divided doses for 2 days in the normal host. The drug has an overall success rate of about 70–80%, but this varies among different studies (282). Patients who fail initial treatment with thiabendazole often respond to another course of therapy.

The clinical response to treatment of strongyloidiasis is readily discernible, but assessment of parasitological cure is more elusive. Factors such as low organism burden, pattern of larval excretion, and autoinfection cycle have contributed to the difficulty in detecting *S. stercoralis* on routine stool examination. The success of various therapeutic regimens can thus be related to the diligence with which the parasite is sought during the follow-up period. In one study of chronic strongyloidiasis, larvae could be demonstrated in 7% of post-treatment specimens, yet skin manifestations (urticaria, larva currens) recurred in 29% of patients, suggesting treatment failure (283).

It is prudent to follow the patient for several months after completion of therapy of *S. stercoralis* infection. At least three stool specimens should be collected on different days and examined microscopically for the presence of larvae. Additional specimens should be obtained, or more sensitive techniques (examination of small intestinal contents, fecal culture, baermanization) should be employed if residual infection is suspected. Serum antibodies to *S. stercoralis* and peripheral eosinophils usually fall after successful treatment (98,283,284) and may thus be helpful in guiding clinical management. Total serum IgE levels vary widely among patients, and little information is available about specific IgE antibodies following therapy.

Less clear-cut guidelines exist for the treatment of uncomplicated strongyloidiasis in the immunocompromised host or in a person with achlorhydria or impaired gastrointestinal mobility. Parasite eradication may be more difficult in these patients than in the normal host, but controlled studies are lacking. We feel that thiabendazole should be used initially in conventional doses, although some authors have favored a longer (5-7 day) duration of therapy (232). Regardless of which approach is used, these patients will require close follow-up. Since corticosteroids or the immunosuppressive drugs may impair the antibody or eosinophil response, parasitological examination assumes increased importance. Patients in whom *S. stercoralis* larvae are found should be treated with a 5-7 day course of therapy. In some cases, repeated courses or longer duration of treatment will be required. There are several case reports of persistent *S. stercoralis* infection in patients with immune deficiency diseases or blind loop of bowel that respond only after the administration of large doses of thiabendazole or other antiparasitic drugs for weeks to months or after direct installation of these agents into the affected area of the intestine (208,255,256).

Disseminated strongyloidiasis or the hyperinfection syndrome is a life-threatening condition. Optimal management requires prompt diagnosis and early institution of thiabendazole therapy. The drug should be administered in the same dose for simple *S. stercoralis* infection for a minimum of 5-7 days. Patients with disseminated strongyloidiasis may respond slowly to therapy, sometimes not for several days or even longer. We find that frequent examination of stools and fluids from other body sites (e.g., sputum when there is pneumonia) for the presence and morphological characteristics of larvae is helpful in monitoring this response. It is prudent to continue thiabendozale for several days after a clinical and parasitological effect has been achieved.

Vigorous supportive measures are an important part of management, including attention to fluid and electrolyte balance, nutrition, and oxygenation if pneumonia is present. Sepsis with gram-negative bacteria, a frequent complication of disseminated strongyloidiasis, should be treated with appropriate broad-spectrum antibiotics. Vigilance should also be maintained for nosocomial infection with other opportunistic pathogens. Corticosteroids and other immunosuppressive drugs should be tapered to the lowest dose allowed by the patient's underlying condition. Even with all these measures, the mortality of disseminated strongyloidiasis remains high (30–40%) (127).

Clinical experience in the therapy of human infection with other *Strongyloides* species is sparse. Thiabendazole has been used to treat *S. fulleborni* infection in individual patients and in community parasite eradication programs (285).

Thiabendazole is rapidly absorbed from the gastrointestinal tract and appears to be widely distributed throughout the body, even reaching detectable levels in cerebrospinal fluid (286). The drug is largely metabolized to its 5-hydroxy derivative (which has no antiparasitic activity) and is excreted in the urine. Limited studies suggest that thiabendazole can be given safely in the standard dose for up to 5 days in anephric patients; however, caution should be used for larger periods of administration because of possible accumulation of metabolites (287,288). Thiabendazole may also compete with other drugs (e.g., theophylline) for metabolic sites in the liver, thereby raising serum levels of these agents (289).

Adverse reactions to thiabendazole vary considerably both among individuals and among population groups. According to standard references, side effects occur in about 5–30% of patients (282); our own experience with patients encountered in a general medical service suggests that most people tolerate the drug reasonably well. In contrast, studies of chronic strongyloidiasis in former prisoners of war have noted a frequency of side effects of 75–90%; in many instances, drug administration had to be curtailed or altered (102,282). Gastrointestinal symptoms (nausea, vomiting, anorexia) are the most common adverse reactions. Neuropsychiatric manifestations (dizziness, lethargy, hallucinations, feelings of unreality) can be especially troublesome; rarely, convulsions have occurred (290). A variety of other manifestations (visual and auditory disturbances, skin rash, leukopenia, malodorous urine) have also been reported. Strategies such as administering thiabendazole over several days have been employed in attempts to improve patient tolerance of the drug.

Alternatives to thiabendazole are quite limited. In experimental models of strongyloidiasis, other benzimidazole derivatives have greater activity against some life-cycle stages of the parasite and hence might offer therapeutic advantages (181). Of these compounds, mebendazole (Vermox) has had the most clinical use (291–295) but has never been directly compared with thiabendazole in a controlled trial. Mebendazole has mainly been used to treat other intestinal helminths (e.g., *Ascarsis*, *Trichuris*), and the optimal dose for *S. stercoralis* has not yet been established. Therapeutic regimens have ranged from 100–300 mg twice daily for 3–8 days to 500 mg daily for 21 days. Mebendazole, which acts mainly within the intestine with little systemic absorption, is usually well tolerated. Very large doses of the drug (40 mg/kg per day) have been used in attempts to treat echinococcosis. Promising anti-*S. stercoralis* results have been found with two other benzimidazole compounds, albendazole and cambendazole (296-299), but the latter drug has apparently been withdrawn from further human use by the manufacturer.

Pyrvinium parmoate (Povan), a luminal antihelminthic drug used to treat pinworm infection, has shown some activity against *S. stercoralis* is limited clinical trials (282). The adult dose is 50 mg three times daily for 7 days. However, there has been little recent interest in investigating pyrvinium parmoate further.

New forms of therapy of strongyloidiasis are needed. Ideally, oral preparations should be able to act at intestinal and extraintestinal sites and be suitable for treatment of individual patients and community parasite eradication campaigns. None of the alternative anti-*S. stercoralis* agents currently in use has been shown to be effective in the treatment of disseminated infection. Parenteral drug preparations would be helpful in patients with impaired gastrointestinal function. Compounds such as ivermectin, which have broad-spectrum systemic antihelminthic activity, offer promise, but there is little available published information about their use in the treatment of *S. stercoralis* in humans.

XIII. PREVENTION

Persons visiting or residing in endemic areas can prevent infection with *S. stercoralis* by avoiding skin contact with soil and materials contaminated with human or animal excreta. In most circumstances, wearing closed shoes at all times and using appropriate sanitary facilities will effectively limit the inter-human spread of this nematode.

Animal caretakers and zoo personnel dealing with primates, dogs, and cats should exert great care when handling biological specimens and excreta from these animals. Reports of human infections acquired from animals have been rare (114,115), but the prevalence of strongyloidiasis in asymptomatic dogs (194,195) and primates (187-189,192) suggests that these animals should be considered potentially infected unless proved otherwise. Rubber gloves, overshoes, and protective clothing should be used when handling the animals and their excreta and while cleaning the cages.

Technicians working in clinical parasitology laboratories should always use rubber gloves when processing fecal specimens. Although in most cases only noninfective rhabditiform larvae are found in the feces of infected persons, some patients pass infective filariform larvae (300). In addition, larvae may molt rapidly in unfixed stool specimens left at room temperature. Therefore, all fecal specimens are best treated as infective. All larval stages of *S. stercoralis* are rapidly killed by contact with 90% alcohol, which should be easily available in the laboratory to immediately rub the skin in case of accidental contact.

Filariform larvae are not resistant to dessication or heat, but in a moist environment they can live for several days and maintain their infectivity. Therefore, all specimens containing *S. stercoralis* as well as equipment and supplies used to process and examine them should be autoclaved before disposal or reuse. If this is not feasible, they may be soaked or washed in a solution of 10% chlorine bleach.

Patients with chronic uncomplicated strongyloidiasis do not normally pose a threat to others, provided that they are continent and that contact with their stools is avoided.

In contrast, patients with extraintestinal infections may have infective filariform larvae in all their body fluids. Most of these patients are severely ill, and they often require intensive care. Catheters, respirators, intravenous lines, and monitoring devices can all become contaminated with infective larvae. Therefore, when the diagnosis of extraintestinal strongyloidiasis is established, these patients should be placed in contact isolation, and all personnel should wear gloves and gowns when attending to them. All fresh specimens collected from these patients should be labeled as infective, and laboratory personnel should handle them according to the guidelines outlined above.

REFERENCES

1. Normand, A. Sur la maladie dite diarrhee de Cochin-Chine. *C. R. Acad. Sci. 83*:316–318 (1876).
2. Scaglia, M., Brustia, R., Gatti, S., Bernuzzi, A. M., Strosselli, M., Malfitano, A., and Cappelli, D. Autochthonous strongyloidiasis in Italy: an epidemiological and clinical review of 150 cases. *Bull. Soc. Pathol. Exot. 77*:328–332 (1984).
3. Walzer, P. D., Milder, J. E., Banwell, J. G., Kilgore, G., Klein, M., and Parker, R. Epidemiologic features of *Strongyloides stercoralis* infection in an endemic area of the United States. *Am. J. Trop. Med. Hyg. 31*:313–319 (1982).
4. Milder, J. E., Walzer, P. D., Kilgore, G., Rutherford, I., and Klein, M. Clinical features of *Strongyloides stercoralis* infection in an endemic area of the United States. *Gastroenterology 80*:1481–1488 (1981).
5. Longworth, D. L., and Weller, P. F. Hyperinfection syndrome with strongyloidiasis. In *Current Clinical Topics in Infectious Diseases* (J. S. Remington and M. N. Swartz, eds.). McGraw-Hill, New York, 1986, pp. 1–26.
6. Bavay, A. Sur l'anguillule stercorale. *C. R. Acad. Sci. 83*:694–695 (1876).
7. Hira, P. R., and Patel, B. G. Human strongyloidiasis due to the primate species *Strongyloides fulleborni*. *Trop. Geogr. Med. 32*:23–29 (1980).
8. Ashford, R. W., Hall, A. J., and Babona, D. Distribution and abundance

of intestinal helminths in man in western Papua New Guinea with special reference to *Strongyloides*. *Ann. Trop. Med. Parasitol.* 75:269–279 (1981).

9. Penner, L. R. Concerning threadworm (*Strongyloides stercoralis*) in great apes-lowland gorillas (*Gorilla gorilla*) and chimpanzees (*Pan troglodytes*). *J. Zoo Animal Med.* 12:128–131 (1982).

10. Cox, D. D., and Todd, A. C. Survey of gastrointestinal parasitism in Wisconsin dairy cattle. *J. Am. Vet. Assoc.* 141:706–711 (1962).

11. Lyons, E. T., Drudge, J. H., and Tolliver, S. C. On the life cycle of *Strongyloides westeri* in the equine. *J. Parasitol.* 59:780–787 (1973).

12. Neilson, J. T. M., and Nghiem, N. D. The dynamics of *Strongyloides papillosus* primary infections in neonatal and adult rabbits. *J. Parasitol.* 60:786–789 (1974).

13. Little, M. D. Comparative morphology of six species of *Strongyloides* (Nematoda) and redefinition of the genus. *J. Parasitol.* 52:69–84 (1966).

14. Levine, N. *Nematode Parasites of Domestic Animals and of Man.* Burgess, Minneapolis, 1980.

15. Little, M. Experimental studies on the life cycle of *Strongyloides*. *J. Parasitol.* 48:41–47 (1962).

16. Faust, E. C. Experimental studies on human and primate species of *Strongyloides*. IV. The pathology of *Strongyloides* infection. *Arch. Pathol.* 29:769–806 (1935).

17. Faust, E. C. Experimental and clinical strongyloidiasis. *Rev. Gastroenterol.* 5:154–158 (1938).

18. Genta, R. M. *Strongyloides stercoralis*: immunobiological consideration on an unusual worm. *Parasitol. Today* 2:241–246 (1986).

19. Chitwood, B. G., and Chitwood, M. B. (eds.). *An Introduction to Nematology*, rev. ed. Chitwood, Baltimore, 1950.

20. Bird, A. F. Further observations on the structure of nematode cuticle. *Parasitology* 48:32–37 (1958).

21. Lee, D. L. An electron microscope study of the body wall of the third-stage larva of *Nippostrongylus brasiliensis*. *Parasitology* 56:127–135 (1966).

22. Grove, D. I., Warton, A., Northern, C., and Papadimitriou, J. M. Electron microscopical studies of *Strongyloides ratti* infective larvae: loss of surface coat during skin penetration. *J. Parasitol.* 73:1030–1034 (1987).

23. Jamuar, M. P. Electron microscope studies on the body wall of the nematode *Nippostrongylus brasiliensis*. *J. Parasitol.* 52:209–232 (1966).

24. Maizels, R. M., Philipp, M., and Ogilvie, B. M. Molecules of the surface of parasitic nematodes as probes of the immune response in infection. *Immunol. Rev.* 61:109–136 (1982).

25. Brumpt, E. Recherches sur le determinisme des sexes et de l'evolution des anguillules parasites (*Strongyloides*). *C.R. Soc. Biol.* 85:149–152 (1921).

26. Faust, E. C. The Panama strains of human *Strongyloides*. *Proc. Soc. Exp. Biol. Med.* 28:253–255 (1930).

27. Galliard, H. Unicite ou pluralite des *Strongyloides*. *C. R. Soc. Biol.* 130:413–416 (1939).

28. Galliard, H. Les types de developpement exogene de *Strongyloides stercoralis* Leur transformation par passages experimentaux. *C. R. Soc. Biol. 141*: 102–105 (1947).
29. Galliard, H. recherches sur l'infestation experimentale a *Strongyloides stercoralis* au Tonkin. *Ann. Parasitol. Hum. Comp. 26*:221–227 (1951).
30. Harper, J. S., Genta, R. M., Gam, A. A., London, W. J., and Neva, F. A. Experimental disseminated strongyloidiasis in *Erythocebus patas*. Part I. Pathology. *Am. J. Trop. Med. Hyg. 33*:431–443 (1984).
31. Genta, R. M. unpublished observations.
32. McRury, J., deMessias, I. T., Walzer, P. D., Huitger, T., and Genta, R. M. Specific IgE responses in human strongyloidiasis. *Clin. Exp. Immunol. 65*: 630–638 (1986).
33. Genta, R. M., Weesner, R., and Walzer, P. D. Strongyloidiasis in Vietnam veterans (letter). *JAMA 258*:3259 (1987).
34. Dafalla, A. A. The indirect fluorescent antibody test for the serodiagnosis of strongyloidiasis. *J. Trop. Med. Hyg. 75*:109–111 (1972).
35. Genta, R. M., and Weil, G. J. Antibodies to *Strongyloides stercoralis* larval surface antigens in chronic strongyloidiasis. *Lab. Invest. 47*:87–90 (1982).
36. Genta, R. M., Frei, D. F., and Linke, M. J. Demonstration and partial characterization of parasite-specific IgA responses in human strongyloidiasis. *J. Clin. Microbiol. 25*:1505–1510 (1987).
37. Genta, R. M., Schad, G. A., and Hellman, M. E. *Strongyloides stercoralis*: parasitological, immunological and pathological observations in immunosuppressed dogs. *Trans. R. Soc. Trop. Med. Hyg. 80*:34–41 (1986).
38. Grove, D. I., and Blair, J. Diagnosis of human strongyloidiasis by immunofluorescence using *Strongyloides ratti* and *S. stercoralis* larvae. *Am. J. Trop. Med. Hyg. 30*:344–349 (1981).
39. Rege, A. A., personal communication, 1986.
40. Lewert, R. M., and Lee, C. Studies on the passage of helminth larvae through host tissues. *J. Infect. Dis. 95*:13–38 (1954).
41. Crompton, D., and Tulley, J. How much ascariasis is there in Africa? *Parasitol. Today 3*:123–127 (1987).
42. Fulmer, H. S., and Huempfner, H. R. Intestinal helminths in eastern Kentucky: a survey in three rural counties. *Am. J. Trop. Med. Hyg. 14*:269–275 (1965).
43. Walker, R. B., Staub, H. B., and Buscho, R. O. Strongyloidiasis in West Virginia. *W. V. Med. J. 78*:57–60 (1982).
44. Berk, S. L., Verghese, A., Alvaryz, S., Hall, K., and Smith, B. Clinical and epidemiological features of strongyloidiasis. A prospective study in rural Tennessee. *Arch. Intern. Med. 147*:1257–1261 (1987).
45. Davidson, R. A. Strongyloidiasis: a presentation of 63 cases. *NC Med. J. 43*:23–25 (1982).
46. Vermund, S. H., Lafleur, F., and McLeod, S. Parasitic infections in a New York City hospital: trends from 1971 to 1984. *Am. J. Public Health 76*: 1024–1026 (1986).
47. Hoffman, S., Barret, E., Norcross, W., et al. Intestinal parasites in Indochinese immigrants. *Am. J. Trop. Med. Hyg. 30*:340–346 (1981).

48. Nutman, T.B., Ottesen, E. A., Ieng, S., Samuels, J., Kimball, E., Lutoski, M., Gam, A. A., and Neva, F. A. Eosinophilia in Southeast Asian refugees: evaluation at a referral center. *J. Infect. Dis. 155*:309–313 (1987).
49. Gyorkos, T. W., Genta, R. M., Viens, and McLean, J. D. Seroepidemiology of *Strongyloides* infection among newly-arrived southeast Asian refugees to Canada. (Submitted for publication, 1988.)
50. Vernes, A., Abdellatifi, M., Dei-Cas, E., Poirriez, J., Abdelmalek, R. Y., Leroux, N., Colin, J. J., and Fourrier, A. Parasitoses et hemoglobinopathies chez 1170 refugies due Sud-Est Asiatique. *Nouv. Presse Med. 11*:2687–2691 (1982).
51. Sampson, I. A., and Grove, D. I. Strongyloidiasis is endemic in another Australian population group: Indochinese immigrants. *Med. J. Aust. 146*: 580–582 (1987).
52. Gonzales, C., and Guevara, G. Parasitismo intestinal humano por helmintos en la provincia de Granada (de 1957 a 1963). Indices globales de parasitizacion. *Rev. Iber. Parasitol. 26*:377–381 (1966).
53. Vieira, R. A. O *"Strongyloides stercoralis"*. Um nematodo de relevante importancia em medicina humana. *J. Med. C-138*:109–126 (1979).
54. Capell-Font, S., Pujol-Farriols, R., Garau-Alemany, J., Pallares-Giner, R., and Campo-Guerri, E. Hiperinfestacion por *Strongyloides stercoralis*. *Med. Clin. (Barcelona)* 79:232–235 (1982).
55. Coulaud, J. P., LeMercier, Y., Tessier, S., and Mechali, D. Analyse epidemiologique, clinique et therapeutique de 427 cas d'anguilluloses observes a Paris. *Bull. Soc. Pathol. Exot. 73*:100–108 (1980).
56. Bouree, P., Taugourdeau, A., Barthelemy, M., Paquignot-Ricome, H., Passeron, J., and Bouvier, J. B. Anguillulose: analyse clinique, biologique et epidemiologique de 350 observations. *Nouv. Presse Med. 10*:679–681 (1981).
57. Cadranel, J. F., Eugene, C., and Quevauvilliers, J. Anquillulose autochtone chez une malade suivie pour une maladie de Hodgkin (letter). *Presse Med. 15*:1831 (1986).
58. Sutter, F., Scaglia, M., Minoli, L., Capra, A., and Carosi, G. La strongiloidosi in provincia di Pavia: attuali aspetti di epidemiologia, clinica e terapia. *Giorn. Mal. Inf. Parass. 33*:30–36 (1981).
59. Giannoulis, E., Arvanitakis, C., Zaphiropoulos, A., Nakos, V., Karkavelas, G., and Haralambidis, S. Disseminated strongyloidiasis with uncommon manifestations in Greece. *J. Trop. Med. Hyg. 89*:171–178 (1986).
60. Jokovic, B., Nikilic, B., and Petkovic, M. O rasprostranjenosti strongiloidoze u SFRJ. Zbornik Vojni Medicinska Akademija, Beograd 1973, pp. 53–54.
61. Breitenfeld, V., and Iskra, M. Strongiloidoza u nas i u svijetu. *Lijek. viesnik 106*:33–38 (1984).
62. Lupascu, G., Dancescu, P., Tintareaunu, J., and Smolinski, M. Aspects of the epidemiology of strongyloidiasis in Romania. *Streszcz. mat. IX Zjazdu PTP, Katowice 18–20*:112–113 (1967).
63. Dancescu, P. Recherches sur un foyer endemique de strongyloidose de la zone temperee. *Bull. Soc. Pathol. Exot. 61*:651–661 (1968).
64. Soroczan, W. *Strongyloides stercoralis* in eastern and southeastern Poland. *Wiad. Parazytol. 22*:515–516 (1976).

65. Soroczan, W. Wegorek jelitowy (*Strongyloides sterocoralis*) we wschodniej i poludniowo-wschodniej Polsce. *Wiad. Parasytol.* 22:261–272 (1976).
66. Soroczan, W. The life cycle of *Strongyloides stercoralis* in the temperate zone. *Acta Parasitol. Polon.* 24:269–267 (1977).
67. Kuliew, N. K rasprostranieniu strongiloidoza w ankilostomidoznych rejjonach Axerbajdzanskoj SSR. *Med. Parasizotol. Parazitarn. Boezni.* 37:622–623 (1968).
68. Sprott, V., Shelby, C. D., Ispahani, P., and Toghill, P. J. Indigenous strongyloidiasis in Nottingham. *Br. Med. J.* 294:741–742 (1987).
69. Fraisse, J. L., Douhet, M., Derrida, J. P., and Lancastre, F. Decouverte d'une strongyloidose persistant depuis au moins 35 ans. *Nouv. Presse, Med.* 7:209 (1978).
70. Lapierre, J. Aspects epidemiologuiques, cliniques et therapeutiques de l'anguillulose. A propos de 150 cas observes a Paris, dont trois autochtones. *Evol. Med.* 13:19–25 (1969).
71. Develoux, M., Datry, A., and Mogahed, A. Larva currens relevant une anguillulose cinquante ans apres le retour de zone d'endemie. *Nouv. Presse Med.* 10:2906–2907 (1981).
72. Junod, C. Etude retrospective de 1934 cas de strongyloidose diagnostiques a Paris (1970–1986). I Epidemiologic. *Bull. Soc. Pathol. Exp.* 80:357–369 (1987).
73. Cook, G. C. *Strongyloides stercoralis* hyperinfection syndrome: how often is it missed? (editorial). *Q. J. Med.* 244:625–629 (1987).
74. Royle, G., Fraser-Moodie, A., and Jones, M. W. Hyperinfection with *Strongyloides stercoralis* in Great Britain. *Br. J. Surg.* 61:498–500 (1974).
75. Berhoud, F., and Berthoud, S. A propos de 18 cas d'anguillulose diagnostiques a Geneve. *Schweizer. Med. Wochensch.* 105:1110–1115 (1975).
76. Flensted-Jensen, J. Kutan strongyloidiasis. *Ugeskr. Laeg.* 144:721–722 (1982).
77. Moesgaard, F., Steven, K., and Engbaek, K. A case with severe diarrhea and *Strongyloides stercoralis* infection. *Acta Med. Scand.* 209:333–334 (1981).
78. Pettersson, T., Stenstrom, R., and Kyrjonseppa, H. Disseminated lung opacities and cavitation associated with *Strongyloides stercoralis* and *Schistosoma mansoni* infection. *Am. J. Trop. Med. Hyg.* 23:158–162 (1974).
79. Faria, J. Prevalencia de *Strongyloides stercoralis* em escolares de 7–14 anos na cidade do Salvador. *Gaz. Med. Bahia* 72:59–63 (1972).
80. Coutinho, J. O., Croce, J., Camros, R., Amato-Neto, V., and Fonseca, L. C. Contribucao para o conhecimento da estrongiloidose humana em Sao Paulo. *Folia Clin. Biol.* 20:141–176 (1953).
81. deMessias, I. T., Telles, F. Q., Boaretti, A. C., Sliva, S., Guimarres, L. M., and Genta, R. M. Clinical, immunological and epidemiological aspects of strongyloidiasis in an endemic area of Brazil. *Allergol. Immunopathol.* 15:37–41 (1987).
82. Avagnina, M. A., Elsner, B., Iotti, R. M., and Re, R. *Strongyloides stercoralis* in Papanicolaou-stained smears of ascitic fluid. *Acta Cytol.* 24:36–39 (1980).

83. Bezares, R. F., Carrares, L. O., Marin, C. A., Rodriguez, O. A., Tezanos-Pinto, M., and Nunez, E. N. Fatal *Strongyloides stercoralis* hyperinfection in acute leukemia. *Lancet 1*:481 (1983).

84. Garcia, F. T., Sessions, J. T., Strum, W. B., Tripathy, K., Balanos, O., Duque, E., Ramelli, D., and Mayoral, L. G. Intestinal function and morphology in strongyloidiasis. *Am. J. Trop. Med Hyg. 26*:859–865 (1977).

85. Lopez, J. E., Marciano-Torres, M., Pena, R. J., Qunitni, A., Malpica, C. C., Lopez, J. E., and Salazar, Y. L. Hepatitis granulomatosa producida por el *Strongyloides stercoralis*. Presentacion de un caso con confirmacion histopatologica. *Rev. Soc. Venez. Gastroenterol. 38*:133–143 (1984).

86. Arroyo, R., Troper, L., and Vargas, G. Estrongiloidiasis fatal. Estudio de ocho casos de autopsia. *Pathologia (Mex.) 23*:135–146 (1985).

87. Carreon-Moldir, J. Bolivian Society of Pathology, La Paz, personal communication. 1985.

88. Bras, G., Richards, R. C., Irvine, R. A., Milner, P. F., and Ragbeer, M. M. Infection with *Strongyloides stercoralis* in Jamaica. *Lancet 2*:1257–1260 (1964).

89. Quinones-Soto, R. A., Harrington, P. T., Gutierrez-Nunez, J. J., Ramirez-Ronda, C. H., and Bermudez, R. H. Estrongiloidiasis en el paciente immunocomprometido. *Bol. Asoc. Med. Puerto Rico 73*:562–566 (1981).

90. Bartholomew, C., Bhaskar, A. G., Butler, A. K., and Jankey, N. Pseudo-obstruction and sprue-like syndrome from strongyloidiasis. *Postgrad. Med. J. 53*:139–142 (1977).

91. Fowler, C. G., Lindsay, I., Lewin, J., Sweny, P., Fernando, O. N., and Moorhead, J. F. Recurrent hyperinfestation with *Strongyloides stercoralis* in a renal allograft recipient. *Br. Med. J. 285*:1394 (1982).

92. Smallman, L. A., Young, J. A., Shortland-Webb, W. R., Carey, M. P., and Michael, J. *Strongyloides stercoralis* hyperinfestation syndrome with *E. coli* meningitis: report of two cases. *J. Clin. Pathol. 39*:366–370 (1986).

93. Brumpt, L. C., Sang, H. T., and Jaeger, G. Quelques reflexions a propos du parasitisme sanguin et intestinal dans deux villages d'Afriques Centrale. *Bull. Soc. Pathol. Exot. 65*:263–270 (1972).

94. Ejezie, G. C., and Otigbuo, I. N. The stabilizing factors of parasitic infections in Nigeria. *J. Hyg. Epidemiol. Microbiol. Immunol. 31*:45–51 (1987).

95. Ilardi, I., Shiddo, S. C., Mohamed, H. H., Mussa, C., Hussein, A. S., Mohamed, C. S., Leone, F., and Amiconi, G. The prevalence and intensity of intestinal parasites in two Somalian communities. *Trans. R. Soc. Trop. Med. Hyg. 81*:336–338 (1987).

96. Leelarasamee, A., Nimmannit, S., Nankorn, S., et al. Disseminated strongyloidiasis: report of seven cases. *Southeast Asian J. Trop. Med. Public Health 94*:539–542 (1978).

97. Keittivuti, B., Agnes. T. D., Keittivuti, A., and Viravaidya, M. Prevalence of schistosomiasis and other parasitic diseases among Cambodian refugees residing in Bang-Kaeng holding center, Prachinburi Province, Thailand. *Am. J. Trop. Med. Hyg. 31*:988–990 (1982).

98. Douce, R. W., Brown, A. E., Khambooruang, C., Walzer, P. D., and Genta, R. M. Seroepidemiology of strongyloidiasis in a Thai village. *Int. J. Parasitol.* *17*:1343–1348 (1987).

99. Fujita, K., Tajima, K., Tominaga, S., Tsukidate, S., Nakada, K., Imai, J., and Hinuma, Y. Seroepidemiological studies on *Strongyloides* infection in adult T-cell leukemia virus carriers in Okinawa Island, Japan. *Trop. Med.* *27*:203–209 (1985).

100. Gill, G. V., and Bell, D. R. *Strongyloides stercoralis* infection in former Far East prisoners of war. *Br. Med. J.* *2*:572–574 (1979).

101. Grove, D. I. *Strongyloides* in Allied ex-prisoners of war in South-East Asia. *Br. Med. J.* *1*:598–601 (1980).

102. Pelletier, L. L. Chronic strongyloidiasis in World War II Far East ex-prisoners of war. *Am. J. Trop. Med. Hyg.* *33*:55–61 (1984).

103. Genta, R. M., Weesner, R., Douce, R. W., Huitger-O'Connor, T., and Walzer, P. D. Strongyloidiasis in United States veterans of the Vietnam and other wars. *JAMA 258*:49–52 (1987).

104. Proctor, E. M., Isaac-Renton, J., Robertson, W. B., and Black, W. A. Strongyloidiasis in Canadian Far East war veterans. *Can. Med. Assoc. J.* *133*:876–878 (1985).

105. Hoy, W. E., Roberts, N. J., Bryson, M. F., Bowels, C., Lee, J. C., Rivero, A. J., and Ritterson, A. L. Transmission of strongyloidiasis by kidney transplant? Disseminated strongyloidiasis in both recipients of kidney allografts from a single cadaver donor. *JAMA 246*:1937–1939 (1981).

106. Brumpt, L. C. Peut-on contracter l'anguillulose dans une piscine? *Nouvelle Presse Med.* *5*:434–435 (1975).

107. Wilson, P. A. G., Cameron, M., and Scott, D. S. Patterns of milk transmission of *Strongyloides ratti. Parasitology 77*:87–96 (1978).

108. Brown, R. C., and Girardeau, M. H. Transmammary passage of *Strongyloides* sp. larvae in the human host. *Am. J. Trop. Med. Hyg. 26*:215–219 (1977).

109. Yoeli, M., Most, H., Hammond, J., et al. Parasitic infections in a closed community. Results of a 10-year survey in Willowbrook State School. *Trans. R. Soc. Trop. Med. Hyg. 66*:764–776 (1972).

110. Sargent, R. G. Parasitic infection among residents of an institution for mentally retarded persons. *Am. J. Mental Defic. 87*:566–569 (1983).

111. Proctor, E. M., Muth, H. A. V., Proudfoot, D. L., Allen, A. B., Fisk, R., Isaac-Renton, J., and Black, W. A. Endemic institutional strongyloidiasis in British Columbia. *Can. Med. Assoc. J. 136*:1173–1176 (1987).

112. Grove, D. I. Strongyloidiasis: is it transmitted from husband to wife? *Br. J. Vener. Dis. 58*:271–272 (1982).

113. Quinn, C., Stamm, W., Goodell, S., Mkrtichian, E., Benedetti, P., Corey, L., Schuffler, M., and Holmes, K. The polymicrobial origin of intestinal infections in homosexual men. *New Engl. J. Med. 309*:576–582 (1983).

114. Galliard, H. Recherches sur la strongyloidose au Tonkin. Role des animaux domestiques dans l'etiologie de l'infestation humaine. *Ann. Parasitol. 17*:533–541 (1940).

115. Georgi, J. R., and Sprinkle, C. L. A case of human strongyloidosis apparently contracted from asymptomatic colony dogs. *Am. J. Trop. Med. Hyg.* *23*:899–901 (1974).

116. Golgi, C., and Monti, A. Sulla storia naturale e sul significato clinico-patologico delle cosiddette anguillule intestinali e stercorali. *Arch. Sci. Med. 10* (3), 93–107 (1886).

117. DePaola, D. Patologia de estrongiloidiase. *Bol. Cent. Est. Hosp. Serv. Est. 14*:3–98 (1962).

118. DePaola, D., Braga-Dias, L., and daSilva, J. R. Enteritis due to *Strongyloides stercoralis. Am. J. Dig. Dis.* *7*:1086–1098 (1962).

119. Caymmi-Gomes, M. Mecanismos patologicos relacionados a autoendo-infeccao na estrongiloidose humana fatal. *Rev. Patol. Trop.* *9*:165–261 (1980).

120. Alcorn, M. O., and Kotcher, E. Secondary malabsorption syndrome produced by chronic strongyloidiasis. *South. Med. J.* *54*:193–197 (1961).

121. Milner, P. F., Irvine, R. A., Barton, C. J., Bras, G., and Richards, R. Infestinal malabsorption in *Strongyloides stercoralis* infestation. *Gut 6*:574–581 (1965).

122. Ruiz-Macia, J. A., Pons-Minano, J. A., Bermejo-Lopez, J., Felices-Abad, F., Serra-Sevilla, J. A., and Felices-Abad, J. M. Estrongloidiasis diseminada: estudio clinico-patologico de un caso diagnosticado en autopsia. *Rev. Clin. Espanola 180*:381–384 (1987).

123. Berry, A. J., Long, E. G., Smith, J. H., Gourley, W. K., and Fine, D. P. Chronic relapsing colitis due to *Strongyloides stercoralis. Am. J. Trop. Med. Hyg. 32*:1289–1293 (1983).

124. Noodleman, J. S. Eosinophilic appendicitis. Demonstration of *Strongyloides stercoralis* as a causative agent. *Arch. Pathol. Lab. Med. 105*:148–149 (1981).

125. Williford, M. D., Foster, W. L., Halvorsen, R. A., and Thompson, W. M. Emphysematous gastritis secondary to disseminated strongyloidiasis. *Gastrointest. Radiol. 7*:123–126 (1982).

126. Lintermans, J. P. Fatal peritonitis, an unusual complication of *Strongyloides stercoralis* infestation. *Clin. Pediatr. 14*:974–975 (1975).

127. Igra-Siegman, Y., Kapila, R., Sen, P., Kaminski, Z. C., and Louria, D. B. Syndrome of hyperinfection with *Strongyloides stercoralis. Rev. Infect. Dis. 3*:397–407 (1981).

128. Rassiga, A. L., Lowry, J. L., and Forman, W. B. Diffuse pulmonary infection due to *Strongyloides stercoralis. JAMA 230*:426–427 (1974).

129. Scoggin, C. H., and Branson-Call, N. Acute respiratory failure due to disseminated strongyloidiasis in a renal transplant patient. *Ann. Intern. Med. 87*:456–458 (1977).

130. Seabury, J. H., Abadie, S., and Savoy, F. Pulmonary strongyloidiasis with lung abscess. Ineffectiveness of thiabendazole therapy. *Am. J. Trop. Med. Hyg. 20*:209–211 (1971).

131. Owor, R., and Wamkota, W. M. A fatal case of strongyloidiasis with *Strongyloides* larvae in the meninges. *Trans. R. Soc. Trop. Med. Hyg. 70*: 497–499 (1976).

132. Neefe, L. I., Pinilla, O., Garagusi, V. F., and Baur, H. Disseminated strongyloidiasis with cerebral involvement. A complication of steroid therapy. *Am. J. Med.* 55:832–837 (1973).

133. Masdeu, J. C., Tantulavenich, S., Gorelick, P. P., Maliwan, N., Heredia, S., Mertinez-Lage, J. M., Ross, E., and Mamdani, M. Brain abscess caused by *Strongyloides stercoralis. Arch. Neurol.* 39:62–63 (1982).

134. Poltera, A. A., and Katsimbura, N. Granulomatous hepatitis due to *Strongyloides stercoralis. J. Pathol.* 113:241–246 (1974).

135. Hakim, S. Z., and Genta, R. M. Fatal strongyloidiasis in a Vietnam veteran. *Arch. Pathol. Lab. Med.* 110:809–812 (1986).

136. Smith, J. D., Goette, D. K., and Odom, R. B. Larva currens. Cutaneous strongyloidiasis. *Arch. Dermatol.* 112:1161–1163 (1976).

137. Kalb, R. E., and Grossman, M. E. Periumbilical purpura in disseminated strongyloidiasis. *JAMA* 256:1170–1171 (1986).

138. Crump-Brannon, M. J., and Faust E. C. Preparation and testing of a specific antigen for diagnosis of human strongyloidiasis. *Am. J. Trop. Med.* 29:229–239 (1949).

139. Pelegrino, J., Chaia, G., and Pompeu-Memoria, J. M. Observacose sobre a reacao intradermica com antigeno de *Strongyloides ratti* em pacientes com estrongiloidose. *Rev. Inst. Med. Top. Sao Paulo* 3:181–185 (1961).

140. Tribouley-Duret, J., Tribouley, J., and Paturizel, R. Interet de tests d'allergie cutanee pour le diagnostic de la strongyloidose. *Bull. Soc. Pathol. Exot.* 69:360–367 (1976).

141. Sato, Y., Otsura, M., Takara, M., and Shiroma, Y. Intradermal reactions in strongyloidiasis. *Int. J. Parasitol.* 16:87–91 (1986).

142. Sato, Y., Takara, M., and Otsuru, M. Detection of antibodies in strongyloidiasis by enzyme-linked immunosorbent assay (ELISA). *Trans. R. Soc. Trop. Med. Hyg.* 79:51–55 (1985).

143. Carroll, S. M., Larthigasu, K. T., and Grove, D. I. Serodiagnosis of human strongyloidiasis by an enzyme-linked immunosorbent assay. *Trans. R. Soc. Trop. Med. Hyg.* 75:706–709 (1981).

144. Neva, F. A., Gam, A. A., and Burke, J. Comparison of larval antigens in an enzyme-linked immunosorbent assay of strongyloidiasis in humans. *J. Infect. Dis.* 144:427–432 (1981).

145. Genta, R. M., Ottesen, E. A., Poindexter, R. W., Gam, A. A., Neva, F. A., Tanowitz, H. B., and Wittner, M. Specific allargic sensitization to *Strongyloides* antigens in human strongyloidiasis. *Lab. Invest.* 48:633–638 (1983).

146. Ottesen, E. A., Kumaraswami, V., Paranjape, R., Poindexter, R. W., and Tripathy, S. P. Naturally occurring blocking in human filariasis. *J. Immunolog.* 127:2014–2019 (1981).

147. Hofstetter, M., Poindexter, R. W., Ruiz-Tiben, E., and Ottesen, E. A. Modulation of the host response in human schistosomiasis. III. Blocking antibodies specifically inhibit immediate hypersensitivity responses to parasitic antigens. *Immunology* 46:777–782 (1982).

148. Genta, R. M., Douce, R. W., and Walzer, P. D. Diagnostic implications

of parasite-specific immune responses in immunocompromised patients with strongyloidiasis. *J. Clin. Microbiol. 23*:1099–1103 (1986).

149. Carvalho, E. M., Andrade, T. M., Andrade, J. A., and Rocha, H. Immunological features in different clinical forms of strongyloidiasis. *Trans. Soc. Trop. Med. Hyg. 77*:346–349 (1983).

150. Badaro', R., Carvalho, E. M., Santos, R. B., Gam, A. A., and Genta, R. M. Parasite-specific humoral responses in different clinical forms of strongyloidiasis. *Trans. R. Soc. Trop. Med. Hyg. 81*:149–150 (1987).

151. Genta, R. M., Ottesen, E. A., Gam, A. A., Neva, F. A., Wittner, M., Tanowitz, H. B., and Walzer, P. D. Cellular responses in human strongyloidiasis. *Am. J. Trop. Med. Hyg. 32*:990–994 (1983).

152. Ottesen, E. A. Immunopathology of lymphatic filariasis in man. *Springer Semin. Immunopathol. 2*:373 (1980).

153. Butterworth, A. E., Taylor, D. W., Veith, M. C., et al. Studies on the mechanisms of immunity in human schistosomiasis. *Immunol. Rev. 61*: 5–39 (1982).

154. Schad, G. A., and Anderson, R. M. Predisposition to hookworm infection in humans. *Science 228*:1537–1539 (1985).

155. Sheldon, A. J. Specificity of artificially acquired immunity to *Strongyloides ratti. Am. J. Hyg. 29*:47–50 (1939).

156. Abadie, S. The life cycle of *Strongyloides ratti. J. Parasitol. 49*:241–248 (1963).

157. Wertheim, G., and Lengy, J. Growth and development of *Strongyloides ratti* Sandground, 1925, in the albino rat. *J. Parasitol. 51*:636–639 (1965).

158. Olson, E. C., and Schiller, E. L. *Strongyloides ratti* infections in rats. I. Immunopathology. *Am. J. Trop. Med. Hyg. 27*:521–526 (1978).

159. Murrell, K. D. *Strongyloides ratti*:acquired resistance in the rat to the preintestinal migrating larvae. *Exp. Parasitol. 50*:417–425 (1980).

160. Murrell, K. D. Protective role of immunoglobulin G and immunity to *Strongyloides ratti. J. Parasitol. 67*:167–173 (1980).

161. Dawkins, H. J. S., and Grove, D. I. Transfer by serum and cells of resistance to infection with *Strongyloides ratti* in mice. *Immunology 43*:317–322 (1981).

162. Genta, R. M., Ottesen, E. A., Gam, A. A., and Neva, F. A. Immune responses in experimental *Strongyloides ratti* infection in rats. *Parasitol. Res. 69*:667–675 (1983).

163. Genta, R. M., and Schad, G. A. Animal models of human disease: strongyloidiasis. *Comp. Pathol. Bull. 18*:2–4 (1986).

164. Davidson, R. A., Fletcher, R. H., and Chapman, L. E. Risk factors for strongyloidiasis. *Arch. Intern. Med. 144*:321–324 (1984).

165. Dobbins, W. O. Human intestinal intraepithelial lymphocytes. *Gut 27*:972–985 (1986).

166. Allardyce, R. A., and Bienenstock, J. The mucosal immune system in health and disease, with an emphasis on parasitic infection. *Bull. WHO 62*: 7–25 (1984).

167. Batt, R. M., and Peters, T. J. Effects of prednisone on the intestinal mucosa of the rat. *Clin. Sc. Mol. Med. 50*:511–523 (1976).

168. Meyers, S., Sachar, D. B., and Goldberg, J. D. Corticotropin versus hydrocortisone in the intravenous treatment of ulcerative colitis. A prospective randomized double-blind clinical trial. *Gastroenterology 85*:351–357 (1983).

169. Haeney, M. R. Acquired immune deficiency syndrome (AIDS) and the gastrointestinal tract. In *Immunopathology of the Small Intestine* (M. N. Marsh, ed.). Wiley, Chichester, 1987.

170. Sinniah, B. Parasites of some rodents in Malaysia. *Southeast Asian Trop. Med. Public Health 10*:115–121 (1979).

171. Moqbel, R., and Wakelin, D. Immunity to *Strongyloides ratti* in rats. I. Adoptive transfer with mesenteric lymph node cells. *Parasite Immunol. 3*: 181–188 (1981).

172. Wilson, P. A. G., Cameron, M., and Scott, D. S. *Strongyloides ratti* in virgin female rates: studies of oestrous cycle effects and general variability. *Parasitology 76*:221–227 (1978).

173. Wilson, P. A. G., Steven, G. E., and Simpson, N. E. *Strongyloides ratti* (homogonic): the time-course of early migration in the generalized host deduced from experiments in lactating rats. *Parasitology 85*:533–542 (1982).

174. Moqbel, R., and Denham, D. A. *Strongyloides ratti*: the effect of betamethasone on the course of infection in rats. *Parasitology 76*:289–298 (1978).

175. Olson, E. C., and Schiller, E. L. *Strongyloides ratti* infection in rats. II. Effects of cortisone treatment. *Am. J. Trop. Med. Hyg. 27*:527–531 (1978).

176. Tada, I., Mimori, T., and Nakai, M. Migration route of *Strongyloides ratti* in albino rats. *Jap. J. Parasitol. 28*:219–227 (1979).

177. Goldgraber, M. B., and Lewert, R. M. Immunological injury of mast cells and connective tissue in mice infected with *Strongyloides ratti*. *J. Parasitol. 51*:169–174 (1965).

178. Dawkins, H. J. S., Grove, D. I., Dunsmore, J. D., and Mitchell, G. F. *Strongyloides ratti*: susceptibility to infection and resistance to reinfection in inbred strains of mice as assessed by excretion of larvae. *Int. J. Parasitol. 10*:125–129 (1980).

179. Dawkins, H. J. S., Thomason, H. J., and Grove, D. I. The occurrence of *Strongyloides ratti* in the tissue of mice after percutaneous infection. *J. Helminthol. 56*:45–50 (1982).

180. Dawkins, H. J. S., Grove, D. I., Dunsmore, J. D., and Mitchell, G. F. Kinetics of primary and secondary infections with *Strongyloides ratti* in mice. *Int. J. Parasitol. 11*:89–96 (1981).

181. Grove, D. I. *Strongyloides ratti* and *Strongyloides stercoralis*: the effects of thiabendazole, mebendazole, and cambendazole in infected mice. *Am. J. Trop. Med. Hyg. 31*:469–476 (1982).

182. Mojon, M., Saura, C., Roojee, N., and Tran Manh Sung, R. Albendazole and tiabendazole in murine strongyloidiasis. *J. Antimicrob. Chemother.* *19*:79–85 (1987).

183. Dawkins, H. J. S., and Grove, D. I. Attempts to establish infection with *Strongyloides stercoralis* in mice and other laboratory animals. *J. Helminthol.* *56*:23–26 (1982).

184. Grove, D. I., Northern, C., and Heenan, P. *S. stercoralis* infections in the muscles of mice: a model for investigating the systemic phase of strongyloidiasis. *Pathology 18*:72–76 (1986).

185. Genta, R. M., and Ward, P. A. Histopathology of experimental strongyloidiasis. *Am. J. Pathol. 99*:208–220 (1980).

186. Moqbel, R. Histopathological changes following primary, secondary, and repeated infections of rats with *Strongyloides ratti*, with special reference to tissue eosinophils. *Parasite Immunol. 2*:11–27 (1980).

187. Liebegott, F. Pericarditis verminosa (*Strongyloides*) beim schimpanse. *Virchows Arch. Pathol. Anat. 335*:211–225 (1962).

188. McClure, H. M., Strozier, L. M., Keeling, M. E., and Helay, G. R. Strongyloidosis in two infant orangutans. *J. Am. Vet. Med. Assoc. 163*:629–632 (1973).

189. De Paoli, A., and Johnsen, D. O. Fatal strongyloidiasis in gibbons (*Hylobates lar*). *Vet. Pathol. 15*:31–39 (1978).

190. Fulleborn, F. On the larval migration of some parasitic nematodes in the body of the host and its biological significance. *J. Helminthol. 7*:15–44 (1929).

191. De Paoli, A. Strongyloidiasis: a comparative study in the gibbon and man. Doctoral dissertation, George Washington University, Washington, DC, 1974.

192. Harper, J. S., Rice, J. M., London, W. T., Sly, D. L., and Middleton, C. Disseminated strongyloidiasis in *Erythrocelsus patas* monkeys. *J. Primatol. 3*:89–98 (1982).

193. Genta, R. M., Harper, J. S., Gam, A. A., London, W. J., and Neva, F. A. Experimental disseminated strongyloidiasis in *Erythrocebus patas*. Part II. Immunology. *Am. J. Trop. Med. Hyg. 33*:444–450 (1984).

194. Jaskoski, B. J., Barr, V., and Borges, M. Intestinal parasites of well-cared-for dogs: an area revisited. *Am. J. Trop. Med. Hyg. 31*:1107–1110 (1982).

195. Prosl, H. Zum Vorkommen von *Strongyloides stercoralis* bein Hunden in Osterreich. *Mitt. Osterr. Ges. Tropenmed. Parasitol. 7*:129–134 (1985).

196. Nishigori, M. The factors which influence the external development of *Strongyloides stercoralis* an on auto-infection with this parasite. *J. Formosa Med. Assoc. 276*:1–28 (1928).

197. Sandground, J. H. Some studies on susceptibility, resistance, and acquired immunity to infection with *Strongyloides stercoralis* (Nematoda) in dogs and cats. *Am. J. Hyg. 8*:507–538 (1928).

198. Galliard, H., and Berdonneau, R. Strongyloidose experimentale chez le chien. Effets de la cortisone. Resultats du test de Thorn à l'hormone corticotrope (ACTH). *Ann. Parasitol. 23*:163–171 (1953).

199. Grove, D. I., and Northern, C. Infection and immunity in dogs infected with a human strain of *Strongyloides stercoralis*. *Trans. R. Soc. Trop. Med. Hyg.* 76:833–838 (1982).

200. Grove, D. I., Heenan, P. J., and Northern, C. Persistence and disseminated infections with *Strongyloides stercoralis* in immunosuppressed dogs. *Int. J. Parasitol.* 13:483–490 (1983).

201. Schad, G. A., Hellman, M. E., and Muncey, D. W. *Strongyloides stercoralis*: hyperinfection in immunosuppressed dogs. *Exp. Parasitol.* 57:287–296 (1984).

202. Carvalho-Filho, E. Strongyloidiasis. *Clin. Gastroenterol.* 7:179–200 (1978).

203. Junod, C. Etude retrospective de 1934 cas de strongyloidose diagnostiques a Paris (1970–1986). II. Diagnostic, eosinophilie, traitement. *Bull. Soc. Pathol. Exp.* 80:370–382 (1997).

204. Jones, C. A. Clinical studies in human strongyloidiasis. I. Semeiology. *Gastroenterology* 16:743–756 (1950).

205. Smith, S. B., Schwartzman, M., Mencia, L. F., Blum, E. B., Krogstad, D., Nitzkin, J., and Healy, G. R. Fatal disseminated strongyloidiasis presenting as acute abdominal distress in an urban child. *J. Pediatr.* 91:607–609 (1977).

206. Brasitus, T. A., Gold, R. P., Kay, R. H., Magum, A. M., and Lee, W. M. Intestinal strongyloidiasis. A case report and review of the literature. *Am. J. Gastroenterol.* 73:65–69 (1980).

207. Rubenstein, M. Strongyloidiasis associated with ulcerative colitis. *J. Med. Soc. New Jersey* 67:779–780 (1970).

208. Wilson, K. H., and Kauffman, C. A. Persistent *Strongyloides stercoralis* in blind loop of the bowel. *Arch. Intern. Med.* 143:357–358 (1983).

209. Amir-Ahmadi, H., Brown, P., Neva, F. A., Gottlieb, L. S., and Zamcheck, N. Strongyloidiasis at the Boston City Hospital. *Am. J. Dig. Dis.* 13:959–973 (1968).

210. Corsini, A. C. Strongyloidiasis and chronic urticaria. *Postgrad. Med. J.* 58:247–248 (1982).

211. Arthur, R. P., and Shelly, W. B. Larva currens. A distinct variant of cutaneous larva migrans due to *Strongyloides stercoralis*. *Arch. Dermatol.* 78:186–190 (1958).

212. Cunliffe, W. J., and Silva, L. G. Linear urticaria due to larva currens—strongyloidiasis. *Br. J. Dermatol.* 80:108–110 (1968).

213. Stone, O. J., Newell, G. B., and Mullins, J. F. Cutaneous strongyloidiasis: larva currens. *Arch. Dermatol.* 105:734–736 (1972).

214. Brumpt, L. C., and Sang, H. T. Larva currens seul signe pathognomonique de la strongyloidose. *Ann. Parasitol. (Paris)* 48:319–328 (1973).

215. Nwokolo, C., and Imohiosen, E. A. Strongyloidiasis of respiratory tract presenting as "asthma." *Br. Med. J.* 2:153–154 (1973).

216. Bocanegra, T. S., Espinoza, L. R., Bridgeford, P. H., Vasey, F. B., and Germain, B. F. Reactive arthritis induced by parasitic infection. *Ann. Intern. Med.* 94:207–209 (1981).

217. Akoglu, T., Tuncer, I., Erken, E., Gurcay, A., Ozer, F. L., and Ozcan, K.

Parasitic arthritis induced by *Strongyloides stercoralis. Ann. Rheum. Dis.* 43:523–525 (1984).

218. Bequet, R., Dutoit, E., Poirriez, J., Dutoit, A., and Vernes, A. Forme cardiaque de l'anguillulose. *Presse Med.* 12:1366–1367 (1983).

219. Kane, M. G., Luby, J. P., and Krejs, G. J. Intestinal secretion as a cause of hypokalemia and cardiac arrest in a patient with strongyloidiasis. *Dig. Dis. Sci.* 29:768–772 (1984).

220. Haggerty, J. J., and Sandler, R. Strongyloidiasis presenting as depression: a case report. *J. Clin. Psychiatry* 43:340–341 (1982).

221. Gage, J. G. A case of *Strongyloides intestinalis* with larvae in the sputum. *Arch. Intern. Med.* 7:561–579 (1911).

222. Ophuls, W. A fatal case of strongyloidosis in man, with autopsy. *Arch. Pathol.* 8:1–8 (1929).

223. Faust, E. C., and DeGroat, A. Internal autoinfection in human strongyloidiasis. *Am. J. Trop. Med.* 20:359–375 (1940).

224. Hartz, P. H. Human strongyloidiasis with internal autoinfection. *Arch. Pathol.* 41:601–611 (1946).

225. Leite-Dias, G. Fatal infection by *Strongyloides stercoralis.* Report of a case. *Gastroenterology* 38:255–258 (1960).

226. Cruz, T., Reboucas, G., and Rocha, H. Fatal strongyloidiasis in patients receiving corticosteroids. *New Engl. J. Med.* 275:1093–1096 (1966).

227. Willis, A. J., and Nwokolo, C. Steroid therapy and strongyloidiasis. *Lancet* 1:1396–1398 (1966).

228. Civantos, F., and Robinson, M. J. Fatal strongyloidiasis following corticosteroid therapy. *Am. J. Dig. Dis.* 14:643–651 (1969).

229. Rivera, E., Maldonado, N., Velez-Garcia, E., Grillo, A., and Malaret, G. Hyperinfection syndrome with *Strongyloides stercoralis. Ann. Intern. Med.* 72:199–204 (1970).

230. Purtilo, D. T., Meyers, W. M., and Connor, D. H. Fatal strongyloidiasis in immunosuppressed patients. *Am. J. Med.* 56:488–493 (1974).

231. Dwork, K. G., Jaffe, J. R., and Lieberman, H. D. Strongyloidiasis with massive hyperinfection. *NY State J. Med.* 75:1230–1234 (1975).

232. Scowden, E. B., Schaffner, W., and Stone, W. J. Overwhelming strongyloidiasis. An unappreciated opportunistic infection. *Medicine (Baltimore)* 57:527–544 (1978).

233. West, B. C., and Wilson, J. P. Subconjunctival corticosteroid therapy complicated by hyperinfective strongyloidiasis. *Am. J. Ophthalmol.* 89:854–857 (1980).

234. Orecchia, G., Pazzaglia, A., Scaglia, M., and Rabbiosi, G. Larva currens following systemic steroid therapy in a case of strongyloidiasis. *Dermatologica* 171:366–367 (1985).

235. Higenbottam, T. W., and Heard, B. E. Opportunistic pulmonary strongyloidiasis complicating asthma treated with steroids. *Thorax* 31:226–233 (1976).

236. Briner, J., Eckert, J., Drei, D., Largiader, F., Binswanger, U., and Blumberg, A. Strongyloidiasis nach nierentransplantation. *Schweiz. Med. Wochenschr. 108*:1632–1637 (1978).

237. Meyrier, A., Sraer, J. D., Kourilsky, O., Jablonsky, J. P., Christol, D., Mayaud, C., and Richet, G. Anguillulose pulmonaire mortelle compliquant une transplantation renale. *Ann. Med. Interne 131*:153–156 (1980).

238. Weller, I. V., Copland, P., and Gabriel, R. *Strongyloides stercoralis* infection in a renal transplant patient. *Br. Med. J. 282*:524 (1981).

239. Morgan, J. S., Schaffner, W., and Stone, W. J. Opportunistic strongyloidiasis in renal transplant recipients. *Transplantation 42*:518–524 (1986).

240. Yim, Y., Kikkawa, Y., Tanowitz, H., and Wittner, M. Fatal strongyloidiasis in Hodgkin's disease after immunosuppressive therapy. *J. Trop. Med. Hyg. 73*:245–249 (1970).

241. McNeely, D. J., Inouye, T., Tam, P. Y., and Ripley, S. D. Acute respiratory failure due to strongyloidiasis in polymyositis. *J. Rheumatol. 7*:745–750 (1980).

242. Buss, D. H. *Strongyloides stercoralis* infection complicating granulocytic leukemia. *NC Med. J. 1971*:269–274.

243. Ajana, F., Lescut, D., Dumont, M., Soots, J., Ayadi, A., Dei-Cas, E., and Vernes, A. Anguillulose a revelation tardive sur terrain tuberculeux. *Sem. Hop. Paris 62*:3851–3853 (1986).

244. Cummins, R. O., Surat, P. M., and Horwitz, D. A. Disseminated *Strongyloides stercoralis* infection. Association with ectopic ACTH syndrome and depressed cell-mediated immunity. *Arch. Intern. Med. 138*:1005–1006 (1978).

245. Klein, R. A., Cleri, D. J., Doshi, V., and Brasitus, T. A. Disseminated *Strongyloides stercoralis*: a fatal case eluding diagnosis. *South. Med. J. 76*:1438–1440 (1983).

246. Chaudhuri, B., Nanos, S., Soco, J. N., and McGrew, E. Disseminated *Strongyloides stercoralis* infestation detected by sputum cytology. *Acta Cytol. 24*:360–362 (1980).

247. Wang, T., Reyes, C. W., Kathuria, S., and Strinden, C. Diagnosis of *Strongyloides stercoralis* in sputum cytology. *Acta Cytol. 24*:40–43 (1980).

248. Smith, B., Verghese, A., Gutierrez, C., Dralle, W., and Berk, S. T. Pulmonary strongyloidiasis. Diagnosis by sputum gram stain. *Am. J. Med. 79*:663–666 (1985).

249. Yassin, S. A., and Garret, M. Parasite in cytodiagnosis: A case report of *Strongyloides stercoralis* in Papanicolaou smears of gastric aspirate with a review of the literature. *Acta Cytol. 24*:539–544 (1980).

250. Silva, O. A., Santos-Amaral, C. F., Bruno, J. C., Lopez, M., and Homem-Pittella, J. E. Hypokalemic respiratory muscle paralysis following *Strongyloides stercoralis* hyperinfection. A case report. *Am. J. Trop. Med. Hyg. 30*:69–73 (1981).

251. Cookson, J. B., Montgomery, R. D., Morhan, H. V., and Tudor, R. W. Fatal paralytic ileus due to strongyloidiasis. *Br. Med. J. 4*:771–772 (1972).

252. Ford, J., Reiss-Levy, E., Clark, E., Dyson, A. J., and Schonell, M. Pulmonary strongyloidiasis and lung abscess. *Chest 79*:239–240 (1981).

253. Meltzer, R. S., Singer, C., Armstrong, D., Mayer, K., and Knapper, W. H. Antemortem diagnosis of central nervous system strongyloidiasis. *Am. J. Med. Sci. 277*:91–98 (1979).

254. Vishwanath, S., Baker, R. A., and Mansheim, B. J. *Strongyloides* infection and meningitis in an immunocompromised host. *Am. J. Trop. Med. Hyg. 31*:857–858 (1982).

255. Shelhamer, J. H., Neva, F. A., and Finn, D. R. Persistent strongyloidiasis in an immunodeficient patient. *Am. J. Trop. Med. Hyg. 31*:746–751 (1982).

256. deOliveira, R. B., Voltarelli, J. C., and Meneghelli, U. G. Severe strongyloidiasis associated with hypogammaglobulinemia. *Parasite Immunol. 3*: 165–169 (1981).

257. Reeder, M., and Palmer, P. E. S. *The Radiology of Tropical Diseases.* Williams & Wilkins, Baltimore, 1981.

258. Paterson, D. E. *Strongyloides* infestation of the jejunum. *Br. J. Radiol. 31*:102–103 (1958).

259. Yoshida, T., Nozaki, F., Tanaka, K., Ebihara, H., Shimayama, T., and Katsuki, T. *Strongyloides stercoralis* hyperinfection: sequential changes of gastrointestinal radiology after treatment with thiabendazole. *Gastrointest. Radiol. 6*:223–225 (1981).

260. Frengley, J. D., and Trewby, P. N. Fatal paraylitic ileus due to strongyloidiasis (letter). *Br. Med. J. 2*:308 (1973).

261. Arantes-Pereira, O., Oliveira, A. D. E., and Barretto-Netto, M. Estrongiloidose intestinal. Correlacao anatomo-radiologica de um caso fatal. *Rev. Brasil. Radiol. 3*:127–142 (1960).

262. Arantes-Perreira, O., Arantes-Pereira, A., and Moraes, J. Caso grave de estrongiloidose curada. Estudo clinico, radiologico, biopsico e terapeutico. *O Hospital 62*:229–252 (1962).

263. Cuni, L. J., Rosner, F., and Chawla, S. K. Fatal strongyloidiasis in immunosuppressed patients. *NY State J. Med. 77*:2109–2113 (1977).

264. Jones, C. A., and Abadie, S. H. Studies in human strongyloidiasis. II. A comparison of the efficiency of diagnosis by examination of feces and duodenal fluid. *Am. J. Clin. Pathol. 24*:1154–1158 (1954).

265. Nielsen, P. B., and Mojon, M. Improved diagnosis of *Strongyloides stercoralis* by seven consecutive stool specimens. *Zentr. Bakteriol. Mikrobiol. Hyg. A 263*:616–617 (1987).

266. Baermann, G. Eine einfache Methode zur Auffindung von Ankylostomum (Nematoden) Larven in Erdproben. *Med. H. Geneesk. Lab. Weltevreden, Feestbundel, Batavia, 1917*:41–47.

267. Pereira-Lima, J., and Delgado, P. G. Diagnosis of strongyloidiasis: importance of Baermann's method. *Am. J. Dig. Dis. 6*:899–904 (1961).

268. Ash, L. R., and Orihel, T. C. *Parasites: A Guide to Laboratory Procedures and Identification*. ASCP Press, Chicago, 1987.

269. Beal, C. B., Viens, P., Grant, R. G., and Hughes, J. M. A new technique for sampling duodenal contents. *Am. J. Trop. Med. Hyg. 19*:349-352 (1970).

270. Goldsmid, J. M., and Davies, N. Diagnosis of parasitic infections of the small intestine by the enterotest duodenal capsule. *Med. J. Aust. 1*:519-520 (1978).

271. Andrade, Z. A., and Caymmi-Gomes, M. Pathology of fatal strongyloidiasis. *Rev. Inst. Med. Trop. Sao Paulo 6*:28-34 (1964).

272. Marcial-Rojas, R. A. Strongyloidiasis. In *Pathology of Protozoal and Helminthic Diseases with Clinical Correlation* (R. A. Marcial-Rojas, ed.). Robert E. Krieger, Huntington, New York, 1975, pp. 711-738.

273. Setia, U., and Bhatia, G. Pancreatic adenocarcinoma associated with *Strongyloides*. *Am. J. Med. 77*:173-175 (1984).

274. Pierce, J. R., and Dyer, E. L. Extreme eosinophilia and strongyloidiasis: an uncommon manifestation of a common disease. *South. Med. J. 74*: 995-996 (1981).

275. Bezjak, B. Immunoglobulin studies in strongyloidiasis with special reference to raised serum IgE levels. *Am. J. Trop. Med. Hyg. 24*:945-948 (1975).

276. Carneiro-Leao, R., Toledo-Barros, M., and Mandes, E. Immunological study of human strongyloidiasis. I. Analysis of IgE levels. *Allergol. Immunopathol. 8*:31-34 (1980).

277. Gill, G. V., Bell, D. R., and Fifield, R. Lack of immunoglobulin E. Response to longstanding strongyloidiasis. *Clin. Exp. Immunol. 37*:292-294 (1979).

278. Genta, R. M. Strongyloidiasis. In *Immunodiagnosis of Parasitic Diseases* (K. Walls, and P. Schantz, eds.). Academic Press, New York, 1986, pp. 183-199.

279. Genta, R. M. Predictive value of an enzyme-linked immunosorbent assay (ELISA) for the serodiagnosis of strongyloidiasis. *Am. J. Clin. Pathol. 89*:391-394 (1988).

280. Drugs for parasitic infections. *Med. Lett. 28*:9-14 (1986).

281. James, D. M., and Gilles, H. M. (eds.). *Human Antiparasitic Drugs: Pharmacology and Usage*. Wiley, Chichester, 1985.

282. Davis, A. Drug treatment in intestinal helminthiases. World Health Organization, Geneva 1973

283. Grove, D. I. Treatment of strongyloidiasis with thiabendazole: an analysis of toxicity and effectiveness. *Trans. R. Soc. Trop. Med. Hyg. 76*:114-118 (1982).

284. Bezjak, B. A clinical trial of thiabendazole in strongyloidiasis. *Am. J. Trop. Med. Hyg. 17*:733-736 (1968).

285. Arroyo, J. C., and Brown, A. Concentration of thiabendazole and parasite-specific IgG antibodies in the cerebrospinal fluid of a patient with disseminated strongyloidiasis. *J. Infect. Dis. 156*:520-523 (1987).

286. Barnish, G., and Barker, J. An intervention study using thiabendazole suspension against *Strongyloides fulleborni*-like infections in Papua New Guinea. *Trans. R. Soc. Trop. Med. Hyg. 81*:60–63 (1987).

287. Schumaker, D., Band, J. D., Lensmeyer, G. L., and Craig, W. A. Thiabendazole treatment of severe strongyloidiasis in a hemodialyzed patient. *Ann. Intern. Med. 89*:644–645 (1978).

288. Leapman, S. B., Rosenberg, J. B., Filo, R. S., and Smith, E. J. *Strongyloides stercoralis* in chronic renal failure. Safe therapy with thiabendazole. *South Med. J. 73*:1400–1402 (1980).

289. Sugar, A. M., Kearns, P. J., Haulk, A. A., and Rushing, J. L. Possible thiabendazole-induced theophylline toxicity. *Am. Rev. Resp. Dis. 122*: 501–503 (1980).

290. Tchao, P., and Templeton, T. Thiabendazole-associated grand mal seizures in a patient with Down syndrome. *J. Pediatr. 102*:317–318 (1983).

291. Keystone, J. S., and Murdock, J. K. Mebendazole. *Ann. Intern. Med. 91*: 582–586 (1979).

292. Mravak, S., Schopp, W., and Bienzle, U. Treatment of strongyloidiasis with mebendazole. *Acta Trop. 40*:93–94 (1983).

293. Boyd, W. R., Campbell, F. W., and Trudeau, W. I. *Strongyloides stercoralis* hyperinfection. *Am. J. Trop. Med. Hyg. 27*:39–41 (1978).

294. Musgrave, I. A., Hawes, R. B., Jameson, J. L., Sloane, R. A., and Quale, P. A. Mebendazole: evaluation of a new antihelminthic for trichuriasis, hookworm, and strongyloidiasis. *Med. J. Aust. 1*:403–405 (1979).

295. Walzer, P. D. Diagnosis and management of strongyloidiasis. *Intern. Med. Spec. 4*:45–57 (1983).

296. Pelletier, L. L., and Baker, C. B. Treatment failures following mebendazole therapy for chronic strongyloidiasis. *J. Infect. Dis. 156*:532–533 (1987).

297. Pene, P., Mojon, M., Garin, J. P., Coulaud, J. P., and Rossignol, J. F. Albendazole: a new broad spectrum anthelminthic. *Am. J. Trop. Med. Hyg. 31*:263–266 (1982).

298. Mojon, M., and Nielson, P. B. Treatment of *Strongyloides stercoralis* with albendazole. A cure rate of 86 per cent. *Zentralb. Bakteriol. Mikrobiol. Hyg. A 263*:619–624 (1987).

299. Bicalho, S. A., Leao, O. J., and Pena, Q. Cambendazole in the treatment of human strongyloidiasis. *Am. J. Trop. Med. Hyg. 32*:1181–1183 (1983).

300. Eveland, L. K., Kenney, M., and Yermakov, V. Laboratory diagnosis of autoinfection in strongyloidiasis. *Am. J. Clin. Pathol. 63*:421–425 (1975).

301. Gam, A. A., Neva, F. A., and Kortoski, W. A. Comparative sensitivity and specificity of ELISA and IHA for the serodiagnosis of strongyloidiasis with larval antigens. *Am. J. Trop. Med. Hyg. 37*:157–161 (1987).

Index

About the Editors

PETER D. WALZER is Chief of the Division of Infectious Diseases at the Cincinnati Veterans Administration Center, and Professor of Medicine as well as of Pathology and Laboratory Medicine at the University of Cincinnati College of Medicine in Cincinnati, Ohio. An authority on *Pneumocystis carinii* pneumonia, he has published nearly 100 articles, book chapters, and proceedings papers, and he has presented numerous papers at conferences throughout the U.S. He is a Fellow of the American College of Physicians and Infectious Disease Society of America, and he is a member of the American Society for Microbiology, American Society of Tropical Medicine and Hygiene, American Society of Parasitologists, American Thoracic Society, American Association of Immunologists, and others. Dr. Walzer received the B.S. degree (1964) from Boston College and M.D. degree (1968) from Albany Medical College in Albany, New York.

ROBERT M. GENTA is Associate Professor of Pathology and Laboratory Medicine at the University of Cincinnati College of Medicine and a Staff Pathologist at the Veterans Administration Medical Center in Cincinnati, Ohio. He is the author or coauthor of some 40 articles and book chapters, many of them concerning his research specialty in *Strongyloides stercoralis*. Among the professional societies he belongs to are the College of American Pathologists, American Public Health Association, American Society of Tropical Medicine and Hygiene, American Society of Parasitologists, and New York Academy of Sciences. Dr. Genta received the M.D. degree (1971) from the University of Turin Medical School in Italy and a diploma (1977) from the University of Liverpool's Liverpool School of Tropical Medicine in the U.K.

CPSIA information can be obtained
at www.ICGtesting.com
Printed in the USA
BVHW031815241119
564715BV00004B/9/P